Psychotropic

Drug

Handbook

7th Edition

Psychotropic
Drug
Handbook

7th Edition

Paul J. Perry, Ph.D.   Professor of Psychiatry, College of Medicine, and Professor, College of Pharmacy, University of Iowa, Iowa City

Bruce Alexander, Pharm.D.   Clinical Pharmacist Specialist, Pharmacy and Psychiatry Services, Department of Veterans Affairs Medical Center, Iowa City, Iowa; Adjunct Associate Professor of Psychiatry, College of Medicine, and Clinical Associate Professor, College of Pharmacy, University of Iowa, Iowa City

Barry I. Liskow, M.D.   Chief of Psychiatry, Department of Veterans Affairs Medical Center, Kansas City, Missouri; Professor, Department of Psychiatry, School of Medicine, University of Kansas Medical Center, Kansas City, Kansas

American Psychiatric Press, Inc.

Washington, DC
London, England

Note: The authors have worked to ensure that all information in this book concerning drug dosages, schedules, and routes of administration is accurate as of the time of publication and consistent with standards set by the U.S. Food and Drug Administration and the general medical community. As medical research and practice advance, however, therapeutic standards may change. For this reason and because human and mechanical errors sometimes occur, we recommend that readers follow the advice of a physician who is directly involved in their care or the care of a member of their family.

Copyright © 1997 American Psychiatric Press, Inc.
ALL RIGHTS RESERVED
Manufactured in the United States of America on acid-free paper
00 99 98 97   4 3 2 1
7th Edition

American Psychiatric Press, Inc.
1400 K Street, N.W., Washington, DC   20005

Library of Congress Cataloging-in-Publication Data
Perry, Paul J.
    Psychotropic drug handbook / Paul J. Perry, Bruce Alexander, Barry I. Liskow. — 7th ed.
        p.   cm.
    Rev. ed. of: PDH. 6th ed. c1991.
    Includes bibliographical references and index.
    ISBN 0-88048-851-4
    1. Psychotropic drugs—Handbooks, manuals, etc.   I. Alexander, Bruce, Pharm. D.   II. Liskow, Barry I.   III. Perry, Paul J. PDH. IV. Title.
    [DNLM: 1. Psychotropic Drugs—handbooks.   QV 39 P464p 1997]
    RM315.P44   1997
    615'.788—dc20
    DNLM/DLC   95-33558
    for Library of Congress   CIP

To George Winokur
We and countless others
will miss his guidance
and wisdom

Contents

Preface

This seventh edition of the *Psychotropic Drug Handbook* has retained the basic format of previous editions. The book remains pocket sized and spiral bound. In the past 5 years, the amount of clinically significant data in the literature that demanded incorporation into the text was extraordinary. New drugs that have been added include the antipsychotics olanzapine, risperidone, and sertindole; the antidepressants mirtazapine, nefazodone, paroxetine, sertraline, and venlafaxine; the hypnotic zolpidem; and the antiobsessional selective serotonin reuptake inhibitor (SSRI) fluvoxamine. The index has been expanded to increase the utility of the text as a rapid-access reference.

Acknowledgments

We are extremely grateful to our editors, Claire Reinburg, Jane Davenport, Pamela Harley, and Rebecca Richters, for their assistance in the preparation of this seventh edition. We wish to express our gratitude to Dr. George Winokur for his encouragement and advice. Additionally, we would like to thank the following members of the University of Iowa Department of Psychiatry who scrupulously reviewed the text: Donald Black, M.D.; William Coryell, M.D.; Raymond Crowe, M.D.; Del Miller, M.D., Pharm.D.; Russell Noyes, M.D.; George Winokur, M.D.; and William Yates, M.D.

Product Lists

The lists provided at the end of Chapters 1 through 7 and 11 contain specific product information for the drugs discussed in those chapters. Where appropriate, each drug is described parenthetically according to a hybrid chemical/therapeutic-use classification system (e.g., dimethylated tricyclic antidepressant [TCA]). The recommended dosages are given. It is noted whether the drug is available as a less-expensive generic product. The average wholesale price (AWP) of the drug appears as the bracketed number after the dosage form description. This figure reflects the average acquisition cost (based on the *1996 Drug Topics® Red Book*[*]) of that dosage formulation rounded to the next whole dollar. The AWP represents the cost of 100 tablets or capsules or of oral liquid doses of the indicated volume. For injectable preparations, the AWP reflects the cost per vial or ampule, as specified. It may be used for cost comparisons between agents of similar efficacy within the same therapeutic category. The generic cost index corresponds to the maximum allowable cost (MAC) for generic drug reimbursement by Medicaid divided by the AWP for the brand-name drug. Finally, a description of each tablet/capsule formulation's color and markings is provided. This information is intended for use as an aid in obtaining a patient's psychiatric drug history. The product list information for nortriptyline is presented below as an example.

Nortriptyline (monomethylated tricyclic antidepressant)
- Daily dose range: 20–150 mg; generically available
- Generic cost index: ≈ 0.31

Capsules:	Pamelor®
10 mg	[$47] Sandoz Pamelor 78–86, orange/white
25 mg	[$95] Sandoz Pamelor 78–87, orange/white
50 mg	[$178] Sandoz Pamelor 78–79, white
75 mg	[$272] Sandoz Pamelor 78–79, orange

Syrup:	Pamelor®
10 mg/5 mL	[$54/480 mL]

---

[*] Cardinale V: *1996 Drug Topics® Red Book.* Montvale, NJ, Medical Economics, 1996.

Generic Drugs

One-third of all prescriptions are filled with generic drugs. Consumers generally pay 30%–50% less when an equivalent generic drug is dispensed rather than the brand-name drug. Since 1970, the U.S. Food and Drug Administration (FDA) has reviewed and approved more than 9,000 generic drug products that may be dispensed interchangeably with the brand-name products. However, it is our experience that the psychiatric patient population is the patient group most resistant to the use of generic drugs. The points listed below should be conveyed to patients in simple and straightforward language before the clinician writes a prescription using the generic name of the medication. It is hoped that this patient-education intervention will put to rest any concerns patients might have regarding the use of generic drugs.

- To be approved by the FDA as a generic equivalent, a drug must have the same active ingredient(s), dosage form, and strength as the brand-name product.
- The manufacturer of the generic drug must demonstrate to the FDA that the drug is bioequivalent to the brand-name product. Bioequivalency is critical in order for the FDA to conclude that the generic drug will produce therapeutic effects similar to those of the brand-name drug.
- Manufacturers of generic drugs must fully document to the FDA their manufacturing methods.
- Both the raw materials used and the finished dosage formulation for the generic drug must meet the same specifications set forth for the brand-name product in the U.S.'s official drug compendium, *The United States Pharmacopoeia.*[*]
- The manufacturing facility for the generic drug must have been inspected and approved by the FDA.

[*] Halpern JA, Grady LT, Allen LV, et al: *The United States Pharmacopoeia—The National Formulary, 1995.* Taunton, MA, Rand McNally, 1994.

Antipsychotics

Members of antipsychotic classes (e.g., phenothiazine, butyrophenone, thioxanthene, dihydroindolone, dibenzoxazepine) introduced in the United States between 1954 and 1979 are referred to as "typical" antipsychotics. In 1984, pimozide, an antipsychotic, was approved by the U.S. Food and Drug Administration (FDA) as an orphan drug for the second-line treatment of Gilles de la Tourette's syndrome (see **Pimozide** section later in this chapter). The availability of the "atypical" antipsychotics has resulted in a new classification system (see **Clozapine, Olanzapine, Risperidone,** and **Sertindole** sections later in this chapter). Although *typical* and *atypical* are common terms in the literature, the use of *first-generation* and *second-generation*, respectively, to refer to typical and atypical antipsychotics is gaining acceptance. The first-/second-generation dichotomy has been suggested as the result of differences in pharmacology within the atypical class of antipsychotics.

These drugs are best referred to as *antipsychotics* because the symptoms they reduce are typical of schizophrenia in particular, and of psychosis in general. Older terms describing antipsychotics include *major tranquilizer, neuroleptic,* and *ataractic.* Use of the term *major tranquilizer* is inappropriate, because these drugs do not produce a state of tranquillity in either healthy or psychotic persons. In fact, nonpsychotic subjects often find the effects unpleasant. The general term *neuroleptic* refers to the ability of these drugs to produce specific neurological effects (i.e., drug-induced parkinsonism). This term likewise is not appropriate because it emphasizes the nontherapeutic effects of this class of drugs.

All antipsychotics ameliorate symptoms of psychosis, which include hallucinations, delusions, formal thought disorder, bizarre behavior, agitation, and/or hyperactivity.

Typical Antipsychotics

■ Indications

Antipsychotics have been used in a variety of disorders, including schizophrenia, schizoaffective and schizophreniform disorder, mania, major depressive disorder with psychotic features, cognitive delusional disorder, and substance-induced cognitive disorders (Black et al. 1985; Kane 1989).

Nonpsychiatric uses of these agents include prevention of vomiting (except that produced by vestibular stimulation [i.e., motion sickness]), control of intractable hiccups, and management of Huntington's chorea and Tourette's syndrome (Black et al. 1985).

■ Efficacy

Schizophrenia

First-episode treatment/nonrefractory schizophrenia.   The primary use of antipsychotics is in the management of schizophrenia. Studies report improvement rates of 40%–75% in schizophrenic patients treated with *oral* phenothiazines (Black et al. 1985; Kane 1989; Kane and Marder 1993; Wolkowitz 1993). All antipsychotics are equal in overall therapeutic efficacy and produce consistent changes of the same symptoms in groups of patients (Davis and Casper 1977; Kane 1989; Kane and Marder 1993; Kane and McGlashan 1995). Four comparison studies of the *long-acting injectable* preparations (i.e., fluphenazine, haloperidol decanoate) revealed no differences in efficacy (Davis and Casper 1977).

The major therapeutic effect of antipsychotics is to ameliorate psychotic symptoms. These agents reduce—but rarely eliminate—such fundamental "core" target symptoms (i.e., "positive symptoms") as thought disorder (e.g., loose associations, conceptual disorganization), hallucinations, and delusions. Normalization of psychomotor behavior in both withdrawn and hyperactive patients can occur (Black et al. 1985; Davis and Casper 1977).

Attempts to predict a response to a specific antipsychotic or to reliably predict a response based on a patient's demographics (e.g., sex, socioeconomic or marital status) or psychiatric history (e.g., age at onset, duration of illness, family history, premorbid characteristics) have not been consistently successful (Beresford and Ward 1987; Kane 1989; Remington 1989). Many studies report that "negative symptoms" (e.g., emotional and social withdrawal, poverty of thought, flat affect, ambivalence, poor self-care) usually do not respond as well as positive symptoms (Awad 1989; Kane and Marder 1993; Kinon et al. 1993a, 1993b; Ortiz and Gershon 1986; Remington 1989). However, several studies indicate equal improvement of positive and negative symptoms (Awad 1989; Daniel et al. 1995; Kay and Singh 1989). The presence of acute extrapyramidal side effects (EPS) may be associated with a less-favorable response (Kinon et al. 1993b; J. A. Lieberman et al. 1996). Antipsychotics are usually chosen on the basis of adverse effects, a patient's past history of response, and cost (Kane and McGlashan 1995; Marder et al. 1993).

The *rate of improvement* can vary among patients, with some improving within several hours or days of initiation of the antipsychotic (Kane and McGlashan 1995; Keck et al. 1989a). Early literature reported that most of the therapeutic gain occurred within the first 4 weeks of antipsychotic treatment, although 12–24 weeks were sometimes needed (Davis and Casper 1977; Levinson et al. 1992). However, it has since been noted that many of these earlier studies had methodological flaws (Breier et al. 1987; Keck et al. 1989a). A more recent study reported that at least a 2-week trial would be necessary to even begin to distinguish antipsychotic responders from nonresponders (Levinson et al. 1992). A subsequent, controlled study reported that only 8% of patients who failed to respond after 4 weeks of treatment responded when given an additional 4-week antipsychotic trial (Kinon et al. 1993a). Thus, an antipsychotic, in order to be considered to have received an adequate trial (i.e., a *therapeutic trial*) in a patient with a first-time diagnosis of psychosis or with an acute exacerbation of chronic psychosis, must be administered for 4 weeks at a sufficient dosage (see *Schizophrenia, Mania, and Schizoaffective and Schizophreniform Disorders* [page 13] under "Dosage"). A recent study reported that maximum symptomatic improvement occurs within the first 6 months of treatment (Szymanski et al. 1996).

The pharmacoeconomic benefit-to-cost ratio for typical antipsychotics has not been extensively studied (Hargreaves and Shumway 1996). These agents need to be studied in comparison with atypical antipsychotics to demonstrate differences, if any, between drugs.

There is evidence that early antipsychotic treatment in newly diagnosed patients improves long-term outcome (Hegarty et al. 1994; J. A. Lieberman et al. 1996; Szymanski et al. 1996). However, the relapse rate when antipsychotics were discontinued in patients with a diagnosis of *first-time psychosis* (e.g., first-episode schizophrenia) ranged from 60% to 90% in 2- to 3-year follow-up studies (Kissling et al. 1991; Marder et al. 1993). Although this rate is high, patients might be given a trial off antipsychotics after a 1- to 2-year period to determine continuing need. Continuous symptomatology while receiving drug treatment or relapse after the drug is discontinued would indicate the need for a longer maintenance period. The patient and family members should be informed that the risk of relapse is high, and that clinical stability might be maintained with continued treatment (Kissling et al. 1991).

Maintenance treatment.   The positive effect of maintenance antipsychotic treatment in patients who have experienced two or more relapses has been demonstrated in four studies (Hegarty et al. 1994; Johnson 1985; Kissling et al. 1991; Marder et al. 1993). For schizophrenic patients who meet this criterion, 68% on placebo will relapse within the first year after hospitalization. An additional 65% of patients who do not relapse the first year on placebo will relapse the following year. This compares with a first- and second-year relapse rate of 41% and 15%, respectively, in patients treated with maintenance antipsychotics for 2 years. The studies noted that the risk of relapse declined further for treated patients over the subsequent years. No clear-cut predictors exist that can distinguish patients who will maintain remission from those who will relapse (Davis and Casper 1977; Johnson 1985). Antipsychotics are extremely important in preventing symptom relapse and possible rehospitalization, but the high percentage of patients on drug treatment who do relapse suggests that nonpharmacological factors (e.g., social and family environment) are also important (Kane and McGlashan 1995). In seven studies, an average of 35% of patients treated from 6 weeks to 2 years relapsed when treated with pharmacotherapy alone, compared with 21% when antipsychotic treatment was combined with social therapies (Davis et al. 1993) (for dosage-reduction strategy, see *Maintenance Dosing* [page 15]). Antipsychotic prophylaxis in combination with social intervention offers the best prognosis for these patients (Davis et al. 1993; Johnson 1985).

Core symptoms of schizophrenia may decrease as patients age. Although a small number of studies support the efficacy of antipsychotics in older persons with schizophrenia, these patients deserve a dosage-reduction or drug-discontinuation trial to determine their continuing need for maintenance antipsychotic treatment (Marder and Van Putten 1988). It has been suggested that long-term use of antipsychotics may actually exacerbate previously controlled positive symptoms of schizophrenia (i.e., "supersensitivity psychosis");

however, sufficient data are not available to confirm or reject this hypothesis (J. A. Lieberman et al. 1996; Ortiz and Gershon 1986).

Refractory schizophrenia. Management of the *nonresponding* or *partially responding patient* after a 4-week treatment course includes the following strategies (Kane and Marder 1993; Kinon et al. 1993a; Miller et al. 1996; Wolkowitz 1993):

1. Continuing the same antipsychotic at the same dose.
2. Increasing the dose of the current antipsychotic (see *Megadosing* [page 15]).
3. Switching to a different class within the typical antipsychotic group (e.g., a butyrophenone to a phenothiazine).
4. Adding a second drug to the current antipsychotic (i.e., adjunctive treatment).
5. Switching to an atypical antipsychotic (see "Efficacy" under **Clozapine, Olanzapine, Risperidone,** and **Sertindole** sections in this chapter).

The relative efficacies of these strategies have not been directly compared (Kane 1989; Keck et al. 1989a; Tandon and Greden 1989).

A recent study directly evaluated the first three strategies (Kinon et al. 1993a). Forty-seven patients who failed to respond to a 4-week trial of fluphenazine 20 mg/day were randomized to receive 4 additional weeks of fluphenazine 20 mg/day ($n = 18$), fluphenazine 80 mg/day ($n = 16$), or haloperidol 20 mg/day ($n = 13$). Overall, there was no difference between the treatment groups, as only 5% ($n = 1$), 13% ($n = 2$), and 8% ($n = 1$) of patients, respectively, responded after receiving the additional 4 weeks of treatment. Although these strategies do not significantly increase the rate of response in patients, they should be considered for an individual patient who fails to respond to a 4-week trial. If the patient is experiencing EPS, the dosage could be maintained for an additional 4 weeks or the patient could be switched to another antipsychotic. However, if no EPS are present, the dosage could be increased.

No studies have directly compared the first three strategies (i.e., *continuing* or *increasing* the dosage of the current antipsychotic, or *switching* to a different antipsychotic class) with *adjunctive treatments.* The use of adjunctive treatments in combination with antipsychotics in treatment-resistant patients has been reviewed (Christison et al. 1991; Wolkowitz 1993). Of all adjunctive agents used, lithium, carbamazepine, benzodiazepines, and reserpine have been associated with more positive outcomes.

Lithium levels of 0.9–1.3 mEq/L for 3–5 weeks have been reported to produce improvement in 30%–50% of patients. No clear predictors of lithium response have been identified; however, those patients with concurrent affective symptoms might respond preferentially. Neurotoxicity has been reported when lithium has been combined with antipsychotics (see *Neurological* adverse effects [page 248] of **Lithium** in Chapter 3).

Carbamazepine-responsive symptoms have included excitement, hostility, aggressive behavior, and temporal lobe or nonspecific electroencephalographic (EEG) abnormalities. An adequate therapeutic trial consists of antimanic doses administered for 4–6 weeks (see "Dosage" [page 261] under **Carbamazepine** in Chapter 3). It is important to note that carbamazepine may lower antipsychotic serum levels by 50% or more through enzyme induction (see **Antipsychotic–Carbamazepine** drug interaction [page 461] in Chapter 8).

Of 16 blinded studies of **benzodiazepines** used adjunctively, 7 reported positive results. The overall improvement rate was 30%–50%. Patients with prominent psychotic symptoms early in their illness, panic or significant anxiety symptoms, or motor disturbances of either agitation or retardation have been reported to respond favorably. The typical dose was diazepam 20–50 mg/day or its equivalent administered for 2–3 weeks (see benzodiazepine equivalent doses in Table 10–3 [page 570]). Some studies report that tolerance develops to the effect of benzodiazepines over several weeks of treatment. However, other studies report continued improvement after months of treatment. If patients are to have a benzodiazepine discontinued after months of treatment, a tapering schedule should be devised (see Benzodiazepine Taper under *Low-Dose Withdrawal* [page 577] in Chapter 10).

Reserpine has been shown to have antipsychotic properties, but it is less effective than typical antipsychotics in the treatment of schizophrenia. Several reports suggest that 50% of patients refractory to typical antipsychotics may improve when reserpine 0.5–6.0 mg/day is added to their regimens (Wolkowitz 1993). Specific symptoms reported to improve include psychosis, hyperactivity, agitation, and assaultiveness. Initial doses should be 0.25 mg/day, which could be increased by 0.25 mg twice daily every week, depending on side effects (e.g., sedation, hypotension). As a result of early dopamine release, patients may experience an initial worsening of symptoms, followed by improvement.

Other adjunctive treatments that have been reported to be useful but overall less effective than the agents discussed thus far include *clonidine, propranolol, valproate, verapamil,* and *levodopa*) (Wolkowitz 1993). If primary adjunctive treatments are not successful, a 4-week trial using standard doses of these drugs might be considered. However, propranolol doses typically consist of 400–4,000 mg/day. Also, levodopa (L-dopa) has been reported to produce or exacerbate psychosis in some patients.

There is no evidence to suggest that *multiple typical antipsychotics* administered simultaneously are better than one if equivalent doses are used (see "Dosage" [page 12]) (Davis and Casper 1977). The combined use of risperidone with clozapine—or of these two drugs individually with other typical antipsychotics—has not been extensively studied, and, therefore, the efficacy and safety of this approach is unknown at present.

Mania

Antipsychotics serve an adjunctive role in the *acute* treatment of mania, as lithium is the primary drug for mania (see "Efficacy" under **Lithium** in Chapter 3). Although any antipsychotic can be used alone or in combination with lithium for mania, most research has been with chlorpromazine and haloperidol. Studies indicate that antipsychotics, at least until therapeutic lithium levels are achieved, are better than lithium in suppressing psychomotor activity, hostility, excitement, grandiosity, and suspiciousness (Johnson 1985). Once lithium levels are therapeutic and clinical response is attained, the antipsychotic dose can be tapered and ultimately discontinued. Several studies report that the addition of a benzodiazepine will reduce antipsychotic dose requirements in mania (see *Lithium or lithium/antipsychotic plus a benzodiazepine* [page 223] in Chapter 3) (Chou 1991; Raskind and Risse 1986).

The efficacy of antipsychotics in the *prophylactic,* or maintenance, treatment of bipolar illness has not been extensively evaluated in controlled trials (Chou 1991; Goodwin and Zis 1979; Prien and Gelenberg 1989; Sernyak and Woods 1993). However, a survey of the literature indicates that such use is common practice (Gelenberg and Hopkins 1996; Sernyak and Woods 1993). Two studies that used a depot antipsychotic not available in the United States reported that some patients benefited from long-term treatment (Sernyak and Woods 1993). Antipsychotics are generally not recommended for long-term management of bipolar illness because of concerns about late-onset side effects (e.g., tardive dyskinesia) (Gelenberg and Hopkins 1996; Keck et al. 1996b; Sernyak and

Woods 1993). If these agents are used in long-term treatment, the rationale should be documented in the clinical record.

Schizoaffective Disorder
As a result of diagnostic ambiguity, it is difficult to draw conclusions regarding the efficacy of antipsychotics in the treatment of schizoaffective disorder (Busch et al. 1989).

Although lithium is the primary treatment for schizoaffective disorder (see Schizoaffective Disorder [page 224] under "Efficacy" of **Lithium** in Chapter 3), antipsychotics are used in combination with lithium when psychotic symptomatology is prominent. Most studies report improvement in psychotic symptoms in schizoaffective patients receiving antipsychotics (Keck et al. 1996a). Because of diagnostic variability among studies and, generally, small sample sizes, the response rate is not known. The principles regarding the use of antipsychotics in schizophreniform illness should be followed in treating patients with schizoaffective disorder (see below).

Schizophreniform Disorder
Schizophreniform disorder is treated the same as schizophrenia (see *First-episode treatment/nonrefractory schizophrenia* [page 2]). The treatment guidelines for patients with first-time psychosis (e.g., first-episode schizophrenia) should be followed (Kissling et al. 1991).

Personality Disorders
Borderline.   Six blind studies and one open report have investigated antipsychotics (e.g., chlorpromazine, haloperidol, loxapine, thiothixene, trifluoperazine, thioridazine) in borderline personality disorder (BPD) (Brinkley 1993; Cowdry and Gardner 1988; Delva and Letemendia 1982; S. C. Goldberg et al. 1986; Kane 1988; Leone 1982; Soloff et al. 1989; Teicher and Glod 1989; Zanarini et al. 1988). Several but not all of the early studies reported that antipsychotics were effective for the broad range of borderline symptoms (e.g., affective, schizotypal, impulsive-behavioral). However, a more recent study was unable to demonstrate a positive effect of haloperidol (Soloff et al. 1993). It is important to note that overall improvement in patients' symptoms was modest, as the rating-scale score often declined (i.e., improved) from severe to moderate impairment (Soloff et al. 1989). Typical doses of antipsychotics consisted of chlorpromazine 100–300 mg/day or its equivalent (see "Dosage" [page 12]); however, several patients received doses equivalent to chlorpromazine 800 mg/day. Most treatment studies had a duration of 5 weeks or less. One 16-week study reported that haloperidol was ineffective in the long-term

treatment of borderline patients, except in alleviating the symptoms of irritability (Cornelius et al. 1993a, 1993b). The dropout rate due to side effects was 64%. In view of the potential for long-term adverse effects (e.g., tardive dyskinesia), a trial discontinuation of the antipsychotic should be considered in order to determine continued benefit in patients who demonstrate an early response.

Because only a limited number of direct-comparison studies have been conducted, the relative differences in efficacy among the antipsychotics—if, in fact, such differences do exist—cannot be specified. Five of seven studies using different populations and medications reported that antipsychotics were more effective than an antidepressant (Zanarini et al. 1988).

Schizotypal. Specific indications for antipsychotics in the treatment of schizotypal disorder await clinical trials.

Psychotic Depression
Major depressive disorder with psychotic features is sometimes treated with a combination of an antidepressant and an antipsychotic (see Major Depression With Psychotic Features [page 134] under "Efficacy" of **Tricyclic Antidepressants** in Chapter 2) (Nelson 1993; Serban and Siegel 1984). There is no evidence to suggest that one antipsychotic is superior to another for this purpose.

Commercially available fixed combinations of an antidepressant and antipsychotic are not recommended because of inflexibility in an individual drug's dosing (Soloff et al. 1986).

Cognitive Disorders
Antipsychotics have been extensively used in the management of patients with cognitive disorders (i.e., dementia) or delirium (Kunik et al. 1994; Riker et al. 1994; Risse and Barnes 1986; Sunderland 1996; Wragg and Jeste 1988; Yudofsky et al. 1990). Drug therapy is often necessary to control psychotic symptoms and/or behavioral disturbances when patients become agitated, aggressive, hostile, or otherwise disruptive and dangerous to themselves or those around them (Wragg and Jeste 1988). Psychotic symptoms may or may not lead to behavioral disturbances (Wragg and Jeste 1988).

▶ Dementia
Concern about inappropriate use and potential adverse effects (i.e., tardive dyskinesia, orthostatic hypotension, and anticholinergic delirium) of antipsychotics led to regulations for their use in long-term care facilities (Druckenbrod et al. 1993; Sunderland 1996).

The Omnibus Budget Reconciliation Act (OBRA) of the Health Care Financing Administration, a government agency that regulates Medicare and Medicaid recipients, went into effect October 1, 1990. This act stated that appropriate indications for antipsychotics would include dementia and delirium with associated psychotic and/or agitated behaviors that 1) are quantitatively and objectively documented, 2) are not the result of preventable factors, and 3) are causing the patient to present a danger to him- or herself or to others. In addition, antipsychotics may be used in patients with psychotic symptoms that are not exhibited as dangerous but that cause them distress or impairment in functional capacity.

In a meta-analysis of double-blind, placebo-controlled studies of inpatients with dementia and severe behavioral disturbances, the average response rates to antipsychotics and placebo were 59% (range 0%–67%) and 41%, respectively (Schneider et al. 1990; Sunderland 1996). Although the specific symptoms responding to antipsychotics could not be determined, it was concluded that agitation, uncooperativeness, and hallucinations were more likely to improve with medication. All antipsychotics are equally effective for treating psychosis or behavioral disturbances (Schneider et al. 1990). Therefore, drug selection is usually determined by individual response and the fewest undesirable effects (see "Adverse Effects" [page 31]).

There is no evidence to suggest that antipsychotics are effective for reversal of memory impairment, confusion, or intellectual deterioration, even if a patient is demonstrating psychosis (Black et al. 1985; Whalley 1989). The efficacy of antipsychotics for a treatment period longer than 6 months has not been determined, as most studies lasted 4–8 weeks (range 3–18 weeks) (Sunderland 1996).

▶ Delirium
Agitation secondary to acute delirium affects almost 60% of patients with a critical illness (Riker et al. 1994). Pharmacological management has been recommended to reduce injury to patients and health professionals (Riker et al. 1994). A first-line treatment has not been determined as no controlled trials have directly compared antipsychotics, benzodiazepines, or their combination. Likewise, the relative efficacy and safety of individual agents within each class has not been determined. The use of benzodiazepines alone in the management of delirium is addressed in Chapter 4. Reports of the use of antipsychotics alone and in combination with benzodiazepines are presented.

Antipsychotics alone.   Most reports recommend the use of high-potency antipsychotics (i.e., haloperidol, fluphenazine), as these are less likely to adversely affect blood pressure and cardiac conduction compared with low-potency antipsychotics (i.e., chlorpromazine, thioridazine) (see *Cardiovascular* adverse effects [page 35]) (Riker et al. 1994; Tesar 1993). The most extensively studied antipsychotic is haloperidol, with more than 700 reports involving more than 2,000 patients (Riker et al. 1994; Santos et al. 1992). Droperidol, a butyrophenone similar to haloperidol, has also been used in agitated medical/surgical patients; however, it produces a greater degree of sedation and orthostatic hypotension than does haloperidol (Tesar 1993). (For a discussion of drug doses and administration, see "Dosage" [page 12].)

Antipsychotic/benzodiazepine combination.   Although lorazepam has been combined with haloperidol, fewer reports exist for this combination than for haloperidol alone (Adams 1988; Adams et al. 1986). In a study involving 25 delirious cancer patients, mild to moderate levels of sedation were achieved in 24 of the patients (Adams et al. 1986). Arterial blood gases and tidal volume improved significantly in seven respirator-assisted patients after they were adequately sedated. Most patients responded within the first 90 minutes of treatment initiation; however, some responded between 10 and 60 minutes (Adams 1988). In most cases, blood pressure and pulse returned to normal limits after the first one or two doses of the combination. No patient experienced any respiratory, cardiac, or hemodynamic adverse effects during treatment. (For a discussion of drug doses and administration, see "Dosage" [page 12].)

Use of high-dose intravenous combination drugs should be considered only in patients refractory to standard doses of the individual drugs administered either orally or intramuscularly (Gelenberg 1988). The relative rate of oversedation associated with haloperidol alone versus the combination of haloperidol and lorazepam has not been studied. Also unaddressed is the question of tolerance to the long-term use of the benzodiazepines.

Drug-Induced Psychosis
The role of antipsychotics in drug-induced psychosis—an adverse reaction associated with lysergic acid diethylamide (LSD), phencyclidine (PCP), and central nervous system (CNS) stimulants—is discussed in Chapter 9.

The management of ***alcoholic hallucinosis*** with antipsychotics is appropriate if the psychosis persists past the period of acute alcohol withdrawal (Petrie et al. 1982). After 7–14 days of antipsychotic drug treatment, the patient usually remains symptom free once the drug is discontinued. Rare chronic cases, however, may require drug therapy indefinitely.

Anxiety Disorders

Although antipsychotics have been used to treat anxiety not re-lated to psychotic disorders, such use is not recommended because of potential long-term adverse effects (e.g., tardive dyskinesia) (Black et al. 1985). Other safer and comparably effective treat-ments are available for these disorders (see "Efficacy" [page 304] under **Benzodiazepines** in Chapter 4).

Evidence is lacking with regard to the superiority of the antipsy-chotic/antidepressant combination over antidepressants alone in the treatment of major depressive disorder with prominent symp-toms of anxiety or hostility unrelated to psychosis (Morris and Beck 1974). Four of six studies reported that the combination was equiv-alent in efficacy to tricyclic antidepressants (TCAs) alone. Of the remaining two studies, one found the combination superior, and the other concluded that the combination was inferior to the TCA alone.

■ Mechanism of Action

Excess dopamine activity in the mesolimbic and mesocortical areas of the CNS has been postulated to cause psychoses. Typical anti-psychotics are hypothesized to act by blocking postsynaptic dopa-mine–2 (D_2) receptors in these specific areas of the CNS, thus leading to an amelioration of psychotic symptoms (Marder et al. 1993; Peterson and Bongar 1989).

■ Dosage

All antipsychotics are equally effective in treating psychotic disor-ders when given in equipotent doses (Kane and McGlashan 1995). Therapeutically *equivalent doses* of antipsychotics are listed in the category "relative oral potency" under the individual agents in the Product List (page 104). For example, chlorpromazine 100 mg is approximately equal therapeutically to trifluoperazine 4 mg or halo-peridol 2 mg (Davis and Casper 1977; Surawicz 1980).

Antipsychotics can be divided into **low-** and **high-potency** cate-gories based on their relative oral potency (Black et al. 1985; Meltzer et al. 1989). This classification is important in predicting some adverse effects (e.g., hypotension, early-onset EPS) (see Ta-ble 1–1 and "Adverse Effects" [page 31]). It is important to note

Table 1–1. Potency classification of antipsychotics

Low potency[a]	High potency[b]
chlorpromazine	acetophenazine
mesoridazine	fluphenazine
thioridazine	haloperidol
	loxapine
	molindone
	perphenazine
	prochlorperazine
	thiothixene
	trifluoperazine

[a]Equivalent dose >15. [b]Equivalent dose <15.
Source. Black et al. 1985; Rhoades and Overall 1984.

that many antipsychotics have not been directly compared in regard to adverse effects. Table 1–1 is based on both in vitro and clinically derived data.

Schizophrenia, Mania, and Schizoaffective and Schizophreniform Disorders

Nonagitated patient. A dose of chlorpromazine 300 mg/day po or its equivalent is considered the minimal therapeutic dose for treatment of acute psychosis. Dose-response studies in patients with schizophrenia have indicated that the peak response occurs at approximately chlorpromazine 600 mg/day or its equivalent (Kane and McGlashan 1995; McIntyre and Gershon 1985). In general, doses larger than chlorpromazine 1,200 mg/day or its equivalent do not produce substantially greater improvement than smaller doses (Baldessarini et al. 1988; Davis and Casper 1977; McIntyre and Gershon 1985). One study comparing haloperidol 5, 10, and 20 mg/day reported that patients receiving the 20-mg/day dose deteriorated in the areas of blunted affect, motor retardation, and emotional withdrawal (Van Putten et al. 1990). However, it is important to remember that patients respond to widely differing dosages. By focusing on the patient's symptoms in order of clinical importance, the best dosage level for the target symptoms may be found more readily.

As a general rule, an acutely psychotic patient who is not uncontrollably agitated can be started on chlorpromazine 100 mg or its equivalent administered two or three times daily. This dosage is gradually increased at a rate of chlorpromazine 100–200 mg/day or its equivalent until clinical response is achieved, the upper limit of the recommended dose range is reached, or intolerable side effects occur. One week after a stable dose is achieved, the medication can be given once daily, usually at bedtime. Because of the slow response time associated with these agents, an antipsychotic must be given an adequate therapeutic trial (see "Efficacy" and "Rational Prescribing" [pages 2 and 59, respectively]).

Although the FDA has set the maximum daily dose of thioridazine at 800 mg, no absolute daily maximum dose exists for any other antipsychotic drugs (see *Ophthalmological* adverse effects [page 53]).

Recent studies demonstrated no significant difference in degree or speed of improvement when oral loading doses of chlorpromazine greater than 800 mg/day or its equivalent were compared with doses less than 800 mg/day (Baldessarini et al. 1988). It is recommended that patients initially receive chlorpromazine doses of less than 800 mg/day or its equivalent, although an exception could be made in the case of an individual patient in whom higher doses had previously been shown to be effective (Ortiz and Gershon 1986).

Agitated patient. The immediate goal of treatment of acutely psychotic agitated patients is to reduce agitation, irritability, and/ or hostility so that patients are not a physical danger to themselves or others. Alleviation of the delusions and/or hallucinations that are assumed to be the basis of the agitated behavior is the ultimate goal.

The technique of titrating the *antipsychotic* dosage against the patient's psychotic symptomatology by administering a series of closely spaced *parenteral* doses over a period of hours is termed "rapid neuroleptization" (Ortiz and Gershon 1986). Because of the risk of mental status impairment and significant EPS associated with high-dose antipsychotic treatment, this technique should be reserved for agitated patients who do not respond to conventional doses of antipsychotics (see *Megadosing* and "Pharmacokinetics" [pages 15 and 26, respectively]).

Rapid neuroleptization was first used in 1963 and has been extensively reported since 1974. The patient receives chlorpromazine 100 mg po or 25 mg im or its equivalent every 1–2 hours until agitation and psychosis are under control. Seldom is more than chlorpromazine 800 mg or its equivalent recommended or required within a 24-hour period (Baldessarini et al. 1988). Because of chlorpromazine's cardiovascular side effects (e.g., hypotension), administration of haloperidol 2–10 mg po or im every 30 minutes– 2 hours has been recommended. Although haloperidol has been used most extensively, there is evidence to suggest that other high-potency antipsychotics are equally effective and safe (Ortiz and Gershon 1986). After intramuscular treatment, the oral dose of the antipsychotic administered should be equivalent to the total parenteral dose administered over the preceding 24 hours, corrected for bioavailability differences (see individual antipsychotics in the Product List [page 104] for intramuscular:oral bioavailability ratios) (Ortiz and Gershon 1986).

A number of uncontrolled trials have recommended ***benzodiazepines*** as a sole treatment or as an adjunct to antipsychotics for control of an agitated psychotic patient (Ortiz and Gershon 1986; Rhoades and Overall 1984). The authors of these studies have reported both an improvement in agitation and hostility and a reduction of positive symptoms with diazepam 30–40 mg/day or lorazepam 2–30 mg/day. One study reported that symptoms initially improved with benzodiazepine treatment alone, but noted that they usually returned after 1 week of use. Antipsychotics are the preferred treatment for controlling psychotic symptoms in the agitated patient. However, benzodiazepines may play a role in the early (i.e., typically ≤1 week) control of agitation if recommended doses of antipsychotics are ineffective for this symptom. Elucidation of the exact role of anxiolytics in agitated psychotic patients awaits the results of controlled trials.

Megadosing

Uncontrolled trials using supranormal doses of antipsychotics have suggested that some patients respond better to high than to low doses of antipsychotics. Daily doses of chlorpromazine 5,000 mg, fluphenazine 1,500 mg, and haloperidol 100 mg, as well as depot injections of fluphenazine enanthate starting at 250 mg, have been used. However, a review of 11 double-blind studies failed to demonstrate a significant superiority of megadosing as compared with conventional dosing (Aubree and Lader 1980). Seven of 11 studies reported that EPS were more common in the high-dose group. A more recent review of 33 studies agreed with the earlier recommendations (Baldessarini et al. 1988). Patients who tolerate standard doses without significant clinical improvement might be considered for a high-dose treatment protocol before changing antipsychotics (Brotman and McCormick 1990; Gelenberg 1986).

Maintenance Dosing

(The following information applies to the management of schizophrenia and schizoaffective disorder diagnoses.) Once patients have demonstrated a relapse of symptoms with drug discontin-

uation, they may be considered candidates for long-term antipsychotic treatment (see *First-episode treatment/nonrefractory schizophrenia* and *Maintenance treatment* [pages 2 and 4, respectively]).
Because antipsychotics have a slow onset of action, a direct correlation between a given dose and therapeutic outcome is difficult to
make. Therefore, many patients will receive higher than necessary
doses during acute exacerbations of their illness, which will produce
an increase in some side effects (e.g., extrapyramidal) (Kane and
McGlashan 1995).

Oral antipsychotics.   Two oral dosing strategies—intermittent, or
"targeted," treatment and continuous minimal dosing—have been
recommended for maintenance treatment (Kane and McGlashan
1995; Marder et al. 1993). Intermittent treatment's strategy is to
reduce total drug exposure by treating the patient only when active
symptoms are present. Under this approach, after an initial response, the antipsychotic is discontinued and the patient is closely
followed. The antipsychotic is reinstituted once the patient demonstrates prodromal symptoms of exacerbation. Older literature on
a similar approach, termed "drug holidays," reported that patients
would not relapse with a 2- or 3-day-per-week drug discontinuation
from oral antipsychotics (Davis and Casper 1977). More recent
studies report that some patients may remain off an antipsychotic
for 1 year, although approximately 50% of patients will relapse
within 6 months of drug discontinuation (Davis and Casper 1977;
Herz 1984; Jeste et al. 1979; Kane 1993; McGreadie et al. 1980).

Under the continuous minimal dosing strategy, patients chronically receive much lower doses than were used during acute treatment. The rationale for this approach is based on the observation
that many patients do not relapse when their dose is significantly
reduced after acute treatment (Marder et al. 1993). Five studies
that compared targeted treatment and low-dose continuous dosing
strategies concluded that targeted treatment was associated with
an increased risk of symptomatic relapse (Kane and McGlashan
1995; Marder et al. 1994). In addition, some studies have reported
that drug holidays increase the risk of tardive dyskinesia (Degivity
1969; Glazer et al. 1987; Shenoy et al. 1981), whereas low-dose
continuous treatment may reduce the risk of tardive dyskinesia
(Marder et al. 1993). The continuous low-dose antipsychotic regimen is still recommended (Kane and McGlashan 1995).

One review concluded that the majority of patients can be
maintained on chlorpromazine 300–600 mg/day or its equivalent
(Baldessarini et al. 1988) (see *relative oral potency* under individual

agents in the Product List [page 104]). Two recent studies reported that dosage reduction from an average chlorpromazine equivalent of 1,290 mg/day to 437 mg/day (mean 62%) and an average haloperidol dosage reduction from 63 mg/day to 23 mg/day (mean 63%) resulted in significant improvement in schizophrenia rating scale (e.g., Brief Psychiatric Rating Scale [BPRS]) scores and a reduction in side effects (Liberman et al. 1994; Smith 1994).

Dosage reduction should be considered after a patient has been stabilized on an antipsychotic dose for 3–6 months (Marder et al. 1993). Thereafter, dosage reduction should occur at a rate of 20% every 6 months to achieve the minimal effective dose (Johnson 1985; Marder et al. 1993).

Long-acting parenteral antipsychotics.   A review of five studies that lasted more than 9 months reported that noncompliance with orally administered antipsychotics averaged 33% (Groves and Mandel 1975; Kane 1993). Because constant drug intake is important in preventing symptom relapse and rehospitalization, long-acting parenteral antipsychotics (LAPAs) have been recommended for patients who are repeatedly noncompliant with oral medication. Many studies comparing rates of relapse and rehospitalization with LAPAs versus oral antipsychotic treatment include too few patients or follow them for too short a time to detect significant differences between the two dosage forms. However, six studies have reported that, compared with oral antipsychotics, LAPAs significantly reduced the relapse rate by an average of 16% (Davis et al. 1993). It is probable that the positive effect of LAPAs compared with oral dosage forms is even greater; however, many eligible patients who would benefit from a constant intake of medication do not consent to be studied because they are reluctant to have their compliance monitored.

Several studies have demonstrated that *fluphenazine decanoate* doses of 2.5–5 mg every 2 weeks result in less blunting of affect, less emotional withdrawal, improved interpersonal performance, and less akathisia and retardation than do higher doses (Marder et al. 1994). However, fluphenazine decanoate 10–30 mg every 2 weeks provides the greatest protection against relapse (Baldessarini et al. 1988). Interestingly, a dose of 45 mg every 2 weeks was associated with a worse outcome (Marder et al. 1993).

A review of six studies indicated that the *haloperidol decanoate* maintenance dose ranged from 50 to 150 mg per month (Beresford and Ward 1987). One study reported average doses of 225 mg monthly (Reyntgens et al. 1982). However, a more recent study reported that with haloperidol decanoate monthly maintenance doses of 200 mg, 100 mg, 50 mg, and 25 mg, the relapse rates were 15%, 23%, 25%, and 60%, respectively (Davis et al. 1993). Although a 200-mg monthly dose was associated with the lowest relapse rate, almost 75% of patients treated with 50 mg or 100 mg per month did not relapse. It is important to note that these patients may have been at a low risk of relapse (Kane 1993).

One difficulty in determining the lowest effective maintenance dose for depot antipsychotics is the delay in relapse of symptoms after a dosage reduction. Several studies have demonstrated that a significant level of drug remains in the tissues for weeks to months after drug discontinuation (Chouinard et al. 1989; Gitlin et al. 1988; Nayak et al. 1987). A decrease in serum prolactin levels may take even longer (Gitlin et al. 1988; Wistedt et al. 1981). An undocumented recommendation indicated that dosage reduction of fluphenazine or haloperidol should not exceed 10% every 3 months (Chouinard et al. 1989). However, a dosage reduction period of at least 6 months would be preferable (Marder et al. 1993, 1994). One study of fluphenazine decanoate suggested that if a patient demonstrates initial signs of relapse during dosage reduction or with maintenance doses, oral doses of fluphenazine 10 mg/day might be added (Marder et al. 1994). The fluphenazine decanoate dose could then be increased by 2.5–5 mg every 2 weeks and a trial discontinuation of the oral drug attempted after 1 month. The same strategy could be applied to haloperidol decanoate using supplemental oral haloperidol doses of 10 mg/day while the decanoate dose was increased by 25–50 mg every month.

Major Depressive Disorder With Psychotic Features

An adequate dosage and treatment duration for an antipsychotic/ antidepressant combination in patients with psychotic depression has not been defined (Spiker et al. 1986). It is reasonable to recommend that these patients receive a therapeutic trial of at least chlorpromazine 300 mg/day or its equivalent for 4–5 weeks (see Major Depression With Psychotic Features [page 134] under "Efficacy" of **Tricyclic Antidepressants** in Chapter 2).

Cognitive Disorders

▶ Dementia

Dementia patients may be unusually sensitive to an antipsychotic's therapeutic and adverse effects; therefore, doses of chlorpromazine less than or equal to 300 mg/day or its equivalent are initially used in this population (see the Product List [page 104] for dosage equivalents) (Raskind and Risse 1986; Sunderland 1996; Whalley 1989). In one review, final doses (expressed in chlorpromazine equivalents) ranged from 66 to 267 mg/day (Schneider et al. 1990). Dose titration is dependent on therapeutic response and adverse effects.

Although as-needed dosing is commonly used to manage patients with dementia, no studies have documented the utility of this approach (Druckenbrod et al. 1993). It is recommended that "prn for agitation" orders should specify the severity, quality, and duration of the disruptive behavior before as-needed medication is administered. Orders should specify maximum daily doses and how adverse effects are to be managed.

▶ Delirium

The use of rating scales that both identify behaviors to treat and assess treatment outcome in agitated patients have been recommended (Riker et al. 1994). A rating scale might be used to quickly chart a patient's behavior and response to treatment according to a department's protocol. One such scale, the Sedation-Agitation Scale (Riker et al. 1994), uses a 7-point approach: $+3$ = immediate threat to safety (e.g., patient is climbing over bedrail or striking at staff); $+2$ = dangerously agitated (e.g., patient is requiring physical restraints); $+1$ = agitated (e.g., patient is attempting to sit up but responds to verbal commands); 4) 0 = calm and cooperative; 5) -1 = oversedated; 6) -2 = very oversedated (e.g., patient responds only to noxious stimuli); and 7) -3 = unarousable.

Antipsychotic alone. Although we present dosing recommendations only for haloperidol, equivalent doses of other high-potency antipsychotics could also be considered (see Delirium [page 10] under *Cognitive Disorders*). In one report, haloperidol infusion rates ranged from 3 to 40 mg/hour, with a mean maximum dose of 18 mg/hour (Riker et al. 1994). Continuous infusion lasted a mean of 7 days (range 3–12 days). Total haloperidol doses were as high as 975–1,200 mg/day.

Intermittent injections of haloperidol should initially be used. However, if more than eight 10-mg boluses in a 24-hour period or more than 10 mg/hour for more than 5 consecutive hours are required, continuous infusion is recommended (Riker et al. 1994). Continuous infusion is initiated with a 10-mg bolus, followed by institution of a 10-mg/hour infusion rate. If agitation continues, a repeat 10-mg bolus is administered every 30 minutes and the infusion rate is increased by 5 mg/hour. If the patient remains agitated, the addition of a benzodiazepine might be considered (see *Antipsychotic/benzodiazepine combination*, below). Once control is established and the patient has required few or no bolus injections for 24 hours, the infusion rate is reduced by 50%. Intermittent injections may then be used. The infusion may be discontinued if the patient becomes oversedated (i.e., Sedation-Agitation Scale score ≤ −2). The patient's vital signs and electrocardiogram should be monitored and the patient assessed for the presence of extrapyramidal symptoms (see Extrapyramidal Side Effects [page 45] under *Neurological* adverse effects).

The standard concentration for haloperidol solutions is 200 mg in 160 mL of 5% dextrose in water (Riker et al. 1994). Maximum concentrations with normal saline are 0.75 mg/mL and 3 mg/mL for 5% dextrose in water.

Antipsychotic/benzodiazepine combination.   One suggested protocol (Adams 1988) is as follows:

1. Initial dose is haloperidol 5 mg and lorazepam 0.5 mg administered over 1 minute.
2. If the patient shows an unacceptable response within 20 minutes, give haloperidol 5 mg and lorazepam 0.5–2.0 mg.
3. If the patient shows an unacceptable response within the next 20 minutes, administer haloperidol 10 mg and lorazepam 2–10 mg every 30 minutes until the patient is sedated (i.e., unresponsive to verbal stimuli but responsive to vigorous flexor-extensor movements of the arms).
4. After the patient is sedated, discontinue the lorazepam, and reduce the haloperidol dose by 50%, and double the time between injections.
5. If the patient becomes restless again, restart haloperidol and lorazepam at the previous highest effective dose and administer every 1–3 hours for the next 10–12 hours, at which time the previously described tapering procedure can be performed.

It was noted that most patients responded within 10 to 60 minutes of treatment initiation and that administering doses greater than 10 mg/hour did not usually increase the response rate. Although most patients typically required less than 100 mg/day of each drug, some significantly agitated patients required haloperidol and lorazepam 240 mg each per day. The combination has been given for more than 2 weeks without adverse effects.

Oral-Parenteral Dose Equivalents—
Hydrochloride/Lactate Salts
Some antipsychotics are available for im use; therefore, it is important to know the bioavailability of the oral versus intramuscular

dosage forms for proper dosing. For example, the intramuscular form of chlorpromazine hydrochloride is four times more bioavailable than an equivalent oral dose, so 25 mg im or less would be required to yield the same blood level as chlorpromazine 100 mg po (Perry et al. 1982). (See individual antipsychotics in the Product List [page 104] for intramuscular:oral bioavailability ratios.)

Long-Acting Parenteral Antipsychotics—Decanoate Esters

Products available in the United States include the fluphenazine esters (e.g., decanoate, enanthate) and haloperidol decanoate. Fluphenazine decanoate is preferred to fluphenazine enanthate because of a lower incidence of side effects and a longer duration of action (Hollister et al. 1963; van Praag and Dols 1973). Only the decanoate ester of fluphenazine and haloperidol is discussed here.

▶ Oral-to-Decanoate Conversion

Most clinicians recommend that patients being considered for a decanoate dosage form have their treatment initiated with a po antipsychotic (Del Giudice et al. 1975; Johnson 1984). The rationale is that the po form allows flexibility in daily dosing and the ability to quickly withdraw the drug if "significant" side effects occur. However, this practice requires the patient to be converted from po to decanoate after clinical improvement. Patients receiving po antipsychotics other than fluphenazine or haloperidol should have their po antipsychotic converted to the respective drug based on relative oral potency (see "Dosage" under **Clozapine, Olanzapine, Pimozide, Risperidone,** and **Sertindole** sections in this chapter and individual agents in the Product List [page 104]). Typically, patients are treated with the po antipsychotic for 1–2 weeks before being administered the decanoate (Kane 1993). A patient who responds to the oral drug will be given one or two injections of the decanoate as an inpatient, with plans to taper the po dose as an outpatient over some variable time period. No specific guidelines are available for tapering the po dose. It is possible that the patient, once discharged to an outpatient setting, may be noncompliant with the oral drug. Such an infraction may significantly affect the total serum level of the antipsychotic and may potentially lead to relapse (Kane 1993). In addition, the long-term use of the combination of dosage forms is not recommended, as noncompliance with the po drug may lead to confusion about the required maintenance dose (see *Long-acting parenteral antipsychotics* [page 17]) (Johnson 1985).

Oral fluphenazine–to–decanoate conversion.   The literature on conversion of po fluphenazine to decanoate indicates a wide variability in recommended doses (Nair et al. 1986; Yadalam and Simpson 1988). Recommendations for conversion doses for decanoate and po doses, as well as for management of the po drug during the change to the decanoate, are summarized in Table 1–2 (Yadalam and Simpson 1988). This information is based on clinical experience rather than on comparative serum-level data. Due to assay technical difficulties and significant interpatient variability in oral fluphenazine "first-pass" metabolism, serum-level data comparing po with decanoate doses indicate a poor correspondence (Ereshefsky et al. 1984; Yadalam and Simpson 1988). Therefore, these recommendations should be viewed as guidelines only. The oral dose can be tapered over 1 month or a shorter period if EPS present or worsen after fluphenazine decanoate is started (see Extrapyramidal Side Effects [page 45] under *Neurological* adverse effects).

Although **loading doses** of fluphenazine decanoate might alleviate the need for continuing po fluphenazine during the conversion, this approach has not been extensively investigated. One recent open-design study suggested that patients receiving initial fluphenazine decanoate doses greater than 25 mg (i.e., "loading doses") administered biweekly required a longer time for their psychotic symptoms to be stabilized (Weiden et al. 1993). The reason for this finding is unclear.

Oral haloperidol–to–decanoate conversion.   Usual haloperidol decanoate doses are 75–300 mg/month, although doses of 500 mg/month have been used. Patient conversion from po haloperidol to

Table 1–2.   Conversion schedule for oral fluphenazine to decanoate

Fluphenazine oral dose (mg/day)	Fluphenazine decanoate dose (mg/2 weeks)
5	6.25
10	12.5
20	12.5
30	25.0
40	25.0

Source.   Ereshefsky et al. 1984; Weiden et al. 1993; Yadalam and Simpson 1988.

maintenance doses has been accomplished with and without the use of a haloperidol decanoate loading dose.

The **non–loading-dose approach** involves administering a calculated maintenance dose while the oral dose is tapered. A review of U.S. studies indicated that a maintenance dose of decanoate (mg/month) to po (mg/day) dose ratio of 10–15 was more reasonable than the European literature's ratio of 20 (Kane 1986). For example, using the U.S. studies' recommendations, if a patient was stabilized on 20 mg/day po, the decanoate dose would be 200 mg administered every month. One review reported that 48% of patients received a supplemental po haloperidol dose of 15 mg/day during the first month of decanoate treatment (Ereshefsky et al. 1984). This dose declined to an average of 13 mg/day in 21% of patients after 4 months. Considering that steady-state haloperidol concentrations are not reached for 3 months with the decanoate, a tapering schedule of po haloperidol over a 1-month period might be attempted. If side effects occur during this period, acceleration of the po taper might be considered.

Loading doses of haloperidol decanoate of 20 and 40 times the stabilized po dose have been investigated (Ereshefsky et al. 1993; Kane 1986). Although both doses were effective in maintaining antipsychotic control, the higher loading dose was associated with more EPS.

A **loading dose protocol** for initiating haloperidol decanoate treatment has been recommended (Kane 1993). In the elderly (i.e., persons more than 65 years of age) and in patients stabilized on 10 mg/day or less of oral haloperidol, the recommended loading dose is 10–15 times the po dose (Kane 1993). If a patient is receiving 10 mg/day of po haloperidol, the total loading dose is 20 times the po dose. Although an initial maximum decanoate dose of 100 mg is recommended, higher initial doses can be used (De Cuyper et al. 1986; Ereshefsky et al. 1993; Kane 1993). For example, a 300-mg total loading dose would be administered as 100 mg with the 200-mg dose administered 3–7 days later. The po haloperidol is discontinued at the time of the first injection of the loading dose or, more conservatively, at the time of the final loading dose. The target maintenance dose is 50% of the loading dose. To achieve the maintenance dose, the second month's dose can be reduced by 25% and the third month's dose by an additional 25%. In older patients, the target maintenance dose would still be 50% of the loading dose. The maximum recommended haloperidol decanoate dose is 450 mg/month (Kane 1993).

Haloperidol **serum levels** have been used to calculate a loading dose, because haloperidol's metabolism is less complicated than fluphenazine's (see *haloperidol* [page 29] under "Pharmacokinetics"). A nomogram using data from two reports of po haloperidol and haloperidol decanoate serum-level monitoring has been constructed (see Table 1–3).

The following example illustrates the use of Table 1–3. A patient's symptoms are well controlled on oral haloperidol with a steady-state serum level of 9.3 ng/mL. Achieving a level close to this would require haloperidol decanoate 250 mg/month *(column 1)* to be administered for 3–4 months *(column 3)*. However, a haloperidol decanoate loading dose of 400 mg *(column 1)* would achieve a serum level of 9.3 ng/mL *(column 2)* in 1 month. The 400-mg dose could be divided and administered in three weekly injections (e.g., 100 mg, 150 mg, 150 mg) (see haloperidol *loading dose protocol* under Dosing Intervals, below). To determine the maintenance dose required to achieve a serum level of 9.3 ng/mL after a loading dose, examine column 3. A level of 9.4 ng/mL would be produced by 250 mg *(column 1)* administered every month. This dose would start 1 month after the first loading-dose injection. *Note:* This dosing nomogram is only a guideline. The patient must be continuously monitored for therapeutic response and adverse effects.

Table 1–3.	Projected plasma steady-state haloperidol plasma concentrations based on oral steady-state levels	
Haloperidol decanoate dose (mg/month)	Haloperidol concentration (ng/mL), month 1	Haloperidol concentration (ng/mL), month 3[a]
50	1.1	1.8
100	2.2	3.6
150	3.3	5.5
200	4.5	7.5
250	5.7	9.4
300	6.9	11.4
350	8.1	13.4
400	9.3	15.4

[a] Based on the following equation:
 haloperidol (ng/mL) = $0.0291 \times$ (decanoate dose $^{1.047}$).
Source. Nair et al. 1986; Perry and Alexander 1991; Reyntgens et al. 1982.

▶ Dosing Intervals

Fluphenazine decanoate has typically been administered on a weekly or a biweekly (i.e., every other week) schedule. One study reported that 30% of patients could be successfully maintained on injections at 3-week intervals and 30% on monthly injections for up to 1 year, while another report indicated that 76% of patients could be maintained on monthly injections for up to 2 years (Nayak et al. 1987; Wistedt et al. 1981). In a more recent study, 30% of patients were managed with monthly injections over an 8-month period (Chouinard et al. 1989). One study demonstrated that no relapses were experienced in patients who had their fluphenazine decanoate discontinued for 6 weeks (Belanger and Chouinard 1982). Therefore, patients stabilized on fluphenazine decanoate should be considered for an increased interval between injections as a dose-reduction strategy.

Six of seven **haloperidol** decanoate maintenance studies used monthly intervals (Beresford and Ward 1987). One study reported that patients were divided equally among dosing intervals of 2, 3, and 4 weeks (Chouinard et al. 1989).

Decanoate dose interconversion. Three reports have suggested haloperidol:fluphenazine decanoate dose ratios of 1.4:1, 3:1, and 7:1 (Chouinard et al. 1989; Johnson 1975; Marriott et al. 1984). However, the use of supplemental oral antipsychotics in these reports makes direct comparisons difficult. The 3:1 ratio would be a reasonable starting point. Subsequent dosage adjustment should be based on therapeutic response and adverse effects.

Injection technique. Typically, the decanoates are injected *intramuscularly.* To prevent loss of medication from the injection site and subcutaneous lumps, indurations, and abscesses, the following intramuscular injection procedure for LAPAs has been recommended (Kissling et al. 1985):

> Use a 2-inch needle and inject into the upper outer quadrant of the buttock—no more than 3 mL into one site (2 mL if the deltoid is used) (Wistedt et al. 1984). After drawing the medication into the syringe, add 0.1 mL of air and then change the needle. Wipe the injection site with alcohol and allow it to dry before giving the injection. This is done because alcohol may infiltrate the subcutaneous tissue, causing local irritation. Stretch the skin to one side over the injection site and hold firm (e.g., Z-track technique), then inject the medication and air bubble slowly into the muscle. The air bubble forces the last drop of medication out of the needle. Allow 10 seconds to elapse after the injection before with-

drawing the needle. Do not massage the area, as this may force medication to ooze from muscle.

One study reported that after im administration, patients lost a mean of 13.2% ± 11.2% (range 0.8%–41.5%) of the injected volume (Kissling et al. 1985). However, the Z-track administration method was not used in this study.

A study reported that fluphenazine decanoate could be successfully administered **subcutaneously** at a volume of up to 2.5 mL using a 19-gauge, 0.5-inch needle (Glazer et al. 1987). It was reported that after subcutaneous administration, some patients lost a mean of 3.1% ± 3% (range 0.1%–11.4%) of the injected volume.

Decanoate dosage forms should not be injected **intravenously.** Although specific information is not available on the stability of an open vial of fluphenazine decanoate, it is recommended that any unused drug be discarded within 30 days of the initial puncture (Wasan and Crismon 1990).

■ Pharmacokinetics

Establishing the right dose of antipsychotic has been largely dependent on the trial-and-error approach. Although patient populations varied, most serum-level versus therapeutic response studies were conducted in patients with schizophrenia. The information presented here refers primarily to this diagnosis. Most early positive studies relating antipsychotic blood levels and clinical response need to be replicated with better study designs (e.g., fixed doses, adequate numbers of patients). Present data do not allow a general recommendation for routine blood-level monitoring and subsequent dosage adjustment of any antipsychotic, except possibly haloperidol (Carpenter et al. 1987; Palao et al. 1994; Preskorn et al. 1993). Concentration measurements might be considered for patients who do not respond to a 4-week trial at therapeutic doses (Kane and Marder 1993). If antipsychotic blood levels are obtained, the recommended **sampling time** is just before the next scheduled dose. For most oral antipsychotics, dosage should have been held constant for at least 1 week before sampling is attempted, and for decanoate, a constant dose for 2–3 months should have been received (Preskorn et al. 1993). This recommendation will be useful in the interpretation of subsequent antipsychotic levels. Dosing adjustments to achieve a desired level are made proportionately, as antipsychotics follow linear kinetics with typical doses.

Meaningful concentration information cannot be obtained if the patient is receiving more than one antipsychotic concurrently (see "Rational Prescribing" [page 59]). Studies indicate that measurement of antipsychotic red blood cell, cerebrospinal fluid, or free (i.e., unbound) levels has no clinical benefit (Garver 1989).

Most laboratories measuring antipsychotic concentrations use gas-liquid chromatography (GLC) or high-performance liquid chromatography (HPLC) (Garver 1989; Jolly et al. 1989). Theoretically, the dopamine receptor assay technique detects the parent compound and all metabolites that compete with the dopamine receptor. This technique would separate active from inactive antipsychotic metabolites. Early research suggested that the dopamine receptor assay would provide a better measure of antipsychotic effect than GLC or HPLC assay methods. However, most studies using the receptor assay have failed to demonstrate a relationship between therapeutic response and antipsychotic "concentrations" measured by this technique.

Available preliminary kinetic data for the more commonly prescribed antipsychotics are presented in Table 1–4. The references noted are recommended for reviews of antipsychotic pharmacokinetics and therapeutic response (Balant-Gorgia et al. 1993; Dahl 1986; Garver 1989; Preskorn et al. 1993; Sramek et al. 1988).

Chlorpromazine is only partially absorbed by the gastrointestinal (GI) tract. Differences in formulations, the presence of food in the GI tract, and concomitant therapy with other drugs, such as antacids, may significantly alter the absorption of chlorpromazine. Plasma levels are 4 to 10 times higher after an im injection than those resulting from an equal dose given po. After initial peak plasma levels are achieved, secondary peaks frequently can be observed during the protracted absorptive phase, probably due to the initial precipitation of the drug at the injection site and to the later redissolution and absorption (Dahl 1986).

Chlorpromazine is extensively metabolized by the liver and intestinal wall. Active metabolites have been described in humans. After 2–3 weeks of chronic treatment, a 40% decline in area under the plasma concentration curve has been seen, possibly due to chlorpromazine's inhibition of its own absorption as the result of decreased GI motility or because of the fact that chlorpromazine may accelerate its own metabolism through enzyme induction (Balant-Gorgia et al. 1993).

In psychotic patients receiving typical antipsychotic doses, steady-state plasma levels of the parent drug ranging from 10 to 1,300 ng/mL have been reported (Garattini and Morselli 1978). Several

Table 1–4.   Pharmacokinetics of typical antipsychotics

Drug	Half-life at steady state	Volume of distribution (L/kg)	Plasma protein binding (%)	Peak plasma levels after oral administration	Peak plasma levels after intramuscular administration
Chlorpromazine	3–40 hours	10–35	95–99	2–4 hours	2–3 hours
Fluphenazine decanoate	15–26 days	—	—	—	24 hours, 8–12 days
Fluphenazine enanthate	3.5 days	—	—	—	48 hours
Fluphenazine HCl	8–32 hours	5–60	99	3–5 hours	—
Haloperidol decanoate	21 days	—	—	—	7 days
Haloperidol HCl and lactate	15–30 hours	15–20	—	3 hours	1 hour
Loxapine	6–8 hours	—	—	—	—
Molindone	1.5–6 hours	—	—	30–60 minutes	—
Perphenazine	10–20 hours	10–36	—	3–5 hours	—
Thioridazine	10–30 hours	10	—	2–4 hours	—
Thiothixene	34 hours	—	—	1–3 hours	—
Trifluoperazine	3–40 hours	10–35	95–99	2–4 hours	—

Source.   Balant-Gorgia et al. 1993; Dahl 1986; Garattini and Morselli 1978; Garver 1989; Preskorn et al. 1993; Simpson et al. 1990; Sramek et al. 1988.

studies have demonstrated that good responders have plasma chlorpromazine concentrations in ranges of 30–100 ng/mL, 10–50 ng/mL, and 300–400 ng/mL (Preskorn et al. 1993; Sramek et al. 1988). However, a significant proportion of nonresponding patients outside these ranges may remain unresponsive when placed within these guidelines (Dahl 1986). Consequently, a therapeutic range for chlorpromazine has not been determined (Sramek et al. 1988).

Fluphenazine's oral bioavailability is less than 50% (Balant-Gorgia et al. 1993).

Fluphenazine decanoate peak serum concentrations after a single injection typically occur within 24 hours (Ereshefsky et al. 1984; Davis et al. 1993), although a second peak has been noted 8–12 days after a single injection (Simpson et al. 1990). The half-life of fluphenazine decanoate after a single injection is approximately 8.6 ± 0.2 days (Ereshefsky et al. 1984). Steady-state concentrations of fluphenazine decanoate may not be reached for 1.5–6 months.

Fluphenazine enanthate pharmacokinetics are discussed in detail in the references noted (Curry et al. 1979; Ereshefsky et al. 1984; Garattini and Morselli 1978; Sramek et al. 1988).

Six studies have examined the relationship between fluphenazine serum levels and therapeutic response (Koreen et al. 1994; Preskorn et al. 1993). Two of these studies indicated that a curvilinear relationship (i.e., a "therapeutic window") may exist for fluphenazine between 0.1 and 2.8 ng/mL, whereas two others reported continued improvement up to 4.5 ng/mL. Finally, two studies reported no relationship between plasma levels and clinical response. However, in one of these last two studies, the inability to find a relationship might have been due to differences between first-episode patients and patients with chronic schizophrenia.

Haloperidol tablets have a bioavailability of 60% (range 40%–80%) (Balant-Gorgia et al. 1993). Thus, po doses must be 1.4–1.7 times as large as im or iv doses to result in similar serum concentrations. Intravenous injections of 10 mg produced serum levels of 30 ng/mL (Garattini and Morselli 1978).

It is estimated that 3% of haloperidol is excreted unchanged in the urine. Long-term treatment with the drug did not result in lower serum levels, thus indicating that haloperidol does not induce its own metabolism. The hydroxy metabolite is inactive but may be converted back to haloperidol (Preskorn et al. 1993). Steady-state serum concentrations of po haloperidol are usually achieved within 7 days.

Haloperidol serum concentrations after a single *decanoate* injection typically remain relatively stable over a 4-week interval (Dysken et al. 1981; Kissling et al. 1985; Nayak et al. 1987). Steady state is usually achieved after 3 months (range 1–4 months) of decanoate dosing (Beresford and Ward 1987).

As a result of its relatively simple metabolic profile, haloperidol has been the antipsychotic most extensively investigated in attempts to correlate serum levels with therapeutic response (Preskorn et al. 1993; Sramek et al. 1988). However, research has yielded inconsistent findings. Of 29 studies, 15 reported no relationship, 5 a linear relationship, and 14 a curvilinear relationship (i.e., a therapeutic window of 5–15 ng/mL) (Marder et al. 1989; Mavroidis et al. 1984; Sramek et al. 1988). According to recent literature, maximal response may plateau at 15 ng/mL (Coryell et al. 1990; Kirch et al. 1988; Ko et al. 1989; Palao et al. 1994). Currently, the use of serum haloperidol levels greater than 15 ng/mL is not recommended.

A recent double-blind, fixed plasma-haloperidol-level study assigned 65 patients with schizophrenia or schizoaffective disorder to either a "low" (2 ng/mL)– or a "moderate" (10 ng/mL)–level group for 3 weeks (Volavka et al. 1995). Patients were then randomly assigned to one of four treatment sequences (low→low, low→moderate, moderate→moderate, moderate→low). After the first 3 weeks of treatment, plasma haloperidol levels around 2 ng/mL were less effective than 10-ng/mL levels in reducing positive symptoms. Only a small additional effect on positive symptoms was noted with plasma haloperidol levels higher than 12 ng/mL. In addition, whereas plasma levels greater than 12 ng/mL were associated with an increase in negative symptoms, the 2-ng/mL levels produced improvement of negative symptoms. An additional reduction of plasma levels in the second 3-week treatment period resulted in a further improvement in negative symptoms. More studies are needed that use levels lower than 5 ng/mL and that change a patient's serum level from one range to another to determine whether symptoms respond with improvement or exacerbation.

In a study in which older (average age 60 ± 9 years) patients with schizophrenia were treated with a mean haloperidol dose of 9 ± 13 mg/day, the average plasma haloperidol level was 1.62 ± 2.75 ng/mL (Lacro et al. 1995). This level was similar to that measured in patients with Alzheimer's disease but substantially lower than that reported for younger patients with schizophrenia.

Loxapine is 85%–90% metabolized in the liver (Garattini and Morselli 1978).

Molindone is extensively metabolized in the liver; less than 3% of a dose is excreted unchanged in the urine (Garattini and Morselli 1978). Although the pharmacokinetic half-life of molindone is short, the drug's pharmacodynamic half-life (i.e., the antipsychotic effect) is maintained with once-daily dosing. One study has suggested a linear relationship between molindone serum levels and therapeutic response (Pandurangi et al. 1989). However, this was not a fixed-dose study.

Perphenazine is 60%–80% bioavailable (Balant-Gorgia et al. 1993). Perphenazine levels of 0.8–2.4 ng/mL have been recommended to improve clinical response and to decrease EPS (Dahl 1986).

Thioridazine's bioavailability is only 10%–60% (Balant-Gorgia et al. 1993). It is suggested that thioridazine impairs its own absorption at higher plasma levels, possibly because of its strong anticholinergic effect, which could influence gastric emptying. Like chlorpromazine, thioridazine undergoes extensive side-chain degradation to active (e.g., mesoridazine) and inactive metabolites (Dahl 1982; Garattini and Morselli 1978). About 10%–20% of the drug is excreted unchanged in the urine (Balant-Gorgia et al. 1993). Insufficient data are available to determine a therapeutic range for thioridazine (Sramek et al. 1988).

Thiothixene has a rapid absorption time, with peak plasma levels being reached within 1 to 3 hours of oral administration. The drug disappears from the circulation according to a biexponential decay, with a half-life of 34 hours. Two fixed-dose studies have reported that thiothixene plasma concentrations in the range of 2–15 ng/mL produce the greatest clinical improvement (Preskorn et al. 1993).

One fixed-dose study with *trifluoperazine* in acutely psychotic inpatients reported a therapeutic window of 1–2.3 ng/mL (Dahl 1982).

■ Adverse Effects

The adverse effects of antipsychotic drugs can be classified as allergic, autonomic, cardiovascular, dermatological, endocrinological, hematological, hepatotoxic, metabolic, neurological, ophthalmological, sexual, and teratogenic. Neuroleptic malignant syndrome (NMS) is listed separately.

Common adverse effects involve the autonomic (e.g., hypotension) and neurological (e.g., sedation, EPS) systems. In general, relatively more sedation and vascular effects are seen with low-potency antipsychotics, whereas more EPS occur with high-potency compounds (see "Dosage" and Table 1–1 [pages 12 and 13, respectively]) (Malhotra et al. 1993; Rhoades and Overall 1984).

Allergic

Simple allergic reactions are manifested in three forms. The most common, a maculopapular rash on the face, neck, or upper chest and extremities, occurs in 5%–10% of patients within 14 to 60 days of initiating chlorpromazine therapy. Other reactions include erythema multiforme and localized or generalized urticaria. These effects may be treated with antihistamines and—in the more serious cases—with steroids. Interruption of treatment is usually unnecessary, but if required, the drug may be resumed as the rash subsides. Recurrence of the rash is uncommon. If a patient develops angioneurotic edema or exfoliative dermatitis, treatment is discontinued (Davis and Casper 1977; Shader and DiMascio 1970; Simpson et al. 1981; Malhotra et al. 1993). An antipsychotic in a different chemical class could be administered with caution.

Autonomic

Autonomic nervous system side effects occur secondary to cholinergic blockade (anticholinergic effects) and autonomic hyperactivity (antipsychotic withdrawal).

Anticholinergic effects. Anticholinergic effects of antipsychotics can be divided into peripheral effects (e.g., dry mouth, eyes, and throat; blurred vision; mydriasis; tachycardia; constipation; urinary retention; paralytic ileus) and CNS effects (e.g., delirium) (see Table 1–5, *Anticholinergic potency* column) (Malhotra et al. 1993). Patients who experience *dry mouth, eyes, and throat* can be advised to rinse their mouths with plain water repeatedly or to chew sugarless gum or candy, as adding sugar to the mouth may lead to fungal infections (e.g., moniliasis) and dental caries. Because patients may develop tolerance to dry mouth and many of the other less troublesome anticholinergic side effects, these may present problems only at the beginning of treatment (Davis and Casper 1977; Janicak et al. 1989; Pandurangi et al. 1989). However, some patients continue to experience these effects and may require long-term management, especially if they are concomitantly receiving anticholinergics.

The cause of *blurred vision* is ciliary muscle paresis that results primarily in difficulty in focusing on close objects (Davis and Casper 1977; Shader and DiMascio 1970; Simpson et al. 1981). If a patient is particularly alarmed about the visual disturbance, the dosage may

Table 1–5. Pharmacological profile

Class	Sedation	Cardiovascular	Extrapyramidal side effects (EPS)[a]	Anticholinergic potency
Phenothiazine (aliphatic)				
chlorpromazine	3	3	2	2
Phenothiazine (piperidine)				
thioridazine	2	2	1	3
mesoridazine	2	2	1	2
Phenothiazine (piperazine)				
fluphenazine	1	1	3	1
perphenazine	1	1	3	1
prochlorperazine	1	1	3	1
acetophenazine	1	1	3	1
trifluoperazine	1	1	3	1
Butyrophenone				
haloperidol	1	1	3	1
Thioxanthene				
thiothixene	1	1	3	1
Dihydroindolone				
molindone	1	1	3	1
Dibenzoxazepine				
loxapine	2	2	3	1

Note. 1 = least relative incidence; 3 = greatest relative incidence.
[a] Refers to dystonia, akathisia, and parkinsonism, not to tardive dyskinesia (see Neurological adverse effects [page 45] under **Typical Antipsychotics**).
Source. Black et al. 1985; Malhotra et al. 1993; Rhoades and Overall 1984.

be reduced for a short period. Usually, however, no special treatment is necessary, although reading glasses may be of some benefit (Malhotra et al. 1993).

Constipation is a common complaint of psychiatric patients, particularly the elderly, and may be aggravated by antipsychotics. It should be managed with proper education concerning bowel habits, diet, and activity. Routine or chronic use of laxatives, especially the irritant or stimulant type (e.g., bisacodyl), should be discouraged. Attention should be paid to patients' complaints, and patients' bowel habits should be monitored, as constipation may progress to adynamic ileus. Adynamic ileus requires discontinuation of the offending anticholinergic agent(s) (Black et al. 1985; Davis and Casper 1977; Malhotra et al. 1993; Shader and DiMascio 1970; Simpson et al. 1981).

Urinary retention is probably due to competitive inhibition of acetylcholine at the neuromuscular junction of the detrusor muscle, resulting in increased sphincter tone and more fluid being required to evoke detrusor contraction. Retention is usually noted within 2 to 4 weeks of initiation of the drug and may result in overflow incontinence. The effect is dose related, and men over 60 years of age who have prostatic hypertrophy are at greatest risk (Black et al. 1985; Davis and Casper 1977; Malhotra et al. 1993; Shader and DiMascio 1970; Simpson et al. 1981). Acute urinary retention requires the offending agent to be discontinued.

Withdrawal reactions.   Antipsychotics are not considered to have abuse potential. However, a variety of withdrawal symptoms, such as insomnia, headache, hypersalivation, diarrhea, nausea, and vomiting, have been reported after abrupt discontinuation of these agents. The incidence of withdrawal symptoms ranges from 10% to 75% (average 38%). The symptoms generally begin 2–3 days after abrupt termination of antipsychotic treatment and may last for up to 14 days. No relationship has been demonstrated between antipsychotic dose or chemical group and withdrawal symptoms. Some studies indicate that the low-potency antipsychotics (i.e., aliphatic phenothiazines, aliphatic thioxanthenes, piperidine phenothiazines) may produce the highest incidence of withdrawal symptoms. Although high-potency antipsychotics (e.g., piperazine phenothiazines, piperazine thioxanthenes, butyrophenones) alone can lead to withdrawal symptoms, they appear to do so most often when anticholinergic drugs are being taken concomitantly and are simultaneously withdrawn. Much less information is available on abrupt discontinuance of molindone and loxapine. Patients who have received an antipsychotic alone or in combination with an anticholinergic at therapeutic doses for 1 month or more should have the antipsychotic tapered. Outpatients should be tapered over a 2-week period. For inpatients, the dose can be tapered over a 1-week period, as patients can be closely monitored and dose and schedule adjusted if necessary. The anticholinergic may be discontinued 5 days after stopping the antipsychotic (Dilsaver 1994; Gallant et al. 1964; Simpson et al. 1965).

Cardiovascular
Postural, or **orthostatic, hypotension** is postulated to be due to the α-adrenergic–blocking effect of the antipsychotics, which creates exaggerated venous pooling by inhibiting the reflex vasoconstriction that normally occurs upon assuming an upright posture (Malhotra et al. 1993). Calcium channel blocking effects may also contribute to this effect (Simpson et al. 1981). Aliphatic derivations of phenothiazines and thioxanthenes are potent α-receptor antagonists, whereas piperazine derivatives and butyrophenones are weak antagonists. Although hypotensive effects are rare, some patients experience them after receiving iv haloperidol (Riker et al. 1994).

Postural hypotension is usually seen during the first few hours or days of treatment and is defined as a drop in systolic pressure of 20 mm Hg or an increase of 20 beats/minute in the pulse rate upon changing from a lying to a standing position. Any patient can develop hypotension, but the elderly seem more susceptible. Hypotension after parenteral antipsychotics may be more pronounced than that after oral administration. Hypotensive episodes can occur unexpectedly, with sudden fainting and falling, during which injury can result. Patients prone to hypotension who are receiving antipsychotics should be given cautionary instructions: rise from bed gradually, sit at first with legs dangling, wait for a minute, and then rise only if no feeling of dizziness or faintness is experienced. Knee-length elastic or support stockings may be used for adjunctive management of orthostatic hypotension. When postural hypotension does occur, patients can be properly managed in most cases by keeping their feet above their heads when they are supine. Only rarely is volume expansion or a vasopressor agent (e.g., norepinephrine) indicated, since patients generally do not develop a shock-like syndrome. Epinephrine is contraindicated because antipsychotics effectively block the α-adrenergic receptor–stimulating properties of epinephrine while allowing the β-stimulation (e.g., vasodilatation) to continue, thereby creating a more pronounced hypotension. Although patients may develop a compensatory subjective tolerance to hypotension, it is best to monitor lying and standing blood pressure for the low-potency antipsychotics for the first few days of treatment. If hypotension is severe or tolerance does not develop, the therapy may be changed to another antipsychotic less likely to cause hypotensive effects (see *Cardiovascular* column in Table 1–5 [page 33]). Lowering the dose of the antipsychotic might be tried empirically (Black et al. 1985; Davis and Casper 1977; Malhotra et al. 1993; Shader and DiMascio 1970; Simpson et al. 1981).

Electrocardiogram (ECG) changes similar to those seen with the antiarrhythmic agent quinidine have been reported. Phenothiazines—in particular, chlorpromazine and thioridazine—have been commonly reported to produce broadened, flattened T waves and an increase in the QR interval; this effect is of uncertain clinical significance. Similar effects with thioxanthenes, dihydroindolones, and dibenzoxazepines have also been reported. Several case reports of death, possibly related to cardiac effects, have been reported with antipsychotics (Black et al. 1985; Davis and Casper 1977; Huyse and Van Schijndel 1988; Malhotra et al. 1993; Riker et al. 1994; Shader and DiMascio 1970; Simpson et al. 1981). However, it is important to note that sudden, unexplained death in psychiatric patients receiving no psychotropics has also been reported. Often, a clear relationship between the antipsychotic and the cause of death cannot be established.

High-dose intravenous haloperidol appears to be relatively free of cardiac effects (Riker et al. 1994). However, three cases of torsade de pointes that developed during treatment with iv haloperidol have been reported (Metzger and Friedman 1993). Total haloperidol doses of 115, 490, and 825 mg were associated with a 28%, 31%, and 22% increase, respectively, in the QTc interval. All three patients had cardiac disease and dilated ventricles on echocardiogram. Five additional cases of torsade de pointes were associated with the use of oral haloperidol. Patients with torsade de pointes may develop either ventricular fibrillation or tachycardia.

A predrug baseline ECG, serial monitoring, and use of an agent less likely to produce cardiac effects are warranted in patients with significant cardiac disease.

Dermatological
Photosensitivity reactions have been reported to occur in 3% of patients taking antipsychotics, with most cases related to chlor-

promazine. Lesions are usually confined to light-exposed areas and are most often sunburn-like and erythematous. Patients should be warned about this side effect, especially during the summer months. Protective clothing, as well as use of a sunscreen with a maximum sunblock rating, is recommended. Patients who have increased sensitivity to light should limit their sun exposure, regardless of which antipsychotic they are receiving (Black et al. 1985; Davis and Casper 1977; Malhotra et al. 1993; Shader and DiMascio 1970; Simpson et al. 1981).

Long-term skin effects include *pigmentary skin changes* involving a tan color that progresses to a slate-gray, metallic blue, or purple color over areas exposed to sunlight. Skin biopsy has demonstrated golden-brown pigment granules similar but not identical to melanin.

Bluish pigmentation appears at a frequency of approximately 1% with all antipsychotics. However, the incidence of the effect depends on the antipsychotic used, its dosage, and the extent of the patient's exposure to the sun. Pigmentation was found in 30% of patients on chlorpromazine who had received a total dose of 600 g, a daily dose of 600 mg or greater for 1 year, or a total yearly dosage of 200 g. Because pigmentation is related to the total dose ingested, the less-potent phenothiazines (e.g., chlorpromazine) will be associated with a higher incidence of pigmentation effects than will the potent ones (e.g., fluphenazine). These skin disorders are thought to occur less frequently today than in the 1950s, possibly because of the use of lower dosages and the preferential use of high-potency antipsychotics. Haloperidol reportedly does not cause this side effect (Black et al. 1985; Davis and Casper 1977; Malhotra et al. 1993; Shader and DiMascio 1970; Simpson et al. 1981).

Endocrinological

Amenorrhea, galactorrhea, and gynecomastia. These effects are possibly related to an elevation of prolactin levels secondary to blockage of dopamine, which inhibits pituitary prolactin secretion directly (Davis and Casper 1977; Gould et al. 1984; Shader and DiMascio 1970; Simpson et al. 1981; Sullivan and Lukoff 1990). The differential diagnosis should include pituitary abnormalities.

Amenorrhea is reported to occur in 18%–95% of women receiving antipsychotics, as compared with 3%–5% of women in the general population (Zito et al. 1990).

Galactorrhea occurs in both men and women and is frequently accompanied by some degree of breast enlargement or engorgement (Sullivan and Lukoff 1990). One study reported an incidence of 57% in females (Huyse and Van Schijndel 1988). Galactorrhea can occur at varying dosage levels, may appear as early as 8 days after onset of treatment, and is more commonly found in premenopausal women. However, it often occurs with high-dose, long-duration regimens and is frequently accompanied by amenorrhea.

Gynecomastia (breast enlargement) of any etiology is uncommon; therefore, other medical causes should be considered. Gynecomastia in females as well as males has been reported (Sullivan and Lukoff 1990). Although there is concern that prolonged elevated prolactin levels may be associated with an increased incidence of breast cancer, at present such an association has not been proven (Zito et al. 1990).

Management of endocrinological effects.   Endocrinological adverse effects appear to persist with continued antipsychotic treatment (Zito et al. 1990). Upon discontinuation of an oral antipsychotic, elevated prolactin levels may subside within 48 to 72 hours (Inoue et al. 1980). However, some reports indicate that normalization of prolactin levels and elimination of breast symptoms may require as long as 3 weeks. Four to 6 months may be needed to reach normal prolactin levels after discontinuation of a LAPA (e.g., fluphenazine decanoate) (Overall 1978).

Because all typical antipsychotics may cause elevated prolactin, switching to another drug in this class may not be effective but may empirically be tried (Sullivan and Lukoff 1990). Dosage reduction may also be beneficial (Sullivan and Lukoff 1990; Zito et al. 1990). Limited experience suggests that amantadine and bromocriptine may control hyperprolactinemia, gynecomastia, and amenorrhea (Zito et al. 1990).

Water dysregulation.   Although polydipsia and intermittent hyponatremia have been reported to improve with antipsychotic treatment, many case reports and studies suggest that antipsychotics contribute to water dysregulation (Leadbetter and Shutty 1994). Future controlled trials of antipsychotics in short- and long-term treatment of patients with hyponatremia are necessary. Management has included behavioral approaches and successful pharmacological treatment with propranolol, lithium, phenytoin, angiotensin-converting enzyme inhibitors (e.g., captopril, enalapril), and naloxone (Burnakis 1992; Godleski et al. 1989; Goldstein 1986; Nishikawa et al. 1994). The relative efficacy of these treatments has not been determined. Substitution of clozapine for a typical antipsychotic has resulted in improved water handling (see *Water Dysregulation* [page 66] under "Efficacy" of **Clozapine**).

Hematological

Transient **leukocytosis** or **leukopenia** and an **eosinophilia** have been reported with all antipsychotics; these effects do not require treatment or discontinuation of the drug.

Agranulocytosis usually begins after a latent period ranging from 20 to 35 days. Ninety percent of cases occur within the first 8 weeks. The incidence of agranulocytosis is estimated to be less than 1 in 10,000 patients. It has been suggested that older patients are at a greater risk for agranulocytosis than are younger patients (i.e., <40 years of age). The condition usually begins with symptoms of a local infection, usually in the pharynx. Examination reveals fever, pharyngeal erythema and ulcerations, cervical and submandibular adenopathy, and systemic symptoms of malaise and prostration. The leukocyte count drops rapidly at the beginning of the illness and reaches a low point in 2–5 days. The complete blood count (CBC) shows a severe leukopenia and essentially no granulocytes; red blood cell and platelet counts are unchanged. The marrow reveals a selective aplasia of the granulocytic series. Upon discontinuation of the antipsychotic, recovery should occur within 2 weeks if the patient is placed in reverse isolation and appropriate antibiotics are instituted in the event of an infection. The use of granulocyte colony–stimulating factor (G-CSF) might hasten recovery of neutrophils (Gerson 1994). Although mortality has decreased significantly within the last 10 years, 10%–20% of patients still die from fulminating infections.

Agranulocytosis has been implicated in case reports with all antipsychotics; however, most reports involve patients receiving aliphatic and piperidine phenothiazines. Whether phenothiazines actually differ in causing this adverse effect is not known. Management of psychosis with an antipsychotic of a different chemical class is recommended (Black et al. 1985). It has been suggested that antipsychotic-induced agranulocytosis is caused by inhibition of the enzymes responsible for DNA synthesis in sensitive individuals who cannot compensate for this toxic effect (Shader and DiMascio 1970). The condition is so rare that regular blood counts are not necessary (Malhotra et al. 1993). However, clinical signs or symptoms of an infection, especially during the first 3 months of treatment, should be investigated.

Hepatotoxicity

Reports indicate that mild and transient elevations in liver enzymes after initiation of therapy can occur with any of the antipsychotics. This side effect does not require drug discontinuation.

A more specific hepatotoxic reaction has been reported with phenothiazines, especially chlorpromazine. However, no adequate studies exist to confirm that chlorpromazine causes liver damage more often than do other phenothiazines. The clinical findings described are characteristic of the reports of chlorpromazine-induced liver disease. Jaundice usually appears within the first month of treatment. Prodromal symptoms may begin abruptly and include fever, chills, nausea, epigastric pain, right upper quadrant pain, and malaise preceding the onset of jaundice by approximately 5 days. Laboratory findings resemble those for cholestatic jaundice, with alkaline phosphatase and conjugated bilirubin commonly elevated. Aspartate and alanine transferase are usually only mildly elevated. Biopsy reveals bile stasis maximally located in the centrilobular region, which is infiltrated with mononuclear cells, lymphocytes, and eosinophils. Age, sex, dosage, and preexisting liver disease have not been related to antipsychotic-induced jaundice. Chlorpromazine-induced hepatitis is a short, self-limiting illness, and the jaundice usually clears within 2 to 8 weeks. Cross-sensitivity between chlorpromazine and other phenothiazines rarely occurs. Some studies have found that liver function returns to normal even if the drug is continued. However, it is recommended that the offending drug be discontinued if possible (Black et al. 1985; Shader and DiMascio 1970). Although routine monitoring of liver function tests are unnecessary, a baseline value might be obtained (Malhotra et al. 1993). If signs or symptoms of hepatitis are present, liver tests should be performed. The incidence of jaundice associated with phenothiazines is estimated to be less than 0.5%. The mechanism of this effect is unknown.

Metabolic
Weight gain averaging 6 kg in a 6-week treatment period has been reported in patients receiving antipsychotics (Davis and Casper 1977; Meltzer and Fang 1976; Shader and DiMascio 1970). Whether this effect is due to the drug alone or to a combination of factors such as lack of activity or increased dietary intake is unknown. Management includes exercise and dietary restriction. Molindone and loxapine have been associated with weight loss during treatment, but differences in weight gain with these drugs have not been conclusively demonstrated (Parent et al. 1986). These drugs may be tried in selected patients with weight problems who do not respond to other management. Prescribing amphetamine or amphetamine-like appetite suppressants is unwarranted because of these agents' potential to exacerbate psychosis.

Neuroleptic Malignant Syndrome

A syndrome characterized by muscular rigidity, hyperthermia, altered consciousness, and autonomic dysfunction has been reported in patients primarily receiving typical antipsychotics (Caroff and Mann 1993). NMS or a NMS-like picture has also been associated with metoclopramide, tetrabenazine, amphetamine, cocaine, lithium, phencyclidine, monoamine oxidase inhibitor overdoses or interactions, reserpine, amoxapine, risperidone, and clozapine (see *Neurological* adverse effects under **Clozapine** and **Risperidone** sections [pages 76 and 96, respectively]) antipsychotics (Caroff and Mann 1993). Discontinuation of levodopa, amantadine, bromocriptine, or TCAs has been reported to produce a NMS-like syndrome (Parent et al. 1986; Wistedt et al. 1981). Lithium in combination with antipsychotics may increase the risk of NMS (Caroff and Mann 1993).

The reported incidence of NMS varies from 0.02% to 3.23% (Caroff and Mann 1993). Prospective studies report the lowest incidence, and pooled data from 16 studies yielded an incidence of 0.2%.

Several authors have suggested the use of *diagnostic criteria* for NMS (Caroff and Mann 1993). One set of criteria proposed is as follows: 1) treatment with po antipsychotics within 7 days or with long-acting agents within 2 to 4 weeks; 2) hyperthermia greater than or equal to 38°C; 3) muscle rigidity; 4) five of the following: change in mental status, tachycardia, hyper- or hypotension, tachypnea or hypoxia, diaphoresis or sialorrhea, tremor, incontinence, creatine phosphokinase elevation or myoglobinuria, leukocytosis, or metabolic acidosis; and 5) exclusion of other drug-induced, systemic, or neuropsychiatric illnesses (Caroff and Mann 1993). The differential diagnosis of NMS has been reviewed (Caroff and Mann 1993).

The *onset* of NMS may occur as early as 45 minutes or as late as 65 days after initiation of the antipsychotic (Caroff and Mann 1993; Keck et al. 1989b; O'Brien and Young 1989; Rosenberg and Green 1989). Sixteen percent of patients developed signs within 1 day, 66% within 1 week, and 96% by 1 month of starting treatment. Once initiated, the syndrome develops rapidly over 24–72 hours.

Clinical presentation includes hyperthermia with significant diaphoresis in 98% of cases (Caroff and Mann 1993). Ninety-seven percent of patients will have generalized (i.e., "lead pipe") rigidity, which may be accompanied by coarse tremors and myoclonus. Prolonged rigidity is often associated with myonecrosis. Body temperature will exceed 38°C in 87% of patients, and 40% will have temperatures higher than 40°C. Mental status changes occur in 97% of cases; typically, the patient is dazed and mute but alert. However, the patient may be delirious and agitated or in a coma. Tachycardia is present in 88% of patients, and fluctuating blood pressure (i.e., hypo- or hypertension) is noted in 61%. About one-third of cases have tachypnea and moderate to severe respiratory distress secondary to aspiration pneumonia, pulmonary emboli, metabolic acidosis, hyperthermia, or chest-wall restriction. Prodromal signs are often difficult to identify.

Laboratory findings are not diagnostic (Caroff and Mann 1993). However, 97% of patients will have a leukocytosis of 15,000–30,000 with or without a left shift, while myoglobinuria and an elevated creatine phosphokinase (up to 15,400 IU) will be present in 67% and 95% of patients, respectively. Myonecrosis may lead to elevations of lactic acid dehydrogenase, transaminases, and aldolase. Blood-gas results are consistent with metabolic acidosis or hypoxia in 75% of patients. An EEG suggestive of diffuse metabolic encephalopathy has been reported in 54% of cases. Computed tomographic (CT) scans are negative in 95% of patients, as is examination of the cerebrospinal fluid.

The mean *duration* of uncomplicated NMS varies from 6.8 to 10.6 days (Caroff and Mann 1993). Twenty-three percent of patients recovered within 2 days, 63% within 1 week, and 97% by 1 month of antipsychotic discontinuation. Ten to 40 days may be required for recovery after cessation of fluphenazine and haloperidol decanoate (Caroff and Mann 1993; Rosenberg and Green 1989).

A 1987 review indicated *mortality rates* of 76%, 23%, and 15% for periods before 1970; from 1979 to 1980; and after 1980, respectively (Keck et al. 1989c; Shalev et al. 1988). More recent reports have not mentioned any NMS-related fatalities, probably because of earlier recognition, which leads to antipsychotic discontinuation and institution of supportive and/or pharmacological treatment (Caroff and Mann 1993). Patients with myoglobinemia and renal failure have a mortality rate of 47% and 56%, respectively (Shalev et al. 1989). Other complications, such as seizures, pulmonary embolus, cardiac infarction or failure, or disseminated intravascular coagulation, may lead to death. Long-term sequelae are rare and may be related to the severity of the hypoxia or hyperthermia (Caroff and Mann 1993).

Predisposing factors have been difficult to determine (Caroff and Mann 1993). Age, sex, psychiatric diagnosis, and environmental situation (e.g., hot climate) do not predict the occurrence of NMS (Addonizio et al. 1987). The potency (i.e., low versus high) and dosage form (i.e., oral versus long acting) of the antipsychotic do not increase the risk of NMS. Psychomotor agitation, dehydration, exhaustion, and the number of intramuscular injections received have been identified as risk factors (Caroff and Mann 1993). Although antipsychotic daily dose has not consistently been demonstrated to be a risk factor, the interrelationship of dose and the aforementioned risk factors has not been prospectively determined. It is possible that higher doses may be the most significant predictor of NMS. The acutely agitated psychotic patient is more likely to experience exhaustion and dehydration and also more likely to receive higher antipsychotic doses.

It has been suggested that patients with a personal or family history of malignant hyperthermia (MH) or NMS might be at a significantly increased risk of developing the alternate syndrome if exposed to precipitating agents (Keck et al. 1995). However, although MH and NMS are clinically similar, a review of the literature indicates that cross-reactivity between offending agents for each disorder is unlikely to occur.

Management of NMS. When NMS is suspected, the antipsychotic should be discontinued and *supportive care* instituted immediately to reduce the risk of morbidity and mortality (Caroff and Mann 1993). Intubation, mechanical ventilation, fever reduction, and other supportive measures may be required until the muscular rigidity and fever begin to resolve (Rosenberg and Green 1989). Hydration is especially important to counteract renal tubular necrosis (Kellam 1987). An attempt must be made to rule out other causes of fever, such as infection (Shalev et al. 1989).

The exact *pharmacological treatment* of NMS is not established, as prospective, controlled trials have not yet been performed (Caroff and Mann 1993; Eiser et al. 1982; Rosenberg and Green 1989; Shalev et al. 1989). Muscle relaxants, dopamine agonists, anticholinergics, calcium channel blockers, and electroconvulsive therapy (ECT) have all been used. Studies have not consistently found that pharmacological management reduces morbidity, mortality, or duration of signs and symptoms (Caroff and Mann 1993). However, some form of pharmacological management is usually instituted (Caroff and Mann 1993).

The muscle relaxant *dantrolene* produces a mean response time and a time to complete symptom resolution of 1.7 and 9 days, respectively (Shalev et al. 1989). Recommended doses are 2–

3 mg/kg/day administered intravenously. Hepatotoxicity has often been noted with repeated doses above 10 mg/kg, but this effect may also occur with much lower doses (Rosenberg and Green 1989). Once the patient recovers sufficiently, oral treatment can be used, which is a much less costly route.

The use of dopamine agonists is based on the hypothesis that NMS results from excessive dopaminergic blockade in predisposed individuals (Guerrero and Shifrar 1988; V. W. Henderson and Wooten 1981; Pearlman 1986). Dopamine agonists include bromocriptine, amantadine, and levodopa. *Bromocriptine*'s recommended dosage is 7.5–40 mg/day po in three to four divided doses (Shalev et al. 1989). It is reported to produce a clinical response and resolution of symptoms in a mean time of 1 and 10 days, respectively (Rosenberg and Green 1989). The pharmacological effects of bromocriptine result from stimulation of dopamine receptors in the CNS. *Amantadine* facilitates the release of dopamine from presynaptic storage sites. This drug has been used in 18 patients, and a typical dose is 100 mg po bid (Hamburg et al. 1986; Shalev et al. 1989). *Levodopa* has been employed in only one case, and this was in combination with amantadine (Pearlman 1986).

In three cases in which *diazepam* was used alone, 3–6 weeks of treatment were required for clinical response. Overall, benzodiazepines appear to have limited usefulness in NMS (Guerrero and Shifrar 1988).

Anticholinergics often are reported as ineffective in NMS, but this finding may be due to inadequate doses or a delay in their use (Tollefson and Garvey 1984; Toru et al. 1981).

Experience is limited with *calcium channel blockers.* These agents may exert their effect by displacing the antipsychotic from dopamine receptors or by reducing intracellular calcium (Toru et al. 1981).

The use of *ECT* in NMS has been associated with an overall improvement rate of 74%–83% (Bamrah 1988; Caroff and Mann 1993; Hughes 1986; Lazarus 1986; Schulte-Sasse and Eberlein 1986). ECT should be reserved for patients who are unresponsive to pharmacological management.

Treatment recommendations. Until adequate studies have been performed, pharmacological treatment with dantrolene or bromocriptine is recommended for NMS (Caroff and Mann 1993). No support exists for using these drugs in combination. If treatment with one of these agents fails, other listed drugs or ECT should be tried. Once the patient responds, drug treatment should continue for an additional 8–12 days (D. A. Casey 1987).

Antipsychotic rechallenge. This treatment issue has been the subject of several review articles (Caroff and Mann 1993; Jessee and Anderson 1983; Rosenberg and Green 1989; Susman and Addonizio 1988). Rates of recurrence in these investigations varied from 13% to 64%. The time between symptom resolution and antipsychotic rechallenge influences the likelihood of a recurrence. One study reported a recurrence rate with antipsychotic rechallenge of 64% when the antipsychotic was re-started within 5 days or less of symptom resolution. This result was in contrast to approximately 30% of patients who were re-started after more than 5 days (Susman and Addonizio 1988; Wells et al. 1988). It is recommended that antipsychotics not be reinstituted until at least 2 weeks after the patient's symptoms are completely resolved and he or she is no longer receiving treatment for NMS (Rosenberg and Green 1989). The effect of age, sex, and diagnosis did not appear to play a role in predicting recurrence of NMS upon rechallenge (Susman and Addonizio 1988). Rechallenge was reportedly more successful with a low-potency antipsychotic and a lower antipsychotic dose (Caroff and Mann 1993). If a patient develops NMS on a high-potency drug, a trial with a low-potency antipsychotic is recommended (see "Dosage" and Table 1–1 [pages 12 and 13, respectively]). If an antipsychotic of the same or similar potency is started, low doses should be used. Close monitoring is recommended if the patient is receiving lithium.

Neurological

▶ **Cognition**
A recent review concluded that typical antipsychotics do not have significant positive or negative effects on memory, except for potentially adverse effects in certain patients (see *Psychiatric* adverse effects [page 55]) (P. E. Goldberg and Weinberger 1996). However, these agents may have a mediating effect on vigilance or response readiness.

▶ **Extrapyramidal Side Effects**
EPS are divided into early-onset and late-onset types. Early-onset EPS usually occur within the first 4 weeks of treatment and include dystonia, akathisia, and parkinsonism. (See Chapter 6 for additional information on the management of early-onset EPS.) Late-onset EPS occur after 6 months of treatment and consist of tardive dyskinesia, tardive dystonia, and tardive akathisia.

Estimates of the incidence of *early-onset EPS* with antipsychotics vary widely, ranging from 2.2% to 95%. Much of the variation in the reported percentages may be explained by differences in the antipsychotic prescribed (e.g., low- versus high-potency), length of treatment, dosage, individual sensitivity, and definitions of EPS. The rates of early-onset EPS for fluphenazine decanoate and haloperidol decanoate were equal in two studies, whereas in another two trials, haloperidol's rate was lower (Davis et al. 1993). However, exact dosage equivalents between these two agents have not been determined (see *Decanoate dose interconversion* [page 25] under Dosing Intervals).

Early-onset EPS are reportedly less common with intravenous haloperidol—as compared with oral or intramuscular administration—in critically ill, delirious patients (Menza et al. 1987; Riker et al. 1994). Theories proposed to explain the lower rate include the following: 1) intravenous administration produces lower levels of the metabolites that may be responsible for EPS; 2) critically ill patients have low levels of acetylcholine, and the dopamine-blocking properties of the antipsychotic reestablish a relative balance; and 3) the use of a benzodiazepine in combination with an antipsychotic reduces the risk of dystonia and akathisia. However, in a prospective study of 38 acquired immunodeficiency syndrome (AIDS) patients treated with intravenous haloperidol and lorazepam, a 50% rate of EPS was detected (Fernandez et al. 1989). There is a suggestion that a combination of lithium and antipsychotic might increase the incidence of EPS (Addonizio et al. 1988).

All EPS wax and wane over time, disappear during sleep, and are exacerbated by emotionally disturbing experiences.

The differences between the low- and high-potency classes of antipsychotics in causing early-onset EPS have historically been attributed to the intrinsic anticholinergic effects of this drug group. Thus, the potent anticholinergic piperidine phenothiazines (e.g., thioridazine) are less likely to cause acute-onset EPS than are the weakly anticholinergic butyrophenones (e.g., haloperidol) (Rhoades and Overall 1984) (see Table 1–5 [page 33]). However, an alternative explanation suggests that certain antipsychotics cause fewer EPS because of differences in dopamine-receptor-site specificity (Borison 1985). Drugs responsible for a lower incidence of these side effects may interact less with extrapyramidal dopamine receptors while having relative site specificity for limbic and/or cortical receptors (i.e., an antipsychotic effect) (see "Mechanism of Action" [page 12]).

Dystonia.   Dystonic reactions consist of involuntary tonic contractions of skeletal muscles of virtually any striated muscle group

(Black et al. 1985; D. E. Casey 1993; Davis and Casper 1977; Shader and DiMascio 1970; Simpson et al. 1981). The most common dystonias involve the muscles of the head and face, producing buccal spasms, oculogyric crisis, facial grimacing, tics, or trismus. Involvement of the neck musculature produces torticollis or retrocollis. If the trunk is involved, shoulder shrugging, tortipelvis, opisthotonus, or scoliosis may occur. Carpopedal spasms, dorsiflexion of the toes, contraction of muscle groups of arms or legs, or a dystonic gait may be seen if the limbs are involved. Rare complications include chipped teeth, dislocation of the temporomandibular joint, tongue injuries, and respiratory distress secondary to involvement of the pharyngeal muscles (Koek and Pi 1989). Ninety percent of dystonic reactions develop the fourth day of antipsychotic treatment. They may also occur after a single dose of an antipsychotic, regardless of the route of administration. Dystonias may appear abruptly or in a stuttering fashion over several hours. Usually they occur only once, but occasionally they recur with an increase in dosage. Although all antipsychotics may produce these reactions, their incidence is greater with certain drugs in this class (see Tables 1–1 and 1–5 [pages 13 and 33, respectively]). The reported incidence of dystonia ranges from 2.3% to 64%, depending on the antipsychotic(s) studied (Borison 1985). Although a dystonic reaction may occur at any age, it is 15 times more common in patients under 35 years of age (Addonizio and Alexopoulos 1988). Men less than 50 years old are twice as likely as women of this age to develop dystonia (Swett 1975). The dystonic reaction rate in patients over 50 years of age is the same for men and women. A retrospective study indicated that dystonia affects 26% and 6% of manic and schizophrenic patients, respectively (Nasrallah et al. 1988). More recent prospective studies have reported no differences in the rates of dystonic reactions in those diagnoses (Khanna et al. 1992; Remington et al. 1990). However, in one of these studies, patients were treated with high doses of intramuscular haloperidol (e.g., average 26–42 mg), which may have obscured a possible diagnosis-related difference (Remington et al. 1990); in the other study, the number of subjects in each group may have been too small to detect a difference (Khanna et al. 1992).

Dystonias are usually benign and disappear without treatment. However, because of the extreme discomfort to the patient and the possibility of serious sequelae, dystonic reactions should be treated as soon after their appearance as possible. Although many agents have been recommended for this purpose, intravenous diphenhydramine (Benadryl®) 50 mg or benztropine (Cogentin®) 2 mg produce rapid reversal of dystonia, usually within 2 minutes. If no relief occurs within 5 minutes, the dose should be repeated. The intramuscular route has been successfully used, but resolution of the dystonia by that route may take 20–40 minutes (Gelenberg 1987). (See Chapter 6 for additional information on the management of dystonias.)

The exact etiology of dystonia is unknown, although it is hypothesized to be the result of an initial hypodopaminergic state followed by a hyperdopaminergic state that occurs within the first few days of treatment (D. E. Casey 1993). This hyperdopaminergic state gradually returns to baseline, thus explaining the symptom's self-limited nature.

Akathisia. *Akathisia* refers to a subjective experience of motor restlessness (D. E. Casey 1993). Patients may complain of an inability to sit or stand still or a compulsion to pace. They may also complain of being restless and having to be in constant motion. When standing, they may rock to and fro or shift their weight from one leg to another. Patients may also suffer from initial insomnia because they cannot lie motionless in bed long enough to fall asleep.

Typically, akathisia appears within 2 to 3 weeks of initiation of an antipsychotic (Van Putten et al. 1984). Ninety percent of cases develop within the first 73 days of treatment (Ayd 1961); however, some patients develop this effect within hours of their first antipsychotic dose. Estimates of the incidence of akathisia range from 21% to 75% (Sachdev and Loneragan 1991). The etiology is unknown (D. E. Casey 1993). Women are approximately twice as likely as men to develop akathisia, and the syndrome demonstrates equal prevalence across all age groups (Ayd 1961; D. E. Casey 1994; Ganzini et al. 1991). An accurate diagnosis is important because misdiagnosis may lead to an unnecessary increase in antipsychotic dose, with potential worsening of akathisia (D. E. Casey 1994).

Nonpharmacological management of antipsychotic-induced akathisia includes drug discontinuation (if indicated), dosage reduction, or switching the patient to an agent less likely to produce EPS (i.e., a low-potency drug) (see Tables 1–1 and 1–5 [pages 13 and 33, respectively]). Upon discontinuation of the antipsychotic, akathisia symptoms generally resolve within 7 days, but may take several weeks. (See Chapter 6 for additional information on the pharmacological management of akathisia.)

Parkinsonism. Parkinsonian side effects manifest as tremor, rigidity, and hypokinesia or akinesia, both individually or in combination (Black et al. 1985; D. E. Casey 1993; Davis and Casper

1977; Shader and DiMascio 1970; Simpson et al. 1981). Drooling, festinant gait, oily skin, dysarthria, and dysphagia may accompany the symptoms. Antipsychotic-induced parkinsonism may be clinically indistinguishable from postencephalitis or idiopathic parkinsonism. Akinesia may originally present as slowness when initiating motor tasks and fatigue when performing activities requiring repetitive movements (e.g., bradykinesia). Affected persons appear apathetic, with little facial expression, and may have difficulty walking; their handwriting may take on a cramped appearance (i.e., micrographia). This drug-induced condition should not be misinterpreted as depressive symptomatology. The typical antipsychotic-induced parkinsonian tremor can be present during movement as well as at rest. Usually, tremor begins in one or both upper extremities; in severe cases, it may involve the tongue, jaw, and lower extremities. "Rabbit syndrome"—tremor involving the mouth, chin, and lips—is very responsive to anticholinergic treatment (Black et al. 1985; D. E. Casey 1993). Cogwheel rigidity, in which a ratchet-like phenomenon can be elicited upon passive movement of a limb, results from the presence of both rigidity and tremor.

As with all drug-induced EPS, there is a wide variance in the reported incidence of parkinsonian effects. The range is 2.2% to 56%. Parkinsonism can develop at various intervals after initiation of antipsychotic drug therapy but usually occurs within the first 4 weeks. Like akathisia, parkinsonism is usually dose related. Drug-induced parkinsonism tends to appear most often in the elderly, with women twice as likely to develop it. Of all the EPS, drug-induced parkinsonism is best explained by the dopaminergic-cholinergic balance hypothesis, its symptoms being due to a relative imbalance of the system in favor of the cholinergic pathway as the result of antipsychotic-induced dopamine blockade (D. E. Casey 1993). Interestingly, cigarette smoking is associated with a lower incidence of antipsychotic-induced parkinsonism; in one study, approximately 43% of nonsmokers were affected, compared with 10% and 30% of male and female smokers, respectively (Decina et al. 1990). Nonpharmacological management of antipsychotic-induced parkinsonism includes drug discontinuation (if indicated), dosage reduction, or switching to an agent less likely to produce EPS (i.e., a low-potency drug) (see Tables 1–1 and 1–5 [pages 13 and 33, respectively]). The condition disappears upon termination of drug therapy, but complete reversal may take several weeks to months, depending on the dosage and the individual patient. (See Chapter 6 for additional information on the pharmacological management of parkinsonism.)

Tardive dyskinesia.   This syndrome is also referred to as *terminal extrapyramidal insufficiency, complex dyskinesia,* and *persistent dyskinesia.* Tardive dyskinesia is a complex syndrome of hyperkinetic involuntary movements of the mouth, lips, and tongue, and is sometimes accompanied by choreiform movements of the limbs or trunk (Black et al. 1985; D. E. Casey 1993; Davis and Casper 1977; Donlon and Stenson 1976; Jeste et al. 1979; Shader and DiMascio 1970; Simpson et al. 1981). Differential diagnoses include Huntington's disease and other basal ganglia disorders (D. E. Casey 1993). The most widely described symptoms comprise the buccolinguomasticatory triad, which consists of 1) sucking and smacking movements of the lips, 2) lateral jaw movements, and 3) puffing of the cheeks, with the tongue thrusting, rolling, or making fly-catching movements. Such movements may occur with the mouth closed, with biting of the tongue and the inside of the cheek as well as chewing motions often being observed. It has been suggested, although not established, that the fine vermicular movements of the tongue may be an early sign of tardive dyskinesia. The extremities may show choreiform movements that are variable, purposeless, involuntary, and quick. Frequently associated with these symptoms are athetoid movements—continuous, arrhythmic, wavelike, slow movement in the distal parts of the limbs. Axial hyperkinesia (i.e., to-and-fro clonic movement of the spine in an anterior-posterior direction) and ballistic movements (i.e., rhythmical side-to-side swaying) may also be present. All involuntary movements disappear during sleep and are exacerbated by emotionally upsetting situations. Drug-induced parkinsonism is present in 30%–40% of patients with tardive dyskinesia (Ambrosini and Nurnberg 1980).

Although tardive dyskinesia usually develops after more than 1 year of treatment, onset within 6 months of initiation of antipsychotics has been reported. Typically, dyskinesia has an insidious onset while patients are still taking antipsychotics, although abnormal movements often appear for the first time or increase dramatically in the few weeks following a reduction in dose or discontinuation of the drug (Feltner and Hertzman 1993).

The *incidence* of tardive dyskinesia is estimated at 2%–5% per year over 5–6 years of treatment (D. E. Casey 1993; Jeste and Caligiuri 1993; Kane 1989). The *prevalence,* corrected for a spontaneous dyskinesia rate of 1%–5%, averages 15%–20% (range 0.5%–80%) (D. E. Casey 1993). Age, gender, psychiatric diagnosis, antipsychotic dose, and duration of antipsychotic exposure are associated with an increased prevalence of tardive dyskinesia. Tardive dyskinesia is present in 5%–10% of patients over 40 years of age but may occur in 50%–80% of the elderly. The female-to-male ratio is 1.7:1. The prevalence of tardive dyskinesia in patients with affective disorder and/or medical diagnoses receiving dopamine-blocking agents was 26% compared with an 18% rate in patients with schizophrenia (Jeste and Caligiuri 1993).

The following have not been identified as risk factors for tardive dyskinesia: antipsychotic type (i.e., low- versus high-potency agents), antipsychotic plasma levels, long-acting injectable dosage forms, concomitant use of anticholinergic agents, and a diagnosis of organic brain disease (D. E. Casey 1993). Although an association is often reported, it is unknown whether prolonged anticholinergic treatment in conjunction with antipsychotics will increase the likelihood of developing the disorder (D. E. Casey 1993). The use of anticholinergics in patients with combined parkinsonism and/or akathisia and tardive dyskinesia might be justified. However, antipsychotic dosage reduction should be attempted to minimize the need for long-term anticholinergics.

Although tardive dyskinesia may be potentially irreversible, recent evidence suggests that with antipsychotic continuation, the syndrome's course in the majority of patients will be stabilization of signs over time or complete symptom resolution (D. E. Casey 1993; D. E. Casey et al. 1986; Chouinard et al. 1986; Fornazzari et al. 1989; Gardos et al. 1983, 1994; Jeste and Caligiuri 1993; Kane 1989; Kane et al. 1986; Wirshing et al. 1989). It is uncommon for dyskinetic symptoms to increase with antipsychotic continuation. After drug withdrawal, the dyskinesia may appear and/or increase in severity over several weeks. This flareup of symptoms may be followed by slow, gradual improvement over a period of many weeks, months, or years.

The exact mechanism of tardive dyskinesia is unknown (D. E. Casey 1993; Jeste and Caligiuri 1993); however, it has been postulated that the condition is caused by a functional hyperactivity of CNS dopaminergic and noradrenergic activity associated with reduced γ-aminobutyric acid (GABA) and cholinergic activity. This effect is a result of prolonged blockade of receptors by antipsychotics.

There is currently no satisfactory treatment for tardive dyskinesia other than discontinuation of the drug (Feltner and Hertzman 1993; Jeste and Caligiuri 1993). Increasing the dosage or changing to another antipsychotic might produce short-term suppression of the dyskinesia, which will then in some patients reappear and require ever-increasing doses to be controlled. Pharmacological agents studied for the treatment of tardive dyskinesia include levodopa/carbidopa, benzodiazepines, calcium channel blockers, α-tocopherol (vitamin E), clonidine, and propranolol (Feltner and Hertzman 1993). However, no one agent clearly emerges as the treatment of choice. Seven recent studies of vitamin E in doses of 400–1,600 IU/day reported conflicting results (Adler et al. 1993; Dabiri et al. 1994; Jeste and Caligiuri 1993; Lohr and Caligiuri 1996). On average, 50% of patients with tardive dyskinesia experienced a 20%–46% reduction in their symptoms. Trials of vitamin E at 1,600 IU/day for more than 12 weeks and in patients who been diagnosed with dyskinesia for less than 5 years might produce more promising and consistent results.

Tardive dystonia, a form of tardive dyskinesia characterized by sustained or slow involuntary twisting movements of the face, neck, trunk, or limbs, has been described. This condition may coexist with tardive dyskinesia (Black et al. 1985; Remington 1989). Tardive dystonia has been estimated to occur in 2% of patients treated long-term with antipsychotics. Anticholinergic treatment might be attempted because of positive treatment reports, although negative reports exist.

Tardive akathisia, another form of tardive dyskinesia, has also been described. Specific treatment recommendations for this condition are not available.

Treatment recommendations.   The prolonged use of antipsychotics should be restricted to situations in which there are compelling indications (e.g., schizophrenia). Whether to discontinue antipsychotics in patients with schizophrenia is a matter of clinical judgment. However, patients who have a long history of homicidal and/or suicidal behavior when psychotic or who have fragile support systems that would be upset by a relapse should discontinue antipsychotics with extreme caution, if at all. Long-term antipsychotic treatment of anxiety disorders, depression, mania, and personality disorder should be avoided, except in unusual clinical circumstances (Black et al. 1985). Thus, the use of antipsychotics should be supported with appropriate indications, demonstrated response (preferably with drug discontinuation), dose minimization, informed consent, and performance of a structured assessment (e.g., Abnormal Involuntary Movement Scale) at least yearly for tardive dyskinesia (Applebaum 1985; Bergen et al. 1989; D. E. Casey 1993; Davis et al. 1983; Gerlach and Casey 1988; Kleinman et al. 1989; Munetz and Benjamin 1988). In addition, clozapine, which rarely has been associated with tardive dyskinesia, might be considered (see *Neurological* adverse effects under **Clozapine, Olanzapine, Risperidone,** and **Sertindole** sections in this chapter).

▶ Sedation
Sedation occurs within the first few days of treatment, and patients may develop tolerance to this effect over several weeks. Although all available antipsychotics can cause sedation, they differ in their tendency to do so (see Table 1–5 [page 33]). This side effect can be minimized by administering the total antipsychotic dose at bedtime (Simpson et al. 1981).

▶ Reduction of Seizure Threshold
All available antipsychotics reduce the seizure threshold (Malhotra et al. 1993). Reports that use of low-potency antipsychotics (see Table 1–1 [page 13]) is associated with a high incidence of seizures are not well documented, and both thioridazine and chlorpromazine have been reported to lower the frequency of seizures in patients with convulsive disorders (Sovner and DiMascio 1978). Generalized and focal motor seizures have been reported, but their incidence is less than 1%. The factors predisposing to antipsychotic-induced seizures include 1) preexisting seizure disorder, 2) abnormal EEG activity without a history of seizures, 3) preexisting CNS pathology, and 4) rapid increases in antipsychotic dosage. In general, antipsychotic-induced seizures do not pose a management problem. It has been observed that patients develop tolerance to this effect, and seizures will continue to occur only if higher doses are used. All that may be required as management is the lowering of the antipsychotic dose and/or the addition or adjustment of an anticonvulsant medication. The exact etiology of seizures is unknown but may be related to depletion of the inhibitory neurotransmitter GABA, activation of latent epileptic focus, or alteration in the balance of dopamine and acetylcholine. Seizure activity usually occurs as an early complication in treatment (Davis and Casper 1977; Simpson et al. 1981).

Ophthalmological
Corneal and lens changes have been noted with chlorpromazine, trifluoperazine, perphenazine, fluphenazine, chlorprothixene, and thiothixene. Chlorpromazine is most clearly associated with these effects, which are related to a total lifetime dose of 1–3 kg . The eye changes are described as whitish-brown granular deposits concentrated in the anterior subcapsular area; in more severe cases, the deposits may also be found in the anterior and posterior lens cortex. Generally, these changes are visible only by slit-lamp examination.

They progress to opaque, white, or yellow-brown granules, often stellate in shape. In some patients, the conjunctiva is discolored by a brown pigment. Vision usually is not impaired. These lens changes differ from and are unrelated to the lens changes of senile cataracts, as they involve depositions in—not loss of transparency of—the lens. The overall incidences of these effects vary from 27% to 90%. If skin pigmentation is present, it is almost always associated with simultaneous depositions in the eye. Cornea and lens changes appear to be positively correlated with a severe photosensitivity response to chlorpromazine; thus, patients who develop photosensitivity reactions should have eye examinations if exposed to high doses of chlorpromazine for many years. Treatment of skin, corneal, and lens changes includes lowering the dose of the antipsychotic, assigning drug holidays, and changing to an antipsychotic that has not been reported to cause such reactions (Black et al. 1985; Davis and Casper 1977; Malhotra et al. 1993; Shader and DiMascio 1970; Simpson et al. 1981).

An acute attack of *angle-closure glaucoma,* which may be precipitated by drugs that dilate the pupil, is caused when the periphery of the iris bulges forward to obstruct the trabecular meshwork, thereby preventing the aqueous humor from reaching the outflow channel. This effect is of greatest concern in patients with narrow-angle-closure glaucoma (i.e., <5% glaucoma patients). If angle-closure glaucoma is adequately treated pharmacologically, the patient may receive anticholinergic-type drugs (E. Lieberman and Stoudemire 1987; Simpson et al. 1981). However, intraocular pressures should be obtained after initiation of any psychotropic agent with anticholinergic effects in high-risk patients. Open-angle glaucoma is not a contraindication to the use of antipsychotics.

Pigmentary retinopathy is primarily associated with thioridazine, although this effect has also been reported with chlorpromazine. Pigment deposits start in the middle zone of the retina, and, over a 3- to 4-week period, the deposits coalesce and edema appears. A drastic reduction in visual acuity or even blindness may result. It is believed that the retinal pigment deposition is irreversible; however, the pigment sometimes recedes upon drug discontinuation. The majority of reports indicate that visual acuity returns when thioridazine is discontinued, but some reports indicate progression after discontinuation. Retinal changes have occurred following administration of thioridazine 1,200 mg/day for a period of 4–8 weeks. The relationship appears to be a function of time and dose rather than of dose accumulation. Thioridazine doses of 800 mg/day or less have been defined as safe. Treatment is discontinuation and substitution of another antipsychotic (Black et al. 1985; Davis and Casper 1977; Simpson et al. 1981; Shader and DiMascio 1970).

Psychiatric

Delirium secondary to therapeutic doses of antipsychotics may occur infrequently. However, this effect is more common when an antipsychotic is used in combination with an anticholinergic agent, especially in elderly patients. Suspected drug-induced cognitive disease should be treated by discontinuing the offending agent(s) (Raskind and Risse 1986).

Although *supersensitivity psychosis* after long-term antipsychotic use and *rebound psychosis* after drug discontinuation have been reported, conclusive evidence that these effects are primarily related to antipsychotic drugs is lacking (Kahne 1989; Ortiz and Gershon 1986).

Sexual Dysfunction

Antipsychotics have been associated with sexual dysfunction. The role in the etiology of sexual dysfunction of anticholinergics used in combination with antipsychotics has not been extensively studied. One study reported no relationship between use of a combined antipsychotic/anticholinergic and sexual dysfunction (Sullivan and Lukoff 1990). However, one case report indicated that sexual dysfunction worsened when the anticholinergic was discontinued (Sullivan and Lukoff 1990).

▶ Men

Erectile and/or ejaculatory disturbances are reported in 30%–60% of men (Sullivan and Lukoff 1990). Erectile dysfunction may include difficulty in achieving or maintaining an erection. Also, changes in libido (typically reduction) and changes in the quality of orgasm may occur in 40%–70% of patients.

Ejaculatory disturbances have been associated with haloperidol, perphenazine, trifluoperazine, fluphenazine, thiothixene, thioridazine, chlorpromazine, mesoridazine, and chlorprothixene (Sullivan and Lukoff 1990). At lower antipsychotic doses, ejaculation may be delayed or completely blocked without interfering with erection. Patients report absence of ejaculation on masturbation or sexual intercourse and, occasionally, suprapubic pain on orgasm. Evidence suggests that the ejaculatory dysfunction may be due to the calcium channel–blocking effects of the antipsychotic, although antiadrenergic effects may be involved (Gould et al. 1984). Because this effect may be dose related, dosage reduction might be tried. Because sexual side effects are less often reported with thio-thixene, perphenazine, and haloperidol, a trial of these agents has been suggested (Shader and DiMascio 1970; Simpson et al. 1981; Sullivan and Lukoff 1990). Neostigmine 7.5–15 mg po 30 minutes before intercourse has reversed ejaculatory dysfunction (Sullivan and Lukoff 1990).

Impotence, decreased libido, and *changes in the quality of orgasm* have been associated with chlorpromazine, fluphenazine decanoate, haloperidol, pimozide, thioridazine, and thiothixene (Gould et al. 1984; Sullivan and Lukoff 1990). The exact mechanism of these effects is not known. However, phenothiazines have been reported to reduce testosterone levels in male schizophrenic patients (Sramek et al. 1990). Management might include dosage reduction and drug substitution as indicated for ejaculatory disturbances (see above) (Segraves 1989). Pharmacological management to alleviate erectile dysfunction and anorgasmia includes bethanechol 10–20 mg po tid and cyproheptadine 4 mg po qid (Sullivan and Lukoff 1990). Bromocriptine 2.5 mg po bid or tid has been reported to increase libido in patients with antipsychotic-induced hyperprolactinemia (Sullivan and Lukoff 1990). Concern that bromocriptine, a dopamine agonist, might exacerbate psychosis in these patients has not been borne out in several studies (Sullivan and Lukoff 1990).

A case of nonpainful, pleasurable *prolonged erection* has been reported (Sullivan and Lukoff 1990). However, most cases of anti-psychotic-induced erections involve *priapism,* which is prolonged *painful* erection. This effect has been reported with chlorpromazine, fluphenazine, haloperidol, mesoridazine, molindone, perphenazine, thioridazine, and thiothixene in a total of 17 cases (Chan et al. 1990; Segraves 1989; Sullivan and Lukoff 1990). Typically, priapism occurs within 12 to 48 hours of the first antipsychotic dose (range 2 hours to 8 months) It does not appear to be dose related. Priapism is considered a medical emergency. Prompt discontinuation of the antipsychotic is absolutely necessary, although the reaction may not reverse upon drug termination. Without rapid resolution of the erection, 18%–80% of patients will become impotent. Acute treatment may include intracavernosal injection of an α-adrenergic agonist (e.g., metaraminol, ephedrine, epinephrine), aspiration of the corpora cavernosa, or placement of a copora cavernosa–to–corpus spongiosum shunt. Alternative management of the patient's psychosis might include substitution of an antipsychotic of a different chemical class and close monitoring. The suggested mechanism of antipsychotic-induced priapism is not known but may be related to α-adrenergic blocking properties of the antipsychotic. However, in cases in which a more potent α-adrenergic blocking antipsychotic was substituted for the causative antipsychotic, priapism did not recur.

▶ Women

The prevalence of sexual dysfunction in women is estimated at 25%–30% (Sullivan and Lukoff 1990). Side effects include anorgasmia, changes in the quality of orgasm, difficulty in achieving orgasm, and decreased libido. These symptoms may be associated with menstrual irregularities (see *Endocrinological* adverse effects [page 37]).

Orgasmic dysfunction and *reduced libido* have been reported with fluphenazine, mesoridazine, thioridazine, and trifluoperazine (Sullivan and Lukoff 1990). Dosage reduction or switching to a different antipsychotic might be empirically tried (Sullivan and Lukoff 1990).

Pharmacological management for anorgasmia includes bethanechol 10–20 mg po tid and cyproheptadine 4 mg po qid (Sullivan and Lukoff 1990). Neostigmine 7.5–15 mg po 30 minutes before intercourse has enhanced libido. In addition, bromocriptine 2.5 mg po bid or tid has been reported to increase libido in patients with antipsychotic-induced hyperprolactinemia. That bromocriptine, a dopamine agonist, might exacerbate psychosis in patients with schizophrenia has been suggested; however, this has not occurred in several studies (Sullivan and Lukoff 1990).

Temperature Regulation

Temperature regulation may be altered by an antipsychotic's inhibition of the hypothalamic control area. It has been demonstrated in patients receiving antipsychotics that normal body temperature cannot be maintained on exposure to heat or cold (Caroff and Mann 1993). Subjects become hyperthermic or hypothermic, depending on the surrounding temperature (Beaumont et al. 1974; Caroff and Mann 1993; Levinson and Simpson 1986; Shader and DiMascio 1970; Simpson et al. 1981). Severe or fatal **hyperpyrexia** has been reported in antipsychotic-treated patients during hot weather or strenuous exercise. It is likely that impairment of cutaneous heat elimination due to cholinergic blockade is a contributing factor. This impairment is aggravated if the patient is concurrently receiving an anticholinergic.

Hypothermia has been reported in phenothiazine-treated patients, particularly during cold weather. Elderly patients and those with hypothyroidism may be particularly susceptible.

Teratogenicity and Excretion Into Breast Milk

Antipsychotics have not been clearly documented to cause *congenital anomalies* (Calabrese and Gulledge 1985; Marken et al. 1989; Nurnberg and Prudic 1984; Shader and DiMascio 1970; Simpson et al. 1981). However, they should not be prescribed during the first trimester of pregnancy, if they can be avoided (Calabrese and Gulledge 1985). Low-dose, high-potency antipsychotics might be preferred because low-potency drugs (see Tables 1–1 and 1–5 [pages 13 and 33, respectively]) have the potential to produce maternal hypotension and uteroplacental insufficiency (Marken et al. 1989).

Because phenothiazines can produce a significant degree of α-adrenergic blockade, nonshivering thermogenesis may be impaired in neonates delivered by mothers receiving these drugs (L. S. Cohen 1989). Also, EPS lasting as long as 9 months have been reported in infants of mothers exposed to antipsychotics during their pregnancy (Nurnberg and Prudic 1984). One report recommended discontinuation of the antipsychotic 5–10 days before the estimated date of delivery to allow the decline of fetal antipsychotic concentrations (Marken et al. 1989).

Altered neonatal hepatic function, with hyperbilirubinemia, jaundice, and enzyme induction, has been reported subsequent to maternal antipsychotic use during pregnancy (Nurnberg and Prudic 1984).

The clinical significance of antipsychotic levels in **breast milk** is unclear. Chlorpromazine, trifluoperazine, prochlorperazine, thioridazine, haloperidol, and mesoridazine have all been detected in breast milk (Calabrese and Gulledge 1985; Pons et al. 1994). Breast feeding while receiving these drugs is not recommended.

Urinary

Phenothiazines, thioxanthenes, and butyrophenones have been associated with enuresis, or urinary incontinence (Ambrosini and Nurnberg 1980; Nurnberg and Ambrosini 1979). Onset may be within hours but often is during the first 2 weeks of treatment. Patients do not report feelings of urge, dribbling, or stress-related loss. Enuresis appears to decrease with continued treatment, although several months may elapse before it resolves. It is reported not to be responsive to anticholinergic agents. The incidence of this side effect is unknown. Incontinence of urine is believed to result from a central disruption of dopaminergic-cholinergic balance by the antipsychotic, because the condition can be seen in non–drug-induced disorders of the basal ganglia.

Urinary retention may occur, primarily with drugs with higher anticholinergic effects (for additional information, see *Anticholinergic effects* and Table 1–5 [pages 32 and 33, respectively]).

■ Rational Prescribing

1. All typical antipsychotics are therapeutically equivalent when used in equipotent doses. A rational method for selecting an antipsychotic is to narrow the choice to seven drugs (i.e., one from each of the three classes of phenothiazines, a butyrophenone, the piperazine thioxanthene, dihydroindolone, and dibenzoxazepine) and then to select from these seven the drug the patient will tolerate best.
2. In treating schizophrenia, a therapeutic dose of an antipsychotic should be maintained for at least 4 weeks. Hyperactivity and agitation accompanying the psychosis may respond within hours or days, whereas delusions, hallucinations, and negative symptoms may not respond for weeks. Empirically, nonresponders to one drug might be given a trial of another antipsychotic of a different chemical group or an increase in dose of the current antipsychotic if side effects are not a problem.
3. Antipsychotics are indicated in patients with dementia who have psychotic symptoms and/or significant agitation. No antipsychotic is more effective than another. Patients who respond to treatment should receive gradual dosage reduction and trial drug discontinuation to determine ongoing need.
4. A goal of complete resolution of schizophrenic symptoms is unlikely to be met. Some patients indicate that the hallucinations they experience while under the influence of antipsychotics are more tolerable than those they have without drug treatment and that delusions, while still present, are not as pronounced.
5. Attempts should be made to administer the antipsychotic in a single daily dose, usually at bedtime, or in a one-third in the morning/two-thirds at bedtime split if the patient is bothered by side effects. Sustained-release preparations, which are typically more expensive mg for mg, should not be prescribed, because antipsychotics are inherently long acting.
6. Duration of antipsychotic treatment is determined individually, based on the patient's life situation and illness. Prophylactic treatment is continued for 1–2 years after remission of the first psychotic episode. If patients are suicidal, homicidal, and/or disrupt their families' lives to an unacceptable degree when

they are psychotic, continuous medication at the lowest effective dosage is justified. In patients with multiple relapses after drug discontinuation, at least a 5-year period of maintenance treatment should be considered. It is not possible by symptomatology to predict the risk of patient relapse. Studies indicate that relapse may occur up to 1–2 years after discontinuation of drug therapy.

7. Drug holidays have been suggested in order to decrease total drug intake and thereby to decrease the likelihood of long-term side effects (e.g., tardive dyskinesia). There is no evidence, however, that drug holidays are any better than simple dosage reduction in preventing tardive dyskinesia.

8. Multiple antipsychotics administered simultaneously should be avoided. Research has not demonstrated that combination antipsychotics are superior to comparable doses of single antipsychotics in treating schizophrenia.

9. Prescribing a proprietary combination of an antipsychotic and an antidepressant, such as perphenazine-amitriptyline (e.g., Triavil®, Etrafon®), is discouraged. From a treatment perspective, empirical trial and error remains the best approach for deriving the maximal therapeutic benefit from a single drug or drug combination. Although clinical experience indicates that some patients are helped by these combination products, routine polypharmacy is discouraged.

Clozapine

Synthesized in 1960, clozapine is a member of the dibenzodiazepine class of antipsychotics. The drug has a pharmacological profile unlike that of standard antipsychotics and is labeled an atypical antipsychotic. It was synthesized in 1960, and the first clinical trial was completed in 1962. Clozapine was made available in Europe for clinical use in 1971 and for research purposes in the United States in 1972. However, U.S. marketing was delayed until February 1990 as a result of adverse hematological reactions noted worldwide.

■ Indications

Because of clozapine's potential adverse hematological effects, the FDA has restricted its use to patients who are refractory to typical antipsychotics or who have severe, intolerable adverse effects (J. A. Lieberman et al. 1989; Marder and Van Putten 1988).

All typical antipsychotics available in the United States are equally effective in the treatment of schizophrenia (Kane et al.

1988). It is estimated that 20%–30% of people with schizophrenia do not respond to long-term treatment with these agents (Kane et al. 1988). It is recommended that patients undergo trials of at least two antipsychotics to demonstrate "refractoriness" before they are considered candidates for clozapine (Marder and Van Putten 1988). (See "Dosage" and *Schizophrenia* under "Efficacy" of **Typical Antipsychotics** [pages 14 and 2, respectively] for the definition of *adequate [therapeutic] trial.)*

Although not specified in the manufacturer's literature, the adverse effects related to typical antipsychotics that might indicate switching to clozapine include treatment-resistant early-onset (i.e., dystonia, parkinsonism, akathisia) or late-onset (i.e., tardive dyskinesia) EPS (Clozaril® Product Information 1994; J. A. Lieberman et al. 1989; Marder and Van Putten 1988).

■ Efficacy

Schizophrenia

▶ Refractory Schizophrenia

Short-term treatment.   In one open trial of 40 treatment-refractory patients, 18 (45%) met response criteria at 5 weeks of treatment (Stern et al. 1994). In two controlled trials, approximately 38% and 30% of patients responded to clozapine within a 4-week and a 6-week period, respectively (Kane et al. 1988; Miller et al. 1994a). In the Kane et al. trial, only 3.5% of the chlorpromazine patients who had failed four or more different antipsychotic drug trials responded. Negative symptoms responded equally as well as positive symptoms and disorganization. Clozapine appeared to improve negative symptoms both secondarily to improvement in positive symptoms and through a direct effect on primary negative symptoms (Miller et al. 1994b; Ranjan et al. 1995). Significant improvement favoring clozapine over chlorpromazine occurred within 1 to 2 weeks (Kane et al. 1988).

Long-term effects.   In five retrospective reports, the improvement rates after 1 year, an average of 1.6 year, 7 years, 12 years, and 13 years of clozapine were 50%, 83%, 33%, 67%, and 51%, respectively (Banov et al. 1994; Juul Povlsen et al. 1985; Kuha and Mietinen 1986; J. A. Lieberman et al. 1994b; Lindstrom 1988; Safferman et al. 1991). In three open studies, the clozapine response rate was 50% in patients treated for 12 weeks, 57% in patients treated for an average of 4.3 months, and 58% in patients treated for an average of 2½ years (Mattes 1989; Miller et al. 1994b; Owen et al. 1989). Four prospective, controlled trials reported response rates of 48%, 54%, 42%, and 29% in patients treated for 3.5 months (average), 29 weeks, 10 weeks, and 12 weeks, respectively (Breier et al. 1994; Kane 1996; Pickar et al. 1992; Zito et al. 1993).

To reduce exposure to clozapine because of potential long-term side effects and treatment cost, the *time course* of a patient's response to clozapine is an important clinical question. In an open study, 25 of 31 (81%) clozapine patients met response criteria within 6 months of treatment initiation (Meltzer 1989). The percentage of patients who responded at 9 and 12 months was 16% ($n = 5$) and 3% ($n = 1$), respectively. In another open trial, 14 of 14 (100%) patients met response criteria by 6 months of clozapine treatment (Miller et al. 1994b). In two prospective, controlled trials, 4% and 0% of patients responded after 12 weeks of treatment (Breier et al. 1994; Lindenmayer et al. 1994).

Discharge rates, rehospitalization rates, quality of life, employment rates, and treatment costs.   In a retrospective study of 96 patients with refractory schizophrenia or significant EPS that were treated with clozapine for 1 year, 85% were *discharged* from the hospital (Lindstrom 1989).

A review of four recent reports indicated reduced *rehospitalization rates* of 50%–87% after 2–2½ years of clozapine treatment (Meltzer and Cola 1994; Reed et al. 1994).

A study involving 64 patients who completed 2 years of clozapine treatment found that 64% were able to *live independently* (Revicki et al. 1990). In another study, 6 of 8 patients receiving clozapine for 1 year were able to be discharged to nonfamilial, supervised residential care (Davies et al. 1991).

Employment in a full- or part-time position was reported in 24 of 62 (39%) patients still receiving clozapine at 2 years (Lindstrom 1989), whereas the employment rate prior to clozapine initiation was 3%. In another report, 3 of 6 patients treated with clozapine for 1 year were attending school at the end of that period, although all remained unemployed (Davies et al. 1991; Green 1996a).

Cost savings through reduced hospitalizations in clozapine responders per patient per year were estimated to be $934–$7,505, $17,402, $9,000–$14,000 (range –$1,000–$28,000), and $33,000–$55,250 (Meltzer 1996b; Meltzer and Cola 1994; Revicki et al. 1990).

Response predictors.   The majority of early studies were unable to identify any predictors of clozapine response (Honigfeld and Patin 1989). However, later studies have suggested that in treatment-resistant patients, an older age at onset and/or the presence of typical antipsychotic–induced EPS are predictive of a response to clozapine (J. A. Lieberman et al. 1994a; Osser 1990; Pickar et al. 1992; Stern et al. 1994). A retrospective report suggested that 76% of treatment-intolerant patients responded to clozapine within 1 year (J. A. Lieberman et al. 1994b). These findings were replicated in a recent study, which also reported a shorter duration of illness, male gender, and paranoid schizophrenia subtype as response predictors (J. A. Lieberman et al. 1994b). In addition, an open study has reported that a significant change in BPRS scores at 1 week predicted a response at 5 weeks with 75% accuracy (Green 1996b; Stern et al. 1994).

Although some studies have reported that weight gain was correlated with a better clinical outcome, others have not found this association (Leadbetter et al. 1992; Umbricht et al. 1994).

One study reported that the rate of response to clozapine in patients with a history of previous or current substance abuse was no different from that in their non–substance-abusing peers (Buckley et al. 1994).

Cognitive effects. In uncontrolled trials, clozapine has been demonstrated to improve impairments in cognitive functioning (Meltzer 1996c).

Suicidality. Uncontrolled reports suggest that clozapine reduces the suicide rate among patients with schizophrenia to one-fourth of the rate that would be expected based on the annual published rate of suicide in schizophrenia (Meltzer 1996a).

◗ Nonrefractory Schizophrenia

Of antipsychotic agents available in the United States, clozapine has been compared with chlorpromazine, perphenazine, haloperidol, and trifluoperazine (Bublenis et al. 1989; J. A. Lieberman et al. 1989; Marder and Van Putten 1988; Stephens 1990). In 8 of 12 studies, clozapine was more effective than the reference antipsychotic according to clinical and/or statistical criteria. Three studies demonstrated equal efficacy, whereas one found clozapine less effective than the standard antipsychotic. Overall, clozapine and typical antipsychotics produce a similar response in patients with "acute schizophrenia." However, in patients with "chronic schizophrenia," clozapine is often more effective.

◗ Childhood-Onset Schizophrenia

Preliminary data from open trials and case reports suggest that clozapine may be beneficial in this age group (Piscitelli et al.

1994). Clozapine is not currently indicated in patients less than 16 years of age.

Borderline Personality Disorder

Fifteen patients with a diagnosis of BPD and a DSM-III-R (American Psychiatric Association 1987) psychotic disorder who had not responded to pharmacotherapy with three or more typical antipsychotics were treated with clozapine for 2–9 months (Frankenburg and Zanarini 1993). On the average, these patients improved significantly in positive and negative symptoms and in their social functioning. These findings need to be confirmed in double-blind, placebo-controlled trials. Only patients who clearly have not responded to or who do not tolerate standard treatments for BPD should be considered for clozapine (see *Borderline* personality disorder [page 8] under "Efficacy" of **Typical Antipsychotics**).

Mood Disorders

Almost all patients included in the reviewed studies were considered treatment-refractory to standard antipsychotic, antimanic, and/or antidepressant agents. Most studies were of open or retrospective design (Zarate et al. 1995). Chart documentation of failure to respond to more standard pharmacological treatments are necessary before clozapine is prescribed.

Mania.   In a retrospective trial of 14 patients with bipolar disorder with psychotic features, 43% of patients had a moderate and 43% had a marked response (McElroy et al. 1991). In a retrospective study involving 18 patients, 55%–70% had moderate or marked improvement (Naber and Hippius 1990). All 7 patients with dysphoric mania in another study responded within the first few weeks of clozapine treatment (Suppes et al. 1992). In one retrospective and two prospective reports involving 52, 52, and 10 patients, respectively, patients were reported to be clozapine responders, although percentages were not given (Kimmel et al. 1994). In a long-term follow-up report, the response rates among bipolar subtypes were 73% (manic), 58% (mixed), and 44% (depressed) (Banov et al. 1994).

Major depressive disorder.   A clozapine trial in patients with depression with psychotic features reported improvement (Kimmel et al. 1994). In a retrospective study, it was reported that of 29 patients, 55%–70% had moderate or marked improvement on clozapine (Naber and Hippius 1990).

Schizoaffective disorder.   A retrospective study reported that 70% and 15% of patients demonstrated moderate and marked improvement, respectively, on clozapine (McElroy et al. 1991). In another retrospective study, 65% of patients had a moderate to marked response to clozapine (Naber and Hippius 1990). Although no response rates were provided in a retrospective report and a prospective study involving 81 and 15 patients, respectively, improvement on clozapine was reported (Kimmel et al. 1994). In a nonblind comparison trial, 12 patients with schizoaffective disorder responded significantly better to clozapine than did 25 patients with schizophrenia (Owen et al. 1989). In a follow-up study of patients treated for an average of 20 months, the response rate was 70% for bipolar type I and 50% for depressed patients (Banov et al. 1994).

Neurological Disorders

Currently, clozapine is not FDA-approved for the treatment of psychotic symptoms associated with Parkinson's or Huntington's disease or other movement disorders (Safferman et al. 1994). These findings need to replicated in double-blind, placebo-controlled trials.

▶ Huntington's Disease

Psychotic and depressive symptoms. In one Huntington's disease patient, psychotic and depressive symptoms improved with clozapine 175 mg/day (Sajatovic et al. 1991).

Choreoathetoid movements. Of four patients treated with clozapine 60, 175, 200, or 500 mg/day, only the patients on the two higher doses experienced improvement in their choreoathetoid symptoms (Caine et al. 1979; Sajatovic et al. 1991).

▶ Parkinson's Disease

Psychosis. One hundred and eight Parkinson's patients with and without drug-induced psychosis have been treated with clozapine (Safferman et al. 1994). The overall response rate varied from 40% to 100%. The average clozapine dosage in 90 patients was 62 mg/day (range 6.25–400 mg/day). The recommended starting dose was 6.25 mg per day or every other day, with slow dosage escalation to minimize side effects. A 2-year follow-up report indicated that 10 of 12 patients had sustained improvement in psychotic symptoms with clozapine (Chacko et al. 1995).

Tremor. Twenty-eight patients experienced at least moderate improvement in tremor when treated with clozapine 18–75 mg/day, according to a review of reported cases (Safferman et al. 1994).

Nocturnal akathisia. Nine patients treated with an average clozapine dosage of 26.4 mg/day (range 12.5–100 mg/day) for an average of 1 year experienced marked improvement in this symptom (Linazasoro et al. 1993).

Motor fluctuations.   Six patients treated with clozapine 25 mg/day for 1 month experienced significant reductions in their parkinsonian signs during interdose "off" periods (Marsden and Parkes 1976).

Levodopa-induced dyskinesia.   Significant reductions in both dyskinetic and parkinsonian signs were demonstrated in six patients treated with an average clozapine dose of 320 mg/day (J. P. Bennett et al. 1993).

▶ Gilles de la Tourette's Syndrome
In a double-blind, placebo-controlled trial in which seven patients with Tourette's syndrome were treated with an average clozapine dose of 370 mg/day (range 150–500 mg/day) for 7 weeks, only one patient had a significant decrease in tics (Caine et al. 1979).

Water Dysregulation
Overall, in 17 patients with polydipsia and intermittent hyponatremia, a significant decrease in diurnal weight gain, a reduction in urine volume, and an increase in serum sodium were noted after clozapine treatment (Leadbetter and Shutty 1994; Munn 1993; Spears et al. 1993). These initial findings of case reports and a small open study need to be confirmed with controlled trials.

■ Mechanism of Action

Clozapine possesses dopamine receptor–blocking effects (Ereshefsky et al. 1989; Meltzer et al. 1989). The exact differences between clozapine and typical antipsychotics in receptor interactions remain to be determined (Meltzer 1988). However, it appears that clozapine has a lower affinity for D_1, D_2, and D_3 receptors and binds proportionately more to D_4 receptors (Meltzer 1994). The drug may also have partial dopamine-agonist effects (Meltzer 1994).

Clozapine appears to act selectively at dopamine sites in the cortical and limbic regions in preference to the nigrostriatal and tuberoinfundibular regions (J. A. Lieberman et al. 1989; Meltzer 1988, 1991; Meltzer et al. 1989). Historically, blockade of the *cortical* and *limbic* receptors has been used to explain antipsychotic drug effect. All antipsychotics, including clozapine, block these receptors. Disruption of *striatal* receptor activity may be more marked with typical antipsychotics than with clozapine. Therefore, typical drugs would be expected to produce more acute and, possibly, long-term EPS as compared with clozapine.

It has been further speculated that clozapine's low affinity for D_2 receptors and high affinity for serotonin-2 (S_2) receptors, which produces a high $S_2:D_2$ ratio, is responsible for its improved efficacy and decreased rate of EPS (Farde et al. 1992; Meltzer 1994).

In addition, clozapine significantly increases noradrenergic function by blocking the reuptake of norepinephrine (Breier 1994). Similar to typical antipsychotics, clozapine has significant inhibiting effects on adrenergic, histamine, and acetylcholine receptors (Meltzer 1991).

Unlike typical antipsychotics, clozapine produces minimal disruption of the ***tuberoinfundibular*** tract. This would explain clozapine's negligible effect on prolactin levels (see *Endocrinological* adverse effects [page 73]).

■ Dosage

In refractory schizophrenia, initiate treatment with doses of 12.5 mg once or twice daily. Increase doses by 12.5–50 mg/day, if tolerated, to a usual dose of 300–450 mg/day, administered on a bid or tid basis by the end of 2 weeks. Subsequent dose increases might be made on a once- or twice-weekly basis in increments of less than 100 mg. A maximum dose of 900 mg/day is recommended, which might be accomplished within a 5-week period. The average clozapine dose in U.S. trials was about 450 mg/day (Fleischhacker et al. 1994). Although maintenance doses of clozapine have not been determined, gradual dosage reduction to minimize adverse effects might be attempted every 6 months to determine the lowest effective dose (Fleischhacker et al. 1994). (See *plasma concentration* and *therapeutic response* under "Pharmacokinetics," below.)

If a patient misses more than 24 hours of clozapine, the drug should be reinitiated with the recommended starting dose to reduce the risk of syncope. Dosage titration might occur more rapidly than with the initial exposure, depending on the patient's previous adverse effects (Clozaril® Product Information 1994).

(For clozapine dosages for nonpsychiatric indications, see individual uses under "Efficacy" [page 61].)

■ Pharmacokinetics

Clozapine is rapidly absorbed, with peak plasma concentrations occurring within 1–6 hours. The systemic bioavailability of clozapine is not affected by food and is reported to be 27%. The drug is 95% plasma protein bound, and the average distribution volume varies from 1.6 to 7.3 L/kg. Clozapine is extensively metabolized by the liver and generates three primary metabolites, of which des-methylclozapine is slightly active. The terminal elimination half-life in humans has a range of 9–17 hours (Byerly and DeVane 1996; Clozaril® Product Information 1994; Jann et al. 1993).

An investigation of 148 adult patients receiving clozapine noted the effect of smoking, sex, and age on serum drug concentration (Haring et al. 1989). Plasma concentrations in males were 69% of females' levels adjusted for weight. The average plasma concentration for male and female smokers was 82% of nonsmokers' concentrations. Male smokers' clozapine levels were only 68% of nonsmokers', whereas smoking status did not affect clozapine levels in females. A more recent report confirmed that clozapine levels in smokers were 77% of those in nonsmokers (Hasegawa et al. 1993). Interestingly, schizophrenia patients with tardive dyskinesia have an average clozapine plasma level that is 70% higher than that in patients without tardive dyskinesia (Pollack et al. 1993). Clozapine concentrations in patients 18–26 years of age were approximately double those in patients 45–54 years of age. Plasma concentrations have not been reported in patients more than 60 years of age (Jann et al. 1993).

A relationship between body weight (mg/kg) and clozapine concentrations has not been consistently demonstrated (Jann et al. 1993). Therefore, it is not possible to dose clozapine on a mg/kg/day basis to achieve a desired plasma concentration (Jann et al. 1993).

Although three early studies did not demonstrate a relationship between clozapine *plasma concentrations* and *therapeutic response,* these studies were not well designed (Potkin et al. 1994). Five recent studies have reported response rates of 60% and 74% in patients with threshold levels above 350 ng/mL and 420 ng/mL, respectively (Kronig et al. 1995; Perry et al. 1991; Potkin et al. 1994). One study reported a response rate of 8% if clozapine plasma concentrations at 4 weeks were less than 420 ng/mL, which compared with a 60% rate if the clozapine concentrations was greater than 420 ng/mL (Potkin et al. 1994). Additionally, 73% of nonresponders were converted to responders at 12 weeks of treatment if their plasma clozapine concentration was increased to more than 420 ng/mL. Conversely, if the clozapine concentration remained less than 420 ng/mL at 12 weeks, only 29% of 4-week nonresponders eventually responded.

In children with schizophrenia who were treated with an average clozapine dose of 6 mg/kg/day, an average clozapine concentration of 378 ng/mL (range 77.5–1,050 ng/mL) was generated (Piscitelli et al. 1994). Clinical response was linearly related to clozapine.

Assay methods for clozapine have been reviewed (Jann et al. 1993). Technical assay difficulties may significantly affect laboratory results. One study reported an average split-sample difference of 61% (range −85% to +127%) between two laboratories (Potkin et al. 1994). Accurate measurement of clozapine plasma concentrations is extremely important if plasma levels are to be routinely used in adjusting clozapine doses.

■ Adverse Effects

The attention paid to clozapine's hematological effects and lack of early-onset (i.e., dystonia, akathisia, parkinsonism) and late-onset (i.e., tardive dyskinesia) EPS has overshadowed the drug's other common and troublesome side effects (see Table 1–6). Besides hematological effects, these primarily include CNS, cardiovascular, GI, and metabolic effects (Ereshefsky et al. 1989). Adverse effects of clozapine have been reviewed (Clozaril® Product Information 1994; Jann et al. 1993; Kane et al. 1988; J. A. Lieberman et al. 1989; Meltzer 1988; Safferman et al. 1991).

Table 1–6.   Early comparisons of clozapine's common adverse effects (%)

Adverse effect	Worldwide (N = 13,000)	Manufacturer (N = 842)	U.S.–Multicenter (N = 268)
Agranulocytosis	N/R	1.0	0.0
Constipation	1.9	14.0	16.0
Dizziness/vertigo	19.0	1.7	14.0
Headache	0.9	7.0	10.0
Hyperthermia	3.3	5.0	13.0
Hypotension	2.2	9.0	13.0
Leukopenia	0.3	3.0[a]	4.9
Nausea/vomiting	1.64	8.0	10.0
Salivation	5.7	31.0	13.0
Sedation	9.0	39.0	21.0
Seizures	0.4	3.0[a]	N/R
Syncope	0.6	6.0	N/R
Tachycardia	25.0	5.3[a]	17.0
Weight gain	0.73	4.0	N/R

N/R = Not reported. [a]Based on 1,700 patients.
Source.   Clozaril® Product Information 1994; Kane et al. 1988.

Allergic

One case of acute dyspnea with stridor and cyanosis requiring intensive-care-unit treatment occurred within 24 hours after a single clozapine 25-mg dose (Stoppe et al. 1992). The patient had been exposed to clozapine 2 years previously without adverse effects. Rechallenge with clozapine 25 and 12.5 mg on two different occasions resulted in the same reaction within 6 hours and 2 hours, respectively.

Autonomic

Autonomic nervous system side effects occur secondary to antiadrenergic blockade (antiadrenergic effects), cholinergic blockade (anticholinergic effects), and autonomic hyperactivity (antipsychotic withdrawal).

Constipation.   Constipation due to the anticholinergic properties of clozapine may be a significant problem in some patients. Increased fluid intake, exercise, and/or the use of a bulk laxative (e.g., psyllium) are recommended. If constipation is significant, dosage reduction might be considered. Prolonged stimulant laxative (e.g., bisacodyl) use is not recommended.

Hypersalivation.   Approximately 6%–31% of clozapine-treated patients will experience some degree of excessive salivation (J. A. Lieberman et al. 1989). Patients may especially complain of significant drooling at night. Also, complaints of gagging and of difficulty swallowing saliva have been reported. Such hypersalivation is not associated with extrapyramidal reactions (e.g., parkinsonism). During long-term treatment, only partial resolution of the problem may occur.

Patients should be forewarned of this side effect. Covering the pillow with a towel at night may decrease patient discomfort. Anticholinergic drugs (e.g., benztropine) have been reported to be either only partially effective or ineffective. One case report suggested that chewing gum reduced a patient's drooling by 60% and that benztropine 2 mg/day produced further improvement (Bourgeois et al. 1991). The authors of this report suggested that chewing gum resulted in more frequent swallowing, which reduced the patient's discomfort from the effect. In another report, four patients given amitriptyline 75–100 mg/day experienced a significant reduction in drooling that was sustained after the drug was discontinued (Copp et al. 1991). Concern has been expressed about adding anticholinergic agents to clozapine because of an increased risk of anticholinergic adverse effects (e.g., delirium, constipation) (see

Delirium [page 77] under *Neurological* adverse effects) (Safferman et al. 1991). Clonidine was reported to markedly reduce salivation in three of four patients treated weekly with a clonidine 0.1-mg transdermal patch (Grabowski 1992). However, in one patient, tolerance developed within 2 weeks. Although the dose was increased to 0.2 mg/week, tolerance again developed within 2 weeks. In patients whose symptoms cannot be managed by any of these strategies, clozapine dosage reduction may be empirically tried. Although some tolerance will develop to hypersalivation within 8 to 12 weeks of the last dosage increase, complete tolerance rarely occurs.

The mechanism of excessive salivation is unknown but might be related to clozapine's augmenting effect on the adrenergic receptors that control saliva production. Sialorrhea is inconsistent with clozapine's anticholinergic properties.

Nausea/vomiting. These symptoms usually occur after several weeks or months of clozapine treatment. Dosage reduction might be considered. Anecdotal reports suggest that metoclopramide may be helpful (J. A. Lieberman et al. 1989). Dopamine-blocking drugs typically are antiemetics; therefore, it is unclear why clozapine would produce these effects. However, possible etiologies include gastric distention secondary to excessive salivation or excessive food intake and delayed gastric emptying time secondary to anticholinergic effects.

Syncope. Infrequent reports of syncope—a sudden loss of muscle tone without a loss of consciousness—have been reported. This effect may be either bodywide or limited to a specific muscle group. It has not been associated with auras, incontinence, or other signs of a seizure; however, a history and workup to rule out such a possibility are recommended. No specific treatment exists for syncope; however, because it may be dose related, dosage reduction should be considered.

Withdrawal reactions. Like typical antipsychotics, clozapine has been associated with withdrawal signs and symptoms that appear with abrupt discontinuation (see *Withdrawal reactions* [page 34] under *Autonomic* adverse effects of **Typical Antipsychotics**) (de Leon et al. 1994). Nausea, vomiting, diarrhea, headache, restlessness, agitation, confusion, and diaphoresis have been reported. The percentage of patients who experience withdrawal effects is unknown. It has been recommended that if abrupt discontinuation of clozapine dosages greater than 600 mg/day is anticipated, 1 mg of trihexyphenidyl could be substituted for each 40 mg of clozapine to treat or prevent withdrawal effects (de Leon et al. 1994). The anticholinergic dose should be administered for 3 days and then tapered over the next 4 days. It is suggested that physical withdrawal results primarily from cholinergic rebound.

Abrupt discontinuation of clozapine has been reported to result in a rapid return of psychotic symptoms; however, this finding has been disputed (for a complete discussion, see *Psychiatric* adverse effects [page 80]).

Cardiovascular

Hypertension.   This effect has been reported in approximately 4% of patients receiving clozapine. Blood pressure should be monitored during the dose titration phase of clozapine dosing. Dosage reduction and/or β-blockers (e.g., atenolol) might be considered.

Hypotension/dizziness.   These effects are primarily observed during treatment initiation (e.g., initial clozapine doses >75 mg) and/or after dose escalation (Ereshefsky et al. 1989; Jann et al. 1993; J. A. Lieberman et al. 1989; Safferman et al. 1991). The estimated incidence is 11%–13%. Orthostatic blood pressure should be monitored, especially during the start of treatment and during dose increases. The rate of dosage increase may be slowed if blood pressure reductions are noted. Patients should be warned of dizziness and instructed how to arise from a lying or sitting position. The use of a liberal sodium diet and support stockings has been recommended, but the utility of these measures is unknown. Although a target dose of fludrocortisone 0.2–0.3 mg/day for 2 weeks has been suggested to be beneficial in hypotensive patients, the use of this agent has not been extensively studied (Testani 1994). Tolerance usually develops to the hypotensive effect within 3–4 weeks. The mechanism is unknown but may be related to clozapine's antiadrenergic blocking effects.

Tachycardia.   An increase of 20–25 beats/minute is typical, although the heart rate may reach 120. Tachycardia can occur in the supine as well as the standing position; thus, it is not solely related to orthostatic blood pressure changes. Sometimes an orthostatic increase in pulse may be present without accompanying changes in blood pressure. The effect is dose related and usually occurs within 7 days of initiation of treatment. Some degree of tolerance to this effect will develop in most patients; however, it rarely completely reverses. If the patient is symptomatic (e.g., palpitations), dosage reduction or the addition of a β-blocker with low CNS penetrability (e.g., atenolol 25–50 mg/day) is recommended. Blood pressure should be monitored for hypotensive effects from the combined use of atenolol and clozapine. Tachycardia is probably related to clozapine's anticholinergic effects.

ECG changes. Reversible nonspecific ST–T-wave changes, T-wave flattening, or inversions have been infrequently reported. These changes are dose related and are similar to those reported with typical antipsychotics (see *Cardiovascular* adverse effects [page 35] of **Typical Antipsychotics**) (Safferman et al. 1991). In U.S. trials, only one patient had a sudden, unexplained death that may have been cardiac in origin (Ereshefsky et al. 1989). Clinicians should use caution when administering clozapine to patients with a history of myocardial infarction or arrhythmias.

Dermatological

Dermatological reactions to clozapine appear to be rare. Urticaria and eczematous exanthema with pruritis have been reported (Stoppe et al. 1992). The drug might be continued with close monitoring and symptomatic treatment, if necessary. Worsening of the condition could necessitate clozapine discontinuation.

Endocrinological

Amenorrhea, galactorrhea, and gynecomastia. Amenorrhea, galactorrhea, and gynecomastia have not been reported in several large studies that used dosages of up to 600 mg/day. Some reports have indicated that clozapine produces no or only minimal elevations in prolactin levels (Ereshefsky et al. 1989; Jann et al. 1993; J. A. Lieberman et al. 1989; Safferman et al. 1991). In one case report, a male patient's gynecomastia reversed when clozapine was substituted for a typical antipsychotic (Uehlinger and Baumann 1991).

Acute pancreatitis. Two cases of acute pancreatitis with onset at 9 and 14 days of treatment have been reported (Frankenburg and Kando 1992; Martin 1992). The patients experienced temperature elevations, nausea, vomiting, abdominal pain, and/or elevated amylase. Symptoms resolved within several days of drug discontinuation. Rechallenge in one patient led to recurrence of the symptoms (Frankenburg and Kando 1992). A third case of asymptomatic pancreatitis was detected in a laboratory screen after a clozapine overdose (Jubert 1994). The rate of asymptomatic pancreatitis is unknown. A serum amylase level should be considered for any patient presenting with acute abdominal symptoms who was recently started on clozapine.

Hematological

Agranulocytosis. The first report of hematological adverse effects occurred in Finland in 1975, with 16 cases of neutropenia ($<1,000/mm^3$). Thirteen of these patients developed agranulocytosis ($<500/mm^3$) and 8 died from secondary infection. In U.S. studies, a cumulative incidence of 0.80% after 1 year and of 0.91% after 1.5 years has been reported for this reaction (Alvir and Lieberman 1994a; Honigfeld 1996). Overall, estimates indicate that the incidence of this adverse effect is higher with clozapine than with typical antipsychotics.

Of the 73 cases of agranulocytosis reported in the United States, 61 (84%) occurred within the first 3 months of treatment, 9 (12%) occurred between 3 and 6 months, and 3 (4%) developed after 6 months (Alvir and Lieberman 1994b). Because the majority of agranulocytosis cases have occurred within 3 months of treatment initiation, arguments have been made for reducing the frequency of white blood cell testing following this critical period (Alvir and Lieberman 1994b; Peacock and Gerlach 1994). After 4.5 months of treatment, testing is performed biweekly in the United Kingdom and at least monthly in Germany, Finland, and Denmark (Alvir and Lieberman 1994a; Peacock and Gerlach 1994). The mortality rate secondary to agranulocytosis is similar in all five countries. However, there are no immediate plans to alter the recommended monitoring practices in the United States (Honigfeld 1996). Reported risk factors in addition to the first 3 months of treatment included female sex, older age, and a 15% or greater spike in the white-cell count, all of which predicted onset of agranulocytosis within 75 days (Alvir and Lieberman 1994a).

A weekly white blood count (WBC) is mandated by the manufacturer. This monitoring schedule is based on the premise that the reduction in granulocytes is gradual and, therefore, advance warning of a potentially serious reduction would be possible. Despite these precautions, 12 fatalities secondary to agranulocytosis have been reported as of January 1, 1994 (Clozaril® Product Information 1994; Honigfeld 1996). Five of these deaths have been reviewed (Gelenberg 1992; Gerson et al. 1991). The patients had been taking clozapine 300–900 mg/day for 5–10 weeks when they developed agranulocytosis. Despite discontinuation of the drug, all of these patients succumbed to sepsis.

A baseline WBC must be obtained before the first dose of clozapine. The WBC must be $3,500/mm^3$ or higher. A WBC with a differential count may be necessary, since the neutrophil count

$(1,000/mm^3)$ can drop while the WBC remains normal $(4,900/mm^3)$ (Cates et al. 1992). If monitoring reveals a total WBC between 3,000 and $3,500/mm^3$ and a granulocyte count greater than $1,500/mm^3$, twice-weekly WBCs with differentials should be performed. Likewise, if the patient's white count decreases by more than $3,000/mm^3$ over a 3-week period or drops by more than $3,000/mm^3$ in a 1-week period but remains above $3,500/mm^3$, a repeat WBC with differential is required. If the WBC falls below $3,000/mm^3$ or the granulocyte count is less than $1,500/mm^3$, clozapine should be discontinued and the patient monitored for an infectious process. Clozapine may be reinitiated if the above criteria are exceeded, but twice-weekly counts should be obtained until the WBC passes $3,500/mm^3$. Likewise, even if the WBC is $3,500/mm^3$ or higher, twice-weekly monitoring is indicated if immature cells are present.

If the WBC falls below $2,000/mm^3$ or the granulocyte count is less than $1,500/mm^3$, clozapine should be discontinued, the patient should be admitted for observation, and hematology and infectious-disease consultations should be obtained. *The patient should not receive clozapine again* (Alvir and Lieberman 1994b). A review of nine cases of leukopenia or agranulocytosis revealed recurrence of the condition when the patient was rechallenged with clozapine (Safferman et al. 1992a). The average time to the event was 24.4 ± 18.2 weeks for the first episode versus 14.6 ± 33.6 weeks for the second. The time interval between the rechallenges ranged from 2 months to 2 years. This finding suggests that the mechanism for agranulocytosis is immune related, which is consistent with other reports (Pfister et al. 1992). Evidence is accumulating that suggests a genetic predisposition to this effect, as human leukocyte antigens (HLAs) in susceptible patients have been identified (Alvir and Lieberman 1994b; Joseph et al. 1992; J. A. Lieberman et al. 1989). However, patients with these HLAs have not developed agranulocytosis on clozapine, whereas patients without these antigens have.

Treatment of agranulocytosis includes hospitalization, reverse isolation, daily CBCs, possibly antibiotics, and consultations with a hematologist, an infectious disease specialist, and/or an internist (Gullion and Yeh 1994). Additionally, the use of granulocyte colony–stimulating factor (G-CSF) is being recommended (Barnas et al. 1992; Chengappa et al. 1995; Geibig and Marks 1993; Gerson 1994; Gerson et al. 1992; Gullion and Yeh 1994; Ryabik et al. 1993; Weide et al. 1992). G-CSF was able to reduce the mean recovery time for an absolute neutrophil count (ANC) of less than $500 \ mm^3$ from 15.7 ± 3.7 days for historical controls to 8.0 ± 2.4 days. A recommended regimen administers 300 μg immediately, followed by doses of 300 μg/day until the agranulocytosis resolves (Gerson 1994; Gullion and Yeh 1994). Although initial reports are encouraging, more experience is needed to fully support the use of G-CSF. Patients should be warned to contact their health professional at any time if they experience lethargy, sore throat, fever, weakness, or other signs of infection.

Eosinophilia.   This effect has been reported to occur in 1% of patients. Onset in two cases occurred between 1 and 5 weeks (Stricker and Tielens 1991; Thhonen and Paanila 1992). In both cases, reversal occurred within 1 week. If the total eosinophil count is higher than 4,000/mm^3, then clozapine should be discontinued until the count is less than 3,000/mm^3 (Clozaril® Product Information 1994).

Leucocytosis.   This effect has been reported in 0.6% of patients. Although leukocytosis is often noted to be a benign condition, it has been suggested that patients with more than a 15% spike in their WBC might be at an increased risk for agranulocytosis (see *Agranulocytosis,* above [page 74]).

Hepatic
Mild increases in liver enzymes have been observed with routine monitoring, but significant clinical consequences (e.g., jaundice) have not been reported. Routine laboratory monitoring for this effect does not appear to be necessary.

Metabolic
Weight gain averaging 9–25 pounds has been reported to occur in 13%–85% of patients (Leadbetter et al. 1992). Two retrospective reports indicated that the average weight gain on clozapine was 14 pounds in 4 months and 17 pounds in 6 months (S. Cohen et al. 1990; Lamberti et al. 1992). In these two reports, 38% and 75% of patients gained at least 10 pounds. A recent 7.5-year prospective study reported that 50% of 82 patients gained more than 20% of their preclozapine weight (Umbricht et al. 1994). The percentage of patients becoming 10%, 20%, 30%, and 40% overweight during the treatment period was 85%, 54%, 23%, and 13%, respectively. Although most patients gained the majority of their weight during the first year of treatment, patients continued to gain weight throughout the treatment period. Patients who were underweight at baseline gained significantly more weight than did patients whose weight was ideal or who were overweight. However, overweight patients gained the most weight of all three groups. Patients

should be informed of this adverse effect. Caloric restriction and/or increased activity should be considered. It is unknown whether this effect responds to dosage reduction. Because excessive weight gain poses significant health risks to patients, the efficacy of behavioral and pharmacological management needs to be investigated. The antihistaminic and antiserotonergic properties of clozapine may be responsible for this effect.

Neuroleptic Malignant Syndrome

Seven cases of NMS have been reported with clozapine (DasGupta and Young 1991; Thornberg and Ereshefsky 1993). Two cases (Muller et al. 1988; Pope et al. 1986) occurred in patients receiving lithium or carbamazepine, while five cases were in patients receiving clozapine alone (Anderson and Powers 1991; Goates and Escobar 1992; Miller et al. 1991; Nopoulos et al. 1990; Viner and Escobar 1994). Although three cases reported NMS-type signs without rigidity, four cases reported its presence. Most cases of clozapine-associated NMS occurred within 2 weeks of clozapine initiation; however, one case occurred after 8 months of treatment (Miller et al. 1991; Thornberg and Ereshefsky 1993). If a patient develops signs of rigidity, autonomic dysfunction (e.g., hypo- or hypertension), significant hyperthermia, leukocytosis, and/or elevated creatine phosphokinase soon after initiation of clozapine, the drug should be discontinued. Supportive therapy and, possibly, pharmacotherapy (e.g., bromocriptine) should be instituted. Although rechallenge did not lead to recurrence of NMS in several cases, caution should be used with reinstitution (S. A. Cohen 1994; Goates and Escobar 1992).

Neurological

▶ Delirium

Four patients have experienced anticholinergic delirium, consisting of disorientation, confusion, agitation, dysarthria, and auditory and/or visual hallucinations, while receiving clozapine (Schuster et al. 1977; Szymanski et al. 1991; Viner and Escobar 1994). In one case, the onset was within 36 hours of a large initial dose (400 mg/day), but the symptom cleared within 9 hours (Szymanski et al. 1991). The patient tolerated a lower dose of 300 mg/day, which was reached with gradual titration. The presentation of these cases is consistent with an "anticholinergic delirium," which is probably due to clozapine's anticholinergic properties (see "Mechanism of Action" [page 66]).

▶ **Extrapyramidal Side Effects**

Acute effects.   Clozapine has not been associated with *dystonia* (Ereshefsky et al. 1989). Although both tremor and rigidity have been reported in 3% of patients, hypokinesia, which is characteristic of *parkinsonism,* has not been reported (Safferman et al. 1991).

Several early reports suggested that *akathisia* occurs in approximately 6% of patients (Chengappa et al. 1994; Safferman et al. 1991). However, one blinded study reported akathisia in 39% of clozapine-treated patients compared with 45% of patients receiving typical antipsychotics (B. M. Cohen et al. 1991). This study's design has been questioned, because clozapine-treated patients may have manifested tardive akathisia, not acute-onset akathisia (Safferman et al. 1992b). A recent prospective trial reported that no patients developed akathisia on clozapine (Safferman et al. 1993). This study also reported that patients with preexisting typical antipsychotic–induced akathisia improved over time after clozapine substitution, primarily during the first 3 months of treatment. Given that most reports of akathisia come from open or retrospective studies, more controlled trials need to be performed to accurately assess the prevalence of akathisia with clozapine.

Long-term effects.   Most literature reviews indicate that clozapine has not been clearly documented to produce tardive dyskinesia (Ereshefsky et al. 1989; J. A. Lieberman et al. 1989; Safferman et al. 1991). However, three recent case reports have associated clozapine with choreoathetoid dyskinesia, jaw dyskinesia, and tardive oculogyric crisis (Dave 1994; de Leon et al. 1991). In one case, the dyskinesia reversed within 3 days of clozapine discontinuation, reappeared within 4 days of the rechallenge, and again reversed with drug discontinuation. In the second case, jaw movements appeared 14 days after drug initiation and continued unchanged for 1 year. The drug was not discontinued, and the dyskinesia did not respond to anticholinergic treatment. The third case of tardive oculogyric crisis responded to benztropine 4 mg/day. A recent prospective, open assessment of 28 patients treated with clozapine for more than 1 year reported possibly two cases of tardive dyskinesia (Kane et al. 1993). More controlled trials are required to assess clozapine's ability to produce tardive dyskinesia.

Uncontrolled studies indicate that clozapine may, like typical antipsychotics, in a dose-related manner suppress dyskinetic movements by more than 50% in approximately 43% of patients (J. A. Lieberman et al. 1991; Small et al. 1987; Tamminga et al. 1994). It is important to note that in these studies, dyskinetic movements were often reported improved but not absent. Dystonic features were said to be most responsive to clozapine. Most of these studies lasted 1 month or less; longer trials with adequate blinding of investigators need to be performed to confirm these reports.

Seizures. A number of case reports have documented primarily tonic-clonic seizures, but myoclonic seizures may also occur (Devinsky and Pacia 1994). A preexisting seizure disorder or history of head trauma increases the risk of seizures (Devinsky and Pacia 1994; Safferman et al. 1991). Although 22%–75% of patients on clozapine will have abnormal EEG findings, significantly fewer patients will have seizures (Devinsky and Pacia 1994). Early reports of 1,418 patients treated in the United States between 1972 and 1988 indicated that this effect was related both to dose and to rate of dosage increase (Devinsky et al. 1991). Daily doses and seizure incidences were as follows: <300 mg/day, 1%; 300–600 mg/day, 2.7%; and >600–900 mg/day, 4.4%. The overall seizure rate was 2.9%, and a cumulative risk of 10% over a 3.8-year period of treatment was calculated. However, a more recent study failed to detect a dose-related association (Devinsky and Pacia 1994).

If a seizure occurs, clozapine should be discontinued. An EEG and a neurology consultation are advised. If the seizure workup is unremarkable, clozapine may be reintroduced at recommended starting doses. A recommended target dose is 50% of the dose at which the seizure occurred. The majority of patients can remain on clozapine with dosage reduction or can be rechallenged with slower dose titration. However, some patients may require the addition of an anticonvulsant. Of 71 patients who had a clozapine-induced tonic-clonic seizure, 24 (34%) had recurrent seizures after clozapine reinitiation. If the workup is abnormal or another seizure occurs upon rechallenge, an anticonvulsant is indicated. After steady-state therapeutic levels of an anticonvulsant are achieved, clozapine may be reinstituted (Devinsky and Pacia 1994; Safferman et al. 1991; Wilson and Claussen 1994). Carbamazepine is not recommended in combination with clozapine because of concerns about additive hematological adverse effects (Safferman et al. 1991). However, phenytoin, valproate, phenobarbital, and primidone might be considered (Devinsky and Pacia 1994). Clozapine may be involved in drug interactions with several anticonvulsants (for management of antipsychotic–anticonvulsant drug interactions, see "Phenytoin" [page 464] under **Antipsychotics** in Chapter 8). The exact mechanism of clozapine-induced seizures is not known (Devinsky and Pacia 1994).

Sedation. This is a dose-related side effect to which most patients develop a degree of tolerance over time; some patients even develop complete tolerance. To minimize sedation, initiate treatment with doses of 12.5 mg once or twice daily (see "Dosage" [page 67]). Administering most or all of the dose at bedtime may also help to mitigate this effect (Ereshefsky et al. 1989; J. A. Lieberman et al. 1989). Because of the potential for respiratory suppression or arrest (see **Antipsychotic–*Benzodiazepine*** interaction [page 460] in Chapter 8), caution should be exercised when clozapine is combined with a benzodiazepine (Cobb et al. 1991). Sedation is probably related to clozapine's antihistaminic and antiadrenergic properties.

Ophthalmological
An ophthalmological examination in 11 patients treated with clozapine from 6 months to 2 years revealed no abnormal pigmentation in the lens or retina (Ayd 1974).

Psychiatric
Obsessive-compulsive symptoms. A retrospective study reported that 5 of 49 patients developed obsessive-compulsive symptoms within 2 to 15 months at clozapine 400–750 mg/day (Baker et al. 1992). It was suggested that clozapine's serotonin-blocking properties may produce these symptoms. However, it is reported that clozapine significantly reduced obsessive-compulsive symptoms in one patient (LaPorta 1994).

Rebound psychosis. There have been reports of rapid return ("rebound") of psychotic symptoms within days after abrupt discontinuation of clozapine (Alphs and Lee 1991; Baldessarini et al. 1995; Breier 1996; Safferman et al. 1991). However, other reports question the existence of such a phenomenon (J. A. Lieberman et al. 1989). Nonetheless, patients should be instructed not to abruptly discontinue clozapine unless directed by a prescriber. Conservatively, if clozapine needs to be discontinued in a nonemergent situation, the drug should be tapered and/or another antipsychotic initiated (Baldessarini et al. 1995) (see *Withdrawal reactions* [page 71]).

Sexual Dysfunction
Anorgasmia, ejaculatory dysfunction, impotence, and decreased libido. The exact incidence of these effects is not known (Safferman et al. 1991). If they occur, dosage reduction or drug discontinuation may be required. Sexual dysfunction effects are probably related to antiadrenergic and/or anticholinergic effects.

Priapism.   Three cases of priapism have been reported (Rosen and Hanno 1992; Seftel et al. 1992; Zeigler and Behar 1992). Onset occurred between 4 and 10 weeks of clozapine initiation. Two cases resulted in impotence despite aggressive treatment. In one case, multiple rechallenges led to recurrences of priapism. Treatment consists of immediate drug discontinuation and injection of intra-corporeal epinephrine, which may provide only temporary relief. Surgical reduction often is necessary. The suggested mechanism of action for this effect is antiadrenergic blockade.

Temperature Regulation

Hypothermia.   This benign effect occurs in 87% of patients (Saf-ferman et al. 1991). The exact mechanism is unknown, but it is believed to be a CNS effect. Hypothermia does not require any specific treatment.

Hyperthermia.   Temperature elevations of 1–2°F have been noted within the first 5–20 days (average 10 days) of treatment (J. A. Lieberman et al. 1989; Safferman et al. 1991). This effect has been reported in 0%–55% of patients, depending on the method of measurement (i.e., po versus rectal) (Ereshefsky et al. 1989). Typi-cally, hyperthermia is a benign effect that resolves either without treatment or with clozapine discontinuation. However, the tem-perature increase might indicate a possible infection secondary to leukopenia (see *Hematological* adverse effects [page 74]). Pa-tients with hyperthermia should have a CBC and sedimentation rate performed to rule out infection. In addition, they should be followed for signs of NMS (see *Neuroleptic Malignant Syndrome* [page 77] under "Adverse Effects"). The mechanism of clozapine-induced hyperthermia is unknown.

Teratogenicity and Excretion Into Breast Milk

Clozapine is classified as a Pregnancy Category B[1] drug (Clozaril® Product Information 1996). The manufacturer recommends that clozapine be used in pregnant women only if clearly indicated. The effect of clozapine on labor and delivery is unknown.

It is unknown whether clozapine or its metabolites appear in human breast milk; therefore, women receiving clozapine should not breast-feed.

---

[1] There is *no* evidence of teratogenicity in animals, but no controlled studies are available in humans.

Urinary

Enuresis, urinary frequency/urgency, urinary hesitancy, or urinary retention may occur in approximately 6% of patients (Frankenburg et al. 1996; Safferman et al. 1991). However, it is believed that these effects are underreported. Cases of enuresis that responded within several days of the addition of desmopressin 10 ug per nostril at bedtime have been reported (Aronowitz et al. 1995; Frankenburg et al. 1996; Steingard 1994). In one study, five of seven patients with clozapine-induced urinary incontinence had complete resolution of symptoms within 24 hours of treatment with ephedrine 50 mg twice daily (Fuller et al. 1995). The remaining two patients had a reduction in frequency of enuresis. Another study reported that five patients with clozapine-induced urinary incontinence experienced symptom resolution without pharmacological management within 3 months of continuous clozapine treatment (Warner et al. 1994). Patients with prostatic hypertrophy may be most susceptible to urinary retention, leading to frequency/urgency or overflow incontinence. Dosage reduction or drug discontinuation may be required (Steingard 1994). These urinary symptoms may occur secondary to anticholinergic effects.

■ Rational Prescribing

1. Clozapine is not indicated as a first-line antipsychotic because of its potential for significant adverse hematological effects and its cost. Prescribers and pharmacists must be registered with the manufacturer before prescribing and/or dispensing clozapine. Patients receiving clozapine must also be registered with the manufacturer (call 1-800-448-5938).
2. Patients with significant early-onset (i.e., dystonia, akathisia, parkinsonism) and/or late-onset (e.g., tardive dyskinesia, tardive dystonia, tardive akathisia) EPS are candidates for clozapine.
3. Patients must be followed closely for adverse hematological reactions with weekly blood counts.
4. An adequate trial of clozapine consists of dosages greater than 450 mg/day administered for at least 3–6 months. If clozapine serum levels are available, the adequacy of a trial might be confirmed by a plasma concentration greater than 420 ng/mL maintained for 3–6 months.
5. Recommendations for combining clozapine with a typical antipsychotic or risperidone await the results of published trials demonstrating efficacy and safety (Safferman et al. 1991).

Olanzapine

Olanzapine is a thienobenzodiazepine antipsychotic that was approved for marketing in September 1996. Its pharmacology is similar to that of clozapine, and it is classified as an atypical antipsychotic.

■ Indications

Olanzapine is indicated for the treatment of schizophrenia. There is very little published literature on this drug.

■ Efficacy

Pharmacoeconomic studies need to be performed to determine the benefit-to-cost ratio for olanzapine.

Schizophrenia

❱ First-Episode Treatment/Nonrefractory Schizophrenia

Olanzapine versus placebo. Patients in a multicenter trial were randomized to receive one of three double-blind treatments: olanzapine 1 mg, olanzapine 10 mg, or placebo (Beasley et al. 1996a). Efficacy measures were based on changes seen in BPRS total, positive, and negative subscale scores; Positive and Negative Syndrome Scale (PANSS) total, positive, and negative subscale scores; and a Clinical Global Impressions severity-of-illness measure. Whereas olanzapine 1 mg and placebo were equal in producing no statistically significant changes in any of the symptom scales, olanzapine 10 mg was statistically significantly superior to placebo on the BPRS total and the PANSS total scores.

Olanzapine versus haloperidol and placebo. Patients were randomized to one of five double-blind treatments: olanzapine 2.5, 5, or 7.5 mg/day (low-dose olanzapine group), olanzapine 7.5, 10, or 12.5 mg/day (medium-dose olanzapine group), olanzapine 12.5, 15, or 17.5 mg/day (high-dose olanzapine group); haloperidol 10, 15, or 20 mg/day; or placebo (Beasley et al. 1996b). Haloperidol and medium- and high-dose olanzapine were superior to placebo and produced comparable improvement on BPRS total scores. The low and high doses of olanzapine were significantly superior to placebo, and the high dose superior to haloperidol, on Scale for the Assessment of Negative Symptoms (SANS) scores.

❱ Refractory Schizophrenia

No reports examining the efficacy of olanzapine in treatment-refractory patients with schizophrenia have been published.

❱ **Maintenance Treatment**

Although studies of patients who had received olanzapine for durations up to 1 year have been conducted, these studies have not been published (Tran et al. 1995b).

Cognitive Disorders

Olanzapine 1–8 mg/day was studied in an 8-week, double-blind, placebo-controlled trial of 238 patients over age 65 with Alzheimer's dementia (Satterlee et al. 1995). No difference between olanzapine and placebo was detected in reduction of psychotic symptoms or behavioral manifestations, although it is possible that higher doses of olanzapine would have demonstrated such a difference. More studies need to be performed to determine olanzapine's efficacy in the treatment of patients with dementia.

■ Mechanism of Action

Olanzapine, like clozapine, has selective effects on the spontaneous firing rate of the dopaminergic neurons of the ventral tegmental area following acute and chronic administration (Stockton and Rasmussen 1995; Tran et al. 1995a). Olanzapine has a high affinity for a variety of receptors. It binds to both the 5-HT_{2A} and the D_4 receptors; however, its binding affinity for the D_2 receptor is three times higher than that for the 5-HT_{2A} and the D_4 receptors (Beasley et al. 1996b; Tollefson et al. 1994). Olanzapine also binds to D_1, D_4, 5-HT_{2C}, muscarinic (especially M_1), α_1-adrenergic, and H_1 histaminic receptors (Beasley et al. 1996b).

■ Pharmacokinetics

Olanzapine plasma levels peak an average of 4.9 hours after oral administration. The average elimination half-life is 27 ± 2 hours. Olanzapine's major metabolite is olanzapine-N-glucuronide; its other metabolites are olanzapine-N-oxide and N-desmethyl olanzapine (Obermeyer et al. 1993). Food does not affect the rate or extent of the drug's absorption (Zyprexa® Product Information 1996).

Renal impairment would be expected to affect the clearance of olanzapine only minimally, since very little active drug is eliminated by this route (Zyprexa® Product Information 1996). Although olanzapine is extensively metabolized by the liver, its clearance from the body was not found to be significantly altered in a study of six patients with cirrhosis. However, caution should be maintained when administering the drug to patients with liver disease (Zyprexa® Product Information 1996). The clearance of olanzapine is three times higher in younger (i.e., ≤65) male smokers than in older (i.e., >65) female nonsmokers (Zyprexa® Product Information 1996). Additionally, in a study of 24 healthy subjects, the mean elimination half-life of olanzapine was 1.5 times greater in subjects over—as opposed to under—65 years of age (Zyprexa® Product Information 1996).

A therapeutic range for olanzapine plasma levels in the treatment of schizophrenia has not been established.

■ Dosage

Schizophrenia
Olanzapine can be administered once daily without regard to meals (Zyprexa® Product Information 1996). Initial doses should be 5–10 mg/day, with a target dose of 10 mg/day. Subsequent dosage increases should be in increments of 5 mg/day and should not be spaced less than 1 week apart. In clinical trials, olanzapine dosages greater than 10 mg/day did not demonstrate greater efficacy in comparison with dosages of 10 mg/day. The safety of olanzapine dosages greater than 20 mg/day has not been established.

For patients over 65 years of age, those with liver disease, and/or those on antihypertensive medications, olanzapine dosages should be initiated at 5 mg/day.

Cognitive Disorders
The one study of olanzapine in patients with Alzheimer's disease did not demonstrate a difference in efficacy between olanzapine dosages less than 8 mg/day and placebo (Satterlee et al. 1995). Whether higher olanzapine dosages may be effective in these patients awaits the results of additional studies.

■ Adverse Effects

Information on olanzapine's adverse effects comes from the manufacturer (Zyprexa® Product Information 1996) and from two multicenter trials involving a total of 480 patients (Beasley et al. 1996a, 1996b).

Autonomic
The anticholinergic effects of constipation and dry mouth occurred in 9% and 7% of patients, respectively (Beasley et al. 1996a). These were dose-related effects.

Cardiovascular

Olanzapine did not significantly affect heart rate, supine systolic blood pressure, supine and standing diastolic blood pressure, or supine and standing heart rate in one multicenter study (Beasley et al. 1996a). Compared with placebo, olanzapine 10 mg/day produced a statistically but not clinically significant increase of 3.6 mm Hg in standing systolic blood pressure. However, orthostatic hypotension has been reported in 5% of subjects (Zyprexa® Product Information 1996). Blood pressure should be monitored during the initial titration phases of olanzapine, especially in elderly patients and those receiving blood pressure–lowering medications.

Olanzapine has not been associated with significant ECG changes (Zyprexa® Product Information 1996).

Hematological

Unlike clozapine, olanzapine has had no leukopenia or agranulocytosis cases reported to date (Beasley et al. 1996a). Information regarding the safety of olanzapine in patients that have experienced clozapine-induced leukopenia and/or granulocytopenia has yet to be published.

Hepatic

Olanzapine was shown to be associated with dose-dependent increases in hepatic transaminases (alanine aminotransferase [ALT], aspartate aminotransferase [AST], γ-glutamyl transpeptidase [GGT]) (Beasley et al. 1996a). In the high-dose olanzapine group (see *Olanzapine versus placebo* [page 83]), an increase in ALT of 24.3 ± 93.5 U/L was seen in 9.2% of the patients. In some patients, transaminases returned to normal upon drug discontinuation; in others, however, transaminase levels normalized despite continued olanzapine treatment.

Metabolic

Olanzapine has been associated with an increase in prolactin levels that is maintained with chronic administration (Zyprexa® Product Information 1996). However, in one study of olanzapine dosages up to 20 mg/day, there were no differences between prolactin levels with olanzapine and those with placebo (Beasley et al. 1996b).

Weight gain has been reported with olanzapine. In the placebo-controlled trial described previously, subjects receiving olanzapine 10 mg gained 2.2 ± 4 kg, whereas those receiving placebo *lost* 0.4 ± 3.1 kg (Beasley et al. 1996a). In the placebo-controlled comparison study of olanzapine and haloperidol, the mean increase in weight was 3.5 ± 3.9 kg (Beasley et al. 1996b).

Unlike clozapine, olanzapine did not cause hypersalivation (Beasley et al. 1996a).

Neuroleptic Malignant Syndrome

Olanzapine has not been associated with NMS (Zyprexa® Product Information 1996). However, this adverse effect is not common, and only a limited number of patients have been exposed to olanzapine.

Neurological

Extrapyramidal side effects. In the haloperidol and placebo-controlled trial, haloperidol and olanzapine did not differ in their effectiveness in producing changes from baseline in extrapyramidal-symptom scores for parkinsonism, akathisia, or dyskinesias (Beasley et al. 1996b). No patients experienced a dystonic reaction. Extrapyramidal-rating-scale scores improved in the subjects receiving olanzapine but deteriorated in those receiving haloperidol (Beasley et al. 1996b).

Although olanzapine would not be expected to produce tardive dyskinesia, patients have not been exposed to the drug for durations sufficient to determine the risk, if any, of this adverse effect.

Sedation. Somnolence has been reported in 26% of patients receiving olanzapine, compared with 15% of patients receiving placebo (Zyprexa® Product Information 1996). This is a dose-related effect. Patients should be warned of possible impairments in driving skills when first taking olanzapine or after dosage increases.

Reduction of seizure threshold. In premarketing studies, seizures occurred in 0.9% of olanzapine-treated patients (Zyprexa® Product Information 1996). Olanzapine should be used cautiously in patients with a seizure history.

Teratogenicity and Excretion Into Breast Milk

Olanzapine is classified as a Pregnancy Category C^2 drug (Zyprexa® Product Information 1996). The drug should not be used during pregnancy unless the potential benefit justifies the potential risk to the fetus. The effect of olanzapine on labor and delivery in humans is unknown.

It is unknown whether olanzapine is excreted in breast milk

---

[2] There is evidence of teratogenicity in animals, but no controlled studies are available in humans.

(Zyprexa® Product Information 1996). Women receiving olanzapine are advised not to breast-feed.

■ Rational Prescribing

1. Because of its relative newness and the limited postmarketing experience regarding its efficacy and safety, olanzapine is not indicated as a first-line antipsychotic.
2. More experience is needed with olanzapine in the maintenance treatment of schizophrenia.
3. Olanzapine has not been studied in the treatment of refractory schizophrenia. The relative efficacies of clozapine, olanzapine, risperidone, and sertindole in this population have not been determined.
4. Patients with significant early-onset (i.e., akathisia, parkinsonism) and/or late-onset (e.g., tardive dyskinesia, tardive dystonia, tardive akathisia) extrapyramidal adverse effects who have not responded to risperidone should be given a trial of olanzapine before clozapine is considered.

Pimozide

Pimozide has been used in Europe for almost 20 years in the treatment of psychosis (Opler and Feinberg 1991; Tueth and Cheong 1993). It was approved in the United States in 1984 as an orphan drug in the treatment of Gilles de la Tourette's syndrome.

■ Indications

Pimozide's only indication in the United States is for the second-line treatment of Gilles de la Tourette's syndrome (Tueth and Cheong 1993). However, it has been used in schizophrenia and delusional disorders and as an augmentation treatment for obsessive-compulsive disorder. Nonpsychiatric uses have included postherpetic and trigeminal neuralgia (Opler and Feinberg 1991).

■ Efficacy

Delusional Disorder
Monosymptomatic delusions (e.g., conjugal paranoia, somatization, dysmorphosis, erotomania, pseudocyesis) have been reported to respond to pimozide 2–12 mg/day in 80% of cases. However, this conclusion is based on case reports rather than on controlled trials (Opler and Feinberg 1991).

Obsessive-Compulsive Disorder

Reports that pimozide, when added to standard antiobsessional treatments, produced significant improvement in patients' symptoms require confirmation in controlled trials (Opler and Feinberg 1991).

Schizophrenia

Four open trials and seven double-blind, controlled trials have examined pimozide's efficacy in *acutely psychotic* patients (Opler and Feinberg 1991). Overall, pimozide was less effective, had a slower onset of action, and produced more EPS than other high-potency typical antipsychotics (e.g., haloperidol).

Ten of 11 studies reported that pimozide was more effective than placebo as a *maintenance* treatment. Of 15 double-blind studies comparing pimozide with typical antipsychotics, 12 reported equal efficacy, while 3 reported more efficacy for pimozide than for the reference antipsychotic.

In seven studies comparing pimozide's effect with that of chlorpromazine, fluphenazine, or trifluoperazine on *negative symptoms* of schizophrenia, the drug did not consistently demonstrate greater efficacy (Opler and Feinberg 1991).

Tourette's Syndrome

Pimozide in dosages up to 20 mg/day has been shown to be as effective as haloperidol and fluphenazine in open and controlled trials (Opler and Feinberg 1991; Tueth and Cheong 1993). Overall, 70%–81% of patients experienced moderate to marked improvement with pimozide. However, concerns about the drug's potential to cause cardiac adverse effects have resulted in its relegation to a second-line treatment (see *Cardiovascular* adverse effects, below).

■ Mechanism of Action

Pimozide has pharmacological properties similar to those of typical antipsychotics (Tueth and Cheong 1993). It acts by blocking postsynaptic D_2 receptors. The drug has minimal effects on noradrenergic and acetylcholine receptors and, therefore, produces few sedative and anticholinergic side effects. Like low-potency antipsychotics, pimozide possesses calcium channel–blocking properties.

■ Dosage

The recommended dose for Tourette's syndrome is 0.3 mg/kg/day or 20 mg/day (Tueth and Cheong 1993). Typical maintenance doses of pimozide in schizophrenia are 20 mg/day or less; however, doses up to 75 mg/day have been used in acutely agitated, psychotic patients (Opler and Feinberg 1991). It is recommended that dose increases not exceed 2-mg increments. The reported dose equivalents vary from 2 to 4 mg (Opler and Feinberg 1991).

Although typically administered once daily, pimozide was successfully administered four times weekly and once a week in a maintenance study (Opler and Feinberg 1991).

■ Pharmacokinetics

Pimozide has not been extensively investigated (Balant-Gorgia et al. 1993). Peak absorption occurs at 4–8 hours, and the drug has a bioavailability of only 15%–25%. It is highly bound to plasma proteins, as less than 1% of the drug is free in the plasma. The volume of distribution is 20–40 L/kg. Pimozide is extensively metabolized by the liver; less than 1% of a dose is excreted unchanged in the urine. The drug's half-life varies from 30 to 150 hours, and it has no active metabolites. A therapeutic range for any indication has not been established.

■ Adverse Effects

The adverse effects of pimozide have been extensively reviewed (Opler and Feinberg 1991; Tueth and Cheong 1993). Only the commonly noted adverse effects are presented here. (For information on management of pimozide's side effects, see relevant adverse effects under sections on typical antipsychotics and clozapine in this chapter.)

It has been suggested that pimozide produces a different side-effect profile in Tourette's patients than in psychotic patients (Opler and Feinberg 1991). Side effects observed in Tourette's patients include irritability, aggression, dysphoria, fearfulness, and impairments in motivation, attention, and memory.

Autonomic
It is uncommon for pimozide to be associated with typical anticholinergic side effects (e.g., dry mouth, constipation, blurred vision, urinary retention).

Cardiovascular
Although early reports suggested that pimozide produced few changes in blood pressure, pulse, or ECG, reports of two deaths possibly secondary to cardiac arrhythmias led the FDA to recommend baseline ECGs and periodic follow-up for patients receiving pimozide (Opler and Feinberg 1991). Both patients were being titrated

to 70–80 mg/day over a 2-week period. Approximately 10% of patients treated with standard doses will experience ECG changes (Tueth and Cheong 1993). It is recommended that pimozide be discontinued or further dose increases be stopped if the QTc interval exceeds 0.47 second in children or 0.52 second in adults or is more than 25% above the patient's baseline value. In addition, T- and U-wave abnormalities have been reported. The risks of significant adverse effects appear to be minimal at pimozide dosages of 20 mg/day or less (Tueth and Cheong 1993). Pimozide should be used cautiously in patients who have preexisting conduction disturbances or who are receiving concurrent TCAs or antiarrhythmic agents.

Dermatological
Photosensitivity has not been reported with pimozide, but patients might be advised to limit sun exposure and/or to use sunscreen products.

Endocrinological
Menstrual irregularities and galactorrhea have been reported with pimozide.

Metabolic
Both weight gain and weight loss have been reported in patients receiving pimozide.

Neuroleptic Malignant Syndrome
One case of NMS has been reported with low-dose pimozide. Use of higher doses may increase the risk for this effect.

Neurological

Extrapyramidal side effects. Although early studies reported few *acute-onset* side effects for dosages of 2–6 mg/day, more recent studies using higher doses have reported an EPS incidence and presentation similar to those found with high-potency typical antipsychotics (e.g., haloperidol, fluphenazine) (see Extrapyramidal Side Effects [page 45] under *Neurological* adverse effects of **Typical Antipsychotics**). Prolonged use of pimozide has been associated with *tardive dyskinesia.* Like typical antipsychotics, pimozide has been reported to suppress dyskinetic movements. Administering the drug once weekly instead of daily led to an increased rate of movements, which is analogous to reports that drug holidays increased the risk of EPS for typical antipsychotics (Kane and McGlashan 1995). The exact incidence or prevalence of tardive dyskinesia secondary to pimozide is not known. There is no known treatment other than drug discontinuation.

Sedation.   In comparison with other typical antipsychotics, including high-potency drugs, pimozide is less likely to produce sedation.

Reduction of seizure threshold.   Although pimozide may lower the seizure threshold, it produces a rate of seizures similar to that produced by typical antipsychotics.

Ophthalmological
Abnormal ocular deposits and pigmentation have not been noted with pimozide.

Sexual Dysfunction
Pimozide use has been associated with decreased libido and impotence, although these effects might be less common with pimozide than with typical antipsychotics.

Teratogenicity and Excretion Into Breast Milk
Pimozide's use during pregnancy and while breast feeding is not recommended.

■ Rational Prescribing

1. Pimozide is recommended as a second-line treatment for Tourette's syndrome if patients do not respond to or tolerate typical antipsychotics.
2. Pimozide is not recommended as a first-line treatment for schizophrenia, as its side effects (e.g., cardiac conduction defects) may be more numerous than those of typical antipsychotics.
3. Pimozide might be considered for a patient who has been unresponsive to more than two trials of typical antipsychotics and risperidone.
4. Although pimozide is a promising treatment for monosymptomatic delusions, an exact determination of the drug's efficacy in these disorders awaits further controlled trials.
5. An ECG is required before prescribing pimozide.

Risperidone

Risperidone is a benzisoxazole derivative that was first marketed in the United States in 1994. It produces a low rate of EPS at recommended doses and therefore might be labeled an atypical antipsychotic; however, because of its ability to produce EPS at higher doses, risperidone resembles high-potency typical antipsychotics. Thus, risperidone might more appropriately be referred to as a "novel" antipsychotic.

■ Indications

Risperidone is indicated in the treatment of schizophrenia.

■ Efficacy

Schizophrenia

Pharmacoeconomic studies need to be performed with risperidone to determine its benefit-to-cost ratio (Carter et al. 1995).

Twenty-six clinical trials of risperidone in schizophrenia have been conducted (Cardoni 1995; L. J. Cohen 1994; Marder 1996). Sixteen studies were open design, 9 were double-blind, and 1 was single-blind. The results of these studies are described in the following paragraphs.

▶ First-Episode Treatment/Nonrefractory Schizophrenia

Risperidone in open reports. In 10 short-term trials of 4 weeks to 3 months in duration, risperidone was reported to improve psychotic symptoms (L. J. Cohen 1994). In two trials lasting 1 year each, risperidone also improved psychotic symptoms.

Risperidone versus placebo. Two double-blind studies and one single-blind study reported that risperidone was more effective than placebo (L. J. Cohen 1994).

Risperidone versus haloperidol. Risperidone has been compared only with the typical antipsychotic haloperidol (Chouinard et al. 1993; L. J. Cohen 1994; Marder et al. 1994). Its efficacy was compared with that of haloperidol alone in three studies and with that of haloperidol and placebo in two studies. The studies varied in length from 4 to 12 weeks. Overall, three of the five studies reported no difference between risperidone and haloperidol, whereas two studies found risperidone to be more effective than haloperidol.

Risperidone versus clozapine. After 1 week of dose titration, 59 patients were treated with risperidone 4 mg/day, risperidone 8 mg/day, or clozapine 400 mg/day at fixed doses for 3 weeks (Heinrich et al. 1990). Patients responded equally to all three treatments. It is important to note that these patients were not refractory.

A double-blind study of clozapine 400 mg/day and risperidone 4 and 8 mg/day for 4 weeks reported improvement rates of 65%, 63.2%, and 52.6%, respectively, for the three treatments (Klieser et al. 1995). These response rates were not significantly different, although there was a trend for risperidone 8 mg/day to be less effective than the clozapine or risperidone 4-mg/day dosages.

▶ **Refractory Schizophrenia**

More double-blind trials are needed that compare risperidone's efficacy with that of clozapine, olanzapine, and sertindole in the treatment of refractory schizophrenia.

Risperidone in open reports.   In a 6-month study, risperidone produced moderate to marked improvement in 11 of 17 patients (L. J. Cohen 1994). Six of 25 (24%) patients hospitalized for a mean of 8.7 years who were treated with risperidone 6–13 mg/day experienced more than a 20% reduction in BPRS scores after 9 months of treatment (Smith et al. 1995). Five of these 6 responders demonstrated improvement as early as month 2 of treatment.

Risperidone versus haloperidol.   In an 8-week study of risperidone 6 mg/day versus haloperidol 15 mg/day in 19 patients, no difference in efficacy was detected between the two treatments (Wirshing et al. 1995). Both groups had, on average, a 10%–15% reduction in positive, negative, and general psychopathology scores. However, all 10 haloperidol-treated patients dropped out of the study early because of adverse effects, whereas all risperidone-treated patients completed the full 2 months of treatment.

A post hoc analysis of a multicenter, double-blind, placebo-controlled study compared risperidone 6 mg/day, haloperidol 20 mg/day, and placebo (Kane 1996). Patients with up to 1 week of current hospitalization were compared with patients hospitalized for up to 1 month, those hospitalized from 1 to 6 months, and those hospitalized for more than 6 months. The latter three groups were considered poor or partial responders to typical antipsychotic drugs. It was concluded that risperidone 6 mg/day was more effective than placebo across all groups in producing improvement in psychopathology rating-scale scores, whereas haloperidol was superior to placebo only in patients hospitalized for up to 1 month. This retrospective analysis suggests that risperidone may be more effective than haloperidol in treatment-resistant patients. This conclusion requires further study.

Risperidone versus clozapine.   In a 10-month open trial in which five patients received risperidone and five received clozapine, the two drugs produced significant and equal improvement in the patients' psychotic symptoms (L.J. Cohen 1994).

A 4-week, double-blind study in 30 patients reported significant improvement in psychotic scores by 1 week with both drugs (Bersani et al. 1990).

In a 3-month, double-blind, unpublished study, a trend for clozapine's superior efficacy on five of six PANSS subscale scores was noted (Lindenmayer 1996). Only in the anxiety/depression subscale score was there a trend for superior efficacy with risperidone compared with clozapine. Information on risperidone dosages, clozapine dosages, and clozapine serum levels were not available.

Eighty-six patients were treated in a double-blind study for 8 weeks with risperidone 3–10 mg/day (mean 6.4 mg/day) or clozapine 150–400 mg/day (mean 291.2 mg/day) (Kane 1996). At the end of the study period, 67% of the risperidone- and 65% of the clozapine-treated patients had improved by 20% or more on the PANSS.

These preliminary data suggest that risperidone might be useful in treatment-refractory patients. It is important to note that clozapine serum levels should be measured and adjusted into the recommended range to optimize treatment (see "Pharmacokinetics" [page 67] under **Clozapine** section). Many studies comparing risperidone with clozapine do not report clozapine serum levels.

Risperidone plus clozapine.   In a 4-week open trial, risperidone 6 mg/day was added to the regimens of 12 patients who had failed to respond to a minimum of 1 year of clozapine treatment (D. C. Henderson and Goff 1996). Ten of the patients had more than a 20% reduction in their total BPRS scores, and all patients tolerated the combination.

Switch from clozapine to risperidone.   In a 3-month prospective, open study, 10 inpatients treated for at least 3 months with clozapine were switched to risperidone 6 mg/day by tapering clozapine from an average dose of 565 mg/day (Still et al. 1995). Five of the 10 patients failed to complete the 3-month trial because of a worsening of psychotic symptoms or intolerable side effects. None of the patients experienced clinical improvement according to standard rating scales after switching to risperidone.

Switch from typical antipsychotics to risperidone.   One study reported that hospital days decreased by 20% per year in 27 patients with schizophrenia when they were switched from typical antipsychotics to risperidone (Addington et al. 1993).

Parkinson's Disease With Psychosis
Six patients treated with risperidone 0.25 to 1.25 mg/day experienced a significant improvement in hallucinations; in three of the patients, the hallucinations completely disappeared (Mecco et al. 1994). Parkinsonian signs and/or symptoms did not worsen on risperidone. However, although another study reported an im-

provement in psychotic symptoms with risperidone 1.5 mg/day, all six patients in this study experienced a worsening of their parkinsonism (Ford et al. 1994). The different findings in these two studies may be attributable to the latter study's use of a higher risperidone dose.

In a report of six cases, five patients experienced an exacerbation of parkinsonism when treated with risperidone 0.5–4.0 mg/day (Rich et al. 1995). However, four of these five patients subsequently improved when treated with clozapine (see Parkinson's Disease [page 65] under "Efficacy" of **Clozapine**).

Mania

Case studies of 30 patients suggest that risperidone dosages of 2–10 mg/day produced a 50%–90% improvement in manic symptoms (Gelenberg and Hopkins 1996; Sajatovic 1995; Schaffer and Schaffer 1996; Tohen et al. 1995). However, in 14 patients, risperidone either did not improve or actually worsened the manic symptoms. Several patients experienced an "activating" effect with risperidone. Risperidone's efficacy in the acute and maintenance treatment of bipolar disorder awaits the results of controlled, prospective trials.

Schizoaffective Disorder

Two open reports involving 84 patients and one double-blind study of 13 patients reported that risperidone was effective in reducing depressive and psychotic symptoms (Keck et al. 1996a). In an open study of 8 patients treated with risperidone, depressive symptoms improved but manic symptoms worsened (see *Mania*, above). These studies ranged in duration from 6 to 24 weeks. More controlled trials of risperidone need to be conducted to determine risperidone's efficacy in the acute and maintenance treatment of schizoaffective disorder.

Mental Retardation

In a placebo-controlled, crossover trial, the addition of risperidone 8–12 mg/day to patients' current drug regimens was significantly more effective than placebo in controlling extreme behaviors (L. J. Cohen 1994).

■ Mechanism of Action

Risperidone is a potent S_2 and D_2 antagonist (L. J. Cohen 1994). In addition, it antagonizes α_1, α_2, and H_1 receptors. It does not bind to cholinergic receptors. Risperidone produces a dose-related increase in prolactin levels.

■ Dosage

Dose-response studies have demonstrated a curvilinear relationship between risperidone and improvement in psychotic symptoms (L. J. Cohen 1994). The optimal dose of risperidone was 6–8 mg/day. The suggested titration schedule is 1 mg bid for 1 day, 2 mg bid for 1 day, and 3 mg bid thereafter. Further dose increases or decreases should be in increments of 1 mg/week. After 4 weeks of treatment, nonresponding patients who are not experiencing EPS might be considered for doses higher than 6 mg/day. Elderly patients may be treated with lower doses (e.g., 4 mg/day), as this population may be sensitive to the drug's hypotensive effects (see *Cardiovascular* adverse effects, below).

■ Pharmacokinetics

Risperidone is rapidly absorbed after oral administration, reaching a peak plasma level within 2 hours (Byerly and DeVane 1996; Cardoni 1995; L. J. Cohen 1994). The drug can be given with or without food, because the extent of absorption is not affected. The half-life of risperidone is 3 hours; however, the active metabolite, hydroxyrisperidone, has a half-life of 24 hours. Risperidone and hydroxyrisperidone are 89% and 77% plasma protein bound, respectively. Risperidone's half-life is longer in elderly patients and in those with renal insufficiency (Cardoni 1995). Although hepatic insufficiency does not lengthen the half-life of risperidone, a more pronounced effect may occur due to the presence of more unbound risperidone (Livingston 1994). Plasma concentrations of the parent drug and its active metabolite are dose proportional in the range of 1–16 mg/day. A therapeutic range has not been established.

■ Adverse Effects

In premarketing studies, approximately 9% of patients treated with risperidone discontinued treatment because of adverse effects, compared with 10% of haloperidol-treated patients and 7% of placebo-treated patients (Cardoni 1995; Chouinard et al. 1993; L. J. Cohen 1994; Marder and Meibach 1994).

Cardiovascular

ECG changes. Risperidone has been reported to lengthen the QTc interval (Risperdal® Product Information 1994).

Hypotension/dizziness. Dizziness was reported by approximately 10% of patients receiving risperidone doses of 6 and 16 mg/day

(Marder and Meibach 1994). Patients complaining of dizziness should have lying and standing blood pressures performed, especially during the first few weeks of treatment. This effect can be minimized by starting the drug at low doses (see "Dosage," above). Elderly patients and patients with significant cardiovascular disease should be closely monitored during the dosage titration phase. Orthostatic hypotension may be related to risperidone's α-adrenergic–blocking properties (L. J. Cohen 1994).

Endocrinological

Prolactin. Risperidone can increase prolactin levels in a dose-related manner. Although no published reports of amenorrhea, galactorrhea, or gynecomastia exist, it is possible that risperidone may be associated with these effects (L. J. Cohen 1994). Prolactin elevation is reversible with drug discontinuation.

Weight gain. Risperidone was reported to produce more than a 7% increase in body weight in 18% of patients (Risperdal® Product Information 1994).

Gastrointestinal

Early studies reported that 18% of patients receiving risperidone 10 mg/day complained of nausea. Administering the dose with food and/or lowering the dose might be empirically tried.

Hematological

No routine hematological laboratory monitoring is currently recommend for risperidone (L. J. Cohen 1994).

Hepatic

No routine hepatic laboratory monitoring is currently recommend for risperidone (L. J. Cohen 1994).

Neuroleptic Malignant Syndrome

Two recent possible cases of NMS have been reported (Webster and Wijeratne 1994). In the first, an 83-year-old man developed blood-pressure changes, urinary incontinence, diaphoresis, an increase in EPS, and hyperpyrexia 5 days after receiving risperidone 1 mg/day. He died 1 week later from pneumonia. In the second report, an 81-year-old woman treated with risperidone 2 mg/day developed a fever of 38.2°C, tachycardia, complete immobility, and an increase in EPS and urinary incontinence 12 hours after the first dose of risperidone. A creatine phosphokinase of 1,200 IU/L was noted. She recovered fully with supportive treatment after risperidone was discontinued.

Neurological

❱ Agitation/Anxiety

Agitation and anxiety were reported in 58% of patients receiving risperidone 16 mg/day, as compared with 45% of patients receiving placebo (Chouinard et al. 1993). It is possible that some of these patients might have been experiencing akathisia. The mechanism of these side effects is unknown.

❱ Cognition

Twenty geriatric patients (age ranging from 57 to 77 years) with schizophrenia were treated in a double-blind design with risperidone up to 6 mg/day or haloperidol up to 10 mg/day (Berman et al. 1995). The patients were evaluated at baseline and on drug treatment with a standard battery of cognitive tests. The study concluded that risperidone at these doses did not significantly alter cognition.

❱ Extrapyramidal Side Effects

The presence of EPS resulted in drug discontinuation in 2.1% of patients (Marder and Meibach 1994).

Early-onset EPS. Risperidone 6 mg/day produces fewer EPS than does haloperidol 10–20 mg/day (L. J. Cohen 1994). However, the incidence and severity of EPS increase proportionally with increasing dose. In one large multicenter study, risperidone 2 mg, 6 mg, and 10 mg/day resulted in EPS treatment (i.e., with anticholinergics) in 25%, 32%, and 46% of patients, respectively (Chouinard et al. 1993). In contrast, the EPS rates for haloperidol and placebo were 74% and 23%, respectively. The U.S. multicenter study (Marder et al. 1994) reported percentages similar to those of the Chouinard et al. study, except that the EPS rate was 38% with risperidone 16 mg/day, as compared with a rate of 46% with haloperidol 20 mg/day.

Tardive dyskinesia. Because risperidone is reported to produce fewer acute EPS than haloperidol, it is possible that it may also be less likely to produce tardive dyskinesia (L. J. Cohen 1994). However, long-term experience with risperidone is limited, and the risk of tardive dyskinesia is unknown at this time.

In several studies in patients with typical antipsychotic–induced tardive dyskinesia, dyskinesia rating scores were lower in patients on risperidone than in those on placebo. It is possible that risperidone, like typical antipsychotics, may temporarily suppress dyskinetic movements.

▶ **Headache**

In one study, headache occurred in 16% of patients receiving risperidone 6 mg/day (Marder and Meibach 1994). Treatment might include a simple analgesic (e.g., acetaminophen).

▶ **Insomnia**

Insomnia was reported in 54%–58% of patients receiving risperidone 2–16 mg/day, as compared with 36% of those receiving placebo (Chouinard et al. 1993). The mechanism of this effect is unknown, but the effect might be related to akathisia.

▶ **Sedation**

Sedation was reported in 9.4% of patients treated with risperidone 16 mg/day. The majority of the daily dose might be administered at bedtime to minimize this effect.

Respiratory

Rhinitis has been reported in approximately 8% and 10% of patients receiving risperidone dosages of 10 mg/day or greater and 16 mg/day, respectively (L. J. Cohen 1994). The mechanism of this effect is unknown.

Teratogenicity and Excretion Into Breast Milk

Risperidone is classified as a Pregnancy Category C drug, as there are no adequate controlled studies in pregnant women (Risperdal® Product Information 1993). One case of agenesis of the corpus callosum in an infant exposed to risperidone in utero has been reported; however, the causal relationship of risperidone to this defect is unknown. The drug's effect on labor and delivery is unknown. Risperidone's use during pregnancy is not recommended.

It is unknown whether risperidone or its metabolites appear in breast milk. For this reason, women taking risperidone should not breast-feed.

Urinary

In one case report, intranasal desmopressin 10 mg/day eliminated nightly enuresis after 4 consecutive days of treatment (J. A. Bennett et al. 1994). When desmopressin was discontinued, the enuresis returned within 2 days. Restarting desmopressin resulted in suppression of the enuresis. At a 3-month follow-up, the patient was still receiving risperidone and desmopressin and had had no recurrences.

■ Rational Prescribing

1. Because of the cost of and the limited U.S. postmarketing experience with risperidone, the drug is not considered a first-line antipsychotic in the treatment of schizophrenia.

2. In patients with refractory schizophrenia who have been unresponsive to two or more trials of typical antipsychotics, a risperidone trial might be considered before initiating clozapine treatment.
3. More double-blind trials are needed that compare risperidone's efficacy relative to those of clozapine, olanzapine, and sertindole in the treatment of refractory schizophrenia.
4. Risperidone might be tried in patients who do not tolerate typical antipsychotics because of EPS.
5. To minimize adverse effects, the initial target dose for risperidone is 6 mg/day and a therapeutic trial is 4 weeks. Doses greater than 6 mg/day might be attempted in nonresponding patients. The maximum recommended dose is 16 mg/day.
6. To avoid exacerbation of psychosis in responding or partially responding patients, it is suggested that typical antipsychotics or clozapine be tapered over at least 1 week while the risperidone dose is being titrated to the target dose. Clozapine should be abruptly discontinued if a hematological abnormality requires the drug's termination.

Sertindole

Sertindole is a new atypical antipsychotic that received FDA approval in October 1996. Very little information has been published on sertindole.

■ Indications

Sertindole is indicated for the treatment of schizophrenia.

■ Efficacy

Open studies. Three trials (M93-061, M92-795, and M94-239) in patients receiving sertindole dosages up to 24 mg/day or placebo demonstrated that sertindole was significantly more effective than placebo in the negative-symptom subscales of the PANSS and the SANS (Sertindole Investigator Consensus Meeting 1995).

Sertindole versus haloperidol and placebo. Two double-blind, placebo-controlled multicenter trials have been conducted with sertindole and haloperidol (Sertindole Investigator Consensus Meeting 1995). The first (M93-113) compared three dosages of sertindole (12, 20, and 24 mg) with three dosages of haloperidol (4, 8, and 16 mg) and placebo. Sertindole and haloperidol at all dosages were comparably effective on PANSS total, PANSS positive-symptom subscale, and BPRS total scores. Sertindole 20 mg/day was significantly more effective than placebo in producing improvement on the negative-symptom subscales of the PANSS and the SANS. The second trial (M93-098) compared two doses of sertindole, 20 and 24 mg/day, with haloperidol 16 mg/day and placebo. All dosages of sertindole and haloperidol were equally effective on the total PANSS, the positive-symptom subscale of the PANSS, and the total BPRS; however, only the 24-mg/day dose of sertindole was statistically significantly more effective than placebo on the PANSS.

■ Mechanism of Action

Sertindole has high affinity for $5-HT_2$ receptors, D_2 receptors, and α_1-adrenoceptors (Hyttel et al. 1992). Its affinity for D_2, α_2, H_1, and σ receptors is low, and it has no affinity for $5-HT_{1A}$, muscarinic, cholinergic, or β-adrenoceptors (Hyttel et al. 1992). Binding experiments indicate a limbic preference versus striatal D_2 receptors (Hyttel et al. 1992).

■ Dosage

It is recommended that sertindole treatment be initiated at 4 mg/day. Dosages can be increased by 4 mg every 2–3 days up to 20 mg/day. Some patients may require sertindole dosages of up to 24 mg/day (Sertindole Investigator Consensus Meeting 1995).

■ Pharmacokinetics

Sertindole is well absorbed; taking the drug with food has no effect on absorption (Sertindole Investigator Consensus Meeting 1995). The mean elimination half-life is 72 hours. Sertindole is 99.3% bound to plasma proteins. Its pharmacokinetics do not appear to be altered in elderly patients and those with renal impairment; at this time, no recommendations exist regarding the need for dosage adjustments. In patients with hepatic impairment, sertindole's clearance is reduced by 50%.

Sertindole is metabolized in the liver by cytochrome P450 (CYP) 3A and CYP2D6 isoenzymes (FDC Reports "pink sheet" July 1996). Potent CYP3A inhibitors such as fluoxetine and paroxetine reduce the clearance of sertindole by 50%, and inducers of CYP3A such as carbamazepine and phenytoin increase the drug's clearance by 100%–200% (FDC Reports "pink sheet" July 1996).

■ Adverse Effects

In the clinical trials described above, the most common side effects were nasal congestion (27%), decreased ejaculatory volume (13%), dizziness (12%), and dry mouth (10%) (FDC Reports "pink sheet" July 1996).

Extrapyramidal side effects. Extrapyramidal symptoms were seen in 15%–25% of both subjects treated with sertindole and those treated with placebo. In contrast, between 40% and 60% of patients treated with haloperidol experienced extrapyramidal symptoms (FDC Reports "pink sheet" July 1996).

QT prolongation/torsade de pointes. The FDA requested that sertindole's manufacturer assemble a panel of cardiologists to assess the drug's cardiovascular risks (FDC Reports "pink sheet" July 1996). Sertindole was reported to increase the QT interval by an average of 21 milliseconds (msec). Of the 1,446 patients in the phase II/III sertindole trials, 4% had QT intervals of more than 500 msec. However, it was noted that nearly 40% of patients in these trials had abnormal ECGs at baseline. The incidence of torsade de pointes from sertindole was calculated to be between 0.13% and 0.21% (95% confidence level). The expert panel concluded that the risk of torsade de pointes from sertindole was relatively low.

■ Rational Prescribing

1. Because of its relative newness and the limited postmarketing experience regarding its efficacy and safety, sertindole is not indicated as a first-line antipsychotic.
2. More experience is needed with sertindole in the maintenance treatment of schizophrenia.
3. Sertindole has not been studied in the treatment of refractory schizophrenia. The relative efficacies of clozapine, olanzapine, risperidone, and sertindole in this population have not been determined.
4. Patients with significant early-onset (i.e., akathisia, parkinsonism) and/or late-onset (e.g., tardive dyskinesia, tardive dystonia, tardive akathisia) extrapyramidal adverse effects who have not responded to risperidone should be given a trial of sertindole before either olanzapine or clozapine is considered.

Product List

Chlorpromazine (aliphatic phenothiazine)
- Relative oral potency: 100
- Oral daily dose range: 25–800 mg
- Oral/intramuscular ratio: 4:1
- Generic cost index: 0.05–0.19

Tablets:	**Thorazine**®
10 mg	[$39] SKFT73, brown
25 mg	[$53] SKFT74, brown
50 mg	[$66] SKFT76, brown
100 mg	[$85] SKFT77, brown
200 mg	[$108] SKFT79, brown

Capsules:	**Thorazine**®
30 mg	[$104] SKFT63, orange/clear
75 mg	[$140] SKFT64, orange/clear
150 mg	[$188] SKFT66, orange/clear

Concentrate:	**Thorazine**®
30 mg/mL	[$34/120 mL]
100 mg/mL	[$184/240 mL]

Syrup:	**Thorazine**®
10 mg/5 mL	[$23/120 mL]

Injection:	**Thorazine**®
25 mg/mL	[$8/1-mL ampule]
25 mg/mL	[$11/2-mL ampule]
25 mg/mL	[$50/10-mL vial]

Suppositories:	**Thorazine**®
25 mg	[$37/12]
100 mg	[$47/12]

Clozapine (dibenzodiazepine)
- Relative oral potency: 50
- Oral daily dose range: 150–900 mg/day

Tablets:[3]	**Clozaril**®
25 mg	[$132] Clozaril 25, yellow
100 mg	[$342] Clozaril 100, yellow

Fluphenazine (piperazine phenothiazine)
- Relative oral potency: 2
- Oral daily dose range: 2–60 mg
- Intramuscular daily dose range: 2.5–10 mg
- Generic cost index: ≈ 0.31

[3] Call 1-800-237-2767.

Tablets:	**Prolixin**®	**Permitil**®
1 mg	[$80] Squibb 863, pink	
2.5 mg	[$113] Squibb 864, yellow	[$104] Schering WDR 442, orange
5 mg	[$146] Squibb 887, green,	[$138] Schering WFF 550, purple-pink
10 mg	[$190] Squibb 956, coral,	[$164] Schering WFG 316, red

Concentrate:	**Prolixin**®	**Permitil**®
5 mg/mL	[$110/120 mL]	[$74/118 mL], 1% ethanol

Elixir:	**Prolixin**®
2.5 mg/mL	[$17/60 mL, $139/473 mL]

Injection:	**Prolixin**®
2.5 mg/mL	[$57/10 mL]

Fluphenazine decanoate (piperazine phenothiazine)
- Intramuscular dosage range: 12.5–100 mg

Injection:	**Prolixin decanoate**
25 mg/mL	[$100/5-mL vial]
25 mg/mL	[$22/1-mL unit dose syringe]

Fluphenazine enanthate (piperazine phenothiazine)
- Intramuscular dosage range: 12.5–100 mg

Injection:	**Prolixin enanthate**
25 mg/mL	[$106/5-mL vial]

Haloperidol (butyrophenone antipsychotic)
- Relative oral potency: 2
- Oral daily dose range: 1–100 mg
- Intramuscular daily dose range: 10–30 mg
- Oral/intramuscular ratio: 2:1
- Generic cost index: ≈ 0.02–0.04

Tablets:	**Haldol**®
0.5 mg	[$43] ½ Haldol/McNeil, white
1 mg	[$63] 1 Haldol/McNeil, yellow
2 mg	[$87] 2 Haldol/McNeil, pink
5 mg	[$143] 5 Haldol/McNeil, green
10 mg	[$183] 10 Haldol/McNeil, aqua
20 mg	[$352] 20 Haldol/McNeil, salmon

Concentrate:	**Haldol**®
2 mg/mL	[$24/15 mL, $97/120 mL], sugar free

Injection:	**Haldol**®
5 mg/mL	[$6/1-mL ampule]
5 mg/mL	[$61/10-mL vial]

Haloperidol decanoate (butyrophenone antipsychotic)
* Intramuscular dosage range: 25–300 mg

Injection:	**Haloperidol decanoate**
50 mg/mL	[$28/1-mL ampule]
100 mg/mL	[$51/1-mL ampule]
50 mg/mL	[$140/5-mL vial]
100 mg/mL	[$256/5-mL vial]

Loxapine (dibenzoxazepine antipsychotic)
* Relative oral potency: 10
* Oral daily dose range: 20–100 mg
* Generic cost index: ≈ 0.56

Capsules:	**Loxitane**®
5 mg	[$82] Lederle L1 5 mg, green
10 mg	[$105] Lederle L2 10 mg, green/yellow
25 mg	[$160] Lederle L3 25 mg, two-tone green
50 mg	[$212] Lederle L4 50 mg, green/blue

Concentrate:	**Loxitane C**®
25 mg/mL	[$235/120 mL]

Injection:	**Loxitane IM**®
50 mg/mL	[$96/10-mL vial]

Mesoridazine (piperidine phenothiazine; metabolite of thioridazine)
* Relative oral potency: 50
* Oral daily dose range: 25–400 mg
* Intramuscular daily dose range: 25–200 mg

Tablets:	**Serentil**®
10 mg	[$56] B10, orange
25 mg	[$75] B125, orange
50 mg	[$84] B150, orange
100 mg	[$103] B100, orange

Concentrate:	**Serentil**®
25 mg/mL	[$49/120 mL] sugar free, 0.61% ethanol

Injection:	**Serentil**®
25 mg/mL	[$4/1-mL ampule]

Molindone (dihydroindolone antipsychotic)
* Relative oral potency: 10
* Oral daily dosage range: 15–200 mg

Capsules:	**Moban**®
5 mg	[$59] Endo 0072, orange
10 mg	[$84] Endo 0073, lavender
25 mg	[$126] Endo 0074, green
50 mg	[$168] Endo 076, blue
100 mg	[$225] Endo 077, tan
Concentrate:	**Moban**®
20 mg/mL	[$119/120 mL], cherry

Olanzapine (thienobenzodiazepine)

- Relative oral potency: 0.5
- Oral daily dose range: 5–15 mg

Tablets:	**Zyprexa**®
5 mg	[$524] Lilly 4115, white
7.5 mg	[$524] Lilly 4116, white
10 mg	[$774] Lilly 4117, white

Perphenazine (piperazine phenothiazine)

- Relative oral potency: 8
- Oral daily dose range: 8–64 mg
- Intramuscular daily dose range: 5–30 mg
- Generic cost index: ≈ 0.49–0.60

Tablets:	**Trilafon**®
2 mg	[$64] Schering ADH or 705, gray
4 mg	[$87] Schering ADK or 940, gray
8 mg	[$106] Schering ADJ or 313, gray
16 mg	[$143] Schering ADM or 077, gray
Concentrate:	**Trilafon**®
16 mg/5 mL	[$36/120 mL], < 0.1% ethanol
Injection:	**Trilafon**®
5 mg/mL	[$5/1-mL ampule]

Prochlorperazine (piperazine phenothiazine)

- Relative oral potency: 15
- Oral daily dose range: 40–150 mg
- Intramuscular daily dose range: 10–80 mg
- Generic cost index: ≈0.19

Tablets:	**Compazine**®
5 mg	[$63] SKFC66, yellow
10 mg	[$93] SKFC67, yellow
Spansules:	**Compazine**®
10 mg	[$110] SKFC44, black/clear
15 mg	[$164] SKFC46, black/clear
Syrup:	**Compazine**®
5 mg/5 mL	[$20/120 mL]

Injection:	**Compazine**®
5 mg/mL	[$7/2 mL ampule]
5 mg/mL	[$14/2-mL vial]
5 mg/mL	[$36/10-mL vial]

Suppositories:	**Compazine**®
2.5 mg	[$26/12]
5 mg	[$29/12]
25 mg	[$36/12]

Risperidone (benzisoxazole)

- Relative oral potency: 1
- Oral daily dose range: 4–16 mg/day

Tablets:	**Risperdal**®
1 mg	[$190] Janssen R 1, white
2 mg	[$316] Janssen R 2, orange
3 mg	[$395] Janssen R 3, yellow
4 mg	[$526] Janssen R 4, green

Sertindole (phenolindole)

(Product information not available at time of publication.)

Thioridazine (piperidine phenothiazine)

- Relative oral potency: 100
- Oral daily dose range: 50–800 mg
- Oral/intramuscular ratio: 3:1
- Generic cost index: ≈ 0.09–0.19

Tablets:	**Mellaril**®
10 mg	[$30] 78-2, chartreuse
15 mg	[$35] 78-8, pink
25 mg	[$42] Mel 25, tan
50 mg	[$51] Mel 50, white
100 mg	[$62] Mel 100, green
150 mg	[$78] Mel 150, yellow
200 mg	[$89] Mel 200, pink

Concentrate:	**Mellaril**®
30 mg/mL	[$32/120 mL], sugar free, 3% ethanol
100 mg/mL	[$84/120 mL], 4.2% ethanol

Suspension:	**Mellaril-S**®
25 mg/5 mL	[$50/480 mL], buttermint
100 mg/5 mL	[$104/480 mL], buttermint

Thiothixene (piperazine thioxanthene)

- Relative oral potency: 3
- Oral daily dose range: 5–120 mg
- Intramuscular daily dose range: 8–30 mg

- Oral/intramuscular ratio: not available
- Generic cost index: ≈ 0.24

Capsules:	**Navane**®
1 mg	[$39] 571, orange/yellow
2 mg	[$53] 572, yellow/green
5 mg	[$83] 573, orange/white
10 mg	[$114] 574, blue/white
20 mg	[$160] 577, green/blue

Concentrate:	**Navane**®
5 mg/mL	[$85/120 mL], 7% ethanol

Powder for injection:	**Navane**®
5 mg/mL	[$36]

Trifluoperazine (piperazine phenothiazine)
- Relative oral potency: 4
- Oral daily dose range: 4–60 mg
- Intramuscular daily dose range: 2–10 mg
- Generic cost index: ≈ 0.32–0.41

Tablets:	**Stelazine**®
1 mg	[$64] SKFS03, blue
2 mg	[$94] SKFS04, blue
5 mg	[$119] SKFS06, blue
10 mg	[$179] SKFS07, blue

Concentrate:	**Stelazine**®
10 mg/mL	[$113/60 mL]

Injection:	**Stelazine**®
2 mg/mL	[$52/10-mL vial]

Triflupromazine (aliphatic phenothiazine)
- Intramuscular daily dose range: 30–150 mg

Injection:	**Vesprin**®
20 mg/mL	[$12/1-mL vial]
10 mg/mL	[$46/10-mL vial]

References

Adams F: Emergency intravenous sedation of the delirious, medically ill patient. J Clin Psychiatry 49 (suppl):22–26, 1988

Adams F, Fernandez F, Andersson BS: Emergency pharmacotherapy of delirium in the critically ill cancer patient. Psychosomatics 27 (suppl 1):33–37, 1986

Addington DE, Jones B, Bloom D, et al: Reduction of hospital days in chronic schizophrenic patients treated with risperidone: a retrospective study. Clin Ther 5:917–926, 1993

Addonizio G, Susman VL, Roth SD: Neuroleptic malignant syndrome: review and analysis of 115 cases. Biol Psychiatry 22:1004–1020, 1987

Addonizio G, Alexopoulos GS: Drug-induced dystonia in young and elderly patients. Am J Psychiatry 145:869–871, 1988

Addonizio G, Roth SD, Stokes PE: Increased extrapyramidal symptoms with addition of lithium to neuroleptics. J Nerv Ment Dis 176:682–685, 1988

Adler LA, Peselow E, Rotrsen J, et al: Vitamin E treatment of tardive dyskinesia. Am J Psychiatry 150:1405–1407, 1993

Alphs LD, Lee HS: Comparison of withdrawal of typical and atypical antipsychotic drugs: a case study. J Clin Psychiatry 52:346–348, 1991

Alvir JMA, Lieberman JA: Agranulocytosis: incidence and risk factors. J Clin Psychiatry 55 (suppl B):137–138, 1994a

Alvir JMA, Lieberman JA: A reevaluation of the clinical characteristics of clozapine-induced granulocytosis in light of the United States experience. J Clin Psychiatry 55 (suppl B):87–89, 1994b

Ambrosini PJ, Nurnberg HG: Enuresis and incontinence occurring with neuroleptics (letter). Am J Psychiatry 137:1278–1279, 1980

American Psychiatric Association: Diagnostic and Statistical Manual of Mental Disorders, 3rd Edition, Revised. Washington, DC, American Psychiatric Association, 1987

Anderson ES, Powers PS: Neuroleptic malignant syndrome associated with clozapine use. J Clin Psychiatry 52:102–104, 1991

Applebaum PS: Must chronic schizophrenic patients who have been stabilized on antipsychotic medication be told of the risk of tardive dyskinesia? J Clin Psychopharmacol 5:364–365, 1985

Aronowitz JS, Safferman AZ, Lieberman JA: Management of clozapine-induced enuresis (letter). Am J Psychiatry 152:472, 1995

Aubree JC, Lader MH: High and very high dosage antipsychotics: a critical review. J Clin Psychiatry 41:341–350, 1980

Awad AG: Drug therapy in schizophrenia—variability of outcome and prediction of response. Can J Psychiatry 34:711–720, 1989

Ayd FJ: A survey of drug-induced extrapyramidal reactions. JAMA 175:1054–1060, 1961

Ayd FJ: Clozapine: a unique new neuroleptic. International Drug Therapy Newsletter 9:5–12, 1974

Baker RW, Chengappa KNR, Baird JW, et al: Emergence of obsessive compulsive symptoms during treatment with clozapine. J Clin Psychiatry 53:439–442, 1992

Balant-Gorgia AE, Balant LP, Andreoli A: Pharmacokinetic optimization of the treatment of psychosis. Clin Pharmacokinet 25:217–236, 1993

Baldessarini RJ, Cohen BM, Teicher MH: Significance of neuroleptic dose and plasma level in the pharmacological treatment of psychoses. Arch Gen Psychiatry 45:79–91, 1988

Baldessarini RJ, Gardner DM, Garver DL: Conversion from clozapine to other antipsychotics (letter). Arch Gen Psychiatry 52:1071–1072, 1995

Bamrah JS: Neuroleptic-induced pyrexia: a benign variant. J Nerv Ment Dis 176:741–743, 1988

Banov MD, Zarate CA, Tohen M, et al: Clozapine therapy in refractory affective disorders: polarity predicts response in long-term follow-up. J Clin Psychiatry 55:295–300, 1994

Barnas C, Zwierzina H, Mummer M, et al: Granulocyte-macrophage colony-stimulating factor (GM-CSF) treatment of clozapine-induced agranulocytosis: a case report. J Clin Psychiatry 53:245–247, 1992

Beasley CM, Sanger T, Satterlee W, et al: Olanzapine versus placebo: results of a double-blind, fixed-dose olanzapine trial. Psychopharmacology 124:159–167, 1996a

Beasley CM, Tollefson G, Tran P, et al: Olanzapine versus placebo and haloperidol: acute phase results of the North American double-blind olanzapine trial. Neuropsychopharmacology 14:111–123, 1996b

Beaumont PJV, Corker CS, Friesen HG, et al: The effects of phenothiazines on endocrine function, II: effects in men and postmenopausal women. Br J Psychiatry 124:420–430, 1974

Belanger MC, Chouinard G: Technique for injecting long-acting neuroleptics (letter). Br J Psychiatry 141:316, 1982

Bennett JA, Keck PE, Wallhausser LJ: Desmopressin for risperidone-induced enuresis. Ann Clin Psychiatry 6:139–140, 1994

Bennett JP, Landow ER, Schuh LA: Suppression of dyskinesias in advanced Parkinson's disease. Neurology 43:1551–1555, 1993

Beresford R, Ward A: Haloperidol decanoate: a preliminary review of its pharmacodynamic and pharmacokinetic properties and therapeutic use in psychosis. Drugs 33:31–49, 1987

Bergen JA, Eyland EA, Campbell JA, et al: The course of tardive dyskinesia in patients on long-term neuroleptics. Br J Psychiatry 154:523–528, 1989

Berman I, Merson A, Allan E, et al: Effect of risperidone on cognitive performance in elderly schizophrenic patients: a double-blind comparison study with haloperidol (abstract). Psychopharmacol Bull 31:552, 1995

Bersani G, Bressa GM, Meco G, et al: Combined serotonin–5-HT2 and dopamine-D2 antagonism in schizophrenia: clinical, extrapyramidal and neuroendocrine response in a preliminary study with risperidone (R 64 766). Human Psychopharmacology 5:225–231, 1990

Black JL, Richelson E, Richardson JW: Antipsychotic agents: a clinical update. Mayo Clin Proc 60:777–789, 1985

Borison RL: Pharmacology of antipsychotic drugs. J Clin Psychiatry 46:25–28, 1985

Bourgeois JA, Drexler KG, Hall MJ: Hypersalivation and clozapine (letter). Hospital and Community Psychiatry 42:1174, 1991

Breier A: Clozapine and noradrenergic function: support for a novel hypothesis for superior efficacy. J Clin Psychiatry 55 (suppl B):122–125, 1994

Breier A: Switching between clozapine and other antipsychotics. J Clin Psychiatry 14:18–19, 1996

Breier A, Wolkowitz OM, Doran AR, et al: Neuroleptic responsivity of negative and positive symptoms in schizophrenia. Am J Psychiatry 144:1549–1555, 1987

Breier A, Buchanan RW, Kirkpatrick B, et al: Effects of clozapine on positive and negative symptoms in outpatients with schizophrenia. Am J Psychiatry 151:20–26, 1994

Brinkley JR: Pharmacotherapy of borderline states. Psychiatr Clin North Am 16:853–884, 1993

Brotman AW, McCormick S III: A role for high-dose antipsychotics. J Clin Psychiatry 51:164–166, 1990

Bublenis E, Weber SS, Wagner RL: Clozapine: a novel antipsychotic. Drug Intelligence and Clinical Pharmacy 23:109–115, 1989

Buckley P, Thompson P, Way L: Substance abuse among patients with treatment-resistant schizophrenia: characteristics and implications for clozapine therapy. Am J Psychiatry 151:385–389, 1994

Burnakis TG: Angiotensin-converting enzyme inhibitors and excessive water consumption. Hospital Pharmacy 27:1097–1098, 1992

Busch FN, Miller FT, Weiden PJ: A comparison of two adjunctive treatment strategies in acute mania. J Clin Psychiatry 50:453–455, 1989

Byerly MJ, DeVane CL: Pharmacokinetics of clozapine and risperidone: a review of recent literature. J Clin Psychopharmacol 16:177–187, 1996

Caine ED, Polinsky RJ, Kartzinel R, et al: The trial use of clozapine for abnormal involuntary movement disorders. Am J Psychiatry 136:317–320, 1979

Calabrese JR, Gulledge AD: Psychotropics during pregnancy and lactation: a review. Psychosomatics 26:413–426, 1985

Cardoni AA: Risperidone: review and assessment of its role in the treatment of schizophrenia. Ann Pharmacother 29:610–618, 1995

Caroff SN, Mann SC: Neuroleptic malignant syndrome. Med Clin North Am 77:185–202, 1993

Carpenter WT: Maintenance therapy of persons with schizophrenia. J Clin Psychiatry 57 (suppl 9):10–18, 1996

Carpenter WT, Heinrichs DW, Hanlan TE: A comparative trial of pharmacologic strategies in schizophrenia. Am J Psychiatry 144:1466–1470, 1987

Carter CS, Mulsant BH, Sweet RA, et al: Risperidone use in a teaching hospital during its first year after market approval: economic and clinical implications. Psychopharmacol Bull 31:719–725, 1995

Casey DA: Electroconvulsive therapy in neuroleptic malignant syndrome. Convuls Ther 3:278–283, 1987

Casey DE: Neuroleptic-induced acute extrapyramidal syndromes and tardive dyskinesia. Psychiatr Clin North Am 16:589–610, 1993

Casey DE: Motor and mental aspects of acute extrapyramidal syndromes. Acta Psychiatr Scand 89 (suppl 380):14–20, 1994

Casey DE, Povlsen UJ, Meidahl B, et al: Neuroleptic-induced tardive dyskinesia and parkinsonism: changes during several years of continuing treatment. Psychopharmacol Bull 22:250–253, 1986

Cates M, Lusk K, Wells BG, et al: Nonleukopenic neutropenia in a patient treated with clozapine (letter). N Engl J Med 326:840–841, 1992

Chacko RC, Hurley RA, Haper RG, et al: Clozapine for acute and maintenance treatment of psychosis in Parkinson's disease. J Neuropsychiatry 7:471–475, 1995

Chan J, Alldredge BK, Baskin LS: Perphenazine-induced priapism. DICP Ann Pharmacother 24:246–249, 1990

Chengappa KNR, Shelton MD, Baker RW, et al: The prevalence of akathisia in patients receiving stable doses of clozapine. J Clin Psychiatry 44:142–145, 1994

Chengappa KNR, Baker RW, Schooler NR, et al: Clozapine associated agranulocytosis: treatment with G-CSF (abstract). Psychopharmacol Bull 31:556, 1995

Chou JC: Recent advances in treatment of acute mania. J Clin Psychopharmacol 11:3–21, 1991

Chouinard G, Annable L, Mercier P, et al: A five-year follow-up study of tardive dyskinesia. Psychopharmacol Bull 22:259–263, 1986

Chouinard G, Annable L, Campbell W: A randomized clinical trial of haloperidol decanoate and fluphenazine decanoate in the outpatient treatment of schizophrenia. J Clin Psychopharmacol 9:247–253, 1989

Chouinard G, Jones B, Remington G, et al: A Canadian multicenter placebo-controlled study of fixed doses of risperidone and haloperidol in the treatment of chronic schizophrenic patients. J Clin Psychopharmacol 13:25–40, 1993

Christison GW, Kirch DG, Wyatt RJ: When symptoms persist: choosing among alternative somatic treatments for schizophrenia. Schizophr Bull 17:217–245, 1991

Clozaril® [clozapine] Product Information. East Hanover, NJ, Sandoz Pharmaceutical Corporation, 1994

Cobb CD, Anderson CB, Seidel DR: Possible interaction between clozapine and lorazepam (letter). Am J Psychiatry 148:1606–1607, 1991

Cohen BM, Keck PE, Satlin A, et al: Prevalence and severity of akathisia in patients on clozapine. Biol Psychiatry 29:1215–1219, 1991

Cohen LJ: Risperidone. Pharmacotherapy 14:253–265, 1994

Cohen LS: Psychotropic drug use in pregnancy. Hospital and Community Psychiatry 40:566–567, 1989

Cohen S, Chiles J, MacNaughton A: Weight gain associated with clozapine. Am J Psychiatry 147:503–504, 1990

Cohen SA: Successful clozapine rechallenge following prior intolerance to clozapine (letter). J Clin Psychiatry 55:498–499, 1994

Copp PJ, Lament R, Tennent TG: Amitriptyline in clozapine-induced sialorrhoea (letter). Br J Psychiatry 159:166, 1991

Cornelius JR, Soloff PH, Perel JM, et al: Continuation pharmacotherapy of borderline personality disorder with haloperidol and phenelzine. Am J Psychiatry 150:1843–1848, 1993a

Cornelius JR, Soloff PH, George A, et al: Haloperidol vs. phenelzine in continuation therapy of borderline disorder. Psychopharmacol Bull 29:333–337, 1993b

Coryell WH, Kelly MW, Perry PJ, et al: Haloperidol plasma levels and acute clinical change in schizophrenia. J Clin Psychopharmacol 10:397–402, 1990

Cowdry RW, Gardner DL: Pharmacotherapy of borderline personality disorder: alprazolam, carbamazepine, trifluoperazine, and tranylcypromine. Arch Gen Psychiatry 45:111–119, 1988

Curry SH, Whelpton R, de Schepper PJ, et al: Kinetics of fluphenazine after fluphenazine dihydrochloride, enanthate and decanoate administration to man. Br J Clin Pharmacol 7:325–331, 1979

Dabiri LM, Pasta D, Karby JK, et al: Effectiveness of vitamin E for treatment of long-term tardive dyskinesia. Am J Psychiatry 151:925–926, 1994

Dahl SG: Active metabolites of neuroleptic drugs: possible contribution to therapeutic and toxic effects. Ther Drug Monit 4:33–40, 1982

Dahl SG: Plasma level monitoring of antipsychotic drugs: clinical utility. Clin Pharmacokinet 11:36–61, 1986

Daniel DG, Kinon BJ, Litman RE, et al: A. Algorithms for the treatment of schizophrenia. Psychopharmacol Bull 31:461–467, 1995

DasGupta K, Young A: Clozapine-induced neuroleptic malignant syndrome. J Clin Psychiatry 52:105–107, 1991

Dave M: Tardive oculogyric crises with clozapine (letter). J Clin Psychiatry 55:264–265, 1994

Davies MA, Conley RR, Schulz SC, et al: One-year follow-up of 24 patients in a clinical trial of clozapine. Hospital and Community Psychiatry 42:628–629, 1991

Davis JM, Casper R: Antipsychotic drugs: clinical pharmacology and therapeutic use. Drugs 14:260–282, 1977

Davis JM, Schyve PM, Pavkovic I: Clinical and legal issues in neuroleptic use. Clin Neuropharmacol 6:117–128, 1983

Davis JM, Kane JM, Marder SR, et al: dose response of prophylactic antipsychotics. J Clin Psychiatry 54 (suppl):24–30, 1993

De Cuyper H, Bollen J, van Praag HM, et al: Pharmacokinetics and therapeutic efficacy of haloperidol decanoate after loading dose administration. Br J Psychiatry 148:560–566, 1986

de Leon J, Moral L, Camunas C: Clozapine and jaw dyskinesia: a case report. Am J Psychiatry 52:494–495, 1991

de Leon J, Stanilla JK, White AO, et al: Anticholinergics to treat clozapine withdrawal (letter). J Clin Psychiatry 55:119–120, 1994

Decina P, Caracci G, Sandik R, et al: Cigarette smoking and neuroleptic-induced parkinsonism. Biol Psychiatry 28:502–508, 1990

Degivity R: Extrapyramidal motor disorders following long-term treatment with neuroleptic drugs, in Psychotropic Drugs and Dysfunctions of the Basal Ganglion (Public Health Service Publ No 1938). Edited by Grave GE, Gardner R. Bethesda, MD, National Institute of Mental Health, 1969, pp 22–32

Del Giudice J, Clark WG, Gocka EF: Prevention of recidivism of schizophrenics treated with fluphenazine enanthate. Psychosomatics 16:32–36, 1975

Delva NJ, Letemendia FJJ: Lithium treatment in schizophrenia and schizoaffective disorders. Br J Psychiatry 141:387–400, 1982

Devinsky O, Honigfeld G, Patin J: Clozapine-related seizures. Neurology 41:369–371, 1991

Devinsky O, Pacia SV: Seizures during clozapine therapy. J Clin Psychiatry 55 (suppl B):153–156, 1994

Dilsaver SC: Withdrawal phenomena associated with antidepressant and antipsychotic agents. Drug Saf 10:103–114, 1994

Donlon PT, Stenson RL: Neuroleptic-induced extrapyramidal symptoms. Diseases of the Nervous System 37:629–635, 1976

Druckenbrod RW, Rosen J, Cluxton RJ: As-needed dosing of antipsychotic drugs: limitations and guidelines for use in the elderly agitated patient. Ann Pharmacother 27:645–648, 1993

Dysken MW, Javaid JL, Chang SS: Fluphenazine pharmacokinetics and therapeutic response. Psychopharmacology 73:205–210, 1981

Eiser AR, Neff MS, Slifkin RF: Acute myoglobinuric renal failure. Arch Intern Med 142:601–603, 1982

Ereshefsky L, Saklad SR, Jann MW, et al: Future of depot neuroleptic therapy: pharmacokinetic and pharmacodynamic approaches. J Clin Psychiatry 45:50–59, 1984

Ereshefsky L, Watanabe MD, Tran-Johnson TK: Clozapine: an atypical antipsychotic agent. Clinical Pharmacy 8:691–709, 1989

Ereshefsky L, Toney G, Saklad SR, et al: A loading-dose strategy for converting from oral to depot haloperidol. Hospital and Community Psychiatry 44:1155–1161, 1993

Farde L, Nordstrom AL, Wiesel FA, et al: Positron emission tomographic analysis of central D_1 and D_2 receptor occupancy in patients treated with classical neuroleptics and clozapine. Arch Gen Psychiatry 49:538–544, 1992

FDC Reports "pink sheet": Serlect U.K. cohort could be analyzed for QT prolongation/torsades—FDA's Leber: extrapyramidal symptoms for Abbott drug equal placebo, less than haloperidol. July 22, 1996, pp 5–7

Feltner DE, Hertzman M: Progress in the treatment of tardive dyskinesia: theory and practice. Hospital and Community Psychiatry 44:25–34, 1993

Fernandez F, Levy JK, Mansell PWA: Management of delirium in terminally ill AIDS patients. Int J Psychiatry Med 19:165–172, 1989

Fleischhacker WW, Hummer M, Kurz M, et al: Clozapine dose in the United States and Europe: implications for therapeutic and adverse effects. J Clin Psychiatry 55 (suppl B):78–81, 1994

Ford B, Lynch T, Greene P: Risperidone in Parkinson's disease (letter). Lancet 344:681, 1994

Fornazzari X, Grossman H, Thornton J, et al: Tardive dyskinesia: a five-year follow-up. Can J Psychiatry 34:700–703, 1989

Frankenburg FR, Kando J: Eosinophilia, clozapine, and pancreatitis (letter). Lancet 340:251, 1992

Frankenburg FR, Zanarini MC: Clozapine treatment of borderline patients: a preliminary study. Compr Psychiatry 34:402–405, 1993

Frankenburg FR, Kando JC, Centorrino F, et al: Bladder dysfunction associated with clozapine therapy (letter). J Clin Psychiatry 57:39–40, 1996

Fuller MA, Borovicka M, Jaskiw GE, et al: Treatment of clozapine-induced urinary incontinence with ephedrine (abstract). Psychopharmacol Bull 31:570, 1995

Gallant DM, Edwards CG, Bishop MP, et al: Withdrawal symptoms after abrupt cessation of antipsychotic compounds: clinical confirmation in chronic schizophrenics. Am J Psychiatry 121:491–493, 1964

Ganzini L, Heintz R, Hoffman WF, et al: Acute extrapyramidal syndromes in neuroleptic-treated elders: a pilot study. J Geriatr Psychiatry Neurol 4:222–225, 1991

Garattini S, Morselli PL: Metabolism and pharmacokinetics of psychotropic drugs, in Principles of Psychopharmacology, 2nd Edition. Edited by Clark WG, del Giudice J. New York, Academic Press, 1978, pp 169–182, 768

Gardos G, Perenyi A, Cole JO, et al: Tardive dyskinesia: changes after three years. J Clin Psychopharmacol 3:315–318, 1983

Gardos G, Casey DE, Cole JO, et al: Ten-year outcome of tardive dyskinesia. Am J Psychiatry 151:836–841, 1994

Garver DL: Neuroleptic drug levels and antipsychotic effects: a difficult correlation; potential advantage of free (or derivative) versus total plasma levels. J Clin Psychopharmacol 9:277–281, 1989

Geibig CB, Marks LW: Treatment of clozapine- and molindone-induced agranulocytosis with granulocyte colony-stimulating factor. Ann Pharmacother 27:1190–1192, 1993

Gelenberg AJ: Lorazepam (Ativan): antipsychotic adjunct? Biological Therapies in Psychiatry 9:37–40, 1986

Gelenberg AJ: Treating extrapyramidal reactions: some current issues. J Clin Psychiatry 48 (suppl):24–27, 1987

Gelenberg AJ: Intravenous haloperidol: uses and cautions. Biological Therapies in Psychiatry 11:45–46, 1988

Gelenberg AJ: Clozapine mortality (abstract). Biological Therapies in Psychiatry 15:25, 1992

Gelenberg AJ, Hopkins HS: Antipsychotics in bipolar disorder. J Clin Psychiatry 57 (suppl 9):49–52, 1996

Gerlach J, Casey DE: Tardive dyskinesia. Acta Psychiatr Scand 77:369–378, 1988

Gerson SL, Lieberman JA, Friedenberg WR, et al: Polypharmacy in fatal clozapine-associated agranulocytosis (letter). Lancet 338:262–263, 1991

Gerson SL, Gullion G, Yeh H, et al: Granulocyte colony-stimulating factor for clozapine-induced agranulocytosis (letter). Lancet 340:1097, 1992

Gerson SL: G-CSF and the management of clozapine-induced agranulocytosis. J Clin Psychiatry 55 (suppl B):139–142, 1994

Gitlin MJ, Midha KK, Fogeson D, et al: Persistence of fluphenazine in plasma after decanoate withdrawal. J Clin Psychopharmacol 8:53–56, 1988

Glazer WM, Maynard C, Berkman CS: Injection site leakage of depot neuroleptics: intramuscular versus subcutaneous injection. J Clin Psychiatry 48:237–239, 1987

Goates MG, Escobar JI: An apparent neuroleptic malignant syndrome without extrapyramidal symptoms upon initiation of clozapine therapy: report of a case and results of a clozapine rechallenge (letter). J Clin Psychopharmacol 12:139–140, 1992

Godleski LS, Vieweg WVR, Leadbetter RA, et al: Day-to-day care of chronic schizophrenic patients subject to water intoxication. Ann Clin Psychiatry 1:179–185, 1989

Goldberg PE, Weinberger DR: Effect of neuroleptic medication on cognition of patients with schizophrenia: a review of recent studies. J Clin Psychiatry 57 (suppl 9):62–65, 1996

Goldberg SC, Schulz C, Schulz PM, et al: Borderline and schizotypal personality disorders treated with low-dose thiothixene vs placebo. Arch Gen Psychiatry 43:680–686, 1986

Goldstein JA: Captopril in the treatment of psychogenic polydipsia (letter). J Clin Psychiatry 47:99, 1986

Goodwin FK, Zis AP: Lithium in the treatment of mania: comparison with neuroleptics. Arch Gen Psychiatry 36:840–844, 1979

Gould RJ, Murphy KMM, Reynolds IJ, et al: Calcium channel blockade: possible explanation for thioridazine's peripheral side effects. Am J Psychiatry 141:352–357, 1984

Grabowski J: Clonidine treatment of clozapine-induced hypersalivation (letter). J Clin Psychopharmacol 12:69–70, 1992

Green AI: Response to clozapine: outcomes. J Clin Psychiatry 14:20–21, 1996a

Green AI: Predictors of response to clozapine. J Clin Psychiatry 14:25–26, 1996b

Groves JE, Mandel MR: The long-acting phenothiazines. Arch Gen Psychiatry 32:893–900, 1975

Guerrero RM, Shifrar KA: Diagnosis and treatment of neuroleptic malignant syndrome. Clinical Pharmacy 7:697–701, 1988

Gullion G, Yeh HS: Treatment of clozapine-induced agranulocytosis with recombinant granulocyte colony-stimulating factor. J Clin Psychiatry 44:401–405, 1994

Hamburg P, Weilburg JB, Cassem NH, et al: Relapse of neuroleptic malignant syndrome with early discontinuation of amantadine therapy. Compr Psychiatry 27:272–275, 1986

Hargreaves WA, Shumway M: Pharmacoeconomics of antipsychotic drug therapy. J Clin Psychiatry 57 (suppl 9):66–76, 1996

Haring C, Meise U, Humpel C, et al: Dose-related plasma levels of clozapine: influence of smoking behavior, sex and age. Psychopharmacology 99:W38–W40, 1989

Hasegawa M, Gutierrez-Esteinou R, Way L, et al: Relationship between clinical efficacy and clozapine concentrations in plasma in schizophrenia: effect of smoking. J Clin Psychopharmacol 13:383–390, 1993

Hegarty JD, Baldessarini RJ, Tohen M, et al: One hundred years of schizophrenia: a meta-analysis of the outcome literature. Am J Psychiatry 151:1409–1416, 1994

Heinrich K, Klieser E, Lehmann E, et al: Experimental comparison of the efficacy and compatibility of risperidone and clozapine in acute schizophrenia, in Risperidone: Major Progress in Antipsychotic Treatment (Satellite Symposium at the 17th Congress of Collegium Internationale Neuro-Pharmacologicum). Edited by Kane JM. Oxford, UK, Oxford Clinical Communications, 1990, pp 37–39

Henderson DC, Goff DC: Risperidone as an adjunct to clozapine therapy in chronic schizophrenics. J Clin Psychiatry 57:395–297, 1996

Henderson VW, Wooten GF: Neuroleptic malignant syndrome: a pathogenetic role for dopamine receptor blockade? Neurology 31:132–137, 1981

Herz MI: Intermittent medication and schizophrenia, in Drug Maintenance Strategies in Schizophrenia. Edited by Kane JM. Washington, DC, American Psychiatric Press, 1984, pp 51–68

Hollister LE, Kanter SL, Wright A: Comparison of intramuscular and oral administration of chlorpromazine and thioridazine. Arch Int Pharmacodyn Ther 144:571–578, 1963

Honigfeld G: The clozapine national registry system: forty years of risk management. J Clin Psychiatry 14:29–32, 1996

Honigfeld G, Patin J: Predictors of response to clozapine therapy. Psychopharmacology 99:S64–S67, 1989

Hughes JR: ECT during and after the neuroleptic malignant syndrome: case report. J Clin Psychiatry 47:42–43, 1986

Huyse F, Van Schijndel RS: Haloperidol and cardiac arrest (letter). Lancet 2:568–569, 1988

Hyttel J, Arnt J, Costall B, et al: Pharmacological profile of the atypical neuroleptic sertindole. Clin Neuropharmacol 15 (suppl 1):267A–268A, 1992

Inoue H, Hazama H, Ogura C, et al: Neuroendocrinological study of amenorrhea induced by antipsychotic drugs (abstract). Folia Psychiatrica et Neurologica Japonica 34:181, 1980

Janicak PG, Javaid JI, Sharma RP, et al: Trifluoperazine plasma levels and clinical response. J Clin Psychopharmacol 9:340–346, 1989

Jann MW, Grimsley SR, Gray EC, et al: Pharmacokinetics and pharmaco-
    dynamics of clozapine. Clin Pharmacokinet 24:161–176, 1993
Jessee SS, Anderson GF: ECT in the neuroleptic malignant syndrome: case
    report. J Clin Psychiatry 44:186–188, 1983
Jeste DV, Caligiuri MP: Tardive dyskinesia. Schizophr Bull 19:303–315,
    1993
Jeste DV, Potkin SG, Sinka S, et al: Tardive dyskinesia-reversible and
    persistent. Arch Gen Psychiatry 36:585–590, 1979
Johnson DAW: Observations on the dose regime of fluphenazine decanoate
    in maintenance treatment of schizophrenia. Br J Psychiatry 126:457–
    461, 1975
Johnson DAW: Observations of the use of long-acting depot neuroleptic
    injections in the maintenance therapy of schizophrenia. J Clin Psychia-
    try 45 (5, sec 2):13–21, 1984
Johnson DAW: Antipsychotic medication: clinical guidelines for mainte-
    nance therapy. J Clin Psychiatry 46 (suppl):6–15, 1985
Jolly AG, Hirsch SR, McRink A, et al: Trial of brief intermittent neuroleptic
    prophylaxis for selected schizophrenic outpatients: clinical outcome at
    one year. BMJ 298:985–991, 1989
Joseph G, Nguyen V, Smith JD: HLA-B38 and clozapine-induced agranu-
    locytosis (letter). Ann Intern Med 116:605, 1992
Jubert P: Clozapine-related pancreatitis (letter). Ann Intern Med 121:722–
    723, 1994
Juul Povlsen U, Noring U, Fog R, et al: Tolerability and therapeutic effect
    of clozapine: a retrospective investigation of 216 patients treated with
    clozapine for up to 12 years. Acta Psychiatr Scand 71:176–185, 1985
Kahne GJ: Rebound psychoses following the discontinuation of a high
    potency antipsychotic. Can J Psychiatry 34:227–229, 1989
Kane JM: Dosage strategies with long-acting injectable neuroleptics includ-
    ing haloperidol decanoate. J Clin Psychopharmacol 6 (suppl):20–23,
    1986
Kane JM: The role of neuroleptics in manic-depressive illness. J Clin Psy-
    chiatry 49 (suppl):12–13, 1988
Kane JM: The current status of neuroleptic therapy. J Clin Psychiatry
    50:322–328, 1989
Kane JM: Depot neuroleptic therapy. Today's Therapeutic Trends 11:93–
    102, 1993
Kane JM: Treatment-resistant schizophrenic patients. J Clin Psychiatry 57
    (suppl 9):35–40, 1996
Kane JM, Marder SR: Psychopharmacologic treatment of schizophrenia.
    Schizophr Bull 19:287–302, 1993
Kane JM, McGlashan TH: Treatment of schizophrenia. Lancet 346:820–
    825, 1995
Kane JM, Woerner M, Borenstein M, et al: Integrating incidence and
    prevalence of tardive dyskinesia. Psychopharmacol Bull 22:254–258,
    1986
Kane JM, Honigfeld G, Singer J, et al: Clozapine for the treatment-resistant
    schizophrenic: a double-blind comparison with chlorpromazine. Arch
    Gen Psychiatry 45:789–796, 1988
Kane JM, Woerner MG, Pollack S, et al: Does clozapine cause tardive
    dyskinesia? J Clin Psychiatry 54:327–330, 1993

Kay SR, Singh MM: The positive-negative distinction in drug-free schizophrenic symptoms. Arch Gen Psychiatry 46:711–718, 1989

Keck PE, Cohen BM, Baldessarini RJ, et al: Time course of antipsychotic effects of neuroleptic drugs. Am J Psychiatry 146:1289–1292, 1989a

Keck PE, Sebastianelli J, Pope HG, et al: Frequency and presentation of neuroleptic malignant syndrome in a state psychiatric hospital. J Clin Psychiatry 50:352–355, 1989b

Keck PE, Pope HG, Cohen BM, et al: Risk factors for neuroleptic malignant syndrome. Arch Gen Psychiatry 46:914–918, 1989c

Keck PE, Caroff SN, McElroy SL: Neuroleptic malignant syndrome and malignant hyperthermia: end of a controversy? J Neuropsychiatry 7:135–144, 1995

Keck PE, McElroy SL, Strakowski SM: New developments in the pharmacologic management of schizoaffective disorder. J Clin Psychiatry 57 (suppl 9):41–48, 1996a

Keck PE, McElroy SL, Strakowski SM, et al: Factors associated with maintenance antipsychotic treatment of patients with bipolar disorder. J Clin Psychiatry 57:147–151, 1996b

Kellam AMP: The neuroleptic malignant syndrome, so called: a survey of the world literature. Br J Psychiatry 150:752–759, 1987

Khanna R, Das A, Damodaran SS: Prospective study of neuroleptic-induced dystonia in mania and schizophrenia. Am J Psychiatry 149:511–513, 1992

Kimmel SE, Calabrese JR, Woyshville MJ, et al: Clozapine in treatment-refractory mood disorders. J Clin Psychiatry 55 (suppl B):91–93, 1994

Kinon BJ, Kane JM, Johns C, et al: Treatment of neuroleptic-resistant schizophrenic relapse. Psychopharmacol Bull 29:309–314, 1993a

Kinon BJ, Kane JM, Chakos M, et al: Possible predictors of neuroleptic-resistant schizophrenic relapse: influence of negative symptoms and acute extrapyramidal effects. Psychopharmacol Bull 29:365–369, 1993b

Kirch DG, Bigelow LB, Korpi ER, et al: Serum haloperidol concentration and clinical response in schizophrenia. Schizophr Bull 14:283–289, 1988

Kissling W, Moller HJ, Walter K, et al: Double-blind comparison of haloperidol decanoate and fluphenazine decanoate effectiveness, side effects, dosage and serum levels during a 6-month treatment for relapse prevention. Pharmacopsychiatry 18:240–245, 1985

Kissling W, Kane JM, Barnes TRE, et al: Guidelines for neuroleptic relapse prevention in schizophrenia: toward a consensus view, in Guidelines for Neuroleptic Relapse Prevention in Schizophrenia. Edited by Kissling W. New York, Springer-Verlag, 1991, pp 155–163

Kleinman I, Schachter D, Koritar E: Informed consent and tardive dyskinesia. Am J Psychiatry 146:902–904, 1989

Klieser E, Lehmann E, Kinzler E, et al: Randomized, double-blind, controlled trial of risperidone versus clozapine in patients with chronic schizophrenia. J Clin Psychopharmacol 15 (suppl 1):45S–51S, 1995

Ko GN, Korpi ER, Kirch DG: Haloperidol and reduced haloperidol concentrations in plasma and red blood cells from chronic schizophrenic patients. J Clin Psychopharmacol 9:186–190, 1989

Koek RJ, Pi EH: Acute laryngeal dystonic reactions to neuroleptics. Psychosomatics 30:359–364, 1989

Koreen AR, Lieberman J, Alvir J, et al: Relation of plasma fluphenazine levels to treatment response and extrapyramidal side effects in first-episode schizophrenic patients. Am J Psychiatry 151:35–39, 1994

Kronig MH, Munne RA, Szymanski S, et al: Plasma clozapine levels and clinical response for treatment-refractory schizophrenic patients. Am J Psychiatry 152:179–182, 1995

Kuha S, Mietinen E: Long-term effect of clozapine in schizophrenia: a retrospective study of 108 chronic schizophrenics treated with clozapine for up to seven years. Nordisk Psykiatrisk Tidsskrift 40:225–230, 1986

Kunik ME, Yudofsky SC, Silver JM, et al: Pharmacologic approach to management of agitation associated with dementia. J Clin Psychiatry 55 (suppl):13–17, 1994

Lacro JP, Roznoski ML, Warren KA, et al: Haloperidol levels in older schizophrenia outpatients (abstract). Psychopharmacol Bull 31:587, 1995

Lamberti JS, Bellnier T, Schwarzkopf SB: Weight gain among schizophrenic patients treated with clozapine. Am J Psychiatry 149:689–690, 1992

LaPorta LD: More on obsessive-compulsive symptoms and clozapine (letter). J Clin Psychiatry 55:312, 1994

Lazarus A: Treatment of neuroleptic malignant syndrome with electroconvulsive therapy. J Nerv Ment Dis 174:47–49, 1986

Leadbetter RA, Shutty MS: Differential effects of neuroleptics and clozapine on polydipsia and intermittent hyponatremia. J Clin Psychiatry 55 (suppl B):110–113, 1994

Leadbetter RA, Shutty MS, Pavalonis D, et al: Clozapine-induced weight gain: prevalence and clinical relevance. Am J Psychiatry 149:68–72, 1992

Leone NF: Response of borderline patients to loxapine and chlorpromazine. J Clin Psychiatry 43:148–150, 1982

Levinson DF, Simpson GM: Neuroleptic-induced extrapyramidal symptoms with fever. Arch Gen Psychiatry 43:839–848, 1986

Levinson DF, Singh H, Simpson GM: Timing of acute clinical response to fluphenazine. Br J Psychiatry 160:365–371, 1992

Liberman RP, Van Putten T, Marshall BD, et al: Optimal drug and behavior therapy for treatment-refractory schizophrenic patients. Am J Psychiatry 151:756–759, 1994

Lieberman E, Stoudemire A: Use of tricyclic antidepressants in patients with glaucoma. Psychosomatics 28:145–148, 1987

Lieberman JA, Kane JM, Johns CA: Clozapine: guidelines for clinical management. J Clin Psychiatry 50:329–338, 1989

Lieberman JA, Saltz BL, Johns CA, et al: The effects of clozapine on tardive dyskinesia. Br J Psychiatry 158:503–510, 1991

Lieberman JA, Kane JM, Safferman AZ, et al: Predictors of response to clozapine. J Clin Psychiatry 55 (suppl B):126–128, 1994a

Lieberman JA, Safferman AZ, Pollack S, et al: Clinical effects of clozapine in chronic schizophrenia: response to treatment and predictors of outcome. Am J Psychiatry 151:1744–1752, 1994b

Lieberman JA, Koreen AR, Chakos M, et al: Factors influencing treatment response and outcome of first-episode schizophrenia: implications for understanding the pathophysiology of schizophrenia. J Clin Psychiatry 57 (suppl 9):5–9, 1996

Linazasoro G, Marti Masso JF, Suarez A: Nocturnal akathisia in Parkinson's disease: treatment with clozapine. Mov Disord 8:171–174, 1993

Lindenmayer JP: Risperidone versus clozapine in treatment refractory state psychiatric inpatients (NR591), in New Research Program and Abstracts, American Psychiatric Association 149th Annual Meeting, New York, NY, May 4–9, 1996, p 231

Lindenmayer JP, Grochowski S, Mabugat L: Clozapine effects on positive and negative symptoms: a 6-month trial in treatment-refractory schizophrenics. J Clin Psychopharmacol 14:201–204, 1994

Lindstrom LH: The effect of long-term treatment with clozapine in schizophrenia: a retrospective study in 96 patients treated with clozapine for up to 13 years. Acta Psychiatr Scand 77:524–529, 1988

Lindstrom LH: A retrospective study on the long-term efficacy of clozapine in 96 schizophrenic and schizoaffective patients during a 13-year period. Psychopharmacology 99:S84–S86, 1989

Livingston MG: Risperidone. Lancet 343:457–460, 1994

Lohr JB, Caligiuri MP: A double-blind placebo-controlled study of vitamin E treatment of tardive dyskinesia. J Clin Psychiatry 57:167–173, 1996

Malhotra AK, Litman RE, Pickar D: Adverse effects of antipsychotics. Drug Saf 9:429–436, 1993

Marder SR: Clinical experience with risperidone. J Clin Psychiatry 57 (suppl 9):57–61, 1996

Marder SR, Meibach RC: Risperidone in the treatment of schizophrenia. Am J Psychiatry 151:825–835, 1994

Marder SR, Van Putten T: Who should receive clozapine? Arch Gen Psychiatry 45:865–867, 1988

Marder SR, Hubbard JW, Van Putten, et al: Pharmacokinetics of long-acting injectable neuroleptic drugs: clinical implications. Psychopharmacology 98:433–439, 1989

Marder SR, Ames D, Wirshing WC, et al: Schizophrenia. Psychiatr Clin North Am 16:567–587, 1993

Marder SR, Wirshing WC, Van Putten T, et al: Fluphenazine vs placebo supplementation for prodromal signs of relapse in schizophrenia. Arch Gen Psychiatry 51:280–287, 1994

Marken PA, Wells BG, Brown CS: Treatment of psychosis in pregnancy. Drug Intelligence and Clinical Pharmacy 23:598–599, 1989

Marriott P, Pansa M, Hiep A: Intervals between long acting neuroleptics: outcome and re-admission variables. Prog Neuropsychopharmacol Biol Psychiatry 8:109–114, 1984

Marsden CD, Parkes JD: "On-off" effects in patients with Parkinson's disease on chronic levodopa therapy. Lancet 2:292–296, 1976

Martin A: Acute pancreatitis associated with clozapine use (letter). Am J Psychiatry 149:714, 1992

Mattes JA: Clozapine for refractory schizophrenia: an open study of 14 patients treated for up to 2 years. J Clin Psychiatry 50:389–391, 1989

Mavroidis M, Kanter DR, Hirschowitz J: Therapeutic blood levels of fluphenazine: plasma or RBC determinations? Psychopharmacol Bull 20:168–170, 1984

McElroy SL, Dessain EC, Pope HG, et al: Clozapine in the treatment of psychotic mood disorders, schizoaffective disorder, and schizophrenia. J Clin Psychiatry 52:411–414, 1991

McGreadie RG, Dingwall JM, Wiles DH, et al: Intermittent pimozide versus fluphenazine decanoate as maintenance therapy for chronic schizophrenia. Br J Psychiatry 137:510–517, 1980

McIntyre IM, Gershon S: Interpatient variations in anti-psychotic therapy. J Clin Psychiatry 46 (suppl):3–5, 1985

Mecco G, Alessandria A, Boniati V, et al: Risperidone for hallucinations in levodopa-treated Parkinson's disease patients (letter). Lancet 343:1370–1371, 1994

Meltzer HY: New insights into schizophrenia through atypical antipsychotic drugs. Neuropyschopharmacology 1:193–196, 1988

Meltzer HY: Duration of a clozapine trial in neuroleptic-resistant schizophrenia (letter). Arch Gen Psychiatry 46:672, 1989

Meltzer HY: The mechanism of action of novel antipsychotic drugs. Schizophr Bull 2:263–287, 1991

Meltzer HY: An overview of the mechanism of action of clozapine. J Clin Psychiatry 55 (suppl B):47–52, 1994

Meltzer HY: Suicidality and clozapine. J Clin Psychiatry 14:13–15, 1996a

Meltzer HY: Cost effectiveness of clozapine treatment. J Clin Psychiatry 14:16–17, 1996b

Meltzer HY: Cognitive and other nonconventional benefits of clozapine treatment. J Clin Psychiatry 14:22–24, 1996c

Meltzer HY, Cola PA: The pharmacoeconomics of clozapine: a review. J Clin Psychiatry 55 (suppl B):161–165, 1994

Meltzer HY, Fang VS: The effect of neuroleptics on serum prolactin in schizophrenic patients. Arch Gen Psychiatry 33:279–286, 1976

Meltzer HY, Bastani B, Ramirez L, et al: Clozapine: new research on efficacy and mechanism of action. European Archives of Psychiatry and Neurological Sciences 238:332–339, 1989

Menza MA, Murray GB, Holmes VF, et al: Decreased extrapyramidal symptoms with intravenous haloperidol. J Clin Psychiatry 48:278–280, 1987

Metzger E, Friedman R: Prolongation of the corrected QT and torsade de pointes cardiac arrhythmia associated with intravenous haloperidol in the medically ill. J Clin Psychopharmacol 13:128–132, 1993

Miller DD, Sharafuddin MJA, Kathol R: A case of clozapine-induced neuroleptic malignant syndrome. J Clin Psychiatry 52:99–101, 1991

Miller DD, Fleming F, Holman T, et al: Plasma clozapine concentration as a predictor of clinical response: a follow-up study. J Clin Psychiatry 55 (suppl B):117–121, 1994a

Miller DD, Perry PJ, Cadoret RJ, et al: Clozapine's effect on negative symptoms in treatment-refractory schizophrenics. Compr Psychiatry 35:8–15, 1994b

Miller DD, Schultz SK, Alexander B: Rational pharmacologic approaches in the management of treatment-resistant schizophrenia, in Psychiatric Clinics of North America: Annual of Drug Therapy, Vol 3. Edited by Jefferson JW, Greist JH. Philadelphia, PA, WB Saunders, 1996, pp 89–118

Morris JB, Beck AT: The efficacy of antidepressant drugs. Arch Gen Psychiatry 30:667–674, 1974

Muller T, Becker T, Fritze J: Neuroleptic malignant syndrome after clozapine plus carbamazepine (letter). Lancet 2:1500, 1988

Munetz MR, Benjamin S: How to examine patients using the Abnormal Involuntary Movement Scale. Hospital and Community Psychiatry 39:1172–1177, 1988

Munn NA: Resolution of polydipsia and hyponatremia in schizophrenic patients after clozapine treatment (letter). J Clin Psychiatry 54:439–440, 1993

Naber D, Hippius H: The European experience with the use of clozapine. Hospital and Community Psychiatry 41:886–890, 1990

Nair NPV, Suranyi-Cadotte B, Schwartz G, et al: A clinical trial comparing intramuscular haloperidol decanoate and oral haloperidol in chronic schizophrenic patients: efficacy, safety, and dosage equivalence. J Clin Psychopharmacol 6 (suppl):30–37, 1986

Nasrallah HA, Churchill CM, Hamdan-Allan GA: Higher frequency of neuroleptic-induced dystonia in mania than schizophrenia. Am J Psychiatry 145:1455–1456, 1988

Nayak RK, Doose DR, Nair NPV: The bioavailability and pharmacokinetics of oral and depot intramuscular haloperidol in schizophrenic patients. J Clin Pharmacol 27:144–150, 1987

Nelson JC: Combined treatment strategies in psychiatry. J Clin Psychiatry 54 (suppl):42–49, 1993

Nishikawa T, Tsuda A, Tanaka M, et al: Decreased polydipsia in schizophrenic patients treated with naloxone (letter). J Clin Psychiatry 151:947, 1994

Nopoulos P, Flaum M, Miller DD: Atypical neuroleptic malignant syndrome with an atypical neuroleptic: clozapine-induced NMS without rigidity. Ann Clin Psychiatry 2:251–253, 1990

Nurnberg HG, Ambrosini PJ: Urinary incontinence in patients receiving neuroleptics. J Clin Psychiatry 40:271–274, 1979

Nurnberg HG, Prudic J: Guidelines for treatment of psychosis during pregnancy. Hospital and Community Psychiatry 35:67–71, 1984

Obermeyer BD, Nyhart EH, Maruz EL: The disposition of olanzapine in healthy volunteers (abstract). Pharmacologist 35:176, 1993

O'Brien RA, Young GB: Neuroleptic malignant syndrome: a review. Canadian Family Physician 35:1119–1122, 1989

Opler LA, Feinberg SS: The role of pimozide in clinical psychiatry: a review. J Clin Psychiatry 52:221–233, 1991

Ortiz A, Gershon S: The future of neuroleptic psychopharmacology. J Clin Psychiatry 47 (suppl):3–11, 1986

Osser DN: Is clozapine response different in neuroleptic nonresponders vs partial responders? (letter). Arch Gen Psychiatry 47:189, 1990

Overall JE: Prior psychiatric treatment and the development of breast cancer. Arch Gen Psychiatry 35:898–899, 1978

Owen RR, Beake BJ, Marby D, et al: Response to clozapine in chronic psychotic patients. Psychopharmacol Bull 25:253–256, 1989

Palao DJ, Arauxo A, Brunet M, et al: Haloperidol: therapeutic window in schizophrenia. J Clin Psychopharmacol 14:303–310, 1994

Pandurangi AK, Narasimhachari N, Blackard WG, et al: Relation of serum molindone levels to serum prolactin levels and antipsychotic response. J Clin Psychiatry 50:379–331, 1989

Parent MM, Roy S, Sramek J, et al: Effect of molindone on weight change in hospitalized schizophrenic patients. Drug Intelligence and Clinical Pharmacy 20:873–875, 1986

Peacock L, Gerlach J: Clozapine treatment in Denmark: concomitant psychotropic medication and hematologic monitoring in a system with liberal usage practices. J Clin Psychiatry 55:44–49, 1994

Pearlman CA: Neuroleptic malignant syndrome. J Clin Psychopharmacol 6:257–273, 1986

Perry PJ, Alexander B: Switching haloperidol from oral to im depot formulation (letter). DICP Ann Pharmacother 25:1270–1271, 1991

Perry PJ, Morgan DE, Smith RE, et al: Treatment of unipolar depression accompanied by delusions. J Affect Disord 4:195–200, 1982

Perry PJ, Miller DD, Arndt SV, et al: Clozapine and norclozapine plasma concentrations and clinical response of treatment-refractory schizophrenic patients. Am J Psychiatry 148:231–235, 1991

Peterson LG, Bongar B: Navane versus Haldol: treatment of acute organic mental syndromes in the general hospital. Gen Hosp Psychiatry 11:412–417, 1989

Petrie WM, Ban TA, Berney S, et al: Loxapine in psychogeriatrics: a placebo and standard controlled clinical investigation. J Clin Psychopharmacol 2:122–126, 1982

Pfister GM, Hanson DR, Roerig JL, et al: Clozapine-induced agranulocytosis in a native American: HLA typing and further support for an immune-mediated mechanism. J Clin Psychiatry 53:242–244, 1992

Pickar D, Owen RR, Litman FE, et al: Clinical and biologic response to clozapine in patients with schizophrenia. Arch Gen Psychiatry 49:345–353, 1992

Piscitelli SC, Frazier JA, McKenna K, et al: Plasma clozapine and haloperidol concentrations in adolescents with childhood-onset schizophrenia: association with response. J Clin Psychiatry 55 (suppl B):94–97, 1994

Pollack S, Lieberman J, Kleiner D, et al: High plasma clozapine levels in tardive dyskinesia. Psychopharmacol Bull 29:257–262, 1993

Pons G, Rey E, Matheson I: Excretion of psychoactive drugs into breast milk. Clin Pharmacokinet 27:270–289, 1994

Pope HG, Cole JO, Choras PT, et al: Apparent neuroleptic malignant syndrome with clozapine and lithium. J Nerv Ment Dis 174:493–495, 1986

Potkin SG, Bera R, Gulasekaram B, et al: Plasma clozapine concentration predict clinical response in treatment-resistant schizophrenia. J Clin Psychiatry 55 (suppl B):133–136, 1994

Preskorn SH, Burke MJ, Fast GA: Therapeutic drug monitoring. Psychiatr Clin North Am 16:611–645, 1993

Prien RF, Gelenberg AJ: Alternatives to lithium for preventive treatment of bipolar disorder. Am J Psychiatry 146:840–848, 1989

Ranjan R, Lee MA, Thompson PA, et al: Effect of clozapine on negative symptoms (abstract). Psychopharmacol Bull 31:607, 1995

Raskind MA, Risse SC: Antipsychotic drugs and the elderly. J Clin Psychiatry 47 (suppl):17–22, 1986

Reed WH, Mason M, Toprac M: Savings in hospital days related to treatment with clozapine. Hospital and Community Psychiatry 45:261–264, 1994

Remington G: Pharmacotherapy of schizophrenia. Can J Psychiatry 34:211–216 (erratum 34:457–461), 1989

Remington GJ, Voineskos G, Pollock B, et al: Prevalence of neuroleptic-induced dystonia in mania and schizophrenia. Am J Psychiatry 147:1231–1233, 1990

Revicki DA, Luce BR, Weschler JM, et al: Cost-effectiveness of clozapine for treatment-resistant schizophrenic patients. Hospital and Community Psychiatry 41:850–854, 1990

Reyntgens AJM, Heykants JJP, Woestenborghs RJH, et al: Pharmacokinetics of haloperidol decanoate. International Pharmacopsychiatry 17:238–246, 1982

Rhoades HM, Overall JE: Side effect potentials of different antipsychotic and antidepressant drugs. Psychopharmacol Bull 20:83–88, 1984

Rich SS, Friedman JH, Ott BR: Risperidone versus clozapine in the treatment of psychosis in six patients with Parkinson's disease and other akinetic–rigid syndromes. J Clin Psychiatry 56:556–559, 1995

Riker RR, Fraser GL, Cox PM: Continuous infusion haloperidol controls agitation in critically ill patients. Crit Care Med 22:433–440, 1994

Risperdal® [risperidone] Product Information. Titusville, NJ, Janssen Pharmaceutica Corporation, 1994

Risse SC, Barnes R: Pharmacologic treatment of agitation associated with dementia. J Am Geriatr Soc 34:368–376, 1986

Rosen SI, Hanno PM: Clozapine-induced priapism. J Urol 148:876–877, 1992

Rosenberg MR, Green M: Neuroleptic malignant syndrome. Arch Intern Med 149:1927–1931, 1989

Ryabik BM, Nguyen VT, Mann RN, et al: Clozapine-induced agranulocytosis and colony-stimulating cytokines. Gen Hosp Psychiatry 15:263–265, 1993

Sachdev P, Loneragan C: The present status of akathisia. J Nerv Ment Dis 179:381–391, 1991

Safferman A, Lieberman JA, Kane JM, et al: Update on the clinical efficacy and side effects of clozapine. Schizophr Bull 17:247–261, 1991

Safferman AZ, Lieberman JA, Alvir JMJ, et al: Rechallenge in clozapine-associated agranulocytosis (letter). Lancet 339:1296–1297, 1992a

Safferman AZ, Lieberman JA, Pollack S, et al: Clozapine and akathisia (letter). Biol Psychiatry 31:749–754, 1992b

Safferman AZ, Lieberman JA, Pollack S, et al: Akathisia and clozapine treatment (letter). J Clin Psychopharmacol 13:286–287, 1993

Safferman AZ, Kane JM, Aronowitz JS, et al: The use of clozapine in neurologic disorders. J Clin Psychiatry 55 (suppl B):98–101, 1994

Sajatovic M: A pilot study evaluating the efficacy of risperidone in treatment-refractory, acute bipolar, and schizoaffective mania (abstract). Psychopharmacol Bull 31:613, 1995

Sajatovic M, Verbanac P, Ramirez LF, et al: Clozapine treatment of psychiatric symptoms resistant to neuroleptic treatment in patients with Huntington's chorea (letter). Neurology 41:156, 1991

Santos AB, Wohlreich MM, Pinosky ST: Managing agitation in the critical care setting. J S C Med Assoc 88:386–391, 1992

Satterlee WG, Reams SG, Burns PR, et al: A clinical update on olanzapine treatment in schizophrenia and in elderly Alzheimer's disease patients (abstract). Psychopharmacol Bull 31:534, 1995

Schaffer CB, Schaffer LC: The use of risperidone in the treatment of bipolar disorder (letter). J Clin Psychiatry 57:136, 1996

Schneider LS, Pollock VE, Lyness SA: A meta-analysis of controlled trials of neuroleptic treatment in dementia. J Am Geriatr Soc 38:553–563, 1990

Schulte-Sasse U, Eberlein HJ: New findings in the field of malignant hyperthermia. Anaesthesist 35:1–9, 1986

Schuster P, Gabriel E, Kufferle B, et al: Reversal by physostigmine of clozapine-induced delirium. Clinical Toxicology 10:437–441, 1977

Seftel AD, De Tejada IS, Szetela B, et al: Clozapine-induced priapism: a case report. J Urol 147:146–148, 1992

Segraves RT: Effects of psychotropic drugs on human erection and ejaculation. Arch Gen Psychiatry 46:275–284, 1989

Serban G, Siegel S: Response of borderline and schizotypal patients to small doses of thiothixene and haloperidol. Am J Psychiatry 141:1455–1458, 1984

Sernyak MJ, Woods SW: Chronic neuroleptic use in manic-depressive illness. Psychopharmacol Bull 29:375–381, 1993

Sertindole Investigator Consensus Meeting. Chicago, IL, Abbott Laboratories, November 13, 1995

Shader RI, DiMascio A (eds): Psychotropic Drug Side Effects: Clinical and Theoretical Perspectives. Baltimore, MD, Williams & Wilkins, 1970, pp 4–9, 63–85, 92–106, 116–123, 149–174, 175–198

Shalev A, Mermesh H, Munitz H: The role of external heat load in triggering the neuroleptic malignant syndrome. Am J Psychiatry 145:110–111, 1988

Shalev A, Mermesh H, Munitz H: Mortality from neuroleptic malignant syndrome. J Clin Psychiatry 50:18–25, 1989

Shenoy RS, Sadler AG, Goldberg SC, et al: Effects of a 6-week drug holiday on symptom status, relapse, and tardive dyskinesia in chronic schizophrenics. J Clin Psychopharmacol 1:141–145, 1981

Simpson GM, Amin M, Kunz E: Withdrawal effects of phenothiazines. Compr Psychiatry 6:347–351, 1965

Simpson GM, Pi EH, Sramek JJ: Adverse effects of antipsychotic agents. Drugs 21:138–151, 1981

Simpson GM, Yadalam KG, Levinson DF, et al: Single-dose pharmacokinetics of fluphenazine after fluphenazine decanoate administration. J Clin Psychopharmacol 10:417–421, 1990

Small JG, Milstein V, Marhenke JD, et al: Treatment outcome with clozapine in tardive dyskinesia, neuroleptic sensitivity, and treatment-resistant psychosis. J Clin Psychiatry 48:263–267, 1987

Smith RC: Lower-dose therapy with traditional neuroleptics in chronically hospitalized schizophrenic patients. Arch Gen Psychiatry 51:427–429, 1994

Smith RC, Lipetsker B, Bhattacharyya A: Risperidone treatment of non-responding chronically hospitalized schizophrenics (abstract). Psychopharmacol Bull 31:618, 1995

Soloff PH, George A, Nathan S, et al: Progress in pharmacotherapy of borderline disorders. Arch Gen Psychiatry 43:691–697, 1986

Soloff PH, George A, Nathan S, et al: Amitriptyline vs. haloperidol in borderlines: final outcomes and predictors of response. J Clin Psychopharmacol 9:238–246, 1989

Soloff PH, Cornelius J, George A, et al: Efficacy of phenelzine and haloperidol in borderline personality disorder. Arch Gen Psychiatry 50:377–385, 1993

Sovner R, DiMascio A: Extrapyramidal syndromes and other neurological side effects of psychotropic drugs, in Psychopharmacology: A Generation of Progress. Edited by Lipton MA, DiMascio A, Killam DF. New York, Raven, 1978, pp 1021–1032

Spears NM, Leadbetter RA, Shutty MS: Influence of clozapine on water dysregulation (letter). Am J Psychiatry 150:1430–1431, 1993

Spiker DG, Dealy RS, Hanin I, et al: Treating delusional depressives with amitriptyline. J Clin Psychiatry 47:243–246, 1986

Sramek JJ, Potkin ST, Hahn R: Neuroleptic plasma concentrations and clinical response: in search of a therapeutic window. Drug Intelligence and Clinical Pharmacy 22:373–380, 1988

Sramek JJ, Gaurana V, Herrera JM, et al: Patterns of neuroleptic usage in continuously hospitalized chronic schizophrenic patients: evidence for development of drug tolerance. DICP Ann Pharmacother 24:7–10, 1990

Steingard S: Use of desmopressin to treat clozapine-induced nocturnal enuresis (letter). J Clin Psychiatry 55:315–316, 1994

Stephens P: A review of clozapine: an antipsychotic for treatment-resistant schizophrenia. Compr Psychiatry 31:315–326, 1990

Stern RG, Kahn RS, Davidson M, et al: Early response to clozapine in schizophrenia. Am J Psychiatry 151:1817–1818, 1994

Still DJ, Dorson PG, Crismon ML: Effects of risperidone in clozapine-treated schizophrenic patients (abstract). Psychopharmacol Bull 31:623, 1995

Stockton ME, Rasmussen K: Olanzapine, a novel atypical antipsychotic, has electrophysiological effects on A9 and A10 dopamine cells similar to clozapine (abstract). Schizophr Res 15:166, 1995

Stoppe G, Muller P, Fuchs T, et al: Life-threatening allergic reaction to clozapine. Br J Psychiatry 161:259–261, 1992

Stricker BH, Tielens JAE: Eosinophilia with clozapine (letter). Lancet 338:1520–1521, 1991

Sullivan G, Lukoff D: Sexual side effects of antipsychotic medication: evaluation and interventions. Hospital and Community Psychiatry 41:1238–1241, 1990

Sunderland T: Treatment of the elderly suffering from psychosis and dementia. J Clin Psychiatry 57 (suppl 9):53–56, 1996

Suppes T, McElroy SL, Gilbert J, et al: Clozapine in the treatment of dysphoric mania. Biol Psychiatry 32:270–280, 1992

Surawicz FG: Alcoholic hallucinosis: a missed diagnosis. Can J Psychiatry 25:57–63, 1980

Susman VL, Addonizio G: Recurrence of neuroleptic malignant syndrome. J Nerv Ment Dis 176:234–240, 1988

Swett C: Drug-induced dystonia. Am J Psychiatry 132:532–534, 1975

Szymanski S, Jody D, Leipzig R, et al: Anticholinergic delirium caused by retreatment with clozapine (letter). Am J Psychiatry 148:1752, 1991

Szymanski SR, Cannon TD, Gallacher F, et al: Course of treatment response in first-episode and chronic schizophrenia. Am J Psychiatry 153:519–525, 1996

Tamminga CA, Thaker GK, Moran M, et al: Clozapine in tardive dyskinesia: observations from human and animal model studies. J Clin Psychiatry 55 (suppl B):102–106, 1994

Tandon R, Greden JF: Cholinergic hyperactivity and negative schizophrenic symptoms. Arch Gen Psychiatry 46:745–753, 1989

Teicher MH, Glod CA: Pharmacotherapy of patients with borderline personality disorder. Hospital and Community Psychiatry 40:887–889, 1989

Tesar GE: The agitated patient, II: pharmacologic treatment. Hospital and Community Psychiatry 44:627–629, 1993

Testani M: Clozapine-induced orthostatic hypotension treated with fludrocortisone (letter). J Clin Psychiatry 55:497–498, 1994

Thhonen J, Paanila J: Eosinophilia associated with clozapine (letter). Lancet 339:488, 1992

Thornberg SA, Ereshefsky L: Neuroleptic malignant syndrome associated with clozapine monotherapy. Pharmacotherapy 13:510–514, 1993

Tohen M, Zarate CA, Centorrino F, et al: Risperidone in the treatment of mania (abstract). Psychopharmacol Bull 31:626, 1995

Tollefson GD, Garvey MJ: The neuroleptic malignant syndrome and central dopamine metabolites. J Clin Psychopharmacol 4:150–153, 1984

Tollefson GD, Beasley CM, Tran PV, et al: Olanzapine: a novel antipsychotic with a broad-spectrum profile (abstract). Biol Psychiatry 35:746–747, 1994

Toru M, Matsuda O, Makiguchi K, et al: Neuroleptic malignant syndrome-like state following a withdrawal of antiparkinsonian drugs. J Nerv Ment Dis 169:324–327, 1981

Tran PV, Beasley CM, Tollefson GD, et al: Olanzapine: a promising "atypical" antipsychotic agent (abstract). Schizophr Res 15:169, 1995a

Tran PV, Beasley CM, Tollefson GD, et al: Olanzapine: an update on recent clinical studies (abstract). Psychopharmacol Bull 31:627, 1995b

Tueth MJ, Cheong JA: Clinical uses of pimozide. South Med J 86:344–349, 1993

Uehlinger C, Baumann P: Clozapine as an alternative treatment for neuroleptic-induced gynecomastia (letter). Am J Psychiatry 148:392–393, 1991

Umbricht DSG, Pollack S, Kane JM: Clozapine and weight gain. J Clin Psychiatry 55 (suppl B):157–160, 1994

van Praag HM, Dols LCW: Fluphenazine enanthate and decanoate: a comparison of their duration of action and motor side effects. Am J Psychiatry 130:801–804, 1973

Van Putten T, May PRA, Marder SR: Akathisia with haloperidol and thiothixene. Arch Gen Psychiatry 41:1036–1039, 1984

Van Putten T, Marder SR, Mintz J: A controlled dose comparison of haloperidol in newly admitted schizophrenic patients. Arch Gen Psychiatry 47:754–758, 1990

Viner MW, Escobar JI: An apparent neurotoxicity associated with clozapine (letter). J Clin Psychiatry 55:38–39, 1994

Volavka J, Cooper TB, Czobor P, et al: Haloperidol plasma levels and clinical effects (abstract). Psychopharmacol Bull 31:586, 1995

Warner JP, Harvey CA, Barnes TRE: Clozapine and urinary incontinence. Int Clin Psychopharmacol 9:207–209, 1994

Wasan S, Crismon ML: Considerations in establishing expiration dates for fluphenazine decanoate multiple-dose vials (letter). DICP Ann Pharmacother 24:889–890, 1990

Webster P, Wijeratne C: Risperidone-induced neuroleptic malignant syndrome (letter). Lancet 344:1228–1229, 1994

Weide R, Koppler H, Heymanns J, et al: Successful treatment of clozapine-induced agranulocytosis with granulocyte colony stimulating activity (letter). Br J Haematol 4:5579, 1992

Weiden P, Schooler NR, Severe JB, et al: Stabilization and depot neuroleptic dosages. Psychopharmacol Bull 29:269–275, 1993

Wells AJ, Sommi RW, Crismon ML: Neuroleptic rechallenge after neuroleptic malignant syndrome: case report and literature review. Drug Intelligence and Clinical Pharmacy 22:475–479, 1988

Whalley LJ: Drug treatment of dementia. Br J Psychiatry 155:595–611, 1989

Wilson WH, Claussen AM: Seizures associated with clozapine treatment in a state hospital. J Clin Psychiatry 55:184–188, 1994

Wirshing WC, Freidenberg DL, Cummings JL, et al: Effects of anticholinergic agents on patients with tardive dyskinesia and concomitant drug-induced parkinsonism. J Clin Psychopharmacol 9:407–411, 1989

Wirshing WC, Ames D, Green M, et al: Risperidone versus haloperidol in treatment-refractory schizophrenia: preliminary results (abstract). Psychopharmacol Bull 31:633, 1995

Wistedt B, Persson T, Hellborn E: A clinical double-blind comparison between haloperidol decanoate and fluphenazine decanoate. Curr Ther Res Clin Exp 53:804–814, 1984

Wistedt B, Wiles DH, Kolakowska T: Slow decline of plasma drug and prolactin levels after discontinuation of chronic treatment with depot neuroleptics (letter). Lancet 1:1163, 1981

Wolkowitz OM: Rational polypharmacy in schizophrenia. Ann Clin Psychiatry 5:79–90, 1993

Wragg RE, Jeste DV: Neuroleptics and alternative treatments: management of behavioral symptoms and psychosis in Alzheimer's disease and related conditions. Psychiatr Clin North Am 11:195–213, 1988

Yadalam KG, Simpson GM: Changing from oral to depot fluphenazine. J Clin Psychiatry 49:346–348, 1988

Yudofsky SC, Silver JM, Jackson W, et al: The overt aggression scale for the objective rating of verbal and physical aggression. Am J Psychiatry 143:35–39, 1986

Yudofsky SC, Silver JM, Hales RE: Pharmacologic management of aggression in the elderly. J Clin Psychiatry 51 (suppl):22–28, 1990

Zanarini MC, Frankenburg FR, Gunderson JG: Pharmacotherapy of borderline outpatients. Compr Psychiatry 29:372–378, 1988

Zarate CA, Tohen J, Baldessarini RJ: Clozapine in severe mood disorders (abstract). Psychopharmacol Bull 31:636, 1995

Zeigler J, Behar D: Clozapine-induced priapism (letter). Am J Psychiatry 149:272–273, 1992

Zito JM, Sofair JB, Jaeger J: Self-reported neuroendocrine effects of antipsychotics in women: a pilot study. DICP Ann Pharmacother 24:176–180, 1990

Zito JM, Volavka J, Craig TJ, et al: Pharmacoepidemiology of clozapine in 202 inpatients with schizophrenia. DICP Ann Pharmacother 27:1262–1269, 1993

Zyprexa® [mirtazapine] Product Information. Indianapolis, IN, Lilly Pharmaceutical Company, 1996

Antidepressants

Antidepressants are used for the treatment of major depressive episodes occurring in patients diagnosed with major depressive disorder, dysthymic disorder, bipolar disorder, mood disorder due to a general medical condition, and/or substance-induced mood disorder. They may also be used when a depressive episode occurs in the context of other Axis I or II disorders.

In regard to efficacy, there are no differences among the various classes of antidepressants. However, the adverse-effect profiles of these agents differ, and these profiles are the primary factor influencing clinicians' decisions of which antidepressant to prescribe. Although in the past, the tricyclic antidepressants (TCAs) were considered the drugs of choice for the treatment of nonpsychotic unipolar depression, the cardiotoxicity associated with tricyclic overdoses, in conjunction with the high rate of suicide and suicide attempts associated with depressive illness, renders these agents less than desirable in many cases. A meta-analysis of the TCA–selective serotonin reuptake inhibitor (SSRI) literature estimated that the discontinuation rate and the dropout rate due to side effects were 10% lower and 25% lower, respectively, with SSRIs than with TCAs (Anderson and Tomenson 1995). However, as expected, there were no significant differences between the two drug classes in dropout rates for treatment failure. The selective serotonin reuptake inhibitors (SSRIs), despite being significantly more expensive than the generically available TCAs, are now nearly as commonly prescribed by physicians, primarily because of their more advantageous adverse-effect profile. In a survey of 216,896 antidepressant prescriptions written for the Iowa Medicaid population in fiscal year 1994–1995, 47% and 40% of the prescriptions were for TCAs and SSRIs, respectively (Pursel and Perry 1995). The monoamine oxidase inhibitors (MAOIs), because of drug and dietary interactions that can lead to hypertensive crisis, accounted for less than 1% of the antidepressant prescriptions. The approximately 13% remaining prescriptions were for miscellaneous antidepressants, of which trazodone accounted for the majority.

Tricyclic Antidepressants

■ Indications

The primary indication for TCAs is the treatment of *major depressive disorder*. The presence of delusions in conjunction with depression is usually a harbinger of an unsatisfactory response to TCAs (Spiker et al. 1986). Numerous other minor indications exist for the TCAs. Of these, the most important are the treatment of *anxiety disorders,* which include panic disorder with or without agoraphobia, obsessive-compulsive disorder, simple and social phobias, posttraumatic stress disorder, and generalized anxiety disorder (Modigh 1987). TCAs are effective in reducing bingeing and purging episodes in patients with *bulimia nervosa* (Fairburn 1990). The TCA imipramine is the drug of choice in the treatment of *nocturnal enuresis* (Miller et al. 1992). TCAs are useful in the treatment of refractory pain syndromes. Specific types of *pain* that have benefited from TCA therapy include diabetic neuropathies, musculoskeletal pain, fibromyalgia or fibrositis, rheumatoid arthritis, and central nervous system (CNS) pain (Magni 1991). The TCAs doxepin and trimipramine effectively inhibit gastric secretions and have been used in the treatment of *peptic ulcer disease* (Ries et al. 1984). TCAs affect *sexual function* and have been used therapeutically to treat premature ejaculation (Hawton 1988). The drugs of choice for the treatment of cataleptic episodes associated with *narcolepsy* are the TCAs imipramine and clomipramine (Aldrich 1990). TCAs have been found to be effective alternatives to the stimulants in the treatment of attention-deficit/hyperactivity disorder (Biederman et al. 1989). Data supporting the use of TCAs or of any other class of antidepressants in the treatment of non–affective disorder diagnoses are less extensive and compelling than the data supporting the use of these agents in depression.

■ Efficacy

The predictors of clinical response for the TCAs in acute depression have been assessed retrospectively by examining double-blind, controlled studies involving imipramine and amitriptyline. According to these data, patients with major depressive disorder or endogenous depression whose presentation includes an insidious onset, anorexia, weight loss, middle or terminal insomnia, diurnal variation in mood, psychomotor retardation, or agitation generally experience a positive response to a TCA (Bielski and Fiedel 1976).

Major Depression

The efficacy of TCAs in the treatment of acute depression is well established. A 1965 review that calculated imipramine response rates in 23 placebo-controlled studies found the overall response rate to be 65% of 540 imipramine-treated patients, compared with 32% of 449 placebo-treated patients (Klerman and Cole 1965). Despite changes in diagnostic criteria for depression over the past 30 years, that figure remains remarkably stable. Later estimates reported a 66% response rate for antidepressant drugs as the initial treatment of depression in a series of studies published between 1974 and 1985 (Feinberg and Halbreich 1986). These rates are based on an adequate treatment exposure time frame of approximately 3–4 weeks. A more recent meta-analysis of antidepressant efficacy studies calculated the antidepressant response rates using an intent-to-treat sample (i.e., all patients randomized to treatment) (Depression Guideline Panel 1993b). The TCA response rate for inpatient and outpatient populations averaged approximately 51%, which was 21%–25% greater than the placebo response rate. No specific TCA or other antidepressant was superior to any other. Thus, the choice of a TCA or of any antidepressant is a function of 1) the drug's adverse-effect profile, 2) the availability of a therapeutic blood level with which to adjust dosing, and 3) the patient's previous response to a particular agent.

Because approximately one-third to one-half of patients with major depression do not respond to TCAs, the management of these *treatment-resistant patients* is an important topic. Numerous treatment alternatives are available for TCA-refractory patients: electroconvulsive therapy (ECT), MAOIs, SSRIs, lithium augmentation, triiodothyronine (T_3) augmentation, trazodone, and bupropion. The effectiveness of **ECT** in TCA nonresponders was illustrated by an investigation of 437 depressed patients who were treated with imipramine 200–350 mg/day; when the 190 patients who failed to respond after 1 month received ECT, a 72% improvement rate was observed (Avery and Lubrano 1979). Overall, the **MAOIs** have been found to be effective in 65% (96 of 147) of TCA treatment–refractory depressed patients (Georgotas et al. 1983; McGrath et al. 1987; Nolen et al. 1988a; Pare 1985; Quitkin et al. 1981). Data from several trials indicated that the **SSRI** fluoxetine was effective in 50%–60% of TCA treatment–refractory depressed patients (Beasley et al. 1990a) and that paroxetine was effective in 64% (23 of 36) of such patients (Gagiano et al. 1989; Peselow et al. 1989). However, another SSRI, fluvoxamine, was effective in only 4% (2 of 56) of patients (Nolen et al. 1988b). Based on these data, the agents comprised in the SSRI antidepressant group cannot be considered equally effective in the management of treatment-refractory depressions. The usefulness of **lithium augmentation of TCA treatment** in patients who have failed to respond to a minimum of 3 weeks of TCA therapy has been demonstrated in seven double-blind, placebo-controlled studies (Heninger et al. 1983; Kantor et al. 1986; Stein and Bernadt 1993; Zusky et al. 1988). Sixty-seven percent of patients (32 of 48) responded to lithium augmentation, in contrast to the 15% (4 of 26) response rate in the control subjects. Response time varied from 2 to 21 days. Some patients may initially respond quickly, relapse within a few days, and then respond to continued lithium treatment. Usually, lithium dosages of 600–1,200 mg/day, producing concentrations greater than 0.3 mEq/L, are sufficient. A controlled study that examined the effectiveness of T_3 **augmentation of TCA therapy** in nonresponding patients suggested that this treatment was no more effective than 4 additional weeks of TCA treatment (Gitlin et al. 1987). However, a direct-comparison study of lithium versus T_3 TCA augmentation in refractory depression found both augmentation regimens to be effective (52% and 59% of patients responded to lithium and T_3, respectively) (Joffe et al. 1993). **Trazodone** 100–600 mg/day for 2–4 weeks was effective in 50% of 22 TCA treatment–refractory patients (Cole et al. 1981). **Bupropion** 300–750 mg/day improved the depressive symptoms of 63% (12 of 19) of the TCA treatment–refractory patients (Stern et al. 1983). Thus, according to the data, all of these therapeutic alternatives appear to be equally effective in the treatment of TCA-nonresponding patients.

Childhood/Adolescent Depression
A meta-analysis of 12 randomized, controlled trials evaluated the efficacy of the TCAs versus placebo in depressed 6- to 18-year-old subjects (Hazell et al. 1995). The analysis concluded that TCAs appear to be no more effective than placebo in the treatment of depression in children and adolescents.

Major Depression With Psychotic Features
Patients with delusional depression often require ECT. A review of the **psychotic depression** literature found that the 82% of patients (104 of 127) with psychotic depression who failed to respond to TCAs responded to ECT (Spiker et al. 1986). In nine of the studies reviewed, 66% of the nondelusional depressed patients

responded to TCAs versus only 34% of the delusional patients. In situations in which ECT is not a viable alternative, the possibly less-effective combination treatment of a TCA with an antipsychotic is recommended. Combination drug treatment can be optimized by prescribing a TCA dose that falls at the higher end of the recommended therapeutic plasma range. Because antipsychotic drugs typically increase TCA concentrations, the ineffectiveness of TCAs in treating delusional depression may be the result of subtherapeutic doses. A 5-week course of amitriptyline was effective in only 41% (7 of 17) of a group of delusional depressive patients, whereas the antipsychotic/antidepressant combination of perphenazine/amitriptyline was effective in 78% (14 of 18) (Spiker et al. 1985). However, after the data were analyzed to take into account the effect of serum concentration, it was found that 64% of the amitriptyline-treated patients with total concentrations greater than 250 ng/mL responded, a response rate similar to that with the combination therapy. Although TCA plasma concentration may be important in treating these patients, duration of the TCA trial is probably more important. A TCA trial in patients with delusional depression resulted in response rates of only 32% after 3 weeks, but this rate increased to 62% after 9 weeks of high-dose treatment with imipramine or amitriptyline (Howarth and Grace 1985). Thus, TCAs alone may be effective in the treatment of delusional depression if dosages titrated to produce high therapeutic blood levels (see *TCA Concentration Versus Antidepressant Response* [page 146] under "Pharmacokinetics") are administered for up to 9 weeks.

Dysthymia

Pharmacological treatment of dysthymia with standard doses of TCAs has been evaluated in three controlled trials (Kocsis et al. 1988; J. W. Stewart et al. 1985; P. Tyrer et al. 1988). The TCAs were effective in this disorder; however, the treatment response was not as robust as that observed in patients with major depression, although those dysthymic patients who responded generally remained in remission on 16- to 20-week follow-up (Kocsis et al. 1995). This reduced treatment response may be related to the finding that socially impaired dysthymic patients have a higher nonresponse rate to pharmacological therapies (Friedman et al. 1995). Thus, the clinical observation that dysthymic patients with personality disorders (e.g., borderline, antisocial) do not derive much benefit from TCA treatment should be considered before initiating pharmacotherapy.

Uncomplicated Bereavement

Few data are available concerning the role of TCAs in the treatment of **bereavement reactions.** Fifteen percent of bereaved spouses meet the criteria for depression 12 months after their loss. Currently, it is recommended that the diagnosis of major depressive episode be made and treatment initiated if symptoms of a major depressive episode are present 2 months after the bereavement (Depression Guideline Panel 1993a). A 10-patient, uncontrolled efficacy study found that 4 weeks of desipramine produced moderate to marked improvement in 70% of the depressed spouses (Jacobs et al. 1987).

Recurrent Major Depression

After an acute depression, a patient should be symptom free for at least 16 weeks before discontinuing TCA treatment. Patients experiencing an acute depression who are not placed on **continuation TCA therapy** have a mean relapse rate of 50% (Prien and Kupfer 1986). Between 50% and 85% of patients experiencing their first episode of major depression will have at least one subsequent episode in their lifetime. Additionally, approximately 50% of these patients will relapse within 2 years, with the greatest risk of relapse occurring within 4 to 6 months of the initial remission. Many of the relapses are the result of early discontinuation of antidepressant medication. Finally, 15%–20% of patients with recurrent depression do not fully recover from any given episode (Prien and Kupfer 1986). Thus, a significant number of depressed patients require **preventive maintenance treatment.** Numerous factors have been associated with an increased risk of recurrence in patients with unipolar illness: the presence of another mental disorder and/or a chronic medical condition, chronic affective symptoms, an older age at onset for the first episode, severe functional impairment while depressed, psychotic affective episodes, a previous serious suicide attempt, and a positive family history for suicide and/or bipolar illness (Consensus Development Panel 1985). If several of these risk factors are present, serious consideration should be given to providing maintenance treatment with either a TCA or lithium. Whereas TCAs and lithium are equally effective in preventing recurrent unipolar illness, lithium is more effective than TCAs in preventing recurrent bipolar illness (Consensus Development Panel 1985). Based on these data, the World Health Organization currently recommends that prophylactic treatment be started in unipolar depression after three episodes, particularly if the episode immediately preceding the present one occurred within the last

5 years. In bipolar illness, prophylactic treatment should be started after the second affective episode (Angst 1981).

Dysphoria With Schizophrenia

It has been determined that early recognition of decompensation in schizophrenic patients is possible and that this clinical strategy can reduce rehospitalization rates (Heinrichs et al. 1985). Prior to decompensation, schizophrenic patients experience a prodromal symptom phase characterized by symptoms of dysphoria, anorexia, insomnia, decreased concentration, and social withdrawal. When patients present with the relapse prodrome, it is important that the depressive symptoms not be treated with antidepressants drugs. Studies consistently demonstrate that the addition of a TCA to the medication regimen of a patient with chronic schizophrenia either has no advantage over antipsychotic treatment alone or can actually result in a worsening of the patient's thought disorder (Kramer et al. 1989; Prusoff et al. 1979). However, unlike the TCAs, the SSRIs, which have no catecholamine agonist activity, may be of benefit in schizophrenic patients (Goff et al. 1995; Spina et al. 1994). Adding an SSRI to a patient's antipsychotic regimen improves negative symptoms without affecting positive symptoms.

Depression With Medical Illness

Depression presenting in the medically ill may represent 1) a *major depressive episode* independent of the medical condition; 2) an *adjustment disorder with depressed mood,* in which the stress of the medical illness precipitates a depressed mood; 3) *secondary depression due to the medical condition,* in which the medical illness precedes the depression and is felt to have an etiological (pathophysiological) relationship to it; 4) *substance-induced depression,* in which alcohol, a drug, or prescription medication produces a depressed mood; or 5) depressive symptoms that are a normal response to being severely ill. These possibilities can be considered under two basic categories: organic mood disorders and secondary depression.

Organic Mood Disorders

Alzheimer's disease.   Studies report that the frequency of depression in Alzheimer's patients ranges from 17% to 31% (Alexopoulos and Abrams 1991). In an 8-week course of subtherapeutic doses of imipramine (mean dose 83 mg/day, total imipramine plasma concentration 119 ng/mL) and placebo, both treatments produced significant improvement in depressed Alzheimer's patients. The CNS anticholinergic effects of the TCA did not affect cognitive functioning (i.e., Mini-Mental Status Examination [MMSE] scores) in the patients (Reifler et al. 1989). Moderate depression in Alzheimer's disease patients appears treatable. It is difficult to judge the significance of this study, given that the adverse-effect profile of the investigators' choice of antidepressant precluded dosing into a therapeutic range.

Epilepsy. Depression is common among individuals with epilepsy. Endogenous depression was reported in 11% of epileptic outpatients, with 30% of these patients describing previous suicide attempts (Mendez et al. 1986). A 6-week controlled trial demonstrated that amitriptyline 75 mg/day and nomifensine 75 mg/day were effective in the treatment of epileptic patients with major depression (Robertson and Trimble 1985). Because of the common occurrence of antidepressant–anticonvulsant drug interactions, it is preferable to confine the selection of antidepressants to those agents for which it is possible to measure therapeutic blood levels.

Multiple sclerosis. Estimates of the prevalence of major depressive episodes in multiple sclerosis patients range from 40% to 70%. This figure is greater than the rate of depression among patients with similar disabling diseases such as amylotrophic lateral sclerosis, temporal lobe epilepsy, spinal cord disorders, and muscular dystrophy (Joffe et al. 1987). A 5-week course of desipramine at doses producing serum concentrations between 125 and 200 ng/mL was moderately effective in ameliorating symptoms of major depression in 86% of patients with multiple sclerosis, in contrast to only 43% of multiple sclerosis patients treated with placebo (Schiffer and Wineman 1990).

Stroke. It was observed that 18% of stroke patients experienced a major depression within 2 months following the stroke (Morris et al. 1990). Two controlled, double-blind trials have documented the effectiveness of antidepressant therapy (i.e., nortriptyline dosages to 100 mg/day and trazodone to 200 mg/day) in dysthymic and depressed poststroke patients (Lipsey et al. 1984; Reding et al. 1986). Antidepressant pharmacotherapy is therefore indicated in patients with a recent stroke who meet the criteria for a major depressive episode.

Secondary Depression With Medical Illness

Cancer. Forty-two percent of patients with cancer experienced major depression; 24% were judged severely depressed. The highest rates occurred in patients with advanced cancer and greater degrees of discomfort and disability (Bukberg et al. 1984). There are as yet no controlled studies documenting the effectiveness of antidepressants in treating the depression of cancer patients. However, it is generally agreed that such depressions should be diagnosed and treated (Depression Guideline Panel 1993a).

Chronic obstructive pulmonary disease.   Estimates of the comorbidity of chronic obstructive pulmonary disease (COPD) and depression exceed 20% (Borson et al. 1992). A controlled trial using nortriptyline 1 mg/kg/day significantly reduced depressive symptoms in a group of 30 severely depressed COPD patients (Borson et al. 1992). Nortriptyline did not affect pulmonary function tests or symptoms of shortness of breath during either day-to-day activities or structured exercise.

Diabetes mellitus.   Although depression is approximately three times more prevalent in diabetic patients than in the general population, it is recognized and treated in less than one-third of such patients. A randomized, controlled trial in 60 insulin-dependent diabetic patients with significant depressive symptoms and diabetic neuropathies found that a 10-week course of imipramine or amitriptyline 100 mg/day was effective in reversing both disorders (Turkington 1980).

Fibromyalgia.   Fibromyalgia is a form of nonarticular rheumatism characterized by diffuse musculoskeletal pain. Major affective disorder occurred in 71% of a group of fibromyalgia patients versus 13% of a rheumatoid arthritis group and 12% of an affective-illness control group (Hudson et al. 1985). However, a controlled 6-week trial found that fluoxetine 20 mg/day was ineffective in reducing either the depressive symptoms or the signs and symptoms of fibromyalgia (Wolfe et al. 1994).

Human immunodeficiency virus seropositivity.   It is estimated that only 4%–14% of human immunodeficiency virus (HIV)–positive patients meet criteria for major depression, a rate similar to that in the general population. A 6-week controlled trial of imipramine (mean 241 mg/day) was effective in 74% of trial completers, whereas placebo was effective in only 26% (Rabkin et al. 1994). There was no difference in the depression response rate of patients with more-severe versus less-severe immunodeficiency, nor was there a difference in the medication dose required or the incidence of adverse drug reactions (ADRs).

Myocardial infarction.   Because of ADRs such as cardiac conduction disturbances, tachycardia, and orthostatic hypotension, TCAs are contraindicated in the first 6 weeks after a myocardial infarction (MI) (Kavan et al. 1991). It has now been found that depression that occurs during hospitalization for an MI is a significant predictor of 18-month post-MI cardiac mortality. The mortality risk associated with depression is greatest among patients with more than 9 premature ventricular contractions (PVCs) per hour. This finding is compatible with the literature suggesting an arrhythmic mechanism as the link between psychological factors and sudden cardiac death and underscores the importance of treatment programs for post-MI depression (Frasure-Smith et al. 1995). An estimated 45% of patients admitted for an MI will develop symptoms of major or minor depression within 8 to 10 days (Schliefer et al. 1989). Although no studies have been conducted to evaluate the safety and efficacy of antidepressants such as fluoxetine or bupropion in the treatment of post-MI depression, these agents appear to have minimal effects on blood pressure, heart rate, and conduction. ECT, despite being considered relatively contraindicated in the first 3 months after an MI, has been used successfully to treat severely depressed patients in the immediate post-MI period. The relationship between depression and increased morbidity and mortality is well documented in both post-MI patients and coronary artery disease patients without MI; hence, the practitioner is advised to treat major depression when it is present in this patient population.

Postpartum depression.   Postpartum depression affects approximately 10%–15% of all childbearing women (Butler and Leonard 1986; Wisner and Wheeler 1994). A 6-week course of 150 mg/ day of nomifensine, an antidepressant no longer available in the United States, was effective in reversing postpartum depressive symptoms (Butler and Leonard 1986). Additionally, prophylactic nortriptyline dosages up to 75 mg/day were successful in preventing recurrence of depression in postpartum patients with a previous history of postpartum affective illness (Wisner and Wheeler 1994). Whereas untreated patients experienced a 63% recurrence rate, the rate was only 7% for treated patients.

■ Mechanism of Action

Animal models demonstrate that a 2- to 3-week exposure to any of the somatic treatments for depression results in the downregulation of β_1-adrenergic, serotonin–2 (5-hydroxytryptamine–2 [5-HT$_2$]), and probably 5-HT$_{1A}$ receptors in the CNS (Stahl 1992). This time frame parallels the onset of antidepressant action in patients with major depression. The somatic therapies include TCAs, MAOIs, SSRIs, lithium, and 5-HT$_{1A}$ agonists. ECT has similar effects except that it upregulates the 5-HT$_2$ receptors.

All recent studies of monoamine neurotransmitters in the cerebrospinal fluid (CSF) suggest that a correlation exists among norepinephrine's metabolite 3-methoxy-4-hydroxyphenylglycol (MHPG), serotonin's metabolite 5-hydroxyindoleacetic acid (5-HIAA), and dopamine's metabolite homovanillic acid (HVA). It has been demonstrated that unipolar and bipolar depressed patients who respond to antidepressants and ECT show small decreases in these three metabolites that correlate with each other both before and after treatment. In contrast, metabolite concentrations in nonresponders show no such correlations. This finding resulted from a study involving administration of a heterogeneous group of antidepressant therapies, including desipramine (a norepinephrine reuptake inhibitor), zimelidine and citalopram (both SSRIs), clorgyline (an MAO-A inhibitor), tranylcypromine (a nonspecific MAOI), ECT, alprazolam (a γ-aminobutyric acid [GABA] agonist), and bupropion (a dopamine reuptake inhibitor) (Katz et al. 1987).

Recently, studies of patients who have responded to desipramine and fluoxetine have suggested that there are two types of depression: that due to a serotonin deficiency and that due to a catecholamine deficiency. A worsening of depressive symptoms was precipitated in patients responsive to fluoxetine (an SSRI) by inducing a dietary 5-HT deficiency; this effect was then reversed by 5-HT dietary supplementation (Delgado et al. 1990). Likewise, depressive symptoms in desipramine (a norepinephrine reuptake inhibitor) and mazindol (a norepinephrine and dopamine reuptake inhibitor) responders have been aggravated by creating a catecholamine-depleted state via administration of the norepinephrine and dopamine synthesis inhibitor α-methyl-*p*-tyrosine (AMPT) (Delgado et al. 1993). AMPT did not exacerbate depressive symptoms in a group of patients who were fluoxetine responders. Clinically, these data suggest that therapy can be optimized by treating patients who do not respond to a 3-week course of an SSRI with a norepinephrine-agonist antidepressant such as desipramine or nortriptyline, and vice versa.

■ **Dosage**

The following empirical dosage schedule is suggested for administration and withdrawal of imipramine and amitriptyline, the two most commonly prescribed TCAs. Treatment with either drug is initiated at a dosage of 25, 50, or 75 mg/day administered as a single dose at bedtime. The dosage is increased by 25–50 mg q1–2d until 150 mg/day is reached. If a response is to occur, the patient will usually show significant clinical improvement in anxiety, physical expression of distress, cognitive impairment, and depressed mood within the first week on this dose (Katz et al. 1987). If these symptoms do not improve and there are no medical contraindications or manifestations of toxicity, the dosage should be raised, at a rate of 25 mg/day, to a maximum dosage of 300 mg/day or until the patient either begins to show improvement or experiences intolerable adverse effects.

This dosing schedule is appropriate not only for imipramine and amitriptyline but also for doxepin, desipramine, and trimipramine. However, the dosage must be adjusted downward for both nortriptyline, which is approximately twice as potent as imipramine, and protriptyline, which is five times more potent than imipramine.

Ten to 20 days of therapy usually are required before improvements in mood and affect become apparent to the physician, the family, and the patient. To increase compliance, this delay in action should be explained in advance to patients and their families. Maximum tolerable dosages should be maintained for at least 3 weeks before it is concluded that the medication is of no benefit. The onset of action of antidepressants is a debatable issue. However, most clinicians believe that 3 weeks is an adequate period of time to determine whether the drug is effective. For amitriptyline and nortriptyline, the steepest gradient for improvement occurred within the first week of treatment, and the second-steepest gradient occurred within the second week of treatment (Ziegler et al. 1977). More specifically, 88% of nondelusional depressed patients who responded to TCAs did so within 3 weeks, whereas a similar percentage (90%) of patients with delusional depression required up to 7 weeks to respond (Howarth and Grace 1985).

As previously noted, the acutely depressed patient should remain on the TCA until asymptomatic for at least 16 weeks. At the end of this period, the patient should be titrated off the drug at a rate of 50 mg q3–7d for amitriptyline, imipramine, desipramine, doxepin, and trimipramine; 25 mg q3–7d for nortriptyline; and 10 mg q3–7d for protriptyline. If the TCA is discontinued abruptly, a withdrawal syndrome, consisting of symptoms such as nausea, headache, malaise, vomiting, dizziness, chills, cold sweats, abdominal cramps, diarrhea, insomnia, anxiety, restlessness, and irritability, may occur. All of these symptoms are probably the result of hypersensitized cholinergic receptors in the CNS and the autonomic nervous system stemming from the TCA's potent anticholinergic activity (Dilsaver et al. 1983). If immediate discontinuation of a TCA is imperative and the patient subsequently experiences TCA withdrawal symptoms, administration of an anticholinergic medication such as diphenhydramine will usually reverse the symptoms.

■ Pharmacokinetics

Table 2–1 presents the pharmacokinetic parameters of bioavailability, free fraction, volume of distribution, and half-life for the heterocyclic antidepressants currently available in the United States.

Absorption
The TCAs are rapidly and completely absorbed from the small intestine after oral administration, with peak blood concentrations usually reached within 2 to 8 hours. The presence of food in the stomach does not delay absorption. Although the TCAs are com-

Table 2–1. Antidepressant pharmacokinetic parameters

Drug	Bioavailability (%)	Free drug (%)	Volume of distribution (L/kg)	Half-life (hour[s])
Amitriptyline	30–60	3–15	6.4–36	9–46
Amoxapine	46–82	—	—	8.8–14
Bupropion	>90	20	27–63	9.6–20.9
Clomipramine	36–62	2–10	9–25	15–62
Desipramine	33–51	8–27	24–60	12–28
Doxepin	13–45	15–32	9–33	8–25
Fluoxetine	≈72	5	12–42	26–220
Fluvoxamine	>90	33	>5	13–19
Imipramine	22–77	4–37	9.3–23	6–28
Maprotiline	79–87	12	16–32	27–50
Nortriptyline	46–70	7–13	15–23	18–56
Paroxetine	>90	5	3–28	7–37
Protriptyline	75–90	6–10	15–31	54–198
Sertraline	—	5	—	≈25
Trazodone	70–90	5–11	0.8–1.5	6.3–13
Trimipramine	18–63	3–7	17–48	16–40
Venlafaxine	13	70	6	4

Source. DeVane 1992; DeVane and Jarecke 1992; Ellingrod and Perry 1995.

pletely absorbed, their systemic bioavailability is incomplete because 30%–70% of the drug is metabolized on the first pass through the liver (DeVane and Jarecke 1992).

Distribution

The TCAs are highly lipophilic agents that distribute widely throughout the body, as evidenced by their volumes of distribution, which can reach 60 L/kg. Distribution studies have suggested that these drugs tend to concentrate to the greatest extent in myocardial and cerebral tissues, with less than 1% of the drug present in the plasma. This distribution, coupled with the TCAs' 63%–98% protein binding, explains why hemodialysis and hemoperfusion are inefficient treatments for TCA overdoses. Hemodialysis, despite removing 75%–95% of the offending TCA from the blood, eliminates only 1% of the ingested drug from the body. Thus, hemodialysis and hemoperfusion are not indicated in TCA overdoses (De Vane and Jarecke 1992).

In the blood, TCAs are extensively but reversibly bound to α_1-acid glycoproteins (AAGs). Efforts to relate the clinical and pharmacological effects of the TCAs with their in vivo plasma levels usually have measured the total (i.e., bound + unbound drug) TCA concentration. However, only the unbound free drug is active, and there is a two- to fourfold interindividual variability in TCA free fractions (DeVane and Jarecke 1992). Thus, measurement of free TCA levels would theoretically seem to be clinically advantageous. Notwithstanding, attempts to prove this hypothesis have been unsuccessful. The correlations of free and total nortriptyline concentrations to antidepressant response have been demonstrated to be similar, thereby obviating the need for free TCA measurements (Nelson et al. 1983). It has been proposed that changes in the concentrations of AAGs might result in significant alterations in the equilibrium between free and bound TCAs in medically ill, depressed patients. AAG is highly labile, with changes in concentration associated with a wide variety of conditions, including renal transplantation, liver disease, MI, pregnancy, malignancy, ulcerative colitis, chronic alcoholism, and rheumatoid arthritis (Piafsky and Borga 1977). Thus, in nonresponding depressed patients with concomitant medical illness, it may be advisable to increase the TCA to the maximum tolerable dose before considering the depression to be treatment refractory. However, in medically healthy, depressed patients, there seems to be no evidence that altered protein binding is a source of altered response to the TCAs.

Metabolism

TCAs are metabolized primarily by the liver. The dimethylated TCAs imipramine, amitriptyline, and doxepin are demethylated to monomethylated tricyclics, which are active metabolites. Thus, when one is interpreting a TCA plasma level for a dimethylated TCA, both the dimethylated and the monomethylated metabolites are measured and their values summed to estimate the concentration of active drug (e.g., for amitriptyline, total plasma concentration = amitriptyline + nortriptyline). Hydroxylation of the mono- and dimethylated TCAs by the hepatic cytochrome P450 (CYP) 2D6 enzyme debrisoquin hydroxylase also occurs. Unlike the monomethylated metabolites, the hydroxylated metabolites, although active, are not assayed routinely, because there is no current evidence to suggest that their measurement yields any useful information for the clinical management of depression (DeVane and Jarecke 1992; Nelson et al. 1983). Glucuronide conjugation of the metabolites is followed by excretion of these inactive metabolites in the urine. Because such a small percentage of a TCA is eliminated as active drug in the urine, no dosage alterations are necessary in patients with decreased renal function (DeVane and Jarecke 1992).

Elimination

As suggested in Table 2–1, the elimination half-life of TCAs can vary from 6 to 198 hours. With the exception of protriptyline, the half-lives are approximately 24 hours for the monomethylated TCAs, thus allowing for single daily dosing, usually at bedtime (DeVane and Jarecke 1992).

Sampling

Absorption and tissue distribution of a TCA may take as long as 5–8 hours. Additionally, it is not known how much time is required for equilibrium to be reached between the receptor site and the TCA in the plasma. However, plasma sampling should be carried out approximately 12 hours after the last dose so as to be reasonably certain that plasma concentrations are being estimated during the more stable elimination phase of the drug concentration-to-time profile for the TCAs. TCA concentrations vary significantly in plasma and erythrocytes. Therefore, plasma samples must be centrifuged within an hour of collection to avoid hemolysis. The plasma sample should be drawn after a *steady state* (the point at which the amount of drug ingested daily equals the amount of drug excreted daily) has been reached (usually 1 week). Thus, the time at which the first meaningful sample can be drawn depends on the half-life of the individual TCA. It must be remembered that five half-lives are required to reach steady state. The pharmacokinetic parameters of the TCAs are summarized in Table 2–1 (DeVane and Jarecke 1992).

TCA Concentration Versus Antidepressant Response

An analysis of the TCA blood-level literature was recently reported (Perry et al. 1994). Table 2–2 presents the recommended therapeutic ranges for amitriptyline, desipramine, imipramine, and nortriptyline from this report.

The desipramine data produced the strongest evidence for the existence of a therapeutic threshold. The response rate above the therapeutic response threshold ($\geq$116 ng/mL) was 51%, whereas below this level the rate was only 15%. There was support for a therapeutic range for imipramine (imipramine + desipramine) between 175 and 350 ng/mL. Nortriptyline produced a robust finding suggesting a therapeutic range between 58 and 148 ng/mL. The response rates were 66% for patients within—versus only 26% for patients outside—the therapeutic range. At concentrations of 175–350 ng/mL, the likelihood of response to imipramine was increased nearly twofold, from 39% outside the range to 67% within the range. The amitriptyline data suggested a therapeutic range between 93 and 140 ng/mL. However, the clinical utility of this range becomes doubtful when one considers that only 37% of the amitriptyline responders had a blood level between 93 and 140 ng/mL, whereas 80% of the nonresponders had blood levels outside the recommended range. For the remaining TCAs, there are insuffi-

Table 2–2.   Therapeutic plasma concentrations for tricyclic antidepressants

Drug	Concentration (ng/mL)	Response rate (% in, % out)	Sensitivity, specificity (%)
Amitriptyline (amitriptyline + nortriptyline)	93–140	50, 30	37, 80
Desipramine	$\geq$116	51, 15	81, 59
Imipramine (imipramine + desipramine)	175–350	67, 39	52, 74
Nortriptyline	58–148	66, 26	78, 61

Source.   Perry et al. 1994.

cient data in the literature to reach firm conclusions as to the validity of plasma concentration measurements.

Retrospective Dosing

TCAs follow first-order linear kinetics. Ordinarily, the only terms in the equation that change with an increase or decrease in maintenance dose are the maintenance dose and the steady-state TCA plasma concentration. Thus, as the dose increases or decreases, the steady-state TCA concentration must increase or decrease proportionately. For example, a patient with a steady-state concentration of 100 ng/mL at a dose of 100 mg/day will have a steady-state level of 200 ng/mL if the dose is increased to 200 mg/day; if the dose is decreased to 50 mg/day, the steady-state level would be 50 ng/mL. It must be remembered that the steady-state TCA concentration in this mathematical relationship is the *mean* plasma concentration, not the peak, 12-hour, or trough plasma level. Notwithstanding, this method can be used clinically as a reasonable approximation of the 12-hour steady-state level (DeVane and Jarecke 1992).

Prospective Dosing

Multiple-point method. A standard prospective dosing protocol for the TCAs using nortriptyline has been evaluated (Browne et al. 1983). This method requires administration of nortriptyline 100 mg, desipramine 200 mg, or imipramine 200 mg, with blood samples drawn at 12 and 36 hours. Plasma levels of the TCA are analyzed and the elimination rate constant determined. From these data, R (the daily accumulation factor) is computed. The kinetic data produced can then be applied to estimate the dosage required by an individual patient to achieve a given steady-state plasma level of the TCA. A total of 22 patients were dosed according to this method. The correlation coefficient r of the observed nortriptyline plasma levels to the predicted nortriptyline levels for these patients was 0.94 ($P < .001$) (Browne et al. 1983). Because the calculations can be time consuming, a Microsoft Excel® spreadsheet has been designed to generate a prospective dosing schedule for individual patients. This program is available from the authors.

Single-point method. A mathematical relationship between the drug concentration in serum or plasma at steady state and a single drug concentration at some time after administration of a test dose has been described (Slattery et al. 1980). The derivation concludes that a direct proportional relationship exists between the mean steady-state drug concentration and the initial drug dose's concentration at some time. This relationship has been found to exist for the TCA nortriptyline (Perry et al. 1984). The nortriptyline dosing nomogram in Figure 2–1 can be used to dose patients. With this

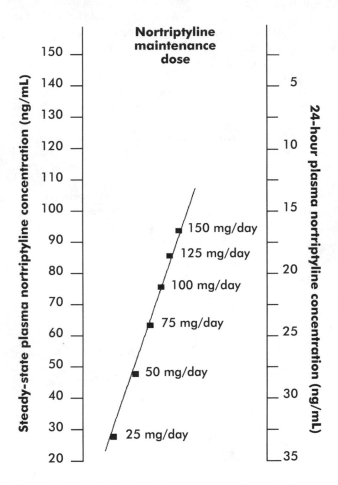

Figure 2–1. Nortriptyline dosing nomogram for predicting steady-state plasma concentrations for 25- to 150-mg/day maintenance doses following a 100-mg nortriptyline test dose and subsequent measurement of the 24-hour plasma nortrip-tyline concentration. The 150-mg/day dose should not be ex-ceeded, because the relationship of nortriptyline plasma concentrations and maintenance doses may not be linear at higher doses.

nomogram, the only information required to predict steady-state doses for maintenance doses of 50–150 mg/day is a plasma nortriptyline concentration measured 24 hours after the administration of a 100-mg test dose of nortriptyline. The sole caveat regarding the use of the nomogram is that a dosage of 150 mg/day should not be exceeded, because the relationship of nortriptyline plasma concentrations to maintenance doses may not be linear at higher doses.

■ Adverse Effects

To estimate potentials for adverse effects, TCAs can be divided into the dimethylated—or tertiary—amine TCAs, which include amitriptyline, imipramine, doxepin, and trimipramine; and the monomethylated—or secondary—amine TCAs, which include nortriptyline, desipramine, and protriptyline. The dimethylated amine TCAs primarily block serotonin reuptake, whereas the monomethylated amine TCAs primarily block reuptake of norepinephrine. Because the dimethylated TCAs primarily affect serotonin and histamine, it is not surprising that these drugs are more sedating. The dimethylated TCAs also are more potent anticholinergic agents, and because of their antihistaminic activity, greater weight gain should be expected. Finally, postural hypotension is less common with the monomethylated TCAs.

Anticholinergic

TCA-induced anticholinergic ADRs of blurred vision, urinary retention, constipation, and dry mouth probably occur less frequently than reported, given that constipation and dry mouth are common complaints in untreated depressed patients. The adverse effects are not necessarily dose related. Usually they are mild and remit after a few weeks, but obviously there are exceptions to this generalization (Davis and Casper 1978; Hollister 1975; Kupfer and Detre 1978).

Blurred vision is usually a result of ciliary muscle paralysis, an anticholinergic effect. This effect, which the patient notices when he or she focuses on close objects, is rarely serious and usually lasts about 1 week. Dosage reduction may be helpful if the blurred vision is persistent or serious. Patients should be cautioned against operating motor vehicles if the vision problem is marked (Davis and Casper 1978; Hollister 1975; Kupfer and Detre 1978).

Urinary retention is most commonly manifested as micturition difficulty or hesitancy because of the increase in bladder sphincter tone and volume of fluid necessary to trigger detrusor contraction. Urgency, increased flow, and incontinence may occur but are probably a result of central as well as autonomic effects. Those symptoms that are related to dose, patient age, and duration of treatment may be helped by bethanechol 10–25 mg po tid or qid (Jefferson 1992).

Dry mouth is reported to occur in 60% of depressed patients taking imipramine, although 20% of placebo control patients also complain of this adverse effect (Leipzig 1992). Nevertheless, at least some of the complaints of dry mouth can be attributed to either anticholinergic or adrenergic effects. This adverse effect can be symptomatically helped by increased fluid intake and by agents that stimulate salivation, such as sugarless hard candy or gum (Leipzig 1992). Therapeutic mouthwashes such as Xerolube®, Moi-Stir®, Sale-ease®, and Slivart® have been developed that not only relieve the painful soft-tissue problem but also remineralize tooth surfaces damaged as a result of salivary deprivation (Leipzig 1992).

Constipation is a complaint of approximately 25% of depressed patients before treatment. After treatment, the figure increases to about 40%. This adverse effect has been attributed to increased anticholinergic and/or adrenergic activity. Regardless of the etiology, constipation is best treated with a bulk laxative (e.g., Metamucil®), hydration, and/or exercise. Some cases of constipation have led to paralytic (adynamic) ileus. TCAs reportedly can also either aggravate or possibly induce a hiatal hernia because of their anticholinergic action on the cardiac sphincter (Leipzig 1992).

The literature regarding the use of TCAs in patients with glaucoma urges caution with closed-angle but not open-angle glaucoma. TCAs can increase intraocular pressure. Thus, the use of TCAs or any anticholinergic medication in patients with closed-angle glaucoma requires the supervision of an ophthalmologist (Davis and Casper 1978; Hollister 1975; Kupfer and Detre 1978).

An in vitro estimation of the anticholinergic potency of the TCAs yielded the following order of anticholinergic activity: amitriptyline > protriptyline > trimipramine > doxepin > imipramine > desipramine > nortriptyline (Richelson 1990). Thus, if anticholinergic ADRs are a problem, switching the medication to desipramine or nortriptyline may be beneficial.

Cardiovascular

The most common—and potentially serious—vascular complication of TCA use is orthostatic hypotension (5%–10% incidence), especially in patients with conduction disturbance (32%) and impaired left-ventricular performance (50%) treated with imipramine and the other TCAs (Glassman and Dalack 1992). This effect is both less frequent and less severe with nortriptyline (Glassman et al. 1983; Roose et al. 1986). Nortriptyline's lower propensity to cause orthostasis is a clinically important finding, given that the risk of hip fractures resulting from falls increases two- to threefold among patients receiving TCAs (Glassman and Dalack 1992). In patients with preexisting first-degree atrioventricular (AV) block, there is a small risk of progressive block. The literature suggests that TCAs are not contraindicated in this population, but TCA concentration and electrocardiogram (ECG) monitoring is required. Patients with preexisting bundle branch blocks have a tenfold increased risk of developing a 2:1 AV block compared with patients with normal ECGs (Roose et al. 1987a). A rational treatment approach in this clinical situation would be to use an SSRI or bupropion in ischemic heart disease patients with concomitant mild or moderate depression and to consider a TCA only in patients who fail to respond. However, a TCA or ECT is preferred in patients with cardiovascular disease who have severe, melancholic depression (Glassman et al. 1993). This recommendation is based on balancing the TCA efficacy against the probable increased risk of mortality suggested by Cardiac Arrhythmia Suppression Trial (CAST; Ruskin 1989) data. Therapeutic doses of TCAs do not adversely affect left-ventricular performance (i.e., do not have a negative inotropic effect). Patients with ventricular arrhythmias (i.e., PVCs) experience improvement of their arrhythmias with TCA therapy, since TCAs are quinidine-like (type 1) antiarrhythmic agents. Thus, the dosage of a type 1 antiarrhythmic such as quinidine administered concurrently with a TCA should be reduced to avoid excessive ventricular slowing. Finally, patients receiving antiarrhythmics (e.g., procainamide, quinidine, disopyramide, encainide, flecainide, tocainide) require close ECG monitoring and may need their antiarrhythmic treatment modified if a TCA is added (Roose et al. 1987a).

Dermatological
Dermatitides include cutaneous vasculitis, urticaria, and photosensitivity. Allergic reactions are more commonly reported with amitriptyline than with imipramine. Skin reactions generally occur within the first 2 months of therapy, are usually harmless, and rarely require discontinuation of therapy (Blackwell 1981; Hollister 1975).

Hematological
Transient eosinophilia may occur in the first few weeks of therapy but is not of clinical significance. Leukopenia is also an apparently

benign and transient effect of the TCAs. Agranulocytosis, although rare, is often fatal (10%–20%). This effect is thought to be a hypersensitivity reaction, occurring usually in the second month of therapy and more frequently in elderly women. Routine periodic white blood cell counts seldom are valuable in predicting the occurrence of this rare disorder. Sudden onset of fever and infection are often the first signs. When agranulocytosis occurs, stopping the medication and beginning vigorous antibiotic therapy are necessary. Nonthrombocytopenic purpura has been reported in two patients, both of whom recovered upon discontinuation of the TCA (Blackwell 1981; Hollister 1975).

Hepatic

Elevations of aspartate aminotransferase (AST), serum glutamic-oxaloacetic transaminase (SGOT), alanine aminotransferase (ALT) serum glutamic-pyruvic transaminase (SGPT), alkaline phosphatase, and even bilirubin are not uncommon during TCA treatment. The origin of these abnormalities may not be the liver. Thus, the liver-specific enzyme γ-glutamyl transpeptidase (GGTP) should be measured to determine whether the liver is the tissue of origin. These findings are usually regarded as benign. However, the TCAs are associated with a hypersensitivity reaction that can result in cholestatic jaundice and, very rarely, chronic biliary cirrhosis. Elevated liver enzymes within the upper ranges of normal are not a cause for concern unless signs and symptoms of hepatic dysfunction are present (Blackwell 1981; Hollister 1975; Leipzig 1992). AST or ALT values three times the upper limit of normal are worrisome, and the TCA should be discontinued if values reach these concentrations (Leipzig 1992).

Metabolic/Endocrinological

Galactorrhea and amenorrhea in women and excessive weight gain in both sexes have been reported. The weight gain is not always reversible on TCA discontinuation, whereas the galactorrhea and amenorrhea are often successfully managed by dosage reduction (Blackwell 1981; Tyber 1975). The weight gain is hypothesized to be a function of the antihistaminic potency of the TCA. Thus, desipramine, the least antihistaminic TCA in vitro, would theoretically be the TCA least likely to cause weight gain. Currently, the only clinical data available to support such a distinction have reported that the antihistaminic TCAs amitriptyline, nortriptyline, and imipramine cause weight gains averaging 1.3–2.9 pound(s) per month (Berken et al. 1984). The TCAs are also theorized to cause weight gain by influencing glucose metabolism via an alteration of hypothalamic sensitivity to glucose (Rockwell et al. 1983). Weight gain can result in noncompliance, discontinuation of treatment, and increases the risk of morbidity and mortality. Thus, if this effect is expected to be a significant problem, it is reasonable to use one of the SSRI antidepressants, because they do not cause weight gain.

Neurological/Psychiatric

Acute organic brain syndrome, or delirium, secondary to the anticholinergic activity of the TCAs is characterized by recent memory loss; disorientation; flushed, dry skin; ataxia; dysarthria; and hallucinations. Treatment with physostigmine 0.5–2.0 mg im, a therapy usually reserved for life-threatening TCA overdoses, can produce complete clearing of this effect within 5 minutes to 36 hours; without treatment, clearing is slower (Perry et al. 1978). It is estimated that 8% of patients receiving TCAs experience anticholinergic delirium. Apparently, increased age, black race, and elevated plasma TCA levels contribute equally and independently to the development of the delirium (Livingston et al. 1983). Anticholinergic delirium is most commonly encountered in elderly nursing home patients who are receiving multiple drugs with anticholinergic activity. Discontinuation of these agents can lead to resolution of the delirium within 24 to 48 hours.

A fine, resting tremor caused by the TCAs has a faster frequency than the pseudoparkinsonian tremor produced by antipsychotics and does not respond to antiparkinsonian drug therapy (Sovner and DiMascio 1978). Theoretically, this tremor, classified as a physiologically accentuated tremor, should respond to propranolol, a β-adrenergic–blocking agent (Jankovic and Fahn 1980).

TCAs can lower the seizure threshold. However, because this effect usually occurs only at high therapeutic doses or in overdoses, the drugs can be given to epileptic patients. In persons with no predisposing medical conditions who are receiving therapeutic doses of TCAs, TCA-induced seizures requiring treatment with anticonvulsants are quite rare, probably on the order of 1 per 1,000 or less (Jick et al. 1983). An exception to this low risk is clomipramine, whose risk is dose related, with a seizure incidence of 0.5% and 2.1% in patients receiving dosages of 250 mg/day or less and 300 mg/day or greater, respectively (McTavish and Benfield 1990).

"Switching" from a depressed to a manic or hypomanic state shortly after starting a TCA has been described, most commonly in bipolar depressed patients (Bunney 1977). This phenomenon reportedly occurs in only 1%–2% of unipolar patients (Wehr and Goodwin 1987). It should be noted that the clinical reality of this

switching process has been challenged (Lewis and Winokur 1982). In one study, discontinuation or dosage reduction of the antidepressant and administration of lithium in treatment-refractory rapid-cycling patients was successful in 37% of 51 patients (Wehr and Goodwin 1987).

The TCAs cause a low incidence of erectile dysfunction, according to an 8-year study by the U.S. Food and Drug Administration (FDA). Imipramine, desipramine, clomipramine, amitriptyline, and protriptyline (in descending order of potency) are the TCAs responsible for causing disturbances in sexual functioning. The problems are reversible upon decreasing the dose or discontinuing the drug (DeLeo and Magni 1983; Mitchell and Popkin 1983). Drugs with cholinergic action appear to correct the erectile and ejaculatory impairment caused by agents with adrenergic-blocking activity. Bethanechol 20 mg po taken 1–2 hours before sexual activity has been reported to reverse protriptyline-induced erectile and ejaculatory dysfunction (Yager 1986).

TCA–MAOI Combination Therapy

A 14-day washout period between the discontinuation of an MAOI and the start of a TCA is advised by many authorities to prevent a hypertensive crisis. Conversely, an MAOI may be started 5–10 days after the discontinuation of a TCA, depending on the TCA's half-life. Concomitant administration of a TCA and an MAOI has been used in patients unresponsive to a TCA and an MAOI administered separately and sequentially. Reports of serious adverse effects—such as hyperpyrexia, seizures, and cardiorespiratory collapse—with this combination have been limited to scattered accounts involving overdoses in which other drugs were involved. It is recommended that all antidepressants be discontinued (5–10 days for TCAs and 14 days for MAOIs) before the combination is started and that, preferably, amitriptyline and phenelzine[1] be administered simultaneously at conservative doses. These can be increased gradually to a maximum of amitriptyline 150 mg and phenelzine 15 mg three to four times per day (White and Simpson 1981). This combination treatment has been shown to be less effective than ECT (Davidson et al. 1978). Medicolegal considerations suggest caution when using this regimen.

---

[1] Originally, isocarboxazid was recommended; however, this drug is no longer available.

Teratogenicity and Excretion Into Breast Milk

Because no increase in the incidence of limb deformities or other major anomalies has been recognized in the 40 years that the TCAs have been marketed, it is quite probable that the use of these drugs during pregnancy is safe. However, common sense dictates that TCA use should be avoided in pregnant women, especially during the first trimester, unless the drug is absolutely necessary for the treatment of the patient's depression (Elia et al. 1987).

Despite receiving relatively small amounts of the drug in breast milk, neonates can be exposed to potentially hazardous TCA concentrations because of the immaturity of their livers (Gelenberg 1987). Thus, it is recommended that TCAs be discontinued close to parturition and that mothers not expect to breast-feed while receiving TCAs.

Some of the following symptoms at birth have occasionally been reported in infants born to mothers exposed to TCAs: urinary retention, nonspecific respiratory distress, peripheral cyanosis, hypertonia with tremor, clonus, and spasm (Elia et al. 1987).

■ Rational Prescribing

1. All of the TCAs currently marketed in the United States are therapeutically equivalent when used in equipotent doses.
2. A rational method for selecting a TCA is to narrow the choice to a dimethylated TCA (e.g., imipramine) and a monomethylated TCA (e.g., nortriptyline) and to make the choice between them on the basis of the patient's sedation requirements and ability to tolerate orthostatic hypotension, weight gain, and anticholinergic adverse effects. The dimethylated TCAs tend to be more sedating and to cause more orthostatic hypotension, weight gain, and anticholinergic adverse effects.
3. The TCAs usually are administered as a single dose at bedtime to take advantage of this group's sedating properties. Protriptyline, an exception to this rule, should be taken in the morning. Single daily dosing increases outpatient compliance, decreases inpatient nursing time required medication distribution, and is more economical because larger dosage forms are employed.
4. Sustained-release or long-acting dosage forms should not be prescribed, because TCAs are inherently long acting.
5. The initial empirical TCA dose is amitriptyline 50–75 mg or its equivalent. The dosage is increased at a rate of 25–50 mg q1–7d, depending on the patient's clinical response and toler-

ance of adverse effects. Dosages for inpatients generally are titrated upward at a faster rate and normally do not exceed 300 mg/day. Measuring TCA plasma concentrations for nortriptyline, imipramine, desipramine, and possibly amitriptyline and then adjusting the maintenance dose into therapeutic range increases the probability of patient response. Therapeutic blood levels should also be determined when a patient is suspected to be noncompliant, is unresponsive to usual therapeutic doses without significant ADRs, or is displaying signs or symptoms of toxicity at usual therapeutic doses.

6. Patients should be counseled that although ADRs may appear within a day of starting the drug, the therapeutic effects may require as many as 21 days to become apparent.

7. A therapeutic trial usually is considered to be amitriptyline greater than 100 mg/day or its equivalent for 3 weeks. Patients who are unresponsive after 3 weeks probably will not respond with longer treatment. Norepinephrine agonists (e.g., desipramine, nortriptyline) should be replaced by antidepressants that are primarily serotonin agonists (e.g., an SSRI, clomipramine) or vice versa. If patients fail to respond to this treatment strategy, lithium augmentation, ECT, an MAOI, or bupropion are reasonable treatment alternatives.

8. To prevent relapse, antidepressants are generally continued for at least 16 weeks after the patient has become asymptomatic. When discontinuing treatment, the dosage of amitriptyline is decreased at a rate of 50 mg/week in outpatients and 50 mg q2–3d in inpatients. For patients with recurrent unipolar illness, chronic prophylactic therapy should be considered.

9. It is appropriate to use TCAs in bereavement reactions lasting longer than 3 months.

Monoamine Oxidase Inhibitors

■ Indications

MAOIs have been used in the management of numerous neuropsychiatric conditions. The most common indication is typical (major depressive disorder) and atypical depression. Additional indications include panic disorder with or without agoraphobia, social phobia, neurodermatitis, treatment-resistant narcoleptic states, recalcitrant migraine headaches, and idiopathic orthostatic hypotension (Tollefson 1983).

■ Efficacy

MAOIs are generally not considered to be as effective as TCAs in the treatment of major (typical) depression. However, this is a tenuous generalization, because the early efficacy studies often used subtherapeutic or borderline-therapeutic dosages. Also, the MAOIs' onset of action might be slower than the TCAs', and too short a therapeutic trial was often used in treating endogenous depression.

Major Depression

A recent meta-analysis of antidepressant efficacy studies calculated MAOI response rates in an intent-to-treat sample (i.e., all patients randomized to treatment) (Depression Guideline Panel 1993b). The MAOI response rate—53% for inpatients and 57% for outpatients—was similar to the response rates of TCAs, SSRIs, and heterocyclic antidepressants. The inpatient and outpatient response rates were 18% and 31% better, respectively, than the placebo rate. Thus, it cannot be generalized that MAOIs are less effective than any of the other antidepressants in the treatment of *major depression.*

Additionally, MAOIs are a logical therapeutic alternative for the treatment of patients who have failed to respond to an initial course of TCA treatment. In five studies (Georgotas et al. 1983; McGrath et al. 1987; Nolen et al. 1988a; Pare 1985; Quitkin et al. 1981), MAOIs were effective in 65% (96 of 147) of *treatment-refractory depressed patients.* This response rate is comparable to the rates reported for all other somatic treatments for refractory depression. The response rate of patients treated with phenelzine for delusional or *psychotic depression* is low (21%) (Janicak et al. 1988). The MAOI tranylcypromine is an effective treatment for *bipolar depression,* which is usually not responsive to TCAs (Himmelhoch et al. 1982). A controlled 4-week trial in bipolar depressed patients reported an 81% (21 of 26) response rate for tranylcypromine versus a 48% (10 of 21) response rate for imipramine (Himmelhoch et al. 1991). A study of imipramine and tranylcypromine *treatment–refractory depression* in which patients were crossed over to the other medication midway through the investigation yielded response rates of 75% (9 of 12) for tranylcypromine and 25% (1 of 4) for imipramine (Thase et al. 1992).

Atypical Depression

Atypical depressions have been characterized in various ways, with the following criteria typical of most definitions: 1) presence of frequent and persistent depression with retained emotional reactiv-

ity to outside stimuli and absence of fixed lowering of mood;
2) features that might be particularly MAOI responsive, including
"reverse" vegetative symptoms (evening worsening of mood, initial
insomnia, increased appetite or weight gain, and hypersomnia),
features of dysthymic disorder, and/or preexisting anxiety, particularly agoraphobia; 3) absence of delusional guilt or manic episodes;
and 4) absence of alcoholism, organic brain syndrome, schizophrenia, or long-standing characterological depression (Nies 1984).

Beginning in 1959, there have been a number of reports suggesting that MAOIs are indicated for "atypical" or "hysterical" depressions. The initial large, open-design study with iproniazid reported
a 59% response rate (West and Dally 1959). Responders were
symptomatically characterized as most commonly presenting with
somatic preoccupations and diurnal mood variation distinguished
by evening rather than morning dysphoria. Marked self-reproach,
early-morning awakening, and weight loss generally were not observed. Improvement after initiation of MAOI therapy appeared
sooner than expected in the atypical group (usually within 5 to
8 days); improvement in the typical endogenous group was rarely as
quick or complete (West and Dally 1959).

Since this initial report, other open studies and anecdotal reports
have made similar observations, although a controlled study did not
appear until 1973. Based on this first controlled study (Robinson et
al. 1973) as well as subsequent studies (Davidson et al. 1981;
Liebowitz et al. 1984; Ravaris et al. 1980), a body of evidence has
developed suggesting that a diagnostically definable subgroup exists
of depressed patients who are more likely to respond to MAOIs than
TCAs. As an example, a 67% response rate to 4–6 weeks of phenelzine 60–90 mg/day versus a 43% response rate for imipramine 200–
300 mg/day has been observed (Liebowitz et al. 1984). This 67% rate
was replicated in 46 atypical depressed patients who were refractory
to a course of imipramine treatment (McGrath et al. 1993).

Dysthymia

Two controlled trials (Harrison et al. 1986; Vallejo et al. 1987)
treating dysthymic patients with standard doses of phenelzine (1 mg/
kg/day) have found the MAOI more effective than imipramine
and placebo. For the treatment of dysthymia, MAOIs should be
considered before TCAs.

■ Mechanism of Action

The MAOIs are postulated to act by inhibiting MAO, an enzyme
responsible for intraneuronal breakdown of catecholamine and

indoleamine neurotransmitters (e.g., norepinephrine and 5-HT, respectively). Inhibition of MAO by these agents is believed to relieve the symptoms of depression by allowing an accumulation of catecholamine and indoleamine neurotransmitters in the presynaptic granules. In turn, more of these neurotransmitters are then available to the postsynaptic neurons, such that the hypersensitive postsynaptic receptor sites return to their normal level of sensitivity. Postmortem studies of elderly patients who died while receiving MAOIs suggest that at least 2–3 weeks are required for the drugs to significantly increase 5-HT (Pare 1985).

Two MAO subtypes have been identified according to their respective substrate and inhibitor specificities. MAO type A preferentially deaminates norepinephrine/5-HT and is selectively inhibited by clorgyline. MAO type B selectively deaminates phenylethylamine, dopamine, and benzylamine and is sensitive to selegiline or pargyline inhibition. With the exception of selegiline, which is used to treat parkinsonism, the currently available MAOIs are not substrate specific. Catecholamine theories of affective illness suggest that a type A MAOI would be specific for depression (Tollefson 1983).

■ Dosage

Some evidence has suggested that the starting dose of phenelzine should be 1 mg/kg/day (Robinson et al. 1973). Other evidence indicates that higher dosages improve the probability of response. Because of the variable stimulating and sedating properties of MAOIs, it is recommended that the dosage be adjusted appropriately to avoid drug-induced insomnia or daytime sedation, which is often seen in patients receiving MAOIs. Usually, the drug is administered on a twice-daily dosage schedule.

An adequate therapeutic trial of an MAOI is 6 weeks. Two weeks of therapy are required before the maximum MAO inhibitory effect of phenelzine 30 mg/day is reached, and 4 weeks are required for a 60-mg/day dosage (Robinson et al. 1978). It is estimated that tranylcypromine 0.7 mg/kg/day is equivalent to phenelzine 1.0 mg/kg/day (Grasso et al. 1991).

When a patient is to be switched from an MAOI to another antidepressant, including the MAOI tranylcypromine, a 2-week washout period is advisable because of the potential risk of hypertensive crisis and serotonin syndrome (i.e., given that 14 days are required for MAO to be fully resynthesized) (True et al. 1985). If the patient is being switched from one MAOI to another, at least a 1-week drug-free interval is advised (Sheehan et al. 1980–1981).

Although the rationale for this recommendation is elusive, its wisdom is based on empirical grounds. Gelenberg (1984) described two patients who, because of ADRs in one and lack of response in the other, were switched from phenelzine to tranylcypromine without any drug-free period. One of the patients experienced a stroke, and the other had a hypertensive crisis (Gelenberg 1984). A case report of a patient who was switched without incident is also available (True et al. 1985).

It has been suggested that the 2-week washout period for MAOIs should also be observed before elective surgery or ECT. However, monitoring of the vital signs (blood pressure, pulse, and temperature) of 13 patients on MAOIs who received 22 ECT treatments did not identify a problem (El-Ganzouri et al. 1985). The authors concluded that "discontinuation of chronic MAOI therapy prior to surgery is not necessary" (p. 595). Notwithstanding, it has been noted that phenelzine may decrease plasma pseudocholinesterase (an enzyme needed to metabolize succinylcholine, which is administered during ECT for muscle relaxation), resulting in prolonged muscle paralysis immediately after ECT (Hansten and Horn 1994).

■ Pharmacokinetics

A positive correlation exists between the degree of platelet MAO inhibition and clinical response for phenelzine and isocarboxazid, but not necessarily for tranylcypromine (Giller 1980). With phenelzine dosages of 60 mg/day for 6 weeks, 68% of patients with more than 80% MAO inhibition responded favorably, and 79% of those with more than 90% inhibition improved. However, the response rate was only 44% in patients achieving less than 80% inhibition, a rate not much better than the placebo improvement rate of 32% (Robinson et al. 1978).

For most depressed patients receiving MAOIs, MAO activity levels cannot be determined because the MAO assay is usually unavailable locally and there are problems associated with shipping platelets to outside laboratories. However, ignorance about MAO activity is seldom a clinical problem, given that in most patients dosages of phenelzine 1 mg/kg/day and of tranylcypromine 0.7 mg/kg/day will usually produce the 80% or greater MAO inhibition necessary to attain an antidepressant response.

■ Adverse Effects

Table 2–3A compares the ADR prevalence for phenelzine and tranylcypromine with that for imipramine and placebo. Although

Table 2–3A. **Prevalence (%) of MAOI adverse drug reactions (ADRs)**

ADR	Placebo	Imipramine	Phenelzine	Tranylcypromine
Hypomania	0	0	10	7
Hypertensive crisis	0	0	8	2
Convulsions	0	2	0	0
Syncope	0	9	11	17
Disorientation	0	3	5	2
Edema[*]	0	0	4	0
Rash[*]	2	2	1	2
Weight gain (>15 lb)[*]	0	0	8	0
Urinary retention	0	3	5	2
Paresthesias	0	3	5	2
Drowsiness[*]	0	0	3	0
Anorgasmia/impotence	0	5	22	2
None	96	71	40	56

Note. MAOI = monoamine oxidase inhibitor. [*] Drug discontinued.
Source. Rabkin et al. 1984.

most of these adverse effects occurred with phenelzine, they did not result in more frequent discontinuation of phenelzine than of tranylcypromine. Additionally, the ADRs could not be accounted for by differences in the subjects' age, sex, diagnosis, or duration of treatment. The mean maximum dosages prescribed were 269 mg/day (imipramine), 69 mg/day (phenelzine), and 50 mg/day (tranylcypromine) (Rabkin et al. 1984).

A comparison of the clinical severity of the ADRs commonly seen with the MAOIs currently used as antidepressants is presented in Table 2–3B (Sheehan et al. 1980–1981). A severe ADR can be alleviated by switching the patient from the offending MAOI to another MAOI less likely to cause that specific ADR. As noted, a 14-day washout period between MAOIs is necessary to avoid any risk of a hypertensive crisis (True et al. 1985).

Allergic
The majority of allergic or idiosyncratic reactions reported with the MAOIs occurred when the drugs were introduced into the market in the early 1960s. Skin rashes, primarily maculopapular, are still occasionally reported. The allergic reactions of red/green color blindness with optic atrophy and hepatotoxicity led to the removal of the causative agents, pheniprazine and iproniazid, respectively.

Table 2–3B. Comparative MAOI adverse drug reactions (ADRs) based on physician clinical experience

ADR	Tranyl-cypromine	Phenel-zine	Iso-carboxazid
Hypertension	5	1	1
Hepatotoxicity	1	5	5
Orthostatic hypotension	1	2	2
CNS stimulation	3	2	1
Sedation	1	2	3
Appetite stimulation	1	3	3
Muscle twitching	2	3	2
Edema	2	3	2
Sexual dysfunction	1	3	2
Urinary retention	1	3	2

Note.   5 = most; 1 = least. CNS = central nervous system. MAOI = monoamine oxidase inhibitor.
Source.   Sheehan et al. 1980–1981.

These reactions are rarely reported with the currently available MAOIs (Kupfer and Detre 1978).

Cardiovascular

Heart rate, QTc interval, and blood pressure.   Phenelzine 60 mg/day decreases the QTc interval of the ECG but does not affect the PR interval or the QRS complex. Heart rate and standing and sitting blood pressures are decreased. Orthostatic hypotension may also occur. Most cases (70%) of MAOI-induced orthostatic hypotension occur within the first 2 months of treatment. The orthostatic hypotensive effects of the MAOIs resolve in the majority of patients and are replaced by significant (systolic blood pressure elevation of ≥20 mm Hg) but asymptomatic and transient (1–2 hours after dosing) increases in blood pressure in about one-half of patients (Keck et al. 1989). Hypotension is also associated with MAOIs. Patients over 50 years of age are more likely to experience declines in standing and sitting blood pressure than are younger patients. As the percentage of MAO inhibition and the phenelzine plasma concentration increase, the standing blood pressure shows a greater decrease (Robinson et al. 1982). Because there is a correlation between dose and the occurrence of hypotension, lowering the dose is helpful in alleviating the problem. Increased numbers of doses during the day or single daily dosing at bedtime may also be beneficial (Rabkin et al. 1985). MAOIs probably affect cardiovascular function largely through a central adrenergic and/or sympathetic ganglionic effect. Inhibition of sympathetic tone by MAOIs accounts for many of the observed effects on heart rate, QTc interval, and blood pressure (Robinson et al. 1982).

Hypertensive crisis.   Ingestion of MAOIs, including selegiline (L-deprenyl) (McGrath et al. 1989), followed by foods containing certain pressor amines or by proprietary drugs containing sympathomimetic agents has been associated with potentially serious hyperadrenergic states, including fatal strokes. The interaction is characterized by severe occipital and temporal headache, diaphoresis, mydriasis, elevation of both systolic and diastolic blood pressures, neck stiffness, and neuromuscular excitation generally occurring within 2 hours of ingestion of the food or drug. Although rare, cardiac dysrhythmias, heart failure, or intracerebral hemorrhage can occur. A retrospective analysis of acute hypertensive crisis in 692 patients treated with MAOIs found that the incidence of this effect was 8.4% before and 3.3% after dietary restrictions were imposed (Bethune et al. 1964). A chart review reported hypertensive crisis incidence rates of 8% for phenelzine and 2% for tranylcypromine (Rabkin et al. 1985).

Tyramine is the pressor amine in foods most often implicated in these reactions. It is produced by decarboxylation of tyrosine, which is derived from protein. Tyramine exerts its pressor action by releasing norepinephrine from the storage sites at nerve endings. The pressor action will be potentiated in patients receiving MAOIs because a greater amount of norepinephrine will be present at the nerve ending as the result of interneuronal MAO inhibition. An 8-mg dose of oral tyramine caused a 30-mm Hg increase in the systolic pressure in 50% of subjects taking tranylcypromine (Shulman et al. 1989). A 25-mg ingestion can produce a severe hypertensive crisis (Blackwell et al. 1967). Other amines and amine precursors such as histamine, dopamine, levodopa, and tyrosine may also be involved in these reactions (Raisfeld 1972). In addition, sympathomimetics such as amphetamines, methylphenidate, ephedrine, pseudoephedrine, phenylpropanolamine, and phenylephrine interact with MAOIs (Ponto et al. 1977).

Aged cheeses are the food most often reported to precipitate hypertensive crisis with MAOIs (67 of 80 reported cases, 84%). Certain *alcoholic beverages* (5 of 80 cases, 6%) and *yeast products* are also reported to produce this effect (Ponto et al. 1977; M. M. Stewart 1976). However, not all types of cheeses contain tyramine in sufficient quantities to cause this ADR. As a general rule, any protein-containing food that has undergone degradation may present a hazard (M. M. Stewart 1976). Therefore, nonaged cheeses such as cottage cheese and cream cheese seem safe, as these contain little or no tyramine. There is disagreement in the literature as to the safety of some dairy products, such as American processed cheese, sour cream, and yogurt. It has been stated that processed cheese products and all fresh milk products (e.g., yogurt, ice cream) that have been properly stored are safe to consume (D. M. Gardner et al. 1996).

Of the alcoholic beverages, in the past it was recommended that patients avoid red wine, sherry, and liqueurs, whereas clear spirits (e.g., vodka, white wine) were permitted. Evidence suggests that no alcoholic beverage contains tyramine in amounts sufficient to cause a rise in blood pressure (Shulman et al. 1989). However, anecdotal case reports exist of hypertensive episodes that implicate all alcoholic beverages and even their nonalcoholic counterparts (e.g., alcohol-free beer) (Gelenberg 1988). Another source recommends that no more than two 12-fluid-ounce cans of domestic beer or 4-fluid-ounce glasses of red or white wine be consumed per day. This advice also applies to nonalcoholic beer (D. M. Gardner et al. 1996). Thus, extreme caution is still the best advice to patients regarding the acceptability of alcohol beverages in the diet.

Yeast/protein extracts sometimes found in packet soups as well as yeast vitamin supplements (brewer's yeast, Marmite) are to be avoided, whereas the baker's yeast contained in baked goods is safe. Unacceptable meats and fish include smoked or pickled fish (herring) and shrimp paste, caviar, beef or chicken liver, and fermented sausages (bologna, pepperoni, salami, and summer sausage). Restricted fruits and vegetables include avocados, canned or overripe figs, and stewed whole bananas or banana peel, although small amounts of banana pulp are allowed ("Foods Interacting With MAO Inhibitors" 1989). Products with fermented bean curd (soy beans, soy paste, soy sauce) contain large amounts of tyramine ("Foods Interacting With MAO Inhibitors" 1989).

There are also a number of *non–tyramine-containing foods* that are not permitted. Broad beans (also known as Fava or Italian broad beans), which contain dopamine, are not allowed, whereas the other shelled beans (e.g., lima beans, string beans) are permitted. Large amounts of caffeine can produce enough pressor activity to cause problems. Chocolate contains phenylethylamine, a weak pressor agent that may be dangerous if ingested in large amounts. Some ginseng-containing products have caused headache, tremors, and mania-like symptoms ("Foods Interacting With MAO Inhibitors" 1989). Monosodium glutamate (MSG) has been associated with complaints of headaches and palpitations (Gelenberg 1988).

After a patient discontinues an MAOI, it is recommended that the tyramine-free diet be continued for at least 1 month (Bieck and Antonin 1988).

Two cases of MAOI hypertensive crisis were successfully treated with nifedipine 10-mg capsules (Clary and Schweizer 1987). The patients chewed, then swallowed the capsules, and within 7 to 10 minutes their diastolic blood pressures had decreased by 96 mm Hg and 84 mm Hg. Rather than having patients go to the emergency room to receive phentolamine 5 mg iv, it seems far more practical to have patients carry nifedipine on their persons and treat themselves immediately at the onset of paroxysmal throbbing headache. The antihypertensive effect of nifedipine lasts 4–6 hours.

The most effective prophylaxis is to convince the patient that adherence to dietary restrictions is mandatory. Informed consent, phrased in the following terminology, is also recommended:

> A medically serious side effect can occur after eating the wrong food or taking medicines that are on the restricted list . . . it starts with palpitations, severe headaches and increase in blood pressure. If severe and not treated, it is conceivable that a stroke could develop. (Rabkin et al. 1985, p. 5)

Patient information such as the MAOI monograph contained in Chapter 13 [page 672] should be given to patients as well.

Neurological
Pyridoxine deficiencies secondary to phenelzine have been reported to result in peripheral sensory neuropathies (J. W. Stewart et al. 1984). Patients had low pyridoxine levels, and all patients' symptoms responded to pyridoxine 150–300 mg/day within several weeks. MAOIs at both therapeutic and toxic doses are known to produce neuromuscular effects ranging from muscle tension and muscle twitches to forceful myoclonic jerks. If untreated, pyridoxine deficiency can result in numerous neurological symptoms, including peripheral neuropathy, ataxia, hyperacusis, hyperirritability, muscle tension, myoclonic jerks, depression, carpal tunnel syndrome, and—in extreme cases—seizures, coma, and death.

Anorgasmia and/or impotence were the most frequently reported ADRs with phenelzine; these effects occurred at a median dosage of 75 mg/day after 7–8 weeks of treatment and were more common in male patients (Rabkin et al. 1984, 1985). Sexual-dysfunction ADRs were much less common with tranylcypromine. For some patients, the reaction abates over time; for others, dosage reduction is helpful; and for still others, the use of cyproheptadine 1–4 mg at bedtime has been an effective treatment (DeCastro 1985). Additionally, ejaculatory dysfunction might be responsive to bethanechol 10 mg taken 30 minutes before sexual activity (Segraves 1987); this treatment has been successful for imipramine-induced ejaculatory dysfunction.

Phenelzine and tranylcypromine have been reported to cause severe daytime drowsiness in a small number of patients. Caffeine and vigorous exercise are not helpful. Tolerance to this effect can eventually develop despite its persisting for months. It is suggested that hypersomnolent bipolar depressed patients are at greatest risk for this side effect. The substitution of isocarboxazid is effective in some patients (Teicher et al. 1988). On the other hand, MAOI-induced insomnia is estimated to occur in 4%–17% of patients. Trazodone 50–200 mg/day was effective in treating this problem in 12 of 13 affected patients (Nierenberg and Keck 1989).

Psychiatric
"Switching" from depressive to a manic state, similar to what is observed with the TCAs, may also occur with the MAOIs. The prevalence of this effect is reported as 10% for phenelzine, 7% for tranylcypromine, and 0% each for imipramine or placebo (Rabkin et al. 1985). Bipolar patients are more likely than nonbipolar patients to develop hypomania while receiving MAOIs (Rabkin et al. 1985). Management includes MAOI dosage reduction or lithium augmentation after the fact or lithium prophylaxis before the fact when MAOIs are used in patients with bipolar illness or with positive bipolar family histories.

Withdrawal Reactions
In rare cases, abrupt discontinuation of an MAOI can result in withdrawal symptoms. Two patients who discontinued their phenelzine dosage regimens (45 mg/day for 7 years, 90 mg/day for 5 months) had vivid and frightening dreams for 2–10 nights (Joyce and Walshe 1983). Additionally, patients may experience acute delirium upon discontinuation: one patient had hallucinations and delusions after discontinuing phenelzine, another became catatonic (Liskin et al. 1985) upon phenelzine withdrawal, and a third became delirious and agitated after withdrawal from tranylcypromine (Absher and Black 1988).

Teratogenicity and Excretion Into Breast Milk

The Collaborative Perinatal Project monitored 21 mother-child pairs exposed to MAOIs, of which 13 were exposed to tranylcypromine, 3 were exposed to phenelzine, and 1 was exposed to isocarboxazide during the first trimester (Heinonen et al. 1977). Although an increased risk of malformation was found, details of the cases are unavailable.

■ Rational Prescribing

1. Patients started on MAOIs are placed on tyramine-restricted diets and must not take any proprietary cold preparations containing indirect-acting sympathomimetics, such as phenylephrine, phenylpropanolamine, or ephedrine. Patients may take asthma preparations that contain epinephrine, a direct-acting sympathomimetic. Patients should be instructed to stay on their tyramine-free diet for 3–4 weeks if the MAOI is discontinued.

2. If stimulating, the MAOI dose should be given by 5 P.M. to avoid insomnia. However, if sedating, the majority of the daily dose should be given at bedtime.

3. When switching a patient from one MAOI to another, a washout period of at least 10 days is required to avoid the potential risk of hypertensive crisis.

4. Like TCAs, the MAOIs are best continued prophylactically until the patient has been asymptomatic for at least 16 weeks; this strategy reduces the possibility of relapse.

Selective Serotonin Reuptake Inhibitors

■ Indications

Four SSRIs have been marketed in the United States since 1988: fluoxetine, sertraline, paroxetine, and fluvoxamine. The primary indication for the use of SSRIs is *major depressive disorder.* However, like the TCAs, the SSRIs are also effective in the treatment of the *anxiety disorders,* including panic disorder with or without agoraphobia, obsessive-compulsive disorder, simple and social phobias, posttraumatic stress disorder, and generalized anxiety disorder (Feighner and Boyer 1991). In addition, SSRIs are effective in *eating disorders.* Fluoxetine and sertraline produce dose-dependent weight loss in nondepressed obese patients (Feighner and Boyer 1991). Fluoxetine reduced bingeing and purging episodes in patients with bulimia nervosa (Goldbloom and Olmsted 1993).

SSRIs are of potential value in the treatment of *drug abuse.* Fluoxetine reduced alcohol consumption in both alcoholic patients and heavy social drinkers (Gorelick and Paredes 1992). Fluoxetine has decreased amphetamine and cocaine ingestion in animal studies (Carroll et al. 1990). The severity of nicotine withdrawal was reduced by fluoxetine (Feighner and Boyer 1991). Fluoxetine also reduces impulsive and aggressive behavior in patients with *borderline personality disorder* (Norden 1989; Salzman et al. 1995) and is effective in treating the symptoms of *premenstrual tension syndrome* (Steiner et al. 1995; Wood et al. 1992). In contrast to amitriptyline and desipramine, fluoxetine was not effective as an *analgesic* in relieving the pain of diabetic neuropathy (Max et al. 1992). On the other hand, fluoxetine was effective in preventing migraine headaches (Adly et al. 1992). Fluoxetine was not effective in decreasing obsessional thinking and compulsive behavior in Tourette's syndrome patients (Kurlan et al. 1993).

■ Efficacy

Major Depression

A recent meta-analysis of antidepressant efficacy studies calculated SSRI response rates in an intent-to-treat sample (Depression Guideline Panel 1993b). The response rate was 54% for inpatients and 47% for outpatients, which was similar to the TCA, MAOI, and heterocyclic antidepressant response rates. The inpatient response rate for SSRIs was 26% better than that for placebo, whereas the outpatient response rate for SSRIs was 20% better than the placebo rate. Thus, the SSRIs are as effective as the other classes of antidepressants in the treatment of *major depression.*

SSRIs provide a potential therapeutic alternative for patients with *TCA-refractory depression.* On the basis of data from several trials in TCA treatment–refractory, depressed patients, fluoxetine was effective in 50%–60% (Beasley et al. 1990a), paroxetine in 64% (23 of 36) (Gagiano et al. 1989; Peselow et al. 1989), and fluvoxamine in only 4% (2 of 56) of patients (Nolen et al. 1988b). Of 55 patients who failed to respond to an initial trial of an SSRI, 51% (28 of 55) experienced a marked or complete remission following substitution of a second SSRI (Joffe et al. 1996). In a 5-week trial of fluoxetine combined with perphenazine, 73% of 30 patients with *psychotic depression* responded to the treatment (Rothschild et al. 1993), and a 21-day trial of paroxetine combined with haloperidol or zotepine was effective in 57% of patients (Wolfersdorf et al. 1995). Additionally, a 6-week course of fluvoxamine alone was effective in 84% (48 of 57) of patients with delusional depression (Gatti et al. 1996). The SSRIs are also effective in preventing *relapses of depression.* A yearlong prophylaxis study demonstrated reduced relapse rates favoring fluoxetine (26%) over placebo (57%) (Montgomery et al. 1988). Sertraline administered prophylactically for 44 weeks to 480 patients resulted in a relapse rate of 13%, in contrast to a 46% relapse rate in patients treated with placebo (Doogan and Caillard 1992). Another 1-year study found reduced relapse rates favoring paroxetine (43%) over placebo (16%) (Montgomery and Dunbar 1993).

Childhood/Adolescent Major Depression

It has been hypothesized that childhood and adolescent depression is associated with CNS changes in the serotonergic system and, therefore, that SSRIs may be a more appropriate drug for treatment of this patient population (Ryan et al. 1992). Two double-blind, controlled studies have assessed the utility of the SSRIs in the treatment of childhood/adolescent depression. Despite a 50% response rate, the first trial concluded that fluoxetine 60 mg/day was no more effective than placebo (Simeon et al. 1990). Problems with the study included the small number of subjects studied, the high dose of fluoxetine used, and the higher-than-expected placebo response rate. The second trial studied 96 depressed children and adolescents treated with either fluoxetine 20 mg/day or placebo (Emslie et al., in press). The fluoxetine response rate of 56% was significantly greater than the 33% response rate for placebo. Significant drug effects were not apparent until week 5 of treatment.

Atypical Depression

Studies have suggested that SSRIs vary in effectiveness for some subtypes of depression. Fluoxetine produced a 65% response rate in patients with *atypical depression,* in contrast with imipramine's rate of only 13% (Reimherr et al. 1984). However, some studies suggest that SSRIs may be less effective than the TCAs in the treatment of patients with the *melancholic* subtype of depression (Perry 1996). In one study, the remission rate for clomipramine was 60%, versus only 30% for the SSRI citalopram (Danish University Antidepressant Group 1986). Likewise, in a nearly identical study, the remission rate for clomipramine was 50%, versus only 25% for paroxetine (Danish University Antidepressant Group 1990). In a group of elderly melancholic depressed patients, the treatment-completer response rate for nortriptyline was 83%, versus only 10% for fluoxetine (Roose et al. 1994). There is one dissenting controlled trial regarding SSRI effectiveness in melancholic depressions: A 71% response rate in depressive symptoms was observed in patients treated with fluoxetine 20–60 mg/day for 8 weeks, in contrast to a 37% response rate in the placebo-treated group (Heiligenstein et al. 1993). The effectiveness of lithium augmentation of SSRI treatment in patients unresponsive to a minimum 4-week trial of fluoxetine has been demonstrated (Bauman et al. 1996). Sixty percent of patients randomized to the SSRI citalopram responded within 1 week of the addition of lithium carbonate 800 mg/day.

Dysthymia

One controlled trial (Hellerstein et al. 1993) treating dysthymia with fluoxetine 10–60 mg/day found the SSRI more effective than placebo in the treatment of dysthymia. It appears that many personality-disorder patients may have been excluded because patients with a history of self-mutilation and suicide attempts were not included. Thus, it is unclear whether an SSRI is effective in treating a dysthymic patient with borderline personality disorder.

■ Mechanism of Action

Serotonin neurotransmission appears to be regulated by at least three serotonin receptor systems. The firing rate of the dorsal raphe 5-HT neurons is controlled by somatodendritic 5-HT_{1A} autoreceptors. The release of 5-HT from nerve terminals is governed by 5-HT_{1B} or 5-HT_{1D} autoreceptors. The nonsaturable enzyme serotonin hydroxylase, which ultimately controls the rate of serotonin synthesis from dietary L-tryptophan, is regulated by 5-HT_{1A} and possibly other 5-HT receptors. Prolonged administration of SSRIs desensitizes the three serotonin feedback systems, causing their regulatory effects on serotonin to be weakened or lost. The SSRIs do not bind to any specific neuroreceptor; instead, they produce their pharmacological effect by blocking 5-HT reuptake from the synaptic cleft, thereby allowing increased 5-HT concentrations to be available to act on one or more types of postsynaptic 5-HT receptors (Briley and Moret 1993).

■ Dosage

A 6-week multicenter trial that compared *fluoxetine* 5, 20, and 40 mg/day reported no significant differences in the response rates (54%, 64%, and 65%, respectively) for the three dosages (Wernicke et al. 1988). A second fixed-dose study comparing fluoxetine 20, 40, and 60 mg/day with placebo again found no significant differences in the rates, which were reported as 53%, 61%, and 48%, respectively (Wernicke et al. 1987). Several studies have investigated the effect of dose escalation on the rate of response to fluoxetine (Dornseif et al. 1989; Schweizer et al. 1990). Patients were treated with fluoxetine 20 mg/day for 3 weeks. The nonresponders were randomized to receive an additional 5 weeks of fluoxetine 20 mg/day or to have their dosages increased to 60 mg/day. After the additional 5 weeks, 50% of patients in both groups had responded. Relatively few patients who fail to respond by week 6 will do so by week 8 (Nierenberg et al. 1995). Thus, a therapeutic trial of fluoxetine is considered to be 6–8 weeks.

The usual recommended antidepressant dose for *paroxetine* is 20–50 mg/day. The drug may be taken once daily either in the morning or at bedtime, depending on whether the drug causes sedation or stimulation in the patient. The initial starting dose is 20 mg/day for 2–3 weeks and can be titrated upward in 10-mg weekly increments. The maximum recommended dose in the elderly is 40 mg/day. Food does not affect the drug's absorption and can reduce gastrointestinal disturbances. A direct-comparison study of paroxetine with fluoxetine found equivalent efficacy with mean dosages of 31 mg/day for paroxetine and 42 mg/day for fluoxetine (DeWilde et al. 1993).

The usual recommended antidepressant dose for *sertraline* is 50–200 mg/day. The drug may be taken once daily in either the morning or the evening, depending on ADRs. The initial starting dose is 50 mg/day for 2–3 weeks, which can be titrated upward in 50-mg increments weekly. It is more cost-effective to prescribe the scored 100-mg tablets. Thus, patients should receive ½ of a 100-mg tablet per day. Food does not affect absorption and can reduce gastrointestinal disturbances. A direct-comparison study of sertraline with fluoxetine found equivalent efficacy with mean dosages of 72 mg/day for sertraline and 28 mg/day for fluoxetine (Aguglia et al. 1993).

The usual recommended antidepressant dose for *fluvoxamine* is 50–300 mg/day. A dose of up to 150 mg may be taken once daily, preferably at bedtime to minimize ADRs. Daytime doses should be taken with food to minimize gastrointestinal ADRs (Grimsley and Jann 1992).

Because of the long half-life of fluoxetine, there is a theoretical concern that excessive SSRI ADRs might be encountered if patients are directly switched (i.e., from one day to the next) to another SSRI. A 2-week fluoxetine washout before starting paroxetine was compared with switching the drugs without a washout period (Kreider et al. 1995). There were no differences between the two groups in the ADRs reported or the number of patients who discontinued medication. Thus, patients can be safely switched from fluoxetine to other SSRIs without an intervening washout period.

■ Pharmacokinetics

Table 2–1 (page 143) presents the pharmacokinetic parameters of bioavailability, free fraction, volume of distribution, and half-life for all of the heterocyclic antidepressants, including the SSRIs.

The elimination half-life of *fluoxetine* ranges from 26 to 220 hours, with a mean of 84 hours; the half-life of its active metabolite norfluoxetine ranges from 77 to 235 hours, with a mean of 146 hours (DeVane and Jarecke 1992). Therefore, 6–7 weeks may be required before steady-state serum concentrations are reached. The same period of time is required to completely eliminate the drug in nonresponding patients. The pharmacokinetic parameters of fluoxetine are not altered in patients with decreased renal function (e.g., Cl_{cr} < 10 mL/minute versus > 90 mL/minute). The rate of fluoxetine elimination is reduced in patients with alcohol-induced cirrhosis (Schenker et al. 1988). Patients with liver disease should be treated with lower dosages (e.g., 20 mg every other day) to minimize adverse effects. The pharmacokinetics of fluoxetine, fluoxetine's active metabolite norfluoxetine, and paroxetine in elderly compared with younger patients indicate that elderly individuals develop higher plasma concentrations. However, this is not the case with sertraline (Preskorn 1993). Four studies have investigated the relationship between fluoxetine blood levels and therapeutic response (Beasley et al. 1990b; Kelly et al. 1989; Montgomery et al. 1990; S. P. Tyrer et al. 1990). Two of the studies were unable to find any relationship (Beasley et al. 1990b; Kelly et al. 1989). However, one observed a negative correlation between norfluoxetine concentrations and therapeutic response (Montgomery et al. 1990), and another noted that patients with high ratios of fluoxetine to norfluoxetine were more likely to respond than were patients with low ratios (S. P. Tyrer et al. 1990).

The elimination half-life of *paroxetine* ranges between 7 and 37 hours. Like fluoxetine, paroxetine exhibits nonlinear pharmacokinetics (i.e., doubling the dose may triple or quadruple the plasma concentration). Patients with severe renal impairment (Cl_{cr} < 30 mg/minute) and hepatic dysfunction require dosage reduction (Grimsley and Jann 1992; Preskorn 1993). Plasma paroxetine concentrations were measured in 94 depressed patients. Steady-state concentrations ranged from 1 to 190 ng/mL, with 90% of the responders and nonresponders having plasma concentrations of less than 110 ng/mL. No correlations were found between clinical response or adverse effects and the drug concentrations in the plasma (Tasker et al. 1989).

The mean elimination half-life of *sertraline* is 26 hours, whereas its less active (5–10 times) demethylated metabolite's mean half-life is 66 hours. Unlike fluoxetine and paroxetine, sertraline exhibits linear pharmacokinetics (i.e., doubling the dose doubles the plasma concentration). Because less than 1% of the drug is excreted unchanged in the urine, dose reduction is not necessary in patients with renal failure. Ingestion with food results in plasma concentrations that are 32% greater than concentrations observed in the fasting state (Grimsley and Jann 1992). No studies are currently available examining the relationship of sertraline blood levels to therapeutic response.

The mean elimination half-life of *fluvoxamine* in depressed patients is 23 hours. The drug has no active metabolites. Most clinical trials have reported a lack of any correlation between plasma fluvoxamine concentration and therapeutic response. However, one unreplicated study found that steady-state fluvoxamine plasma concentrations between 160 and 200 ng/mL were more likely to be associated with a beneficial clinical response than were higher or lower levels (Nathan et al. 1990).

■ Adverse Effects

Because the SSRIs have no effect on muscarinic, histaminic, and adrenergic receptors, their ADR profile differs considerably from those of the TCAs and the MAOIs. Anticholinergic ADRs, orthostatic hypotension, and weight gain are not observed with SSRIs. Table 2–4 presents the ADR profiles for this group. These data are based on controlled clinical trials rather than on postmarketing surveillance reports. Despite there being some variation in the ADR frequencies, we remain unconvinced that there are any significant clinical differences in the ADR profiles of the four SSRIs. Two trials that contrasted the efficacy of fluoxetine with that of paroxetine and of sertraline were able to identify some differences in the ADR profiles of the three SSRIs. One study found that fluoxetine caused more agitation, anxiety, and insomnia ADRs than did sertraline (Aguglia et al. 1993). A second trial found more respiratory and dermatological ADRs with fluoxetine than with paroxetine (DeWilde et al. 1993). The most common SSRI ADRs are associated with the autonomic nervous system, the CNS, and the gastrointestinal tract.

Table 2–4. Common adverse drug reactions (ADRs) (%) associated with SSRI antidepressants

(handwritten note: Nefazodone)

ADR	Placebo[a] (n = 182)	Fluoxetine[a] (n = 2,938)	Fluvoxamine[b] (n = 222)	Paroxetine[c] (n = 2,683)	Sertraline[d] (n = 1,902)
Autonomic nervous system					
Dizziness	6	8 (n = 813)	14	12	14
Dry mouth	7	11	26	18	16
Sweating	5	9	11	12	8 (n = 861)
Central nervous system					
Anxiety/agitation	11	13	16	8	11
Drowsiness	3	11 (n = 813)	26	21	10
Headache	22	19	22	19	18
Insomnia	7	16	15	14	15
Tremor	4	11	11	10	12
Gastrointestinal					
Anorexia	2	13 (n = 813)	15	4	3 (n = 861)
Diarrhea	7	12	6	11	15
Nausea	11	23	37	27	21

Note. SSRI = selective serotonin reuptake inhibitor. [a] G. L. Cooper 1988; [b] Benfield and Ward 1986; [c] Dunbar 1989; [d] Doogan 1991.

Cardiovascular

There is no theoretical basis for the suspicion that the SSRIs are cardiotoxic. The most compelling data to support this conclusion are the lack of arrhythmias in overdose cases. In patients without cardiovascular disease, *fluoxetine* has been shown to produce a modest decrease (3 beats/minute) in heart rate. The drug had no effect on PR interval or QRS complex (Fisch 1985). *Fluvoxamine* causes a slight increase in the pulse and in the ECG's R-R and QT—but not QTc—intervals (Benfield and Ward 1986). *Paroxetine* has no significant effect on ECG and blood pressure in depressed patients without cardiovascular disease (Edwards et al. 1989). *Sertraline* has no significant effect on the ECG and pulse in depressed patients without cardiovascular disease (Fisch and Knoebel 1992).

Central Nervous System

The anxiety/agitation, insomnia, and tremor ADRs associated with the SSRIs have been characterized as transient **hyperstimulation or akathisia-like reactions** lasting about 1 month (Lipinski et al. 1989). The estimated incidence rate of these reactions in patients on fluoxetine is 10%–25%. Clinically, the hyperstimulation may be more likely to occur in patients with anxiety disorder–associated depressions whose dosages have been titrated upward too quickly. Slow upward dose titration, dose reduction, and/or a 1-month course of low-dose propranolol (20–40 mg/day) or benzodiazepine are useful treatment options.

A number of case reports have detailed a potentially fatal interaction between the SSRIs fluoxetine and sertraline and the MAOIs phenelzine, selegiline, and tranylcypromine. This interaction, known as the **serotonin syndrome,** consists of a constellation of clinical symptoms and signs triggered by a precipitous increase in CNS concentrations of serotonin as a result of the MAOI's marked inhibition of serotonin metabolism. Signs and symptoms most commonly include confusion, restlessness, myoclonus, hyperreflexia, diaphoresis, shivering, and tremor. Thus, the MAOI should be discontinued for at least 2 weeks before reinitiating therapy with any of the potent serotonin-agonist drugs. Likewise, if a patient has not responded to a serotonin agonist, five half-lives for both the parent SSRI and its active metabolites should elapse before MAOI therapy is begun (Graber et al. 1994). Examination of the SSRI half-lives presented in Table 2–1 (page 143) reveals that whereas a fluoxetine washout could take as long as 2–3 months, a sertraline or paroxetine washout requires only about 2 weeks.

Sexual dysfunction, including ejaculatory disturbances, impotence, decreased libido, and anorgasmia, are associated with the SSRIs. All of the drugs in this class seem equally likely to cause these problems. Yohimbine, cyproheptadine, bethanechol, and amantadine have been used as treatments (Grimsley and Jann 1992). Three-day SSRI drug holidays (from 8 A.M. Thursday to 12 A.M. Sunday) produced improvement in sexual functioning in patients taking sertraline and paroxetine, but not in those receiving fluoxetine (Rothschild et al. 1995). Overall, no significant increases in depressive symptoms were associated with the drug holidays. If the above measures are ineffective, switching to bupropion or tranylcypromine, which are not associated with sexual dysfunction ADRs, might be preferable.

Increases in *suicidal ideation* have been anecdotally associated with fluoxetine (Teicher et al. 1990). However, a meta-analysis of fluoxetine efficacy trials was unable to demonstrate an increased risk of either suicidal acts or of suicidal ideation for fluoxetine or the TCAs as compared with placebo (Beasley et al. 1991).

Fluoxetine, when administered concurrently with *ECT,* does not affect seizure duration or alter stimulus energy requirements (Gutierrez-Esteinou and Pope 1989). Thus, unlike lithium, the SSRIs as well as the TCAs can be administered during a course of ECT treatments.

Withdrawal reactions have been described for all four of the currently available SSRIs. These reactions are most likely to occur with the shorter half-life SSRIs paroxetine, sertraline, and fluvoxamine. Twelve of 14 subjects abruptly withdrawn from a 7- to 8-month course of fluvoxamine developed withdrawal symptoms characterized by dizziness/incoordination, headaches, nausea, and irritability. After discontinuation of the SSRI, symptom onset occurred as early as 24 hours, peaked at day 5, and persisted for more than 2 weeks (Black et al. 1993).

Gastrointestinal

The nausea associated with SSRIs is generally mild, transient, and rarely associated with vomiting. It occurs more frequently with the SSRIs than with either the TCAs or placebo. Fluoxetine-treated patients experience weight loss that is directly proportional to their body weight at the start of therapy. Nonobese patients lost an average of 2 pounds, whereas obese patients lost an average of 7 pounds (G. L. Cooper 1988). Sertraline, unlike fluoxetine, is as likely to cause weight gain as weight loss in patients (Doogan 1991). Long-term use (>6 weeks) of paroxetine is actually associated with weight gain in 9% of patients (Dechant and Clissold 1991). Fluvoxamine was found to cause weight loss in nonvomiting eating-disorder patients (Gardiner et al. 1993).

Renal

Fluoxetine and sertraline can precipitate the *syndrome of inappropriate secretion of antidiuretic hormone (SIADH)* (Blacksten and Birt 1993; Doshi and Borison 1994). This syndrome appears early in treatment and occurs more commonly in elderly than in younger patients. After drug discontinuation, the hyponatremia resolves within 6 days to 2 weeks. Geriatric patients receiving fluoxetine should be monitored for electrolyte changes weekly during the first month of treatment.

Teratogenicity and Excretion Into Breast Milk

Pregnancy outcome in patients with first-trimester fluoxetine exposure was compared with that in two matched control groups receiving TCAs and nonteratogens[2] (Pastuzak et al. 1993). Rates of major malformations were comparable in the three groups and did not exceed those in the general population. However, compared with women exposed to nonteratogens, women treated with fluoxetine tended to have an increased risk for miscarriage (relative risk $= 1.9$; 95% confidence interval $= 0.92–3.92$). The rate of miscarriages in the fluoxetine group (13.5%) was comparable to that in the tricyclic group (12.2%); this rate was 6.8% in the nonteratogen group. The data suggest that the use of fluoxetine during embryogenesis is not associated with an increased risk of major malformations, although women exposed to both fluoxetine and TCAs tended to report higher rates of miscarriage.

Fluoxetine is excreted in breast milk and may produce clinically significant plasma concentrations in the nursing infant, which have been reported to manifest as increased irritability (Isenberg 1990).

Drug Interactions

A number of drug interactions are associated with the ability of the SSRIs to competitively inhibit the liver enzyme CYP2D6, which is responsible for the oxidation of numerous drugs, including TCAs, antipsychotics (e.g., clozapine, thioridazine), carbamazepine, meto-

---

[2] Defined as a medication or environmental agent that, in large studies, has been proven not to increase the baseline teratogenic risk (e.g., acetaminophen, penicillins, dental X rays).

prolol, and flecainide and encainide. Sertraline's inhibition of CYP 2D6 is less than that of fluoxetine or paroxetine (von Moltke et al. 1993). (See Chapter 8 for a summary of the clinically relevant drug interactions associated with the ability of the SSRIs to inhibit this enzyme.)

■ Rational Prescribing

1. All SSRIs are equally effective in treating depression.
2. Fluoxetine and paroxetine have been shown to be effective in TCA-refractory patients.
3. Paroxetine, sertraline, and fluvoxamine have shorter half-lives and are preferable to fluoxetine in situations in which the possibility exists that an MAOI will be used as the second-line treatment (i.e., if the SSRI fails to produce a response).
4. Other available SSRIs may have a faster onset of action than fluoxetine.
5. The SSRIs are expensive antidepressants in comparison with the generically prescribed TCAs.
6. The ADR profiles of the SSRIs are similar.
7. The SSRIs can be administered once daily.

Miscellaneous Antidepressants

■ Indications

The miscellaneous antidepressants consist of amoxapine, bupropion, maprotiline, trazodone, venlafaxine, and nefazodone. All are indicated for the treatment of *major depressive disorder.* Amoxapine is also effective in the treatment of *major depressive disorder with psychotic features* (Anton and Burch 1990). Bupropion is as effective as methylphenidate in the treatment of *attention-deficit/ hyperactivity disorder* (Barrickman et al. 1995).

■ Efficacy

A meta-analysis of antidepressant efficacy studies calculated the response rates for the miscellaneous antidepressants (with the exception of venlafaxine and nefazodone) in an intent-to-treat sample (Depression Guideline Panel 1993b). The overall response rates for amoxapine, bupropion, maprotiline, and trazodone were 55% for depressed inpatients and 62% for depressed outpatients. These findings were similar to the TCA, MAOI, and SSRI response rates (Depression Guideline Panel 1993b). The inpatient and outpatient response rates for the four drugs were 39% and 17% better, respectively, than those for placebo. Thus, the miscellaneous antidepressants are as effective as the other classes of antidepressants in the treatment of *major depression.* These drugs are used as therapeutic alternatives for patients who have not responded to an initial course of TCA or SSRI treatment. A placebo-controlled study found bupropion effective in 63% of TCA-refractory patients (Stern et al. 1983). A 4-week trial of trazodone was effective in 45% (10 of 22) of *treatment-refractory depressed patients* (Cole et al. 1981). A 4-week trial of amoxapine was as effective as an amitriptyline/perphenazine combination in the treatment of *major depressive disorder with psychotic features;* although the combination treatment had slightly better global ratings, these better ratings were at the expense of a higher incidence of extrapyramidal ADRs (Anton and Burch 1990). The miscellaneous antidepressants are effective in preventing *relapses of depression.* Bupropion was equal to amitriptyline in maintaining therapeutic effectiveness in a 6- to 12-month follow-up study (Othmer et al. 1983). Prophylactic administration of maprotiline 75 mg/day to 1,141 patients for 1 year resulted in a 16% relapse rate, in contrast to a 32%–38% relapse rate for patients treated with placebo (Rouillon et al. 1991).

Six clinical studies submitted to the FDA led to its approval of *venlafaxine* for the treatment of depression. The FDA concluded from these studies that 1) venlafaxine is an effective antidepressant; 2) venlafaxine is effective in treating both severely depressed inpatients with melancholia and outpatients with major depression; and 3) venlafaxine is at least as effective as the usual recommended doses of standard antidepressants such as imipramine and trazodone (Ellingrod and Perry 1994).

Nefazodone is more effective than placebo and as effective as imipramine in the treatment of depression, although it is less effective than amitriptyline in treating melancholic depression. The response rates and dropout rates in all trials were comparable for the TCA and nefazodone treatment groups, with the anxiety and sleep disturbance Hamilton Rating Scale for Depression (HAM-D) factors responding best to nefazodone (Ellingrod and Perry 1995).

Mirtazapine is more effective than placebo (Kehoe and Schorr 1996) and trazodone (van Moffaert et al. 1995) and as effective as amitriptyline (Bremner 1995; Smith et al. 1990) in the treatment of major depression.

■ Mechanism of Action

Amoxapine is the demethylated metabolite of the antipsychotic loxapine. Amoxapine and its 8-hydroxy (8-OH) metabolite inhibit synaptosomal uptake of both norepinephrine and 5-HT. However, the inhibitory effect on 5-HT is relatively weak. The second major metabolite, 7-OH-amoxapine, has significant dopamine receptor–blocking activity comparable to that of haloperidol and thus may give amoxapine a degree of antipsychotic activity. Amoxapine has a moderately active affinity for α_1 and D_2 (dopamine 2) and a weak affinity for H_1 (histamine 1) and muscarinic (acetylcholine) receptors (Lydiard and Gelenberg 1981; Rudorfer and Potter 1989).

Bupropion, chemically related to the CNS stimulant diethylpropion, inhibits dopamine reuptake. Unlike the TCAs, bupropion does not significantly inhibit the reuptake of either 5-HT or norepinephrine. It does not inhibit type A or type B MAO or have a significant H_1-receptor–blocking effect in vivo. Postsynaptically, bupropion may downregulate β-receptors and potentiate dopamine activity. The drug has no affinity for α_1, α_2, H_1, or muscarinic receptors (Branconnier et al. 1983; Dufresne et al. 1984).

Maprotiline is a tetracyclic antidepressant with an aliphatic side chain identical to the monomethylated TCAs nortriptyline and desipramine. It inhibits norepinephrine presynaptic uptake across the neuronal membrane, but does not significantly alter 5-HT or dopamine reuptake. This neuropharmacological profile is qualitatively similar to that of the monomethylated TCAs. Maprotiline has a mild affinity for the α_1, muscarinic, and D_2 receptors and a moderate affinity for the H_1 receptor (Rudorfer and Potter 1989; Wells and Gelenberg 1981).

Trazodone is a triazolopyridine antidepressant that is chemically distinct from other antidepressants. It inhibits 5-HT presynaptic reuptake, causes adrenoreceptor subsensitivity, and induces significant changes in 5-HT presynaptic receptor adrenoreceptors. The biochemical actions of trazodone suggest that its antidepressant effect is primarily a result of increased serotonergic sensitivity and decreased adrenergic sensitivity (Coccaro and Siever 1985). It is important to note that the TCAs amitriptyline and imipramine, on a milligram-per-milligram basis, are 6 to 10 times as potent as trazodone in their 5-HT agonistic activity. Trazodone's metabolite, m-chlorophenylpiperazine (m-CPP), is a potent 5-HT agonist (Richelson and Nelson 1984). Unlike the SSRIs, trazodone has a moderate affinity for the α_1 and a weak affinity for the α_2 receptor (Rudorfer and Potter 1989).

Venlafaxine is a potent inhibitor of norepinephrine and 5-HT reuptake and a moderate inhibitor of dopamine reuptake. Binding studies have concluded that venlafaxine has a greater affinity for the imipramine receptor than does desipramine. The drug is weak or inactive at the dopamine and benzodiazepine receptors. It also does not inhibit MAO. Venlafaxine is inactive in inhibiting the binding of ligands to muscarinic, cholinergic, α_1, α_2, and β-adrenergic receptors and is only weakly active at histamine H_1 receptors. O-desmethylvenlafaxine (ODV) is venlafaxine's major metabolite in humans; it is equipotent to venlafaxine in blocking the reuptake of norepinephrine and 5-HT (Ellingrod and Perry 1994).

Nefazodone enhances serotonin synaptic transmission by acting as an antagonist at the 5-HT$_2$ receptor and by inhibiting the reuptake of 5-HT. These two mechanisms in combination may enhance 5-HT$_{1A}$–mediated transmission. In addition, nefazodone weakly inhibits the reuptake of norepinephrine. Nefazodone, although a structural analogue of trazodone, is pharmacologically distinct (Ellingrod and Perry 1995).

Mirtazapine is a selective presynaptic α_2-adrenoceptor antagonist that increases noradrenergic cell firing and norepinephrine release (de Boer 1996). Mirtazapine also blocks 5-HT$_2$ and 5-HT$_3$ receptors, both of which have been associated with deep-sleep–promoting and anxiolytic properties (de Boer 1996). It has a 10-fold higher affinity for central α_2 receptors than for peripheral α_2 receptors (Kehoe and Schorr 1996). Mirtazapine is a potent histamine antagonist, a moderate peripheral α_1-adrenergic antagonist, and a moderate antagonist at muscarinic receptors (Remeron® Product Information 1996).

■ Dosage

The dosage usually recommended for **amoxapine** is 200–300 mg/day. The dosage can be initiated at 150 mg/day and increased in 25- to 50-mg daily increments to 300 mg/day taken as a single dose at bedtime. Doses as high as 400–600 mg/day have been administered on rare occasions. Elderly patients should be started at a dose of 75 mg/day (Lydiard and Gelenberg 1981). The finding that amoxapine has a faster onset of action than do the TCAs has not been consistent. There also have been some reports of a premature loss of efficacy after 6–12 weeks of therapy in some patients (Lydiard and Gelenberg 1981).

Bupropion is instituted at 100 mg bid or 75 mg tid, with doses taken at least 6 hours apart. This dosage may be increased at a rate of 75–100 mg q3d to a maximum daily dose of 450 mg.

The dosage recommendations for **maprotiline** (3.5 mg/kg/day) are identical to those for imipramine, amitriptyline, and desipramine. A daily dose of 150 mg is considered the threshold level for treating acute depressions, and 300 mg/day is considered the maximum dose. The dose can be administered once daily, preferably at bedtime. Additionally, it is recommended that initial and titration dosages be conservative in the elderly, because hallucinations with or without delirium have been reported in patients 60 years of age or older receiving doses of 200 mg/day (Wells and Gelenberg 1981). It has been claimed that maprotiline, like amoxapine, has a more rapid onset of action than the TCAs. However, this claim is inconsistently supported (Wells and Gelenberg 1981).

The initial **trazodone** dose is 150 mg/day; this can be increased at a rate of 50 mg/day every third day to a maximum inpatient dose of 600 mg/day. Many of the patients who do not respond to trazodone are unable to tolerate the drug's sedation, which accounts for its having been prescribed at subtherapeutic doses. Despite trazodone's short half-life, it is preferable to give the entire dose at bedtime to take advantage of the drug's strong sedative action (Georgotas et al. 1982).

The minimum effective dosage of **venlafaxine** is 75 mg/day; the maximum dosage is 375 mg/day. The initial dose is 75 mg/day administered with food; this may be increased to 150 mg/day, depending on the efficacy and tolerability of the drug. When increasing dosage, increments of no more than 75 mg/day should be used, and increases should be at intervals of no less than 4 days. In severely depressed or hospitalized patients, the recommended starting dose is 75–150 mg/day, which may then be further increased over the next 7 days. Patients receiving 300–375 mg/day had the most treatment-emergent ADRs and discontinuations due to study events and the largest changes in blood pressure. Therefore, the usual dosage range is 75–225 mg/day, which appears to be adequate and desirable for most patients (Ellingrod and Perry 1994).

The recommended starting dose of **nefazodone** is 100 mg twice daily. This dosage may be increased by 100–200 mg/day at 1-week intervals based on clinical response and ADRs. The maximum recommended dose of nefazodone is 600 mg administered twice daily. In elderly persons (>65 years old), the recommended starting dose is 100 mg/day (50 mg twice daily). These dosage recommendations should also be followed for patients with severe hepatic impairment, given that the half-life and area under the curve (AUC) of both nefazodone and hydroxynefazodone are approximately doubled. A curvilinear dose-response curve demonstrated that the optimum dose of nefazodone was between 300 and 500 mg/day (Hearst 1993). Other studies have suggested that elderly patients (≥65 years old) may respond to nefazodone doses between 100 and 400 mg/day, although this therapeutic range may be the same as that recommended for healthy younger patients. In clinical trials, the highest dose of nefazodone (600 mg/day) used was safe but was associated with lower response rates than were doses less than 600 mg/day (Ellingrod and Perry 1995).

Most patients in the **mirtazapine** clinical trials were started on dosages of 15 mg/day, increased to 30 mg/day after 1–2 weeks, and then raised to 45 mg/day if needed. Mirtazapine can be dosed once daily, usually at bedtime.

■ **Pharmacokinetics**

Amoxapine is almost completely absorbed after oral administration and achieves peak blood concentrations within 1 to 2 hours of ingestion. It is metabolized in the liver to two active hydroxylated metabolites. The two norepinephrine agonist agents amoxapine and 8-OH-amoxapine have half-lives of 8 and 30 hours, respectively, whereas 7-OH-amoxapine, the dopamine agonist, has a half-life of 4 hours (T. B. Cooper and Kelly 1979). A study of the metabolism of radiolabeled amoxapine recovered 36% as the 8-OH metabolite and 27% as the 7-OH metabolite, with 3% of the drug excreted unchanged (Greenblatt et al. 1979). An acceptable therapeutic blood level has not been established for amoxapine.

Bupropion is absorbed rapidly after oral administration, and serum concentrations peak 2 hours after ingestion. The drug undergoes extensive first-pass metabolism in the liver; less than 1% is excreted in the urine unchanged. Six urinary metabolites have been identified that are less active and slightly more toxic than the parent compound. The drug induces its own metabolism as well as that of other drugs. The half-life ranges from 10 to 21 hours (Dufresne et al. 1984).

Maprotiline is completely absorbed after administration, with peak blood concentrations occurring 9–16 hours after ingestion. The drug is highly protein bound, with 88% being a relatively constant estimate. Its elimination half-life averages 43 hours. Maprotiline follows first-order kinetics, such that dosage increases or decreases are reflected by directly proportional increases or decreases in the drug's blood level. A therapeutic blood level has not been identified. Radiolabeled maprotiline was excreted primarily in the urine (57%), with more than 90% as inactive metabolites. Thirty percent of the drug was recovered in the feces. Maprotiline is metabolized by N-demethylation, deamination, aromatic and aliphatic hydroxylation, and formation of aromatic methoxy derivatives. The N-desmethyl metabolites appear in the blood in greater concentrations than does the parent drug. Maprotiline's volume of distribution is large, estimated to be approximately 23 L/kg (Riess 1976).

Trazodone is well absorbed after oral administration, with concentrations peaking within 2 hours (according to animal data). The drug is 89%–95% protein bound. Trazodone is highly metabolized in the liver by hydroxylation, pyridine ring splitting, oxidation, and N-oxidation, with less than 1% of the unchanged drug appearing in the urine and feces. It is noteworthy that m-CPP is eliminated from the body at a slower rate than trazodone. No data are available correlating trazodone or m-CPP blood concentrations with therapeutic effect. An elimination phase half-life of 7–8 hours has been calculated (Georgotas et al. 1982).

Venlafaxine is quickly absorbed after oral administration and is metabolized extensively in the liver. Food has no effect on either the absorption of venlafaxine drug or the formation of its metabolite, ODV. The mean half-lives for venlafaxine and ODV were 4 hours and 10 hours, respectively. Venlafaxine's mean volume of distribution for all doses was 6 L/kg, whereas that of ODV was 5 L/kg. At venlafaxine dosages between 25 and 75 mg/day, linear kinetics were observed. However, an exponential rather than a linear increase in C_{max} and AUC for the 150-mg dose was noted, suggesting nonlinear kinetics. As hinted by the drug's pKa of 9.4, venlafaxine and ODV are bound to albumins, α-amino glycoproteins, and lipoproteins. However, only 30% of the drug is protein bound. This low level of protein binding independent of drug concentration suggests that drug interactions associated with tissue binding are not expected with venlafaxine. Venlafaxine is extensively metabolized in the liver by a saturable process to one active metabolite (ODV) and two less-active metabolites (N-desmethyl and N,O,-didesmethyl). ODV is 0.2 to 0.33 times as active as the parent compound. Venlafaxine and its metabolites are primarily renally cleared. The urinary excretion profile for 80 or 100 mg of parent drug in five healthy subjects consisted of 1%–10% of unchanged venlafaxine, 30% of ODV, and 20%–60% as the other minor inactive metabolites. Accumulation data suggest that the clearance of the drug at high doses is lower than that with single doses (1.9 L/hrkg), indicating that venlafaxine undergoes saturable metabolism at higher doses (Ellingrod and Perry 1994).

Nefazodone is rapidly absorbed after oral administration, with an absolute bioavailability of 20%. Food delays absorption by 20%. Nefazodone is widely distributed in the body tissues, including the CNS. It is highly (>99%) protein bound, which may cause clinical drug interactions with other medications that are highly protein bound. Nefazodone is extensively metabolized in the liver to three active metabolites—hydroxynefazodone, triazoledione, and m-CPP. At steady state, nefazodone's mean half-life is dependent on dose, varying from 2 hours at 100 mg/day to 4–5 hours at 600 mg/day. No dosage adjustments are required in patients with renal dysfunction. However, because of nefazodone's altered kinetics, caution is warranted in patients with severe—but not moderate—hepatic dysfunction (Ellingrod and Perry 1995).

The bioavailability of *mirtazapine* following single and multiple doses is 50%. Mirtazapine is metabolized in the liver primarily by demethylation and oxidation, with its metabolite, demethylmirtazapine, undergoing conjugation (Kehoe and Schorr 1996). The desmethyl metabolite is three- to fourfold less active than the parent drug; it is not yet known what contribution this metabolite will have on the clinical outcome (Kehoe and Schorr 1996). The average elimination half-life is 21.5 ± 5 hours, with a range of 20–40 hours (Kehoe and Schorr 1996). Mirtazapine is nonspecifically bound to serum proteins and 85% bound in plasma (Kehoe and Schorr 1996). Caution is indicated when administering mirtazapine in patients with compromised renal function or hepatic dysfunction (Remeron® Product Information 1996). Serum concentrations have been reported to be higher in elderly patients, with an increased incidence of certain side effects, such as dry mouth, dizziness, and constipation. Specific dosage adjustments in this population have not yet been suggested.

■ Adverse Effects

Amoxapine
The overall incidence of ADRs observed during clinical trials was similar for amoxapine, amitriptyline, and imipramine when the dosage ratio of amoxapine to these agents was 2:1 (Asendin® Product Information 1981).

▶ Autonomic Nervous System
Anticholinergic ADRs were the most common problems reported by patients receiving amoxapine. The overall incidence was 28%, which was similar to the incidences for amitriptyline and imipramine. Individual incidences included 14% for dry mouth, 12%

for constipation, and 7% for blurred vision (Asendin® Product Information 1981).

▶ **Cardiovascular**

Minor orthostatic decreases in both systolic and diastolic blood pressure occurred in 42% of amoxapine-treated patients, compared with 44% of imipramine- and amitriptyline-treated patients. Dizziness, probably secondary to orthostatic hypotension, was experienced by 5% of the patients receiving amoxapine (Asendin® Product Information 1981). Although no serious ECG abnormalities have been observed, atrial flutter and fibrillation and conduction defects similar to those associated with the TCAs have been reported (Rudorfer and Potter 1989).

▶ **Central Nervous System**

The incidence of sedation for amoxapine was 14%, which was similar to the incidence for imipramine but less than that for amitriptyline (Asendin® Product Information 1981).

Seizures have been reported in patients receiving therapeutic doses of amoxapine (Asendin® Product Information 1981). In overdoses with the drug, seizures are severe and frequent (36%). The estimated prevalence of seizures from TCA overdoses is 4%; the mortality rate from such overdoses is 15% (Litovitz and Troutman 1983).

Extrapyramidal side effects (EPS) noted in clinical trials include pseudoparkinsonism and akathisia. However, amoxapine's inherent clinical anticholinergic action can offset EPS that occur as a result of dopamine blockade. Thus, EPS occur relatively infrequently (Lydiard and Gelenberg 1981).

Tardive dyskinesia has been reported in a patient receiving amoxapine (Lapierre and Anderson 1983). This ADR is predictable for some portion of patients receiving the drug prophylactically over a period of years. Amoxapine-induced withdrawal and tardive dyskinesia account for one-third of all antidepressant-associated dyskinesias (Rudorfer and Potter 1989). Thus, maintenance therapy with this agent is discouraged. Neuroleptic malignant syndrome has been described in a patient taking up to 200 mg/day of amoxapine for 4 months (Madakasira 1989).

▶ **Hematological**

Agranulocytosis has been reported in a patient who received amoxapine 15 g over 57 days. Granulocytes did not appear in the peripheral blood until 15 days after the drug was discontinued (D. J. Cooper et al. 1981; Sedlacek et al. 1986).

▶ **Metabolic/Endocrinological**
Hyperprolactinemia, an ADR usually specific to dopamine-antagonist drugs, has been reported with amoxapine. More pronounced in women, hyperprolactinemia can result in delayed menses, breast engorgement, loss of libido, galactorrhea, and fluid retention (Sedlacek et al. 1986).

▶ **Teratogenicity and Excretion Into Breast Milk**
The teratogenic potential of amoxapine is unknown at this time. The drug is excreted in breast milk; therefore, breast feeding is discouraged (Lydiard and Gelenberg 1981).

Bupropion
Of 28 ADRs recorded in the placebo-controlled studies of bupropion, only dry mouth (14%) occurred in more than 10% of bupropion-treated patients. Objective changes such as in heart rate, blood pressure, ECG, and clinical laboratory values were not significantly different from those with placebo. Of 2,400 patients who participated in preapproval clinical trials, 10% discontinued the drug because of ADRs. The most common ADRs were neuropsychiatric disturbances (3.0%); gastrointestinal disturbances (2.1%), primarily nausea and vomiting; neurological disturbances (2.1%), primarily seizures, headache, and/or sleep disturbances; and dermatological problems (1.4%), primarily rashes. ADRs that occur more often with bupropion are headache, decreased appetite, nausea, vomiting, agitation, insomnia, and decreased libido, whereas those that occur more often with amitriptyline are dry mouth, blurred vision, dizziness, drowsiness, fatigue, tremors, constipation, increased appetite, and nightmares (Wernicke 1985). A follow-up study of 41 patients receiving bupropion prophylactically for 6–12 months found that only two ADRs increased significantly during long-term treatment: dry mouth (4%) and menstrual disturbances (23%) (Othmer et al. 1983).

▶ **Cardiovascular**
No bupropion-induced ECG abnormalities have been reported at therapeutic doses. Bupropion does not cause orthostatic hypotension in patients who experienced significant orthostasis while on a TCA (Farid et al. 1985). It also does not produce a further decrease in the ejection fraction of patients with congestive heart failure (Roose et al. 1987b). However, in one study in depressed patients with cardiovascular disease, bupropion induced increases in blood pressure that resulted in drug discontinuation in an estimated 14% of patients (Roose et al. 1991).

▶ **Dermatological**

Maculopapular lesions and/or pruritus may occur, usually at doses of 300–900 mg/day. The maculopapular rashes clear within 3–4 days after drug discontinuation. Pruritus alone usually clears with a reduction in dosage (Wernicke 1985).

▶ **Endocrinological**

A transient weight loss of at least 5 pounds occurs over a 3- to 6-week treatment period in up to 30% of patients on bupropion. Weight returns to baseline within 6 months (Harto-Truax et al. 1983).

▶ **Neurological**

The relationship between seizure occurrence and bupropion use at therapeutic doses was reviewed on the basis of manufacturer reports involving 4,259 patients. The overall incidence of seizures was found to be 0.80% (37 of 4,259). The incidence rate was 0.44% (15 of 3,395) in patients receiving doses less than or equal to 450 mg/day; for doses greater than 450 mg/day, the rate was 2.2% (19 of 864), a fivefold increase. The length of time subjects had been receiving the dose associated with seizure activity ranged from 1 to 281 days (median 8 days). The risk of seizures associated with the use of TCAs is estimated to be 0.1% in outpatients with no predisposing factors for imipramine dosages of 150 mg/day or less, with an estimated frequency of 0.5%–1% for higher dosages. Risk factors included a history of bulimia, doses greater than 450 mg/day, and a past history of seizures (Davidson 1989).

Bupropion is one of the few antidepressants that does not cause significant sexual function problems in males. Twenty-eight patients with sexual-dysfunction ADRs from TCAs, MAOIs, maprotiline, and trazodone were switched to bupropion. The problems resolved in all but four of the patients, two of whom were diabetic and two who had lifelong impairments of sexual function (E. A. Gardner and Johnston 1985).

▶ **Psychiatric**

In view of the possibility that dopaminergic hyperactivity may exacerbate psychosis, the question has been raised of whether bupropion exacerbates schizophrenia, psychotic depression, and schizoaffective disorders. One report described four patients who variously experienced auditory and visual hallucinations, paranoid delusions, confusion, agitation, and disorientation from 1 day to 3 weeks after starting the medication at doses ranging from 100 to 500 mg/day. The symptoms resolved within 3 to 9 days of discontinuation of the drug (Golden 1985).

▶ **Teratogenicity and Excretion Into Breast Milk**

No reports are available linking the use of bupropion during pregnancy or while breast feeding with adverse effects.

Maprotiline

The incidence of the common adverse effects seen with maprotiline is shown in Table 2–5 (Pinder et al. 1977).

▶ **Autonomic Nervous System**

The anticholinergic adverse effects of dry mouth, constipation, and blurred vision appear to occur with similar frequencies for maprotiline, amitriptyline, and imipramine (Pinder et al. 1977), although in vitro data suggest that maprotiline's intrinsic anticholinergic action is considerably less than that of the two TCAs (Richelson and Nelson 1984).

▶ **Cardiovascular**

ECG abnormalities induced by maprotiline are similar to those observed with amitriptyline, including a lengthened PR interval and a widened QRS complex; however, T-wave changes, sinus tachycardia, and incomplete bundle branch block usually are seen only with maprotiline dosages of 300 mg/day or more. Maprotiline's effect on cardiac arrhythmias is similar to imipramine's, probably because both have a quinidine-like membrane stabilization effect. Postural hypotension is less common with maprotiline than with amitriptyline (Pinder et al. 1977; Wells and Gelenberg 1981).

Table 2–5. Adverse drug reactions (ADRs) occurring during treatment with maprotiline, amitriptyline, or imipramine (150 mg/day for 4 weeks)

ADR	Maprotiline (%) ($n = 368$)	Amitriptyline (%) ($n = 180$)	Imipramine (%) ($n = 81$)
Dry mouth	33	38	22
Constipation	16	24	18
Dizziness/faintness	11	17	15
Blurred vision	12	16	12
Hypotension	9	14	8
Sweating	8	15	16
Nasal congestion	5	11	3
Skin rash	11	5	5
Nausea/vomiting	3	5	10

Source. Pinder et al. 1977.

▶ **Dermatological**

Rashes occur twice as frequently with maprotiline as with amitriptyline or imipramine. These are usually described as small and localized but occasionally as large, exanthemic, and pruritic (Wells and Gelenberg 1981).

▶ **Neurological**

Of the less-common effects, maprotiline-induced seizures have received the most attention. Case reports have indicated that maprotiline, like the TCAs, can cause seizures at therapeutic doses (Pinder et al. 1977; Wells and Gelenberg 1981). In one study, the prevalence of seizures in patients receiving maprotiline was 16% versus 2% in TCA-treated patients (Jabbari et al. 1985).

▶ **Teratogenicity and Excretion Into Breast Milk**

Maprotiline appears in breast milk in concentrations 1.3–1.5 times greater than those in the blood. Thus, breast feeding is not recommended in women receiving the drug for postpartum depression. Dysmorphogenic studies performed in animals have suggested no potential problems (Pinder et al. 1977; Wells and Gelenberg 1981).

Trazodone

The most common adverse effect with trazodone is sedation. Table 2–6 lists other adverse effects reported in more than 1% of patients receiving trazodone (Georgotas et al. 1982).

▶ **Autonomic Nervous System**

The anticholinergic ADRs of dry mouth, blurred vision, constipation, and urinary retention were compared in trazodone, imipramine, and placebo. The incidence of dry mouth was 15%; blurred vision, 6%; constipation, 8%; and urinary retention, 1% in patients on trazodone. These ADRs occurred no more frequently with trazodone than with placebo, and they occurred significantly less frequently with trazodone than with imipramine (Gershon and Newton 1980).

▶ **Cardiovascular**

Trazodone has been shown to exacerbate preexisting myocardial irritability, possibly precipitating ventricular tachycardia (Janowsky et al. 1983). This problem has been reported only in depressed patients with a history of cardiac disease. In addition, one case report noted that trazodone might also cause cardiac conduction delay, which can have serious implications for patients with prolonged PR intervals. Thus, patients with PVCs should be treated

Table 2–6. **Trazodone adverse drug reactions (ADRs) occurring in more than 1% of recipients**

Allergic	dermatitides, edema
Autonomic nervous system	blurred vision, constipation, dry mouth
Cardiovascular	hypertension, hypotension, syncope, palpitations, tachycardia
Central nervous system	agitation, confusion, decreased concentration, disorientation, dizziness, drowsiness, excitement, fatigue, headache, insomnia, impaired memory, nervousness
Gastrointestinal	nausea, vomiting, diarrhea, bad taste, abdominal discomfort
Musculoskeletal	aches, pains
Neurological	incoordination, paresthesias, tremors
Miscellaneous	anorexia; red, tired, or itching eyes; heavy-headedness; malaise; nasal congestion; nightmares, vivid dreams; sweating, clamminess; tinnitus; weight gain or loss

Source. Georgotas et al. 1982.

with TCAs (Irwin and Spar 1983). Patients with cardiac arrhythmias and/or mitral valve prolapse should be carefully monitored when administered trazodone.

Like TCAs, trazodone can cause orthostatic hypotension that is occasionally severe. However, it differs from TCAs in that the hypotension is transient and lasts for approximately 4–6 hours after the dose is taken. Thus, the problem can be circumvented by using single daily dosing at bedtime. Trazodone can also cause bradycardia (Janowsky et al. 1983).

▶ Central Nervous System

Drowsiness, the most commonly experienced ADR with trazodone, has been reported to occur in up to 45% of patients, although an incidence of 9% seems to be a more reasonable approximation (Gershon and Newton 1980). Many of the CNS ADRs noted by the manufacturer may result from the sedation or disinhibition produced by the drug. A number of reports exist of trazodone-associated mania in both bipolar and unipolar patients (Rudorfer and Potter 1989).

▶ Hepatic
Several case reports exist of hepatotoxicity that occurred within the first few weeks of trazodone therapy but reversed after drug discontinuation (Brogden et al. 1981; Chu et al. 1983; Sheikh and Nies 1983).

▶ Neurological
A total of 123 cases of trazodone-associated *priapism* have been reported in the United States to the manufacturer, who estimated the incidence to be 1 in 6,000 men. This figure is conservative because of the voluntary-reporting nature of the system. Forty-nine percent of these patients experienced spontaneous detumescence, 15% required conservative medical management, and 28% required surgical intervention; treatment in the remaining 8% is unknown. At least 41% of the patients had been receiving the drug for 2 weeks or less. Injection of epinephrine or of metaraminol, an α-adrenergic agonist, into the cavernosal space has been effective and obviates the need for surgical shunts from the corpora cavernosa to the corpora spongiosum (Falk 1987). Priapism is most likely to occur within the first 4 weeks of treatment at doses of 150 mg/day (Rudorfer and Potter 1989).

▶ Teratogenicity and Excretion Into Breast Milk
Dysmorphogenic studies in animals have not indicated a teratogenic potential for trazodone. As with the other antidepressants, however, it is best to advise women taking the drug for postpartum depression not to breast-feed their newborns (Georgotas et al. 1982).

Venlafaxine
The ADRs most commonly associated with venlafaxine are presented in Table 2–7 (Ellingrod and Perry 1994). Venlafaxine was administered to 1,902 patients in phase II and III trials. The venlafaxine database consists of 19 worldwide studies involving 2,181 patients. More than 400 of these patients received venlafaxine for a year or more. The ADR statistics are based on 451 patients receiving placebo and 500 patients receiving comparator antidepressants. The most common ADRs associated with venlafaxine are nausea and vomiting. Venlafaxine has a very low incidence rate of serious, rare ADRs. The rates (per 100 patient-years of exposure) for these more-serious events for venlafaxine versus comparator antidepressants, respectively, are seizures (0.4 versus 1.5), death (0.4 versus 3.1), suicide (0.4 versus 0.8), suicide attempts (4.0 versus 3.1), suicidal ideation (0.4 versus 0.8), significant elevations

Table 2–7. Venlafaxine adverse drug reactions (ADRs) (≥ 10%) versus comparators antidepressants and placebo

ADR	Placebo (n = 451)	Venlafaxine (n = 1902)	Imipramine (n = 240)	Trazodone (n = 77)
Autonomic nervous system				
Dizziness	30 (7%)	418 (22%)	60 (25%)	29 (38%)
Dry mouth	50 (11%)	387 (20%)	136 (57%)	20 (26%)
Insomnia	45 (10%)	458 (24%)	43 (18%)	5 (6%)
Nervousness	25 (6%)	295 (16%)	33 (14%)	8 (10%)
Central nervous system				
Asthenia	31 (7%)	302 (16%)	44 (18%)	12 (16%)
Headache	111 (25%)	602 (32%)	68 (28%)	23 (30%)
Somnolence	44 (10%)	468 (25%)	79 (33%)	49 (64%)
Gastrointestinal				
Anorexia	8 (2%)	198 (10%)	20 (8%)	1 (1%)
Constipation	26 (6%)	312 (16%)	59 (25%)	8 (10%)
Urogenital system (male)	(n = 170)	(n = 737)	(n = 95)	(n = 24)
Abnormal ejaculation or abnormal orgasm	0 (0%)	81 (11%)	4 (4%)	3 (13%)

in liver function tests (0.8 versus 3.1), severe rash (0.8 versus 2.3), and mania or hypomania (0.4 versus 0.0). A number of ADRs are dose dependent, including chills, hypertension, anorexia, nausea, agitation, dizziness, somnolence, tremor, yawning, sweating, and abnormal ejaculation.

▶ **Cardiovascular**

A significant mean increase of baseline blood pressure (range 0.7–2.5 mm Hg) was observed in the clinical trials at most time intervals and as early as the first week of treatment. The cumulative probability of having a sustained supine diastolic blood pressure (SDBP) elevation after 12 months of treatment was 7.4% for placebo-, 11.9% for venlafaxine-, 8.0% for imipramine-, and 0% for trazodone-treated patients. Patients who were "mildly" hypertensive at baseline (90–104 mm Hg) were not necessarily predisposed to further increases in SDBP during venlafaxine treatment, regardless of dosage. The percentage of patients who received intervention therapy for hypertension or who discontinued the phase II or III studies because of hypertension did not differ between the groups. For all venlafaxine-treated groups, irrespective of dosage, the crude rate of sustained SDBP was 4.8%, which is comparable to the rate in imipramine-treated patients (4.7%) but higher than that in placebo-treated patients (2.1%). Only 10 patients actually discontinued venlafaxine because of sustained increased SDBP. Therefore, if a patient experiences a clinically significant increase in SDBP while taking venlafaxine, dosage reduction should be tried before discontinuation of the drug. Venlafaxine treatment in patients with hypertension should be instituted cautiously. The incidence of SDBP elevation is higher at dosages greater than 300 mg/day, and venlafaxine is not recommended in hypertensive patients at such elevated dosages (Ellingrod and Perry 1994).

▶ **Teratogenicity and Excretion Into Breast Milk**

No adequate studies in humans exist regarding venlafaxine's teratogenicity. Fifteen pregnancies were reported during the phase II and III clinical trials. Ten of these women were receiving venlafaxine, 3 were receiving placebo, 1 was receiving trazodone, and 1 was receiving placebo. Fetal exposure to venlafaxine ranged from 10 to 60 days. Normal Apgar scores were found in four venlafaxine-exposed infants who were tested. As a result of the outcomes of these four pregnancies, the sponsor concluded that venlafaxine exposure during the first trimester of pregnancy had no adverse effects on the fetus or on the pregnancy in general. However, because of the poor correlation between animal studies and human studies, venlafaxine is assigned to Pregnancy Category C[3] for its pregnancy risk factor. Thus, the drug should be administered to a pregnant woman only if the potential benefits justify the potential risk to the fetus. It is not known whether venlafaxine is excreted in human milk; therefore, caution should be exercised when venlafaxine is used in lactating women (Ellingrod and Perry 1994).

Nefazodone

The most common ADRs associated with nefazodone are dry mouth (25%), somnolence (25%), nausea (22%), dizziness (17%), constipation (14%), asthenia (11%), lightheadedness (10%), blurred vision (9%), confusion (7%), and abnormal vision (7%). Table 2–8 contains a partial listing of the ADRs patients experienced during the placebo controlled trials. These ADRs were found to be dose dependent and to diminish over a 6-week treatment period. ADRs for which there was a difference between nefazodone dosages of 300–600 mg/day and 300 mg/day or less included nausea (23% versus 14%), constipation (17% versus 10%), somnolence (28% versus 16%), dizziness (22% versus 11%), confusion (8% versus 2%), abnormal vision (10% versus 0%), and blurred vision (9% versus 3%) (Ellingrod and Perry 1995).

▶ Cardiovascular

No life-threatening events or clinically important ECG changes have been associated with nefazodone use. The incidence of postural hypotension and sinus bradycardia has been reported as 2.8% and 1.5%, respectively (Ellingrod and Perry 1995).

▶ Drug Interactions

Nefazodone does not inhibit CYP1A2, only weakly inhibits CYP 2D6, and will probably cause few interactions due to inhibition of CYP2D6. Most of the drug interactions observed with nefazodone involve its inhibition of CYP3A4. Because of this effect, caution is recommended when administering alprazolam, triazolam, or midazolam concurrently with nefazodone, and coadministration of terfenadine or astemizole is contraindicated (Ellingrod and Perry 1995).

---

[3] Either 1) studies in animals have revealed adverse effects on the fetus (teratogenic, embryocidal, or both) and there are no controlled studies in women, or 2) studies in women and in animals are not available (Briggs et al. 1994).

Table 2–8. **Treatment-emergent adverse drug reactions (ADRs) (>5%) from nefazodone 300–600 mg/day in 6–8 weeks of placebo-controlled clinical trials**

Body system and ADR	Nefazodone (%) (*n* = 393)	Placebo (%) (*n* = 394)
Body as a whole		
Headache	36	33
Asthenia	11	5
Infection	8	6
Gastrointestinal		
Dry mouth	25	13
Nausea	22	12
Constipation	14	8
Dyspepsia	9	7
Diarrhea	8	7
Increased appetite	5	3
Central nervous system		
Somnolence	25	14
Dizziness	17	5
Insomnia	11	9
Lightheadedness	10	3
Confusion	7	2
Respiratory		
Pharyngitis	6	5
Special senses		
Blurred vision	9	3
Abnormal vision	7	1

▶ Neurological

The incidence of *sexual dysfunction* in men and women receiving nefazodone is reported as comparable to that for placebo. In a 6-week trial, nefazodone (mean dosage 450 mg/day) and the SSRI sertraline (150 mg/day) were compared to determine their relative effects on sexual function. Although nefazodone produced fewer adverse reactions involving sexual functioning, the creditability of this finding is questionable because of the relatively large sertraline dosages used in the study (Feiger et al. 1996). In clinical trials, the most common sexual-dysfunction ADRs reported for nefazodone were impotence (1.5%), decreased libido (1%), abnormal ejaculation (0.2%), and anorgasmia (0.1%). Nefazodone 200 mg has been found to increase total nocturnal penile tumescence time (TTT), whereas the incidence of this effect with nefazodone 400 mg or buspirone 20 mg was equal to that with placebo. The increase in TTT caused by nefazodone was not abnormally prolonged beyond rapid eye movement (REM) sleep, whereas trazodone was found to increase TTT by delaying detumescence onset after cessation of REM sleep. These differences between nefazodone and trazodone suggest that nefazodone, unlike trazodone, may not cause priapism (Ellingrod and Perry 1995).

▶ Teratogenicity and Excretion Into Breast Milk
The use of nefazodone during pregnancy has not been studied in humans. Currently, the drug is categorized as a Pregnancy Category C drug and should be used during pregnancy only if the potential benefit outweighs the potential risk to the fetus. There is no evidence from animal studies to suggest that nefazodone has an effect on human reproduction or fetal development. Animal studies at dosages 8–16 times those used in humans produced a slightly lower fertility rate, although this finding is not considered significant in humans. Nefazodone's effects on labor and delivery in humans is not known. It is likewise unknown whether nefazodone is excreted into human breast milk, and therefore caution should be exercised when nefazodone is administered to pregnant women (Ellingrod and Perry 1995).

Mirtazapine
Mirtazapine has been compared with placebo and amitriptyline in trials involving a total of 1,378 subjects. Compared with persons receiving placebo, those receiving mirtazapine had a significantly higher ($P < .05$) incidence of the following side effects: dry mouth (25% versus 16%), drowsiness (23% versus 14%), excessive sedation (19% versus 5%), increased appetite (11% versus 2%), and weight gain (10% versus 1%). The adverse-effect incidence for subjects taking mirtazapine versus amitriptyline was as follows: dry mouth (34% versus 60%), constipation (16% versus 23%), palpitations (6% versus 11%), tremor (6% versus 15%), vertigo (8% versus 13%), tachycardia (1% versus 5%), and abnormal vision (2% versus 6%). Switching from depression to hypomanic or manic episodes has been reported to occur in 0.25% of bipolar patients; the incidence of seizures with mirtazapine is 0.04%, which is not different from that with placebo (Kehoe and Schorr 1996). In men receiving mirtazapine, impotence and decreased libido have been reported at rates of 2% and 6%, respectively, which also did not differ from the placebo rate (Kehoe and Schorr 1996). Of 2,796 patients receiving mirtazapine, 2 developed agranulocytosis and 1 developed neutropenia, yielding an incidence for severe neutropenia of 1.1 case per

1,000 patients exposed, with a very wide 95% confidence interval of 2.2/10,000–3.1/1,000 (Remeron® Product Information 1996). The incidence of neutropenia, based on patient exposure-years, is 0.062 for mirtazapine, 0.045 for amitriptyline, and 0.014 for placebo (Kehoe and Schorr 1996). Liver-function test abnormalities may also occur; data indicate that the rate of such results with mirtazapine is 1.4 and 1.6 times higher, respectively, than it is with other antidepressants and with placebo (Kehoe and Schorr 1996). In controlled studies, nonfasting cholesterol and triglyceride were found to increase by 20% and ≥ 500 mg/dL in 15% and 6% of patients, respectively (Remeron® Product Information 1996).

▶ Drug Interactions

Mirtazapine is metabolized by the cytochrome P450 system subfamilies of CYP2D6, CYP1A2, and CYP3A4. Drug interaction data for potential interactions between drugs metabolized by these hepatic isoenzymes and mirtazapine are unavailable at this time. When ethanol or diazepam is combined with mirtazapine, an additive effect on cognitive and motor performance is seen (Remeron® Product Information 1996). Mirtazapine should not be used in combination with an MAOI or within 14 days of initiating or discontinuing therapy with an MAOI (Remeron® Product Information 1996).

■ Rational Prescribing

1. The antidepressant effectiveness of amoxapine is apparently equivalent to that of the TCAs. The antidepressant amoxapine is the demethylated metabolite of loxapine, an antipsychotic. The drug does have significant dopamine-antagonist activity and, therefore, should not be prescribed prophylactically because of the risk of tardive dyskinesia. Additionally, amoxapine's extremely high risk of morbidity (i.e., seizures) and mortality after an overdose make it a less-than-ideal drug for use in patients with suicidal ideation.

2. Bupropion is devoid of anticholinergic, cardiovascular, and sedative effects. It does have dopamine-agonist activity that could be responsible for deterioration of mental status in psychotic patients. The drug is as effective as the TCAs in treating depression and causes fewer anticholinergic and cardiovascular adverse effects. Bupropion needs to be studied in patients with cardiac conduction disturbances. At dosages of more than 450 mg/day, the risk of seizures is four times greater with bupropion than with the TCAs.

3. Maprotiline is a monomethylated tetracyclic antidepressant with no obvious advantages over the TCAs. Evidence that this drug has a more rapid onset of action is debatable. Its pharmacological profile is similar to that of the monomethylated TCAs.

4. Trazodone appears to be as effective an antidepressant as the TCAs. Although it does not cause anticholinergic adverse effects, some patients cannot tolerate its sedative action. Patients with cardiac disease who receive trazodone should be closely monitored.

5. Venlafaxine is as effective as comparator antidepressants (i.e., trazodone, imipramine, fluoxetine) in the treatment of major depression. Its reputed shorter latency period for the onset of antidepressant effect cannot be taken seriously until the comparator drug studies are published and the data presented to support this suggestion.

6. Nefazodone is purported to have a lower incidence of anxiety, agitation, insomnia, and sexual ADRs than do all other antidepressants currently available. However, these ADR claims are based on only 393 patients, and it is unknown whether the manufacturer actively inquired about these ADRs or whether patient complaints were used to catalog nefazodone's ADRs. Nefazodone may offer a new treatment option for patients who are inadequately helped by or unable to tolerate ADRs from other antidepressants. As nefazodone is used more in clinical practice, the true incidence of ADRs should be assessed to determine whether the manufacturer's initial claim of a lower incidence of certain ADRs (e.g., sexual dysfunction) can be substantiated.

Benzodiazepines

Seven studies have compared *alprazolam,* a triazolobenzodiazepine, with imipramine, amitriptyline, desipramine, or doxepin in outpatients with mild to moderate depression. The findings suggest that alprazolam may have antidepressant activity (Eriksson et al. 1987; Fawcett et al. 1987; Goldberg et al. 1986; Overall et al. 1987; Rickels et al. 1987; Rush et al. 1985; Warner et al. 1988). One criticism of these studies involved the studies' use of outpatients whose depression was less severe than that of patients in other studies. A German-language study discussed by the authors in one of the studies (Rickels et al. 1987) concluded that whereas in mildly and moderately depressed outpatients (i.e., Hamilton Rating Scale for Depression [HAM-D] means of 15 and 22, respectively) ami-triptyline and alprazolam were equally effective, in severely de-pressed patients (HAM-D mean 32) amitriptyline was more effective than alprazolam. Another study compared alprazolam and amitriptyline in both inpatients and outpatients with Research Diagnostic Criteria (RDC)–diagnosed depression (Rush et al. 1985). These patients also had shortened REM latencies, a possible labo-ratory marker of endogenous depression. The authors of this study concluded that amitriptyline's effects significantly exceeded those of alprazolam as measured with the HAM-D and the Beck Depres-sion Index and induced a more complete degree of symptom remis-sion in more patients. Goldberg et al. (1986) found imipramine to be more effective than alprazolam in reversing depressed patients' neurovegetative signs (i.e., sleep disturbance, loss of appetite, weight loss, motor agitation or retardation, insidious onset). Fi-nally, an investigation that defined response as a HAM-D score of less than 7 concluded that amitriptyline's response rate (87%) was greater than that for alprazolam (60%) (Eriksson et al. 1987). Thus, the benzodiazepines are not indicated in major depression. Additionally, because no continuation or maintenance phase trials have been published, alprazolam is not recommended for affective-disorder prophylaxis (Depression Guideline Panel 1993b).

Central Nervous System Stimulants

A substantial amount of anecdotal literature suggests that CNS stimulants (methylphenidate, amphetamine, dextroamphetamine, methamphetamine, pemoline) may have some utility in depression. The sizable rate of response to stimulants in the treatment of depression reported in uncontrolled studies has not been replicated in 9 of 10 placebo-controlled trials. All but one of the studies were reported between 1958 and 1972. Of similarly designed, controlled studies involving the TCA imipramine, 14 of 23 showed the drug to be clearly superior to placebo. However, according to the find-ings of controlled studies, stimulants may have more therapeutic utility in the treatment of apathetic "senile" geriatric patients who do not have primary depression. Partial improvement but not re-missions have been observed in these patients (Satel and Nelson 1989). A small, placebo-controlled 8-day trial comparing methyl-phenidate 10–20 mg/day with placebo found the stimulant effec-tive in the 63% of elderly debilitated patients with major depression (Wallace et al. 1995). Although some data suggest that stimulants may be useful in physically ill patients with depression, replicated confirmation of this finding in 6-week controlled studies is still necessary (Masand et al. 1991; Pickett et al. 1991).

Finally, the stimulants have been reported in uncontrolled studies to be effective in the treatment of TCA-refractory patients. However, controlled studies in this patient population have reported placebo response rates ranging from 50% to 72% (General Practice Research Group 1964; Robin and Wiseberg 1958; Wheatley 1969).

Overall, fewer adverse effects are reported with the stimulants than with the TCAs. Habituation is commonly described as a risk, but this has not been confirmed in controlled trials. Stimulant adverse effects, in decreasing order of frequency, include insomnia, nausea, tremor, appetite change, palpitations, blurred vision, dry mouth, constipation, and dizziness. Other adverse effects, also in decreasing order of frequency, include blood pressure changes in either direction, dysrhythmias, and tremor (Satel and Nelson 1989).

Product List

Amitriptyline (dimethylated tricyclic antidepressant)
- Daily dose range: 50–300 mg; generically available
- Generic cost index: ≈ 0.08

Tablets:	Elavil®
10 mg	[$19] MSD 23, blue
25 mg	[$39] MSD 45, yellow
50 mg	[$69] MSD 102, beige
75 mg	[$94] MSD 430, orange
100 mg	[$119] MSD 435, mauve
150 mg	[$170] MSD 673, blue
Injection:	Elavil®
10 mg/mL	[$9/10-mL vial]

Amoxapine (piperazine tricyclic antidepressant)
- Daily dose range: 100–600 mg; generically available
- Generic cost index: ≈ 0.54

Tablets:	Asendin®
25 mg	[$77] A13, white
50 mg	[$125] A15, orange
100 mg	[$209] A17, blue
150 mg	[$99/30] A18, peach

Bupropion (monocyclic phenylbutamine of the aminoketone type antidepressant)
- Daily dose range: 300–450 mg

Tablets:	**Wellbutrin**®
75 mg	[$56] Wellbutrin 75, yellow-gold
100 mg	[$75] Wellbutrin 100, red

Clomipramine (dimethylated tricyclic antidepressant)
- Daily dose range: 75–250 mg; generically available

Capsules:	**Anafranil**®
25 mg	[$81] Anafranil 25 mg 115, orange/yellow
50 mg	[$109] Anafranil 50 mg 116, blue-green/ yellow
75 mg	[$144] Anafranil 75 mg 117, yellow/yellow

Desipramine (monomethylated tricyclic antidepressant)
- Daily dose range: 75–300 mg; generically available
- Generic cost index: ≈ 0.15

Tablets:	**Norpramin**®
10 mg	[$50] 68/-7, blue
25 mg	[$61] Norpramin 25, yellow
50 mg	[$114] Norpramin 50, green
75 mg	[$145] Norpramin 75, orange
100 mg	[$191] Norpramin 100, peach
150 mg	[$138/50] Norpramin 150, white

Doxepin (dimethylated tricyclic antidepressant)
- Daily dose range: 75–300 mg; generically available
- Generic cost index: ≈ 0.13

Capsules:	**Sinequan**®
10 mg	[$35] Sinequan Roerig 534, pink/red
25 mg	[$45] Sinequan Roerig 535, blue/pink
50 mg	[$64] Sinequan Roerig 536, pink/white
75 mg	[$106] Sinequan Roerig 539, white
100 mg	[$115] Sinequan Roerig 538, blue/white
150 mg	[$96/50] Sinequan Roerig 537, blue
Concentrate:	**Sinequan**®
10 mg/mL	[$27/120 mL]

Fluoxetine (bicyclic antidepressant)
- Daily dose range: 20–80 mg

Capsules:	**Prozac**®
10 mg	[$219] Dista Prozac 3104 10 mg, green/white
20 mg	[$225] Dista Prozac 3105 20 mg, green/off-white
Oral solution:	**Prozac**®
20 mg/5 mL	[$100/120 mL]

Fluvoxamine (selective serotonin reuptake inhibitor)
- Daily dose range: 50–300 mg

Tablets:	**Luvox**®
50 mg	[$191] Solvay 4205, yellow
100 mg	[$197] Solvay 4210, beige

Imipramine (dimethylated tricyclic antidepressant)
- Daily dose range: 50–300 mg; generically available
- Generic cost index: ≈ 0.07

Tablets:	**Tofranil**®
10 mg	[$27] 32, coral
25 mg	[$45] Geigy 140, coral
50 mg	[$77] Geigy 136, coral

Capsules:	**Tofranil PM**®
75 mg	[$107] Geigy 20, coral
100 mg	[$141] Geigy 40, dark yellow/coral
125 mg	[$176] Geigy 45, light yellow/coral
150 mg	[$201] Geigy 22, coral

Injection:	**Tofranil**®
12.5 mg/mL	[$2/2-mL ampule]

Maprotiline (monomethylated tetracyclic antidepressant)
- Daily dose range: 75–300 mg; generically available
- Generic cost index: ≈ 0.45

Tablets:	**Ludiomil**®
25 mg	[$47] Ciba 110, dark orange
50 mg	[$69] Ciba 26, dark orange
75 mg	[$95] Ciba 135, dark orange

Mirtazapine (tetracyclic antidepressant)
- Daily dose range: 15–45 mg

Tablets:	**Remeron**®
15 mg	[$59/30] Organon TZ3 oval, yellow coated
30 mg	[$61/30] Organon TZ5 oval, red-brown coated

Nefazodone (phenylpiperazine antidepressant)
- Daily dose range: 100–600 mg

Tablets:	**Serzone**®
100 mg	[$52/60] 25 W 701, white
150 mg	[$52/60] 37.5 W 781, peach
200 mg	[$52/60] 50 W 703, light yellow
250 mg	[$52/60] 75 W 704, white

Nortriptyline (monomethylated tricyclic antidepressant)
- Daily dose range: 20–150 mg; generically available
- Generic cost index: ≈ 0.31

Capsules:	**Pamelor**®
10 mg	[$47] Sandoz Pamelor 78–86, orange/white
25 mg	[$95] Sandoz Pamelor 78–87, orange/white
50 mg	[$178] Sandoz Pamelor 78–79, white
75 mg	[$272] Sandoz Pamelor 78–79, orange

Syrup:	**Pamelor**®
10 mg/5 mL	[$54/480 mL]

Paroxetine (selective serotonin reuptake inhibitor)
- Daily dose range: 20–50 mg

Tablets:	**Paxil**®
20 mg	[$198] Paxil 20, pink
30 mg	[$61/30] Paxil 30, blue

Phenelzine (hydrazine monoamine oxidase inhibitor)
- Daily dose range: 15–90 mg or 1 mg/kg/day

Tablets:	**Nardil**®
15 mg	[$40] PD 270, orange

Protriptyline (monomethylated tricyclic antidepressant)
- Daily dose range: 10–60 mg

Tablets:	**Vivactil**®
5 mg	[$47] MSD 26, orange
10 mg	[$67] MSD 47, yellow

Sertraline (selective serotonin reuptake inhibitor)
- Daily dose range: 50–200 mg

Tablets:	**Zoloft**®
50 mg	[$209] Zoloft 50 mg, blue
100 mg	[$215] Zoloft 100 mg, yellow

Tranylcypromine (nonhydrazine monoamine oxidase inhibitor)
- Daily dose range: 20–40 mg

Tablets:	**Parnate**®
10 mg	[$48] Parnate SKF, maroon

Trazodone (triazolopyridine antidepressant)
- Daily dose range: 300–800 mg; generically available
- Generic cost index: ≈ 0.06

Tablets:	**Desyrel**®
50 mg	[$130] Desyrel/MJ 775, orange
100 mg	[$227] Desyrel/MJ 776, white
150 mg	[$196] MJ 778, orange
300 mg	[$348] MJ 796, yellow

Trimipramine (trimethylated tricyclic antidepressant)

- Daily dose range: 50–300 mg; generically available

Tablets:	**Surmontil**®
25 mg	[$66] 4132, blue/yellow
50 mg	[$108] 4133, blue/orange
100 mg	[$157] 4158, blue/white

Venlafaxine (phenethylamine antidepressant)

- Daily dose range: 75–375 mg

Tablets:	**Effexor**®
25 mg	[$95] 25 W 701, peach
37.5 mg	[$98] 37.5 W 781, peach
50 mg	[$101] 50 W 703, peach
75 mg	[$107] 75 W 704, peach
100 mg	[$114] 100 W 705, peach

References

Absher JR, Black DW: Tranylcypromine withdrawal delirium. J Clin Psychopharmacol 8:379–380, 1988

Adly C, Straumanis J, Chesson A: Fluoxetine prophylaxis of migraine. Headache 32:101–104, 1992

Aguglia E, Casacchia M, Cassano GB, et al: Double-blind study of the efficacy and safety of sertraline versus fluoxetine in major depression. Int Clin Psychopharmacol 8:197–202, 1993

Aldrich MS: Narcolepsy. N Engl J Med 323:389–394, 1990

Alexopoulos GS, Abrams RC: Depression in Alzheimer's disease. Psychiatr Clin North Am 14:327–340, 1991

Anderson IM, Tomenson BM: Treatment discontinuation with selective serotonin reuptake inhibitors compared with tricyclic antidepressants: a meta-analysis. BMJ 310:1433–1438, 1995

Angst J: Clinical indications for a prophylactic treatment of depression. Advances in Biological Psychiatry 7:218–229, 1981

Anton RF Jr, Burch EA Jr: Amoxapine versus amitriptyline combined with perphenazine in the treatment of psychotic depression. Am J Psychiatry 147:1203–1208, 1990

Asendin® [amoxapine] Product Information. Pearl River, NY, Lederle Laboratories, American Cyanamid Company, 1981, pp 1–50

Avery D, Lubrano A: Depression treated with imipramine and ECT: the De Carolis study reconsidered. Am J Psychiatry 136:559–562, 1979

Barrickman LL, Perry PJ, Allen AJ, et al: Bupropion versus methylphenidate in the treatment of attention deficit hyperactivity disorder. J Am Acad Child Adolesc Psychiatry 34:649–657, 1995 auman P, Nil R, Souche A, et al: A double-blind, placebo-controlled study of citalopram with and without lithium in the treatment of therapy-resistant depressive patients: a clinical, pharmacokinetic, and pharmacogenetic investigation. J Clin Psychopharmacol 16:307–314, 1996

Beasley CM, Saylor ME, Cunningham TE, et al: Fluoxetine in tricyclic refractory major depressive disorder. J Affect Disord 20:193–200, 1990a

Beasley CM, Bosomworth JC, Wernicke JF: Fluoxetine: relationships among dose, response, adverse effects, and plasma concentrations in the treatment of depression. Psychopharmacol Bull 26:18–24, 1990b

Beasley CM, Dornseif BE, Bosomworth JC, et al: Fluoxetine and suicide: a meta-analysis of controlled trials of treatment for depression. BMJ 303:685–692, 1991

Benfield P, Ward A: Fluvoxamine: a review of its pharmacodynamic and pharmacokinetic properties, and therapeutic efficacy in depressive illness. Drugs 32:313–334, 1986

Berken GH, Weinstein DO, Stern WC: Weight gain: a side effect of tricyclic antidepressants. J Affect Disord 7:133–138, 1984

Bethune HC, Burrell RH, Culpan RH, et al: Vascular crisis associated with monoamine oxidase inhibitors. Am J Psychiatry 121:245–248, 1964

Bieck PR, Antonin KH: Oral tyramine pressor test and the safety of MAOI drugs: comparison of brofaromine and tranylcypromine in healthy subjects. J Clin Psychopharmacol 8:237–245, 1988

Biederman J, Baldessarini RJ, Wright V, et al: A double-blind placebo controlled study of desipramine in the treatment of ADD, I: efficacy. J Am Acad Child Adolesc Psychiatry 28:777–784, 1989

Bielski RJ, Fiedel DO: Prediction of tricyclic antidepressant response: a critical review. Arch Gen Psychiatry 33:1479–1489, 1976

Black DW, Wesner R, Gabel J: The abrupt discontinuation of fluvoxamine in patients with panic disorder. J Clin Psychiatry 54:146–149, 1993

Blacksten JB, Birt JA: Syndrome of inappropriate secretion of antidiuretic hormone secondary to fluoxetine. Ann Pharmacother 27:723–724, 1993

Blackwell B: Adverse effects of antidepressant drugs, I: monoamine oxidase inhibitors and tricyclics. Drugs 21:201–219, 1981

Blackwell B, Marley E, Price J, et al: Hypertensive interaction associated with monoamine oxidase inhibitors and food stuffs. Br J Psychiatry 113:349–365, 1967

Borson S, McDonald GJ, Gayle T, et al: Improvement in mood, physical symptoms, and function with nortriptyline for depression in patients with COPD. Psychosomatics 33:190–201, 1992

Branconnier RJ, Cole JO, Ghazvinian S, et al: Clinical pharmacology of bupropion and imipramine in elderly depressives. J Clin Psychiatry 44 (sec 2):130–133, 1983

Bremner JD: A double-blind comparison of Org 3770, amitriptyline, and placebo in major depression. J Clin Psychiatry 56:519–525, 1995

Briggs GG, Freeman RK, Yaffe SJ: Drugs in Pregnancy and Lactation, 4th Edition. Baltimore, MD, Williams & Wilkins, 1994, p 10

Briley M, Moret C: Neurobiological mechanisms involved in antidepressant therapies. Clin Neuropharmacol 16:387–400, 1993

Brogden RN, Hell RC, Speight TM: Trazodone: a review of its pharmacological properties and therapeutic use in depression and anxiety. Drugs 21:401–429, 1981

Browne JL, Perry PJ, Alexander B, et al: Pharmacokinetic protocol for predicting plasma nortriptyline levels. J Clin Psychopharmacol 3:351–356, 1983

Bukberg J, Penman D, Holland JC: Depression in hospitalized cancer patients. Psychosom Med 46:199–212, 1984

Bunney WE: The switch process in manic-depressive psychosis. Ann Intern Med 87:319–325, 1977

Butler J, Leonard BE: Postpartum depression and the effect of nomifensine treatment. Int Clin Psychopharmacol 1:244–252, 1986

Carroll ME, Lac SR, Asencio M, et al: Fluoxetine reduces intravenous cocaine self-administration in rats. Pharmacol Biochem Behav 35:237–244, 1990

Chu AG, Gunsolly BL, Summers RW, et al: Trazodone and liver toxicity. Ann Intern Med 99:128–129, 1983

Clary C, Schweizer E: Treatment of MAOI hypertensive crisis with sublingual nifedipine. J Clin Psychiatry 48:249–250, 1987

Coccaro EF, Siever LJ: Second generation antidepressants: a comparative review. J Clin Pharmacol 25:241–260, 1985

Cole JO, Schatzberg AF, Sniffin C, et al: Trazodone in treatment-resistant depression: an open study. J Clin Psychopharmacol 1 (suppl):49–54, 1981

Consensus Development Panel: NIMH/NIH Consensus Development Conference Statement—Mood disorders: pharmacologic prevention of recurrences. Am J Psychiatry 142:469–476, 1985

Cooper DJ, Gelenberg AJ, Wojcik JC, et al: The effects of amoxapine and imipramine on serum prolactin levels. Arch Intern Med 141:1023–1025, 1981

Cooper GL: The safety of fluoxetine: an update. Br J Psychiatry 153 (suppl 3):77–86, 1988

Cooper TB, Kelly RG: GLC analysis of loxapine, amoxapine, and their metabolites in serum and urine. J Pharm Sci 68:216–219, 1979

Danish University Antidepressant Group: Citalopram: clinical effect profile in comparison with clomipramine: a controlled multicenter study. Psychopharmacology (Berl) 90:131–138, 1986

Danish University Antidepressant Group: Paroxetine: a selective serotonin reuptake inhibitor showing better tolerance, but weaker antidepressant effect than clomipramine in a controlled multicenter study. J Affect Disord 18:289–299, 1990

Davidson J: Seizures and bupropion: a review. J Clin Psychiatry 50:256–261, 1989

Davidson J, McLeod M, Law-Yone B, et al: A comparison of ECT and combined phenelzine-amitriptyline in refractory depression. Arch Gen Psychiatry 35:639–642, 1978

Davidson JRT, McLeod MN, Turnbull CD, et al: A comparison of phenelzine and imipramine in depressed inpatients. J Clin Psychiatry 42:395–397, 1981

Davis JM, Casper RC: Side effects of psychotropic drugs and their management, in Principles of Psychopharmacology. Edited by Clark WG, DelGiudice J. New York, Academic Press, 1978, pp 479–494

de Boer T: The pharmacologic profile of mirtazapine. J Clin Psychiatry 57 (suppl 4):19–25, 1996

DeCastro R: Reversal of MAOI-induced anorgasmia with cyproheptadine (letter). Am J Psychiatry 142:783, 1985

Dechant KL, Clissold SP: Paroxetine. Drugs 41:225–253, 1991

DeLeo D, Magni G: Sexual side effects of antidepressant drugs. Psychosomatics 24:1076–1081, 1983

Delgado PL, Charney DS, Price LH, et al: Serotonin function and the mechanism of antidepressant action: reversal of antidepressant-induced remission by rapid depletion of plasma tryptophan. Arch Gen Psychiatry 47:411–418, 1990

Delgado PL, Miller HL, Salomon RM, et al: Monoamines and the mechanism of antidepressant action: effects of catecholamine depletion on mood of patients treated with antidepressants. Psychopharmacol Bull 29:389–396, 1993

Depression Guideline Panel: Depression in Primary Care, Vol 1: Detection and Diagnosis (Clinical Practice Guideline No 5; AHCPR Publ No 93-0550). Rockville, MD, U.S. Department of Health and Human Services, Public Health Service, Agency for Health Care Policy and Research, April 1993a

Depression Guideline Panel: Depression in Primary Care, Vol 2: Treatment of Major Depression (Clinical Practice Guideline No 5; AHCPR Publ No 93-0551). Rockville, MD, U.S. Department of Health and Human Services, Public Health Service, Agency for Health Care Policy and Research, April 1993b

DeVane CL: Pharmacokinetics of the selective serotonin reuptake inhibitors. J Clin Psychiatry 53:13–20, 1992

DeVane CL, Jarecke CR: Cyclic antidepressants, in Applied Pharmacokinetics: Principles of Therapeutic Drug Monitoring, Vol 33. Edited by Evans WE, Schentag JJ, Jusko WJ. Vancouver, WA, Applied Therapeutics, 1992, pp 1–47

DeWilde J, Spiers R, Mertens C, et al: A double-blind, comparative, multicentre study comparing paroxetine with fluoxetine in depressed patients. Acta Psychiatr Scand 87:141–145, 1993

Dilsaver SC, Kronfol Z, Sackellares JC, et al: Antidepressant withdrawal syndromes: evidence supporting cholinergic overdrive hypothesis. J Clin Psychopharmacol 3:157–164, 1983

Doogan DP: Toleration and safety of sertraline: experience worldwide. Int Clin Psychopharmacol 6 (suppl 2):47–56, 1991

Doogan DP, Caillard V: Sertraline in the prevention of depression. Br J Psychiatry 160:217–222, 1992

Dornseif BE, Dunlop SR, Potvin JH, et al: Effect of dose escalation after low-dose fluoxetine therapy. Psychopharmacol Bull 25:71–79, 1989

Doshi D, Borison JR: Sertraline-related syndrome of inappropriate secretion of antidiuretic hormone. Am J Psychiatry 1512:779–780, 1994

Dufresne RL, Weber SS, Becker RE: Bupropion hydrochloride. Drug Intelligence and Clinical Pharmacy 18:957–964, 1984

Dunbar GC: An interim overview of the safety and tolerability of paroxetine. Acta Psychiatr Scand 80 (suppl 350):135–137, 1989

Edwards JG, Goldie A, Papayanni-Papasthatis S, et al: The effect of paroxetine on the EEG, ECG, and blood pressure (abstract). Acta Psychiatr Scand 80 (suppl 350):124, 1989

El-Ganzouri AR, Ivankovich AD, Braverman B, et al: Monoamine oxidase inhibitors: should they be discontinued preoperatively? Anesthesia and Analgesia 64:592–596, 1985

Elia J, Katz I, Simpson GM: Teratogenicity of psychotherapeutic medications. Psychopharmacol Bull 23:531–586, 1987

Ellingrod VL, Perry PJ: Venlafaxine: a heterocyclic antidepressant. Am J Hosp Pharm 51:3033–3046, 1994

Ellingrod VL, Perry PJ: Nefazodone: a new antidepressant or another "me too" drug? American Journal of Health-Systems Pharmacy 52:2799–2812, 1995

Emslie G, Rush A, Weinberg W, et al: Efficacy of fluoxetine in depressed children and adolescents. Arch Gen Psychiatry (in press)

Eriksson B, Nagy A, Starmark JE, et al: Alprazolam compared to amitriptyline in treatment of major depression. Acta Psychiatr Scand 75:656–663, 1987

Fairburn CG: Bulimia nervosa. BMJ 300:485–487, 1990

Falk WE: Trazodone and priapism. Biological Therapies in Psychiatry 10:9–10, 1987

Farid FF, Wenger TL, Tsai SY, et al: Use of bupropion in patients who exhibit orthostatic hypotension on tricyclic antidepressants. J Clin Psychiatry 46 (sec 2):170–173, 1985

Fawcett J, Edwards JH, Kravitz HM, et al: Alprazolam: an antidepressant? alprazolam, desipramine, and an alprazolam-desipramine combination in the treatment of adult depressed outpatients. J Clin Psychopharmacol 7:295–310, 1987

Feiger A, Kiev A, Shrivastava RK, et al: Nefazodone versus sertraline in outpatients with major depression: focus on efficacy, tolerability, and effects on sexual function and satisfaction. J Clin Psychiatry 57 (suppl 2):53–62, 1996

Feighner JP, Boyer WF: Selective Serotonin Reuptake Inhibitors: The Clinical Use of Citalopram, Fluoxetine, Fluvoxamine, Paroxetine, and Sertraline. New York, Wiley & Sons, 1991, pp 89–132

Feinberg SS, Halbreich U: The association between the definition and reported prevalence of treatment-resistant depression, in Psychosocial Aspects of Nonresponse to Antidepressant Drugs. Edited by Halbreich U, Feinberg SS. Washington, DC, American Psychiatric Press, 1986, pp 5–34

Fisch C: Effect of fluoxetine on the electrocardiogram. J Clin Psychiatry 46:42–44, 1985

Fisch C, Knoebel SB: Electrocardiographic findings in sertraline depression trials. Drug Investigation 4:305–312, 1992

Foods interacting with MAO inhibitors. Medical Letter 31:11–12, 1989

Frasure-Smith N, Lesperance F, Talajic M: Depression and 18-month prognosis after myocardial infarction. Circulation 91:999–1005, 1995

Friedman RA, Parides M, Baff R, et al: Predictors of response to desipramine in dysthymia. J Clin Psychopharmacol 15:280–283, 1995

Gagiano CA, Muller PGM, Fourie J, et al: The therapeutic efficacy of paroxetine, A: an open study in patients with major depression not responding to antidepressants; B: a double-blind comparison with amitriptyline in depressed outpatients. Acta Psychiatr Scand 80 (suppl 350):130–131, 1989

Gardiner HM, Freeman CP, Jesinger DK, et al: Fluvoxamine: an open pilot study in moderately obese female patients suffering from atypical eating disorders and episodes of bingeing. Int J Obes Relat Metab Disord 17:301–305, 1993

Gardner DM, Shulman KI, Walker SE, et al: The making of a user-friendly MAOI diet. J Clin Psychiatry 57:99–104, 1996

Gardner EA, Johnston JA: Bupropion—an antidepressant without sexual pathophysiological action. J Clin Psychopharmacol 5:24–29, 1985

Gatti F, Bellini L, Gasperini M, et al: Fluvoxamine alone in the treatment of delusional depression. Am J Psychiatry 153:414–416, 1996

Gelenberg AJ: Switching MAOIs. Biological Therapies in Psychiatry 7:37, 1984

Gelenberg AJ: Antidepressants in milk (letter). Biological Therapies in Psychiatry 10:13, 1987

Gelenberg AJ: MAOIs: assorted concerns. Biological Therapies in Psychiatry 11:33–36, 1988

General Practice Research Group: Dextroamphetamine compared with an inactive placebo in depression. Practitioner 192:151–154, 1964

Georgotas A, Forsell TL, Mann JJ, et al: Trazodone hydrochloride: a wide-spectrum antidepressant with a unique pharmacological profile. A review of its neurochemical effects, pharmacology, clinical efficacy, and toxicology. Pharmacotherapy 2:255–265, 1982

Georgotas A, Friedman E, McCarthy M, et al: Resistant geriatric depressions and therapeutic response to monoamine oxidase inhibitors. Biol Psychiatry 18:195–205, 1983

Gershon S, Newton R: Lack of anticholinergic side effects with a new antidepressant—trazodone. J Clin Psychiatry 41:100–104, 1980

Giller EG: Monoamine oxidase inhibitors and platelet monoamine oxidase inhibition. Communication in Psychopharmacology 4:79–82, 1980

Gitlin MJ, Winer H, Fairbank L, et al: Failure of T_3 to potentiate tricyclic antidepressant response. J Affect Disord 13:267–272, 1987

Glassman AH, Dalack GW: Cardiovascular effects of heterocyclic antidepressants, in Adverse Effects of Psychotropic Drugs. Edited by Kane J, Lieberman JA. New York, Guilford, 1992, pp 287–297

Glassman AH, Johnson LL, Giardina EGV, et al: The use of imipramine in depressed patients with congestive heart failure. JAMA 250:1997–2001, 1983

Glassman AH, Roose SP, Bigger JT: The safety of tricyclic antidepressants in cardiac patients: risk-benefit reconsidered. JAMA 269:2673–2675, 1993

Goff D, Midha K, Sarid-Segal O, et al: A placebo-controlled trial of fluoxetine added to neuroleptic in patients with schizophrenia. Psychopharmacology 117:417–423, 1995

Goldberg SC, Ettigi PE, Schulz PM, et al: Alprazolam versus imipramine in depressed outpatients with neurovegetative signs. J Affect Disord 11:139–145, 1986

Goldbloom DS, Olmsted MP: Pharmacotherapy of bulimia nervosa with fluoxetine: assessment of clinically significant attitudinal change. Am J Psychiatry 150:770–774, 1993

Golden RN: Psychoses associated with bupropion treatment. Am J Psychiatry 142:1459–1462, 1985

Gorelick DA, Paredes A: Effect of fluoxetine on alcohol consumption in male alcoholics. Alcohol Clin Exp Res 16:261–265, 1992

Graber MA, Hoehns TB, Perry PJ: Sertraline-phenelzine drug interaction: a serotonin syndrome reaction. Ann Pharmacother 28:732–735, 1994

Grasso RA, Perry PJ, Sherman AD: Relationship between tranylcypromine sulfate dose and monoamine oxidase inhibition (letter). DICP Ann Pharmacother 25:99–100, 1991

Greenblatt EN, Hardy RA, Kelly RG: Amoxapine. Pharmacological and Biochemical Properties of Drug Substances 2:1–19, 1979

Grimsley SR, Jann MW: Paroxetine, sertraline, and fluvoxamine: new selective serotonin reuptake inhibitors. Clinical Pharmacy 11:930–957, 1992

Gutierrez-Esteinou R, Pope HG: Does fluoxetine prolong electrically induced seizures. Convuls Ther 5:344–348, 1989

Hansten PD, Horn JR: Drug Interactions and Updates. Vancouver, WA, Applied Therapeutics, 1994

Harrison W, Rabkin J, Stewart JW, et al: Phenelzine for chronic depression: a study of continuation treatment. J Clin Psychiatry 47:346–349, 1986

Harto-Truax N, Stern WC, Miller LL, et al: Effects of bupropion on body weight. J Clin Psychiatry 44 (sec 2):183–187, 1983

Hawton K: Erectile dysfunction and premature ejaculation. Br J Hosp Med 40:428–436, 1988

Hazell P, O'Connell D, Heathcote D, et al: Efficacy of tricyclic drugs in treating child and adolescent depression: a meta-analysis. BMJ 310:897–901, 1995

Hearst EB: Review and evaluation of clinical data. New drug application. Nefazodone application summary. Rockville, MD, Food and Drug Administration, November 23, 1993 (obtained through the Freedom of Information Act)

Heiligenstein JH, Tollefson GD, Faries DE: A double-blind trial of fluoxetine 20 mg and placebo in outpatients with DSM-III-R major depression and melancholia. Int Clin Psychopharmacol 8:247–251, 1993

Heinonen OP, Slone D, Shapiro S: Birth Defects and Drugs in Pregnancy. Littleton, MA, Publishing Sciences Group, 1977

Heinrichs DW, Cohen BP, Carpenter WT: Early insight and the management of schizophrenic decompensation. J Nerv Ment Dis 173:133–138, 1985

Hellerstein DJ, Yanowitch P, Rosenthal J, et al: A randomized double-blind study of fluoxetine versus placebo in the treatment of dysthymia. Am J Psychiatry 150:1169–1175, 1993

Heninger GR, Charney DS, Sterberg DE: Lithium carbonate augmentation of antidepressant treatment: an effective prescription for treatment of refractory depression. Arch Gen Psychiatry 40:1335–1342, 1983

Himmelhoch JM, Fuchs CZ, Symons BJ: A double-blind study of tranylcypromine treatment of major anergic depression. J Nerv Ment Dis 170:628–634, 1982

Himmelhoch JM, Thase ME, Mallinger AG, et al: Tranylcypromine versus imipramine in anergic bipolar depression. Am J Psychiatry 148:910–916, 1991

Hollister LE: Antidepressant drugs, in Meyler's Side Effects of Drugs, Vol VIII. Edited by Dukes MNG. New York, American Elsevier, 1975, pp 31–46

Howarth BG, Grace MGA: Depression, drugs, and delusions. Arch Gen Psychiatry 42:1145–1147, 1985

Hudson JI, Hudson MS, Pliner LF, et al: Fibromyalgia and major affective disorder: a controlled phenomenology and family history study. Am J Psychiatry 142:441–446, 1985

Irwin M, Spar JE: Reversible cardiac conduction abnormality associated with trazodone administration. Am J Psychiatry 140:945–946, 1983

Isenberg KE: Excretion of fluoxetine in human breast milk (case report). J Clin Psychiatry 51:169, 1990

Jabbari B, Bryan GE, Marsh EE, et al: Incidence of seizures with tricyclic and tetracyclic antidepressants. Arch Neurol 42:480–481, 1985

Jacobs SC, Nelson JC, Zisook S: Treating depression of bereavements with antidepressants: a pilot study. Psychiatr Clin North Am 10:501–510, 1987

Janicak PG, Pandey GN, Davis JM, et al: Response of psychotic and nonpsychotic depression to phenelzine. Am J Psychiatry 145:93–95, 1988

Jankovic J, Fahn S: Physiologic and pathologic tremors: diagnosis, management and treatment. Ann Intern Med 93:460–465, 1980

Janowsky D, Curtis G, Zisook S, et al: Trazodone-aggravated ventricular arrhythmia. J Clin Psychopharmacol 3:372–376, 1983

Jefferson JW: Genitourinary system effects of psychotropic drugs, in Adverse Effects of Psychotropic Drugs. Edited by Kane J, Lieberman JA. New York, Guilford, 1992, pp 431–444

Jick H, Dinan BJ, Hunter JR, et al: Tricyclic antidepressants and convulsions. J Clin Psychopharmacol 3:182–185, 1983

Joffe RT, Lippert GP, Gray TA, et al: Personal and family history of affective illness in patients with multiple sclerosis. J Affect Disord 12:63–65, 1987

Joffe RT, Singer W, Levitt AJ, et al: A placebo-controlled comparison of lithium and triiodothyronine augmentation of tricyclic antidepressants in unipolar refractory depression. Arch Gen Psychiatry 50:387–393, 1993

Joffe RT, Levitt AJ, Sokolov ST et al: Response to an open trial of a second SSRI in major depression. J Clin Psychiatry 57:114–115, 1996

Joyce PR, Walshe J: Nightmares during phenelzine withdrawal (letter). J Clin Psychopharmacol 3:121, 1983

Kantor D, McNevin S, Leichner P, et al: The benefit of lithium carbonate adjunct in refractory depression—fact or fiction? Can J Psychiatry 31:416–418, 1986

Katz MM, Koslow SH, Maas JW, et al: The timing, specificity and clinical prediction of tricyclic drug effects in depression. Psychol Med 17:287–309, 1987

Kavan MG, Elsasser GN, Hurd RH: Depression after acute myocardial infarction. Postgraduate Medicine 89:83–89, 1991

Keck PE Jr, Vuckovic A, Pope HG Jr, et al: Acute cardiovascular response to monoamine oxidase inhibitors: a prospective assessment. J Clin Psychopharmacol 9:203–206, 1989

Kehoe WA, Schorr RB: Focus on mirtazapine: a new antidepressant with noradrenergic and specific serotonergic activity. Formulary 31:455–469, 1996

Kelly MW, Perry PJ, Holstad SG, et al: Serum fluoxetine and norfluoxetine concentrations and antidepressant response. Ther Drug Monit 11:165–170, 1989

Klerman GL, Cole JO: Clinical pharmacology of imipramine and related antidepressant compounds. Pharmacol Rev 17:101–141, 1965

Kocsis JH, Frances AJ, Voss C, et al: Imipramine treatment for chronic depression. Arch Gen Psychiatry 45:253–257, 1988

Kocsis JH, Friedman RA, Markowitz JC, et al: Stability of remission during tricyclic antidepressant continuation therapy for dysthymia. Psychopharmacol Bull 31:213–216, 1995

Kramer MS, Vogel WH, DiJohnson C, et al: Antidepressants in depressed schizophrenic inpatients: a controlled trial. Arch Gen Psychiatry 46:922–928, 1989

Kreider MS, Bushnell WD, Oakes R, et al: A double-blind, randomized study to provide safety information on switching fluoxetine-treated patients to paroxetine without an intervening washout period. J Clin Psychiatry 56:142–145, 1995

Kupfer DJ, Detre TP: Tricyclic and MAO-inhibitor antidepressants, in Affective Disorders: Drug Actions in Animals and Man. Edited by Iverson LL, Iverson SD, Snyder SH. New York, Plenum, 1978, pp 199–232

Kurlan R, Como PG, Deeley C, et al: A pilot controlled study of fluoxetine for obsessive-compulsive symptoms in children with Tourette's syndrome. Clin Neuropharmacol 16:167–172, 1993

Lapierre YD, Anderson K: Dyskinesia associated with amoxapine antidepressant therapy: a case report. Am J Psychiatry 140:493–494, 1983

Leipzig RM: Gastrointestinal and hepatic effects of psychotropic drugs, in Adverse Effects of Psychotropic Drugs. Edited by Kane J, Lieberman JA. New York, Guilford, 1992, pp 348–430

Lewis JL, Winokur G: The induction of mania: a natural history study with controls. Arch Gen Psychiatry 39:303–306, 1982

Liebowitz MR, Quitkin FM, Stewart JW, et al: Phenelzine versus imipramine in atypical depression. Arch Gen Psychiatry 41:669–677, 1984

Lipinski JF, Mallya G, Zimmerman P, et al: Fluoxetine-induced akathisia: clinical and theoretical implications. J Clin Psychiatry 50:339–342, 1989

Lipsey JR, Robinson RG, Pearlson GD: Nortriptyline treatment of poststroke depression: a double-blind study. Lancet 1:297–300, 1984

Liskin B, Roose SP, Walsh BT, et al: Acute psychosis following phenelzine discontinuation. J Clin Psychopharmacol 5:46–47, 1985

Litovitz TL, Troutman WG: Amoxapine overdose: seizures and fatalities. JAMA 250:1069–1071, 1983

Livingston RL, Zucker DK, Isenberg K, et al: Tricyclic antidepressants and delirium. J Clin Psychiatry 44:173–176, 1983

Lydiard RB, Gelenberg AJ: Amoxapine: an antidepressant with some neuroleptic properties? a review of its chemistry, animal pharmacology and toxicology, human pharmacology, and clinical efficacy. Pharmacotherapy 1:163–178, 1981

Madakasira S: Amoxapine-induced neuroleptic malignant syndrome. Drug Intelligence and Clinical Pharmacy 23:50–55, 1989

Magni G: The use of antidepressants in the treatment of chronic pain: a review of the current evidence. Drugs 42:730–748, 1991

Masand P, Pickett-P, Murray GB: Psychostimulants for secondary depression in medical illness. Psychosomatics 32:203–208, 1991

Max MB, Lynch SA, Muir J, et al: Effects of desipramine, amitriptyline and fluoxetine on pain in diabetic neuropathy. N Engl J Med 326:1250–1256, 1992

McGrath PJ, Stewart JW, Harrison W, et al: Treatment of tricyclic antidepressant depression with a monoamine oxidase inhibitor. Psychopharmacol Bull 23:169–172, 1987

McGrath PJ, Stewart JW, Quitkin FM: A possible L-deprenyl–induced hypertensive reaction (letter). J Clin Psychopharmacol 9:310–311, 1989

McGrath PJ, Stewart JW, Harrison W, et al: A double-blind crossover trial of imipramine and phenelzine for outpatients with treatment-refractory depression. Am J Psychiatry 150:118–123, 1993

McTavish D, Benfield P: Clomipramine: an overview of its pharmacological properties and a review of its therapeutic use in obsessive-compulsive disorder and panic disorder. Drugs 39:136–153, 1990

Mendez MF, Cummings JL, Benson DF: Depression in epilepsy: significance and phenomenology. Arch Neurol 43:766–770, 1986

Miller K, Atkin B, Moody ML: Drug therapy for nocturnal enuresis: current treatment recommendations. Drugs 44:47–56, 1992

Mitchell JE, Popkin MK: Antidepressant drug therapy and sexual dysfunction in men: a review. J Clin Psychopharmacol 3:76–79, 1983

Modigh K: Antidepressant drugs in anxiety disorders. Acta Psychiatr Scand 76 (suppl 335):57–74, 1987

Montgomery SA, Dunbar GH: Paroxetine is better than placebo in relapse prevention and the prophylaxis of recurrent depression. Int Clin Psychopharmacol 8:189–195, 1993

Montgomery SA, Dufour H, Brion S, et al: The prophylactic efficacy of fluoxetine in unipolar depression. Br J Psychiatry 153 (suppl 3):69–76, 1988

Montgomery SA, Baldwin D, Shah A, et al: Plasma-level response relationships with fluoxetine and zimelidine. Clin Neuropharmacol 13 (1, suppl):S71–S75, 1990

Morris PLP, Robinson RG, Raphael B: Prevalence and course of depressive disorders in hospitalized stroke patients. Int J Psychiatry Med 20:349–364, 1990

Nathan RS, Perel JM, Pollock BG, et al: The role of neuropharmacologic selectivity in antidepressant action: fluvoxamine versus desipramine. J Clin Psychiatry 51:367–372, 1990

Nelson JC, Bock JL, Jatlow PI: Clinical implications of 2-hydroxydesipramine plasma concentration. Clin Pharmacol Ther 33:183–189, 1983

Nierenberg AA, Keck PE Jr: Management of MAOI-associated insomnia. J Clin Psychopharmacol 4:42–45, 1989

Nierenberg AA, McLean NE, Alpert JE, et al: Early nonresponse to fluoxetine as a predictor of poor 8-week outcome. Am J Psychiatry 152:1500–1503, 1995

Nies A: Differential response patterns to MAO inhibitors and tricyclics. J Clin Psychiatry 45 (sec 2):70–77, 1984

Nolen WA, Van dePutte JJ, Dijken WA, et al: L-tryptophan in depression resistant to reuptake inhibitors: an open comparative study with tranylcypromine. Br J Psychiatry 147:16–22, 1988a

Nolen WA, Van dePutte JJ, Dijken WA, et al: Treatment strategy in depression, I: nontricyclic and selective reuptake inhibitors in resistant depression: a double-blind partial-crossover study on the effects of oxaprotiline and fluvoxamine. Acta Psychiatr Scand 78:668–675, 1988b

Norden MJ: Fluoxetine in borderline personality disorder. Prog Neuropsychopharmacol Biol Psychiatry 13:885–893, 1989

Othmer E, Othmer S, Stern WC, et al: Long-term efficacy and safety of bupropion. J Clin Psychiatry 44 (sec 2):153–156, 1983

Overall JE, Biggs J, Jacobs M, et al: Comparison of alprazolam and imipramine for treatment of outpatient depression. J Clin Psychiatry 48:15–19, 1987

Pare CMB: The present status of monoamine oxidase inhibitors. Br J Psychiatry 146:576–584, 1985

Pastuzak A, Schick-Boschetto B, Zuber C et al: Pregnancy outcome following first-trimester exposure to fluoxetine (Prozac). JAMA 269:2246–2248, 1993

Perry PJ: Pharmacotherapy for major depression with melancholic features: relative efficacy of tricyclic versus selective serotonin reuptake inhibitor antidepressants. J Affect Disord 39:1–6, 1996

Perry PJ, Wilding DC, Juhl RP: Anticholinergic psychosis. Am J Hosp Pharm 35:725–728, 1978

Perry PJ, Browne JL, Alexander B, et al: Two prospective dosing methods for nortriptyline. Clin Pharmacokinet 9:555–563, 1984

Perry PJ, Zeilmann C, Arndt SV: Tricyclic antidepressant plasma concentrations: an estimate of their sensitivity and specificity as a predictor of response. J Clin Psychopharmacol 14:230–240, 1994

Peselow ED, Filippi A, Goodnick P, et al: The short- and long-term efficacy of paroxetine, B: data from a double-blind crossover study and from a year-long trial vs imipramine and placebo. Psychopharmacol Bull 25:272–276, 1989

Piafsky KM, Borga O: Plasma protein binding of basic drugs, II: importance of α_1-acid-glycoprotein to interindividual variation. Clin Pharmacol Ther 22:545–549, 1977

Pickett P, Masand P, Murray GB: Psychostimulant treatment of geriatric depressive disorders secondary to medical illness. J Geriatr Psychiatry Neurol 13:146–151, 1991

Pinder RM, Brogden RN, Speight TM, et al: Maprotiline: a review of its pharmacological properties and therapeutic efficacy in mental depressive states. Drugs 13:321–352, 1977

Ponto LB, Perry PJ, Liskow BI, et al: Tricyclic antidepressant and monoamine oxidase inhibitor combination therapy. Am J Hosp Pharm 34:954–961, 1977

Preskorn SH: Recent pharmacologic advances in antidepressant therapy for the elderly (review). Am J Med 94:2S–12S, 1993

Prien RF, Kupfer DJ: Continuation drug therapy for major depressive episodes: how long should it be maintained? Am J Psychiatry 143:18–23, 1986

Prusoff BA, Williams DH, Weissman MM, et al: Treatment of secondary depression in schizophrenia: a double-blind, placebo-controlled trial of amitriptyline added to perphenazine. Arch Gen Psychiatry 36:569–575, 1979

Pursel M, Perry PJ: Fiscal year 1994–1995 annual report of drug ranking by prescription number. Des Moines, IA, Iowa Medicaid Drug Utilization Review Commission, 1995

Quitkin FM, McGrath P, Liebowitz MR, et al: Monoamine oxidase inhibitors in bipolar endogenous depressives. J Clin Psychopharmacol 1:70–74, 1981

Rabkin JG, Quitkin F, Harrison W, et al: Adverse reactions to monoamine oxidase inhibitors, I: a comparative study. J Clin Psychopharmacol 4:270–278, 1984

Rabkin JG, Quitkin FM, McGrath P, et al: Adverse reactions to monoamine oxidase inhibitors, II: treatment correlates and clinical management. J Clin Psychopharmacol 5:2–9, 1985

Rabkin JG, Rabkin R, Harrison W, et al: Effect of imipramine on mood and enumerative measures of immune status in depressed patients with HIV illness. Am J Psychiatry 151:516–523, 1994

Raisfeld IH: Cardiovascular complications of antidepressant therapy. Am Heart J 83:129–133, 1972

Ravaris CL, Robinson DS, Ives JO, et al: Phenelzine and amitriptyline in the treatment of depression. Arch Gen Psychiatry 37:1075–1080, 1980

Reding MJ, Orto LA, Winter SW, et al: Antidepressant therapy after stroke: a double-blind trial. Arch Neurol 43:763–765, 1986

Reifler BV, Teri L, Raskind M, et al: Double-blind trial of imipramine in Alzheimer's disease patients with and without depression. Am J Psychiatry 146:45–49, 1989

Reimherr FW, Wood DR, Byerley B, et al: Characteristics of responders to fluoxetine. Psychopharmacol Bull 20:20–72, 1984

Remeron® [mirtazapine] Product Information. West Orange, NJ, Organon Inc., 1996

Richelson E: Antidepressants and brain neurochemistry. Mayo Clin Proc 65:1227–1236, 1990

Richelson E, Nelson A: Antagonism by antidepressants of neurotransmitter receptors of normal human brain in vitro. J Pharmacol Exp Ther 230:94–102, 1984

Rickels K, Chung HR, Csanalosi IB, et al: Alprazolam, diazepam, imipramine, and placebo in outpatients with major depression. Arch Gen Psychiatry 44:862–866, 1987

Ries RK, Gilbert DA, Katon W: Tricyclic antidepressant therapy for peptic ulcer disease. Arch Intern Med 144:566–569, 1984

Riess W: The relevance of blood level determinations during the evaluation of maprotiline in man, in Research and Clinical Investigation in Depression. Edited by Murphy JE. Northampton, UK, Cambridge Medical Publications, 1976, pp 19–38

Robertson MM, Trimble MR: The treatment of depression in patients with epilepsy: a double-blind trial. J Affect Disord 9:127–136, 1985

Robin AA, Wiseberg S: A controlled trial of methylphenidate in the treatment of depressive states. J Neurol Neurosurg Psychiatry 21:55–57, 1958

Robinson DS, Nies A, Ravaris CL, et al: The monoamine oxidase inhibitor, phenelzine, in the treatment of depressive anxiety states. Arch Gen Psychiatry 29:407–413, 1973

Robinson DS, Nies A, Ravaris CL, et al: Phenelzine and amitriptyline in the treatment of depression. Arch Gen Psychiatry 35:629–635, 1978

Robinson DS, Nies A, Corcella J, et al: Cardiovascular effects of phenelzine and amitriptyline in depressed outpatients. J Clin Psychiatry 43:8–15, 1982

Rockwell WJK, Ellinwood EH, Trader DW: Psychotropic drugs promoting weight gain: health risks and treatment implications. South Med J 76:1407–1412, 1983

Roose SP, Glassman AH, Giardina EGV, et al: Nortriptyline in depressed patients with left ventricular impairment. JAMA 256:3253–3257, 1986

Roose SP, Glassman AH, Giardina EGV, et al: Tricyclic antidepressants in depressed patients with cardiac conduction disease. Arch Gen Psychiatry 74:360–364, 1987a

Roose SP, Glassman AH, Giardina EGV, et al: Cardiovascular effects of imipramine and bupropion in depressed patients with congestive heart failure. J Clin Psychopharmacol 7:247–251, 1987b

Roose SP, Dalack GW, Glassman AH, et al: Cardiovascular effects of bupropion in depressed patients with heart disease. Am J Psychiatry 148:512–516, 1991

Roose SP, Glassman AH, Attia E, et al: Comparative efficacy of selective serotonin reuptake inhibitors and tricyclics in the treatment of melancholia. Am J Psychiatry 151:1735–1739, 1994

Rothschild AJ: Selective serotonin reuptake inhibitor–induced sexual dysfunction: efficacy of a drug holiday. Am J Psychiatry 152:1514–1516, 1995

Rothschild AJ, Samson JA, Bessette MP, et al: Efficacy of the combination of fluoxetine and perphenazine in the treatment of psychotic depression. J Clin Psychiatry 54:338–342, 1993

Rouillon F, Serrurier D, Miller HD, et al: Prophylactic efficacy of maprotiline on unipolar depression relapse. J Clin Psychiatry 52:423–431, 1991

Rudorfer MV, Potter WZ: Antidepressants: a comparative review of the clinical pharmacology and therapeutic use of the "newer" versus the "older" drugs. Drugs 37:713–738, 1989

Rush AJ, Erman MK, Schlesser JA, et al: Alprazolam versus amitriptyline in depression with reduced REM latency. Arch Gen Psychiatry 42:1154–1159, 1985

Ruskin JN: The Cardiac Arrhythmia Suppression Trial (CAST). N Engl J Med 321:386–388, 1989

Ryan ND, Birmaher B, Perel JM, et al: Neuroendocrine response to L-5-hydroxytryptophan challenge in prepubertal major depression: depressed vs normal children. Arch Gen Psychiatry 49:843–851, 1992

Salzman C, Wolfson AN, Schatzberg A, et al: Effect of fluoxetine on anger in symptomatic volunteers with borderline personality disorder. J Clin Psychopharmacol 15:23–29, 1995

Satel SL, Nelson JC: Stimulants in the treatment of depression: a critical overview. J Clin Psychiatry 50:241–249, 1989

Schenker S, Bergstrom FR, Wolen RL, et al: Fluoxetine disposition and elimination in cirrhosis. Clin Pharmacol Ther 44:353–359, 1988

Schiffer RB, Wineman NM: Antidepressant pharmacotherapy of depression associated with multiple sclerosis. Am J Psychiatry 147:1493–1497, 1990

Schleifer SJ, Macari-Hinson MM, Coyle DA, et al: The nature and course of depression following myocardial infarction. Arch Intern Med 149:1785–1789, 1989

Schweizer E, Rickels K, Amsterdam JD, et al: What constitutes an adequate antidepressant trial for fluoxetine? J Clin Psychiatry 51:8–11, 1990

Sedlacek SM, Rudolf PM, Kaehny WD: Amoxapine-associated agranulocytosis with thrombocytosis occurring early during recovery. Am J Med 80:533–536, 1986

Segraves RT: Reversal by bethanechol of imipramine-induced ejaculatory dysfunction (letter). Am J Psychiatry 144:1243–1244, 1987

Sheehan DV, Claycomb JB, Kauretas N: Monoamine oxidase inhibitors: prescription and patient management. Int J Psychiatry Med 10:99–212, 1980–1981

Shulman KI, Walker SE, MacKenzie S, et al: Dietary restriction, tyramine, and the use of monoamine oxidase inhibitors. J Clin Psychopharmacol 9:397–402, 1989

Simeon J, Dinicola V, Phil M, et al: Adolescent depression: a placebo-controlled fluoxetine treatment study and follow-up. Prog Neuropsychopharmacol Biol Psychiatry 14:791–795, 1990

Sheikh KH, Nies AS: Trazodone and intrahepatic cholestasis (letter). Ann Intern Med 99:572, 1983

Slattery JT, Gibaldi M, Koup JR: Prediction of maintenance dose required to attain a desired drug concentration at steady state from a single determination of concentration after an initial dose. Clin Pharmacokinet 5:77–85, 1980

Smith WT, Glaudin V, Panagides J, et al: Mirtazapine versus amitriptyline versus placebo in the treatment of major depressive disorder. Psychopharmacol Bull 20:191–196, 1990

Sovner R, DiMascio A: Extrapyramidal syndromes and other neurological side effects of psychotropic drugs, in Psychopharmacology: A Generation of Progress. Edited by Lipton MA, DiMascio A, Killam DF. New York, Raven, 1978, pp 1021–1032

Spiker DG, Weiss JC, Dealy RS, et al: The pharmacological treatment of delusional depression. Am J Psychiatry 142:430–436, 1985

Spiker DG, Dealy RS, Hanin I, et al: Treating delusional depressives with amitriptyline. J Clin Psychiatry 47:243–246, 1986

Spina E, DeDomenico P, Ruello C, et al: Adjunctive fluoxetine in the treatment of negative symptoms in chronic schizophrenic patients. Int Clin Psychopharmacol 9:281–285, 1994

Stahl SM: Neuroendocrine markers of serotonin responsivity in depression. Prog Neuropsychopharmacol Biol Psychiatry 16:655–659, 1992

Stein G, Bernadt M: Lithium augmentation therapy in tricyclic-resistant depression: a controlled trial using lithium in low and normal doses. Br J Psychiatry 162:634–640, 1993

Steiner M, Steinberg S, Stewart D, et al: Fluoxetine in the treatment of premenstrual dysphoria (Canadian Fluoxetine/Premenstrual Dysphoria Collaborative Study Group). N Engl J Med 332:1529–1534, 1995

Stern WC, Harto-Truax N, Bauer N: Efficacy of bupropion in tricyclic resistant or intolerant patients. J Clin Psychiatry 44 (sec 2):148–152, 1983

Stewart JW, Harrison W, Quitkin F, et al: Phenelzine-induced pyridoxine deficiency. J Clin Psychopharmacol 4:225–226, 1984

Stewart JW, McGrath PJ, Liebowitz MR, et al: Treatment outcome variation of DSM-III depressive subtypes: clinical usefulness in outpatients with mild to moderate depression. Arch Gen Psychiatry 42:148–153, 1985

Stewart MM: MAOI and food: fact and fiction. Adverse Drug Reactions Bulletin 58:200–203, 1976

Tasker TCG, Kaye CM, Zussman BD, et al: Paroxetine plasma levels: lack of correlation with efficacy or adverse effects. Acta Psychiatr Scand 80 (suppl 350):152–155, 1989

Teicher MH, Cohen BM, Baldessarini RJ, et al: Severe daytime somnolence in patients treated with an MAOI. Am J Psychiatry 145:1552–1556, 1988

Teicher MH, Gold C, Cole JO: Emergence of intense suicidal preoccupation during fluoxetine treatment. Am J Psychiatry 147:207–210, 1990

Thase ME, Mallinger AG, McKnight D: Treatment of imipramine-resistant recurrent depression, IV: a double-blind crossover study of tranylcypromine for anergic bipolar depression. Am J Psychiatry 149:195–198, 1992

Tollefson GD: Monoamine oxidase inhibitors: a review. J Clin Psychiatry 44:280–288, 1983

True BL, Alexander B, Carter BL: Switching monoamine oxidase inhibitors. Drug Intelligence and Clinical Pharmacy 19:825–827, 1985

Turkington RW: Depression masquerading as diabetic neuropathy. JAMA 243:1147–1450, 1980

Tyber MA: The relationship between hiatus hernia and tricyclic antidepressants: a report of five cases. Am J Psychiatry 132:652–653, 1975

Tyrer P, Murphy S, Kingdon D, et al: The Nottingham study of neurotic disorder: comparison of drug and psychological treatment. Lancet 2:235–240, 1988

Tyrer SP, Marshall EP, Griffiths HW: The relationship between response to fluoxetine, plasma drug levels, imipramine binding to platelet membranes and whole-blood 5-HT. Prog Neuropsychopharmacol Biol Psychiatry 14:797–805, 1990

Vallejo J, Gasto C, Catalan R, et al: Double-blind study of imipramine versus phenelzine in melancholias and dysthymic disorders. Br J Psychiatry 151:639–642, 1987

van Moffaert M, de Wilde J, Vereecken A, et al: Mirtazapine is more effective than trazodone: a double-blind, controlled study in hospitalized patients with major depression. Int Clin Psychopharmacol 10:3–9, 1995

von Moltke L, Greenblatt D, Harmatz JS: In vitro inhibition of desipramine oxidation by fluoxetine and norfluoxetine is greater than inhibition by sertraline or desmethylsertraline (abstract). Clin Pharmacol Ther 53:196, 1993

Wallace A, Kofoed LL, West AN: Double-blind, placebo-controlled trial of methylphenidate in older, depressed, medically ill patients. Am J Psychiatry 152:929–931, 1995

Warner MD, Peabody CA, Whiteford HA, et al: Alprazolam as an antidepressant. J Clin Psychiatry 49:148–150, 1988

Wehr TA, Goodwin FK: Can antidepressants cause mania and worsen the course of affective illness? Am J Psychiatry 144:1403–1411, 1987

BG, Gelenberg AJ: Chemistry, pharmacology, pharmacokinetics, adverse effects, and efficacy of the antidepressant maprotiline hydrochloride. Pharmacotherapy 1:121–129, 1981

Wernicke JF: The side effect profile of fluoxetine. J Clin Psychiatry 46 (sec 2):59–67, 1985

Wernicke JF, Dunlop SR, Dornseif BE, et al: Fixed dose fluoxetine therapy for depression. Psychopharmacol Bull 23:164–168, 1987

Wernicke JF, Dunlop SR, Dornseif BE, et al: Low dose fluoxetine therapy for depression. Psychopharmacol Bull 24:183–188, 1988

West ED, Dally PJ: Effects of iproniazid in depressive syndromes. BMJ 1:2491–2494, 1959

Wheatley D: Amphetamines in general practice. Seminars in Psychiatry 1:163–173, 1969

White K, Simpson G: Combined MAOI–tricyclic antidepressant treatment: a reevaluation. J Clin Psychopharmacol 1:264–281, 1981

Wisner KL, Wheeler SB: Prevention of recurrent postpartum major depression. Hospital and Community Psychiatry 45:1191–1196, 1994

Wolfe F, Cathey MA, Hawley DJ: A double-blind placebo-controlled trial of fluoxetine in fibromyalgia. Scand J Rheumatol 23:255–259, 1994

Wolfersdorf M, Barg T, Konig F, et al: Paroxetine as antidepressant in combined antidepressant-neuroleptic therapy in delusional depression: observation of clinical use. Pharmacopsychiatry 28:56–60, 1995

Wood SH, Mortola JF, Chan YF, et al: Treatment of premenstrual syndrome with fluoxetine: a double-blind placebo-controlled, crossover study. Obstet Gynecol 80:339–344, 1992

Yager J: Bethanechol chloride can reverse erectile and ejaculatory dysfunction induced by tricyclic antidepressants and mazindol. J Clin Psychiatry 47:210–211, 1986

Ziegler VE, Clayton PJ, Biggs JT: A comparison study of amitriptyline and nortriptyline with plasma levels. Arch Gen Psychiatry 34:607–612, 1977

Zusky PM, Biederman J, Rosenbaum JF, et al: Adjunct low dose lithium carbonate in treatment-resistant depression: a placebo controlled study. J Clin Pharmacol 8:120–124, 1988

3

Antimanics

Lithium

The calming effect of lithium chloride in mania was first reported in 1949 (Price and Heninger 1994). That same year, the U.S. Food and Drug Administration (FDA) banned lithium in the United States after several deaths occurred secondary to lithium intoxication. The drug had been used as a salt substitute. The FDA did not approve lithium carbonate for psychiatric use until 1970.

■ Indications

The primary indications for lithium carbonate in psychiatry are the treatment of acute mania and depression as well as the prophylactic treatment of patients with recurrent bipolar or unipolar affective illness. Lithium has been successfully used to treat aggression, whether related to a primary psychiatric illness or not (Pabis and Stanislav 1996). Less well-established psychiatric indications for lithium carbonate include anorexia nervosa, premenstrual tension, phobias, and anxiety (D. F. Klein et al. 1980). Nonpsychiatric uses include cluster headaches.

■ Efficacy

Acute Treatment

▶ Mania

An American Psychiatric Association working group and other authors have recommended lithium carbonate as the first-line agent for the acute treatment of mania (Calabrese et al. 1995; Hirschfeld et al. 1994; Price and Heninger 1994; Sachs 1996). A 3-week therapeutic trial is suggested, as lithium's onset of action is often delayed 1–2 weeks (Price and Heninger 1994). Although patients may not be completely well after 3 weeks of treatment, substantial improvement is often noted. Once a patient starts to improve, resolution of symptoms generally occurs quickly. If lithium carbonate is abruptly discontinued during the manic phase, relapse may occur within several days.

Lithium alone.   If a patient is not acutely agitated, he or she might be treated with lithium carbonate alone (see *Lithium plus an antipsychotic*, below, and *Lithium or lithium/antipsychotic plus a benzodiazepine* [page 223]).

Open/single-blind reports.   According to 10 reports involving a total of 413 patients, lithium carbonate produced an average improvement rate of 81% (range 68%–100%) (Goodwin and Zis 1979).

Placebo-controlled trials.   Four studies have compared lithium carbonate's effectiveness with that of placebo (Goodwin and Zis 1979; Hirschfeld et al. 1994); however, only three of these studies reported response rates. Overall, 65 of 80 patients (81%) with typical mania were reported to respond to lithium carbonate. The fourth study, involving 28 patients, reported that lithium carbonate was more effective than placebo. Most of these studies included relatively young patients. A recent review of 55- to 77-year-old patients treated with lithium carbonate for mania reported a response rate similar to that reported for younger patients (Mirchandani and Young 1993). However, some of these older patients did not tolerate typical antimanic lithium carbonate levels (see "Dosage" and *Neurological* adverse effects [pages 230 and 248, respectively]).

Lithium versus antipsychotics.   Nine double-blind, controlled trials have compared lithium carbonate with typical antipsychotics (Chou 1991; Goodwin and Zis 1979). Seven of the nine studies involved chlorpromazine; the other two used haloperidol and pimozide. The study results can be summarized as follows: 1) the percentage of patients experiencing remission or marked improvement after 3 weeks of treatment was greater with lithium carbonate than with the antipsychotic; 2) lithium carbonate was particularly effective in ameliorating the affective and ideational symptoms associated with mania, whereas the antipsychotic was initially superior to lithium carbonate in controlling psychomotor activity; 3) compared with those receiving an antipsychotic alone, inpatients treated with lithium carbonate were more likely to be discharged at the end of the 3-week treatment period.

Lithium plus an antipsychotic.   Often, a lithium carbonate/antipsychotic combination is started immediately, on the rationale that the antipsychotic will control hyperactivity and irritability during the interval before lithium begins to exert its effect (Chou 1991). This common clinical practice has been evaluated in only one study in patients with mania (Chou 1991). The study concluded that lithium carbonate combined with haloperidol produced a slightly greater control of symptoms than did haloperidol alone. As manic symptoms are brought under control and the patient's behavior normalizes, the antipsychotic can be discontinued.

Lithium or lithium/antipsychotic plus a benzodiazepine. When a lithium/antipsychotic combination is used, benzodiazepines have been reported to reduce the daily dosage requirements of the antipsychotic by 33% (Edwards et al. 1991; Gerner 1993).

Case reports/open trials. Clonazepam and lorazepam alone or in combination with antipsychotics have been reported to control agitation when added to lithium carbonate treatment (Aronson et al. 1989; Gerner 1993).

Two open trials involving a total of 11 manic patients reported that lorazepam 9–80 mg/day, when added to lithium carbonate treatment, resulted in control of agitation (Lenox et al. 1986; Modell et al. 1985). Typical doses were difficult to determine, as only dosage *ranges* were given for some patients; however, most patients required more than 20 mg/day. The dosing regimen consisted of lorazepam 2–4 mg po/im q2h prn for agitation. Several patients required the addition of an antipsychotic to control agitation. Sedation and clinical control were reported to occur within the first 2 days of treatment (Modell et al. 1985).

Double-blind studies. In one trial, lithium carbonate plus lorazepam was as effective in overall response rate as lithium carbonate in combination with haloperidol (Lenox et al. 1992). Both treatments produced an onset of effect within 5 to 7 days. More patients dropped out of the lorazepam group because of nonresponse, whereas more patients dropped out of the haloperidol group because of adverse effects.

After manic symptoms have been controlled in a patient receiving lithium/benzodiazepine combined treatment, an attempt should be made to discontinue the benzodiazepine by tapering the dose over 1 week. The patient should be monitored for relapse of manic symptoms.

▶ Atypical Mania

Patients with organic, psychotic, dysphoric, mixed, or rapid-cycling (i.e., more than four episodes in 1 year) features of mania and/or concurrent substance abuse are reported to be less responsive to lithium carbonate than to carbamazepine or valproate (see "Efficacy" subsections for those agents, later in this chapter) (Gerner 1993; Price and Heninger 1994; Solomon and Bauer 1993). However, this conclusion was not derived from controlled studies of lithium carbonate versus carbamazepine or valproate (Janicak et al.

). A review suggested that approximately 10%–35% and 15%–%
of patients with rapid-cycling illness and dysphoric or mixed ania, respectively, will respond to lithium carbonate (Dilsaver et al. 1993; Gerner 1993). Therefore, patients with these features should not be labeled lithium-refractory unless a therapeutic trial has been performed.

Major Depressive Disorder

An antidepressant response to lithium carbonate may occur within 3 weeks; however, up to 6 weeks of treatment may be required for a response to be seen (Mendels et al. 1979). A therapeutic trial consists of 4–6 weeks.

The use of lithium carbonate as an augmentation strategy in treatment-refractory depression is discussed in *Major Depression* (page 133) under "Efficacy" of **Tricyclic Antidepressants** in Chapter 2.

Bipolar depression. In a review of 13 studies, 60%–80% of bipolar patients in the depressive phase responded to lithium carbonate alone (Price and Heninger 1994). A patient admitted with a depressive episode secondary to noncompliance with lithium carbonate should be considered for a treatment trial with lithium carbonate alone. Conversely, if the patient had been compliant with lithium carbonate, adding a standard antidepressant should be considered (Janicak et al. 1995) (see "switching" [page 153] under *Neurological/Psychiatric* adverse effects of **Tricyclic Antidepressants** in Chapter 2).

Unipolar depression. Lithium used alone is less effective than typical antidepressants in the treatment of unipolar depression, as only 30%–40% of patients may respond (Price and Heninger 1994). It is recommended only as an alternative treatment in patients who fail to respond to first-line antidepressants (see Major Depression [page 133] under "Efficacy" of **Tricyclic Antidepressants** in Chapter 2). When lithium is used to treat an acute depressive episode, antimanic lithium levels should be achieved (see "Dosage" [page 230]), and a trial should last 3–4 weeks.

Schizoaffective Disorder

Fourteen studies have investigated lithium carbonate's role in schizoaffective disorder (Goodnick and Meltzer 1984; Keck et al. 1996; Lapensee 1992). Despite the diagnostic ambiguity associated with schizoaffective illness, the available data indicate that lithium carbonate is effective in the initial treatment of schizoaffective mania. Many patients with schizoaffective disorder require lithium carbonate in combination with an antidepressant and/or an antipsychotic (Keck et al. 1996). The onset of response to lithium carbonate is slower for schizoaffective mania than for bipolar mania (Lapensee 1992).

▶ Aggression

Lithium has been successfully used in the management of chronic aggression in a variety of patients studied in double-blind, placebo-controlled trials (Pabis and Stanislav 1996). Subjects have included patients with mania, violent adult prison inmates, aggressive children, mentally retarded individuals, and patients with brain injuries. Treatment trials lasted 3–4 months, and lithium serum levels of 0.7–1.0 mEq/L were typically used. Some subjects did not tolerate lithium serum levels of 1.0 mEq/L because of neurological adverse effects (e.g., sedation, ataxia) (see *Neurological* adverse effects [page 248]).

Continuation Treatment

Continuation treatment is the uninterrupted extension of pharmacological management after resolution of an acute affective episode. It is instituted to prevent **relapse** (defined as an exacerbation of the current episode). (**Maintenance treatment,** in contrast, is geared toward preventing a **recurrence** [defined as a new episode].)

Unless maintenance treatment is to be instituted, lithium carbonate can be stopped when continuation treatment has been completed (see *Maintenance Treatment,* below). It has been suggested that abrupt discontinuation of lithium carbonate may lead to a rapid return of manic symptoms in one-third of patients, typically within 2 to 14 days (Grell and Schmidt 1988). Another study indicated that tapering lithium carbonate over a 2- to 4-week period reduced the recurrence rate (Faedda et al. 1993). Conservatively, if time permits, lithium carbonate should be tapered over a 4-week period, with the daily dose reduced by 25% every week. Investigators in another study reported that when abrupt lithium carbonate discontinuation led to a rapid return of manic symptoms, patients often responded within 2 to 14 days of lithium carbonate reinstitution (Faedda et al. 1993).

▶ Depressive Episode

An untreated episode of depression may last 6–13 months (Winokur 1994). The risk of relapse is highest during the 2- to 3-month period directly after the depressive symptoms have been brought under control. Likewise, the greatest risk of recurrence coincides with the 4–6 months immediately after recovery, and declines thereafter (Solomon and Bauer 1993). When lithium carbonate is used to treat a depressive episode, antimanic plasma levels should be maintained for 4–6 months after the patient responds (Burrows 1992). The need for maintenance treatment depends on the number of previous depressive episodes the patient has experienced (see Unipolar Depression [page 229] under *Maintenance Treatment*, below).

▶ Manic Episode
The mean duration of a manic episode is 3 months (Clayton 1994). Conservatively, antimanic lithium levels should be maintained for 3–6 months after resolution of manic symptoms (Solomon and Bauer 1993) (see *Maintenance Treatment*, below).

▶ Schizoaffective Disorder
See Depressive Episode and Manic Episode, above, for guidelines for treating a current episode of depression and mania, respectively.

Maintenance Treatment
As previously noted, **maintenance treatment** is the extension of pharmacological management to prevent recurrence (i.e., a new affective episode). An American Psychiatric Association working group and other authors have recently recommended that lithium carbonate be used as the first-line agent for the maintenance treatment of affective illness (Calabrese et al. 1995; Hirschfeld et al. 1994; Price and Heninger 1994; Sachs 1996).

In a recent report, factors that reduced the response to maintenance treatment in bipolar patients included number of previous episodes, type of clinical presentation (e.g., mixed states), and presence of dual diagnoses (e.g., alcohol dependence, polysubstance abuse, and borderline, narcissistic, or histrionic personality disorders) (Janicak et al. 1995).

Epidemiological findings in a large series of patients receiving prophylactic lithium carbonate profiled those who responded to lithium carbonate (Abou-Saleh and Coppen 1986). Lithium responders were more likely to have a bipolar diagnosis with a positive family history of either unipolar or bipolar illness. Lithium responders with unipolar depression often had endogenous depression and a positive family history of "pure" depressive disease (i.e., no alcoholism or sociopathy in first-degree relatives). Bipolar patients who responded in less than 6 months and unipolar patients who responded in less than 1 year were more likely to have a successful outcome with maintenance treatment.

Several case reports have suggested that frequent interruption of treatment (e.g., by drug discontinuation or noncompliance) may lead to loss of treatment efficacy in a previously responsive patient (Maj et al. 1995). This phenomenon has been termed "lithium discontinuation–induced refractoriness." A study was recently performed in 54 patients with bipolar illness for whom lithium carbonate prophylaxis had been successful (Maj et al. 1995). All patients were taken off lithium carbonate for reasons other than recurrence of illness or occurrence of significant side effects and had experienced one or more affective episodes while off drug treatment. During the 1-year follow-up period after lithium maintenance treatment had been reinstituted, 10 of the 54 (20%) patients underwent one or more affective episodes. These findings suggest that experiencing an interruption of lithium treatment and a subsequent affective episode may adversely affect future response to lithium carbonate in some patients. This was especially true for patients who had successfully received lithium treatment for more than 2 years. Nonetheless, preliminary evidence was noted to indicate that some patients regained their response to lithium maintenance treatment even after several illness recurrences.

Occasionally, patients may require maintenance treatment with a lithium/antipsychotic combination (Sachs 1990) (see Mania [page 7] under "Efficacy" of **Typical Antipsychotics** in Chapter 1). Benzodiazepines have been used in the maintenance treatment of mania. In one open trial of 12 patients receiving maintenance treatment of lithium plus an antipsychotic, no patient relapsed when clonazepam was substituted for the antipsychotic (Sachs 1990). However, when clonazepam was added to lithium in another open trial, it did not prevent relapse of symptoms in 5 patients with lithium-resistant bipolar illness (Aronson et al. 1989).

▶ Bipolar Disorder

A study of the course of affective illness in 95 bipolar patients reported that 85% of patients experienced more than two episodes of illness over a 19- to 27-year follow-up period (Angst 1981). Of those patients undergoing recurrences, 67% experienced two additional affective episodes within the subsequent 5-year period. A recent study suggested that a patient experiencing one manic episode had a 54% lifetime chance of having an additional episode and a 29% chance of having two or more additional episodes (Solomon and Bauer 1993).

Open reports and 10 prospective, double-blind, placebo-controlled trials have demonstrated the efficacy of lithium carbonate in preventing manic and depressive episodes in bipolar patients (Price and Heninger 1994; Solomon and Bauer 1993). The rate of recurrence and relapse for lithium carbonate and placebo ranged from 0% to 44% (mean 23%) and from 38% to 93% (mean 56%), respectively. Responders in these studies included patients who experienced no recurrent episodes as well as patients who experienced another affective episode "in an attenuated form" (i.e., a reduced number—or intensity or duration—of episodes). An exact definition of lithium carbonate nonresponse is seldom stated in these studies.

An early report recommended that maintenance treatment be initiated after the second affective episode (e.g., mania, depression) if that episode occurred within 4 years of the first episode (Angst 1981). However, a recent study advises that maintenance treatment be instituted after the second affective episode, regardless of the time elapsed between the first and second episodes (Solomon and Bauer 1993). Although a patient has an 85% chance of sustaining at least one additional manic episode, it is important to note that approximately 15% of patients will not experience another episode (Solomon and Bauer 1993). Unfortunately, it is not possible to consistently differentiate patients who are likely to experience recurrent episodes of mania or depression from those who are not.

It is recommended after a response in first-episode mania that lithium carbonate be administered as continuation treatment for 3–6 months to prevent relapse (see Manic Episode [page 226] under *Continuation Treatment,* above). In addition, the patient, in consultation with family members and/or a significant other, may wish to initiate maintenance treatment after resolution of the first manic episode to reduce the possibility of recurrence. Considerations in evaluating which of these treatment approaches should be used include the complications resulting from the first episode (e.g., legal and economic difficulties, sexual indiscretions, suicide attempts) and the high risk of recurrence.

Although maintenance treatment with lithium carbonate alone should be attempted, some patients respond better to a combination of lithium carbonate and a tricyclic antidepressant (Price and Heninger 1994). It has been suggested that antidepressants may induce rapid cycling in bipolar patients; however, evidence for this effect is inconclusive (see *Neurological/Psychiatric* adverse effects [page 153] under **Tricyclic Antidepressants** in Chapter 2).

▶ Schizoaffective Disorder

Follow-up of 150 schizoaffective patients from age 19 to age 27 years revealed that 82% experienced more than two affective episodes during the 8-year period (Angst 1981). Of the patients who experienced recurrent affective episodes, 67% had two additional episodes within the subsequent 5 years.

Lithium prophylaxis can decrease the frequency and duration of relapse in both schizoaffective mania and depression (Goodnick and Meltzer 1984). Often, patients with these disorders will receive lithium in combination with an antipsychotic, as lithium alone may be ineffective in preventing recurrent affective and psychotic episodes, according to three controlled trials (Keck et al. 1996). (For maintenance treatment recommendations for schizoaffective disorder, bipolar type, see Bipolar Disorder [page 227]; for schizoaffective disorder, depressive type, see Unipolar Depression, below.)

▶ Unipolar Depression

A 19- to 27-year follow-up of 159 unipolar patients reported that 63% of patients experienced two or more episodes (Angst 1981). In addition, 40% of the patients with recurrent affective episodes underwent two additional episodes during the subsequent 5-year period. More recent literature suggests that 50%–85% of patients treated for depression at university medical centers will have at least one additional episode of depression during their lifetime (Solomon and Bauer 1993). In those patients experiencing recurrence, 50% will have an additional depressive episode within 2 years. In addition, 10%–15% of unipolar patients will experience manic or hypomanic symptoms and therefore be reclassified as bipolar patients (Price and Heninger 1994; Winokur 1994).

Overall, 10 placebo- and/or antidepressant-controlled trials have concluded that lithium carbonate is more effective than placebo and equal in efficacy to antidepressants in the maintenance treatment of unipolar patients (Price and Heninger 1994; Solomon and Bauer 1993; Souza and Goodwin 1991).

Patients experiencing their first or second episode of depression should receive continuation treatment as previously outlined (see Depressive Episode [page 225] under *Continuation Treatment,* above). In general, it is recommended that maintenance treatment be instituted after three depressive episodes, particularly if the third episode occurred within 5 years of the second episode (Burrows 1992). However, this recommendation may be modified based on discussions with the patient, family, and/or significant other.

▶ Aggression

The efficacy of lithium in the maintenance treatment of aggression has not been extensively studied. To determine ongoing need, a periodic trial off the drug might be considered.

■ Mechanism of Action

Lithium interferes with multiple neurobiological processes (Price and Heninger 1994). The relationship of these changes to mood regulation is not clear. Lithium may exert part of its therapeutic effect by intervening in neuronal regulation. The neuron receptor effects of lithium are as follows: 1) lithium carbonate pretreatment prevents reserpine-induced upregulation of the β-adrenergic receptors in the cerebral cortex; 2) it reduces the number of striatal dopamine receptors; 3) lithium carbonate blocks haloperidol-induced upregulation of dopamine receptors; and 4) it downregulates α_2-adenoreceptor function. Lithium does not prevent imipramine-induced downregulation of β-adrenergic receptors. Lithium produces significant effects on the cyclic nucleotide–generating system. This action may be due to an antagonism of certain magnesium-dependent enzyme activities of β-adrenergic cerebral adenylate cyclase (AC). AC is affected similarly by antidepressants, electrostimulation, and rapid eye movement (REM)–sleep deprivation. Acute and chronic lithium carbonate administration causes inhibition of two of the system's second messengers, inositol 1,4,5-triphosphate and diacylglycerol, thereby compromising neuronal transmission, modifying the activity of AC, and changing the permeability of some ion channels. In addition, lithium may enhance or stabilize acetylcholine function.

■ Dosage

Special Populations

▶ Hemodialysis Patients
Patients undergoing hemodialysis should have their lithium carbonate dose administered after each dialysis treatment (DasGupta and Jefferson 1990). Adjustment of doses should be based on measurement of lithium levels and clinical response.

▶ Pregnant Patients
The effect of pregnancy on lithium pharmacokinetics has not been extensively studied. An early study involving a few patients reported that lithium clearance increased by 50%–100% during gestation (Schou and Amdisen 1973) but returned to baseline at the time of delivery. However, other factors (e.g., sodium and fluid changes secondary to other medical conditions) may affect lithium levels. Therefore, it is recommended that lithium levels be monitored monthly throughout pregnancy to maintain the desired lithium level. Lithium levels should be measured weekly or biweekly

the month before the estimated delivery date and appropriate dosage adjustments made. Lithium should be discontinued at the time of delivery and reinstituted at the prepregnancy dose immediately after delivery (Weinstein and Goldfield 1975). It is recommended that the daily dose be divided into multiple doses to minimize peak lithium levels. However, the safety of once- versus multiple-daily dosing of lithium carbonate in pregnancy has not been studied.

Dosing Techniques

Lithium doses required to achieve target plasma levels may be determined by empirical (i.e., trial and error) or predictive methods using individually derived pharmacokinetic parameters or population-derived equations. Predictive lithium carbonate dosing techniques have been reviewed (Lobeck 1988). Lithium is well suited for predictive approaches because of its large interindividual pharmacokinetic differences, defined concentration-therapeutic relationship, and narrow therapeutic index. Overall, individually determined kinetic parameters identified by a multiple-point assessment method more accurately predicts steady-state lithium concentrations than do population-based methods (Lobeck 1988).

In theory, use of a predictive dosing strategy should reduce the time needed to attain a therapeutic lithium level. However, this hypothesis has not been extensively investigated. A recent study in acutely manic patients found no difference in time to symptom response or patient outcome variables between a single-point predictive method and empirical dosing (Marken et al. 1994). However, patients in the predictive group spent 3–4 fewer days in an acute psychiatric unit than patients dosed with an empirical method. It is possible that sample sizes in this study were not large enough to detect a difference between dosing methods. Reasonably, one would expect that use of a predictive method—as opposed to empirical dosing—would reduce the frequency of lithium-level monitoring, as fewer dosage adjustments would be required. More studies need to be performed to address these questions.

Predictive methods might be useful for patients who have stable—but altered—lithium pharmacokinetics. Patients for whom such dosing methods might be appropriate include those who have reduced renal function, who are older, and/or who are stabilized on interacting drugs (e.g., thiazide diuretics). Identifying a lithium carbonate dose requirement a priori in these patients may help reduce the time needed to reach a therapeutic lithium concentration and/or avoid adverse effects (Lobeck 1988).

▶ **Empirical or Retrospective Dosing**

In the majority of patients, lithium follows first-order kinetics; therefore, as the dosage increases or decreases, the steady-state serum lithium concentration must increase or decrease proportionately, provided that no change occurs in lithium's renal clearance (see *Elimination* [page 238] under "Pharmacokinetics"). Thus, a patient with a steady-state concentration of 0.5 mEq/L at 1,200 mg/day will have a steady-state concentration of 1.0 mEq/L if the dose is increased to 2,400 mg/day. If the dose is decreased to 600 mg/day, the steady-state concentration should be 0.25 mEq/L.

The following dosing recommendations refer to the management of mania, depression, and schizoaffective disorder.

Acute treatment.   The recommended starting dosage for younger patients with normal renal function and no interacting drugs is 1,200–1,800 mg/day (Price and Heninger 1994). However, patients who are older than 50 years of age, have reduced renal function, and/or are taking interacting drugs should receive starting doses of 300–600 mg/day (Hewick et al. 1977; Mirchandani and Young 1993).

Continuation treatment.   Patients' lithium carbonate dosages should be maintained to yield antimanic lithium levels for at least 4 months after an acute episode. If a patient is euthymic, the lithium carbonate dose may be reduced to a maintenance level (see *Maintenance treatment,* immediately below, and Maintenance Treatment [page 241] under *Therapeutic Concentrations).*

Maintenance treatment.   Typical doses consist of 900–1,500 mg/day in healthy patients less than 50 years of age (Price and Heninger 1994). However, in patients who are older than 50 years of age, have reduced renal function, and/or are taking interacting drugs, maintenance doses of 300–600 mg/day may be required to achieve the desired plasma concentration (see *Acute treatment,* above).

▶ **Predictive Dosing**

Note: If the renal clearance of lithium increases or decreases after the administration of the test dose, the accuracy of the prediction will be affected.

Single-point method.   A mathematical relationship between drug concentration in serum at steady state and a single drug concentration after one test dose has been described (Perry et al. 1986). A serum lithium concentration measured 24 hours after a single lithium carbonate 1,200-mg test dose will predict steady-state concentrations for lithium carbonate doses ranging from 600 to 2,400 mg/day (see Figure 3–1) (Perry and Alexander 1987). *Note:*   Steady-

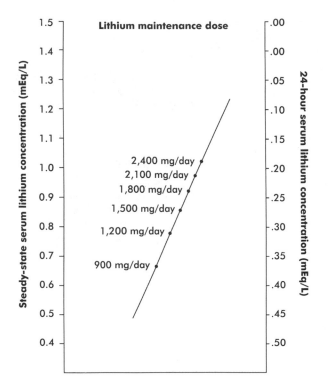

Figure 3–1. Lithium dosing nomogram for predicting steady-state serum concentrations for 900- to 2,400-mg/day maintenance doses following a 1,200-mg lithium carbonate test dose and subsequent measurement of the 24-hour serum lithium concentration.
Source. Reprinted from Perry PJ, Alexander B: "Dosage and Serum Levels," in *Modern Lithium Therapy.* Edited by Johnson FN. Lancaster, UK, MTP Press, 1987, p. 70. Copyright 1987, MTP Press. Used with permission.

state concentrations for patients requiring lithium carbonate dosages less than 900 mg/day or greater than 2,400 mg/day cannot be predicted with this method.

The single-point method has the advantage of requiring only a 24-hour wait before starting regular lithium carbonate dosing. However, it requires that a fixed 1,200-mg test dose be used, which as a single dose may produce adverse effects in some patients. Also, exact timing of the 24-hour sample and accurate assay results are necessary to prevent an inaccurate steady-state level prediction. In addition, limited pharmacokinetic information (e.g., no half-life determination) is available with this method.

Multiple-point method.   With this predictive dosing strategy, the patient is administered a single lithium carbonate 1,200-mg test dose, and serum lithium samples are obtained at two time points separated by 24 hours (Perry et al. 1982). Usually the samples are obtained approximately 12 and 36 hours after the test dose.

The multiple-point method has the advantages of greater accuracy compared with the single-point method and calculation of the patient's half-life, which can be used to determine time to steady state. Disadvantages include the following: 1) the test dose must be scheduled at a time when the laboratory is available to run the samples, 2) a longer delay is required before initiating the target dose because of the need to wait until the 36-hour sample has been obtained and both samples analyzed; and 3) hand-calculation of the steady-state serum lithium concentrations for various doses and dosing schedules is a time-consuming procedure.

A pharmacokinetic interactive computer program to simplify the use of this dosing method has been developed. The program is written in BASIC and is run on either a DOS-based PC or a Macintosh. With the program, the user enters the patient's name, the serum concentrations and sampling times after the test dose, and the number of hours after the target dose that future blood-level measurements will be taken. The screen then displays the patient's lithium half-life, the number of days necessary to reach steady state, and the correlation coefficient (if three or more posttest levels are obtained). This display is followed by a table of steady-state serum lithium concentrations predicted for various doses and dosing schedules. In addition to this information, the printout contains instructions for transforming serum lithium concentrations measured from blood samples drawn other than 12 hours after the last dose to a 12-hour steady-state concentration.[1]

▶ Loading Doses
A 30-mg/kg loading dose of the sustained-release lithium carbonate product Lithobid® was administered to 38 patients (Kook et al.

---

[1] The keystrokes for a hand-held calculator and/or a complimentary copy of the computer program may be obtained from the authors on request. Please include a formatted disk for the computer program.

1985). The total dose was rounded to the nearest 300-mg increment and divided into three doses, which were administered q2h. The total loading doses ranged from 1,200 to 3,000 mg. Twenty-one of the 38 patients (55%) had 12-hour lithium levels less than 0.90 mEq/L, and 4 patients (11%) had levels between 1.28 mEq/L and 1.40 mEq/L. No adverse effects were noted 12 hours after loading dose administration. The authors suggested that for women, ideal rather than actual body weight should be used to determine dosage, because this measure provided a more accurate prediction of lithium blood levels.

Patient diagnoses were not presented in the study. If one assumes that most of the patients in the study were in a manic phase at the time the loading dose was administered, more than half of them would not have received enough medication to control their symptoms (see Acute Treatment, *Mania* [page 240] under *Therapeutic Concentrations*). Therefore, lithium blood levels may need to be adjusted after the initial loading dose. Use of loading doses greater than 30 mg/kg is not recommended until the accuracy and safety of doses of this size can be determined.

Dosing Regimens

▶ Once-Daily Dosing

It is recommended that lithium carbonate treatment be initiated with doses administered two to three times a day (Price and Heninger 1994). In this author's experience, most patients will tolerate twice-a-day lithium carbonate dosing. After the target steady-state lithium level is achieved, once-daily dosing can be considered if the patient's total daily dose is 1,800 mg or lower (Hammond 1994). The safety of once-daily lithium carbonate doses greater than 1,800 mg has not been determined. Once-daily dosing has the advantage of yielding improved compliance and a lower incidence of polyuria (see *Renal* adverse effects [page 249]).

Administration of lithium carbonate once daily will affect the 12-hour steady-state lithium level. Historically, therapeutic lithium levels were determined with lithium carbonate administered three or four times daily; therefore, the standard therapeutic ranges will not apply to once-daily dosing. Table 3–1 was developed by the authors to demonstrate the effect of different dosing regimens on the 12-hour steady-state lithium level (Perry and Alexander 1987).

There is a relatively small difference between the 12-hour serum lithium steady-state concentrations for the q8h and q12h schedules; however, a greater difference exists between these two sched-

Table 3–1.   Effect of dosing regimen on 12-hour steady-state lithium level

Half-life (hours)	Three times daily (q8h)	Twice daily (q12h)	Once daily (q24h)
12	0.54	0.60	0.80
18	0.75	0.81	1.00
24	0.96	1.02	1.20
30	1.18	1.24	1.41
36	1.41	1.46	1.63

Source. Reprinted from Perry PJ, Alexander B: "Dosage and Serum Levels," in *Modern Lithium Therapy.* Edited by Johnson FN. Lancaster, UK, MTP Press, 1987, p. 68. Copyright 1987, MTP Press. Used with permission.

ules and the single-daily-dosing (q24h) schedule. Table 3–1 also demonstrates that as lithium's half-life increases, the rate of increase in the 12-hour steady-state concentration slows. Overall, in a patient with a lithium half-life of 24 hours, switching from twice-daily to once-daily dosing with the same total dose would increase the 12-hour steady-state lithium level by approximately 0.2 mEq/L. Therefore, when converting a patient receiving lithium carbonate twice daily to once-daily dosing, the dosage might be reduced by approximately 20%.

▶ **Every-Other-Day Dosing**

In an open study of 10 patients followed for 13 months and a blinded study of 15 patients followed for 2 years, no patients relapsed with every-other-day lithium carbonate administration (Jensen et al. 1995; Plenge and Mellerup 1992). However, a more recent double-blind study involving 50 patients reported that lithium carbonate administered every second day resulted in a relapse rate three times greater than that resulting from lithium administered every day (Jensen et al. 1995). A general recommendation regarding this dosing strategy awaits the results of additional studies.

■ Pharmacokinetics

Lithium-Level Sampling

Therapeutic lithium levels are determined based on multiple daily dosing of lithium carbonate, steady-state levels, and blood samples obtained in the morning 12 hours after the last dose. Measurement of lithium levels should not be undertaken earlier than 8 hours following a dose, because distribution may not yet be complete and a falsely elevated measurement may result.

Although blood levels of lithium carbonate are the standard for monitoring lithium carbonate therapy, some patients are reluctant to have frequent venipunctures and/or are difficult to obtain blood samples from. One study reported identical steady-state plasma and tear concentrations in 7 patients (Brenner et al. 1982), while another study of 13 patients found a tears-to-plasma ratio of 0.77 ± 0.06 (Jefferson et al. 1984).

The use of *saliva* has been recommended as a noninvasive technique for measuring lithium levels. However, the saliva–to–serum lithium carbonate ratio demonstrates significant interindividual variation, which precludes the use of mean population values for comparing serum and saliva levels. Therefore, the ratio must be individually determined by comparing samples obtained simultaneously (Preskorn et al. 1993).

The availability of methods for measuring lithium in microliter samples of blood obtained from fingertip or ear lobe sites precludes the need for non–blood sample measurement (Jefferson et al. 1984).

▶ **Acute Treatment**

Mania. As lithium carbonate has a half-life of 8–20 hours in most manic patients with normal renal function who are not receiving interacting medications, steady-state lithium carbonate levels will often be reached within 3 to 4 days (i.e., four to five times the half-life) (Perry et al. 1982). Therefore, lithium carbonate concentrations should be obtained twice weekly when treating an acutely manic patient. However, lithium may have a half-life of 2–3 days in patients with reduced renal lithium carbonate clearance and may not reach steady state for several weeks. These patients might have their lithium carbonate levels measured weekly after dosage changes.

A patient experiencing an acute manic episode may require higher lithium carbonate doses due to an increased lithium clearance (Almy and Taylor 1973). However, lithium half-life and blood levels may increase on a stabilized dose once the manic episode begins to abate (Goodnick et al. 1982). Therefore, manic patients who have been discharged following acute treatment should continue to be monitored as outpatients, with lithium levels obtained every 2 weeks for several months, in order to detect any changes in lithium clearance.

Depression. Patients undergoing acute depressive episodes might have their lithium levels measured twice weekly during dosage adjustments and then weekly once a stabilized dose is reached. As described above for mania, there is no evidence that lithium's clearance changes when a patient's depression responds to lithium carbonate (Goodnick et al. 1982).

▶ **Maintenance Treatment**

Inpatients.   Inpatients' lithium levels should be checked on admission and then 1 week later to assess compliance. Thereafter, monitoring should not be necessary unless the clearance of lithium is altered.

Outpatients.   A consensus recommendation for frequency of lithium-level monitoring in a stable outpatient population is not available. One reference advocates a frequency of every 1–2 months (Price and Heninger 1994). However, it is suggested that once a maintenance dose is achieved, very little change in serum lithium levels is expected. Therefore, monitoring more frequently than every 6–12 months would not seem necessary. Monitoring frequency may be increased to every 6 months in patients older than 65 years of age. The addition or deletion of interacting drugs or a change in renal function would indicate the need for a lithium level to be taken within 5 to 10 days.

Pharmacokinetic Parameters

▶ **Absorption**
Lithium is completely absorbed from the gastrointestinal (GI) tract (Amdisen 1980). Lithium absorption takes place over the whole length of the intestine and is not affected by the presence of food.

▶ **Distribution**
Lithium is distributed to various tissues and has a volume of distribution of 0.7–1.0 L/kg, which approximates that of total body water (Amdisen 1980). Lithium's volume of distribution is slightly less in patients older than 65 years, leading to smaller daily dose requirements than in younger patients. Lithium is not bound to plasma proteins. The drug crosses the placenta, and fetal lithium concentrations equal maternal levels (McEvoy et al. 1993) (see *Teratogenicity and Excretion Into Breast Milk* [page 253]).

▶ **Elimination**
Lithium's clearance varies in individuals from about 10 to 40 mL/ minute and is 20% lower at night than during the day (Amdisen 1980; Lauritsen et al. 1981). Lithium is not metabolized; however, it is almost completely eliminated from the body by the kidneys (Carson 1992). Therefore, changes in renal function or in sodium and fluid balance will significantly affect serum lithium concentra-

tions (see **Lithium** drug interactions [pages 473–476] in Chapter 8 and **Lithium** overdose management [pages 519–521] in Chapter 9). The lithium half-life in psychiatric patients has been estimated to range from 15 to 55 hours (Thornhill and Field 1982). However, a half-life range of 8–64 hours has been determined in manic patients with normal renal function (Perry et al. 1982). Therefore, time to steady state may range from 1.5 to 13 days.

Lithium's half-life in euthymic bipolar I, bipolar II, and unipolar depressive patients averages 2.4 days, 1.5 days, and 1 day, respectively (Goodnick et al. 1982).

Lithium follows first-order kinetics in the majority of patients; therefore, as the dosage increases or decreases, the steady-state serum lithium concentration must increase or decrease proportionately (see Empirical or Retrospective Dosing [page 232] under "Dosage," above). However, one report suggests that increasing a lithium carbonate dose may result in an increase or a decrease in lithium clearance in 13% and 9% of patients, respectively (Eggert et al. 1995). Therefore, in approximately 20% of patients, disproportionate changes in serum lithium level may occur with dosage changes.

Lithium clearance may be increased with peritoneal and hemodialysis (see **Lithium** overdose management [pages 519–521] in Chapter 9).

Dosage Forms
Lithium formulations available in the United States include lithium citrate syrup, lithium immediate-release capsules and tablets, and two sustained-release products.

Lithium citrate is 100% bioavailable and is considered the comparison standard for relative bioavailability, as lithium is not administered intravenously (Carson 1992). No clinically significant differences exist between lithium immediate-release capsules and tablets, as both formulations are 95%–100% absorbed, regardless of manufacturer (Needham et al. 1979). Switching among the citrate, capsule, and tablet dosage forms should not result in significantly different 12-hour steady-state lithium levels (McEvoy et al. 1993).

Sustained-release formulations were developed in an attempt to decrease the adverse effects associated with peak and rapidly rising serum lithium concentrations (see "Dosage" [page 230]) (Table 3–2). However, the only comparison study that examined an immediate-release (Lithotabs™) and a sustained-release lithium carbonate product (Lithobid®) was unable to detect any differences in the adverse-effect profiles of the two formulations (Lys-

Table 3–2.   **Comparison of average pharmacokinetic values of various lithium carbonate products derived from a single 900-mg lithium carbonate dose**

Variable	Citrate syrup	Lithotabs™	Eskalith CR®	Lithobid®a
C_{max}[b] (mEq/L)	1.0	0.86	0.51	0.64
T_{max}[c] (hour)	0.38	2.25	5.25	5.17

[a]Ciba-Geigy formulation. Manufacturer as of September 19, 1994, is Solvay Pharmaceutical Company.
[b]Maximum lithium concentration.
[c]Time to maximum lithium concentration.
Source.   Kirkwood et al. 1994; McEvoy et al. 1993.

kowski and Nasrallah 1981). Thus, if slow-release lithium carbonate preparations do cause fewer adverse effects, the difference may be restricted to a minority of patients (see *Gastrointestinal* and *Neuromuscular* adverse effects [pages 246 and 248, respectively]).

The two sustained-release products differ neither in relative bioavailability nor in time required to reach maximum concentration after a single dose (Kirkwood et al. 1994). In one study, Lithobid® produced a statistically significantly higher average peak lithium concentration after a single dose than did Eskalith CR®; however, the difference was only 0.1 mEq/L. The clinical significance, if any, of such a small variance remains to be determined. One bioavailability study reported that the areas under the curve (AUCs) and the 12-hour lithium concentrations of an immediate-release lithium carbonate tablet and the two sustained-release products did not significantly differ (Kirkwood et al. 1994). Therefore, patients may be switched between an immediate-release and a sustained-release lithium product on a mg-for-mg basis. Sustained-release lithium products should be swallowed whole, without crushing or chewing. However, Eskalith CR®, which is scored, may be broken in half before administration (personal communication, A. S. Murabito, SmithKline Beecham Pharmaceutical, July 1993). In one study, the halves resulting after splitting were within 46% to 54% of the intact tablet's weight.

Therapeutic Concentrations

▶ **Acute Treatment**

Mania.   According to an early study, lithium carbonate doses should be adjusted to achieve a steady-state plasma level of 0.9–

1.4 mEq/L (Prien et al. 1972). In this study, some patients experienced significant improvement or remission of symptoms at lithium levels greater than 1.4 mEq/L; however, these patients often developed more adverse effects than did patients with levels less than 1.4 mEq/L. In addition, no patients with serum lithium concentrations less than 0.9 mEq/L had a complete remission of manic symptoms. Typical doses required to achieve a therapeutic level may range from 150 to 4,200 mg/day.

Major depression.   The target lithium carbonate level for acute treatment of major depressive disorder is 0.9–1.4 mEq/L (Price and Heninger 1994).

▶ Continuation Treatment

The recommended lithium-level range for continuation treatment is 0.9–1.4 mEq/L (Price and Heninger 1994).

▶ Maintenance Treatment

Recommended maintenance levels are the same for bipolar and unipolar depression (Price and Heninger 1994). Early lithium carbonate maintenance studies recommended lithium levels from 0.8 to 1.2 mEq/L (Solomon and Bauer 1993). However, three more-recent studies demonstrated equal relapse rates for lithium maintenance levels greater than 0.6 mEq/L and between 0.4 and 0.6 mEq/L (Abou-Saleh and Coppen 1989; Coppen et al. 1983; Hullin 1979). One study reported that patients older than 59 years of age had lower relapse rates at higher lithium levels (Coppen et al. 1983). A U.S. study compared lithium concentration ranges of 0.8–1.0 mEq/L and 0.4–0.6 mEq/L in 94 bipolar patients followed for up to 150 months or until they relapsed (Gelenberg et al. 1989; Suppes et al. 1993). The relapse rate in the high-level group was only 13%, compared with 38% in the low-level group. The effect of age on relapse rate was not examined in this study. Although the authors recommended the high-level range for prophylaxis, it is important to note that 62% of patients in the low-level group did not relapse. Patients should initially be maintained at levels of 0.6–0.8 mEq/L. If dose-related side effects occur (see "Adverse Effects," below), a maintenance level of 0.4–0.6 mEq/L should be attempted. Likewise, if level fails and adverse effects are not a factor, 0.8–1.0 mEq/L should be considered.

■ Adverse Effects

Lithium primarily affects the renal (e.g., thirst, polyuria), nervous (e.g., tremor, memory complaints), metabolic (e.g., weight gain), and GI (e.g., nausea, diarrhea) systems (Vestergaard 1992). The incidence of adverse effects involving these systems ranges from 20% to 40%, depending on the patient's lithium levels. Rare and idiosyncratic side effects occurring in less than 5% of patients involve the skin (e.g., acne, psoriasis), heart (e.g., conduction disturbances), and thyroid gland (e.g., hypothyroidism). Overdose may cause more serious complications (see **Lithium** overdose management [pages 519–521] in Chapter 9).

Approximately 60%–90% of patients maintained on lithium levels of 1.0 mEq/L will experience at least one adverse effect. Achieving lithium levels of 0.4–0.6 mEq/L will significantly reduce the number of patients experiencing adverse effects (Price and Heninger 1994; Solomon and Bauer 1993).

Cardiovascular

Lithium-induced T-wave flattening and inversion and widening of the QRS complex have been reported (Mitchell and Mackenzie 1982). T-wave changes occur in 13%–100% of patients. In healthy individuals, no clinical symptoms are related to these changes, which frequently disappear on continued treatment and are readily reversible with lithium discontinuation. T-wave changes appear to be related to the replacement of intracellular potassium and thus do not represent a direct pharmacological effect on the conduction system. In most patients receiving lithium carbonate, little risk of a significant adverse event exists. However, sinus node dysfunction has infrequently been reported and may be potentially serious. Patients with preexisting conduction abnormalities should be monitored with an electrocardiogram (ECG) after steady-state lithium levels are achieved.

Dermatological

Lithium has been associated with a wide range of dermatological problems of varying clinical significance (Deandrea et al. 1982). *Maculopapular eruptions,* which usually occur 1–3 weeks after lithium carbonate initiation, may clear spontaneously without discontinuing the drug or using any specific therapy. However, the use of diphenhydramine and topical steroids may hasten improvement (DasGupta and Jefferson 1990). *Acneiform eruptions* may emerge or worsen with lithium carbonate therapy (DasGupta and Jefferson 1990). Eruptions are often found on the upper arms and forearms. Although some cases resolve without lithium carbonate termination, management may require a dosage decrease or discontinuation of the drug. Tetracycline and erythromycin have not been consistently effective in improving lesions. Recent case reports suggest that isotretinoin and topical retinoic acid may be useful. *Follicular eruptions* may occur in up to one-third of patients, but these often go unnoticed due to lack of symptoms and spontaneous termination despite continued lithium carbonate treatment (Deandrea et al. 1982). Lithium may induce—or, more commonly, exacerbate—*psoriasis,* which may be intractable to usual treatments and therefore require drug discontinuation (DasGupta and Jefferson 1990). However, lithium carbonate does not necessarily exacerbate psoriasis in patients with a preexisting condition. *Hair loss* secondary to lithium carbonate has been reported, but its relationship to lithium carbonate exposure is difficult to confirm (Das Gupta and Jefferson 1990). Should hair loss occur, thyroid function should be assessed, as lithium carbonate-induced hypothyroidism may play a role (see Thyroid [page 244] under *Endocrinological* adverse effects, below). Lithium does not exacerbate preexisting hair loss. *Exfoliative dermatitis* occurs as a rare but potentially serious reaction to lithium carbonate. The exact mechanism of all lithium-induced dermatological reactions is unknown.

Endocrinological

▶ **Weight Gain**

Six studies have assessed the prevalence of lithium-induced weight gain (Garland et al. 1988). The duration of lithium carbonate treatment ranged from 6 months to 17 years. Four studies reported weight gain of more than 4.5 kg in 11%–64% of patients. Two studies reported that 20% of patients treated with lithium carbonate gained more than 10 kg, as compared with a weight gain of more than 4.5 kg in 8% of affective-disorder patients who received placebo. Overall, the amount of weight gained ranged from 3 to 28 kg, with the average being 8.5 kg. Factors associated with this effect included increased thirst and a previous history of weight problems. Edema was not consistently associated with weight gain. Lithium responders typically gained more weight than nonresponders.

Weight gain can be minimized and reversed by limiting caloric consumption and restricting excessive high-caloric fluid intake (Dempsey et al. 1976). It is important to inform patients of the potential for weight gain and the need to avoid high-calorie soft drinks in replacement of fluid loss secondary to polyuria.

Lithium may have an insulin-like effect in decreasing blood glucose and inhibiting adenylate cyclase to reduce lipolysis. Although lithium is not contraindicated in patients with diabetes, adjustment of antidiabetic treatment may be required because of decreased glucose tolerance.

▶ Thyroid

Hypofunction is the most common thyroid abnormality associated with lithium carbonate. It can present as an abnormal laboratory test (i.e., chemical hypothyroidism), goiter without hypothyroidism, or hypothyroidism. In rare cases, lithium has been associated with thyrotoxicosis (DasGupta and Jefferson 1990; Vestergaard 1992).

The incidence of *chemical hypothyroidism,* including response to thyrotropin-releasing hormone stimulation tests, is approximately 50%. One study measured thyroxine (T_4) and thyroid-stimulating hormone (TSH) at baseline, 6 months, 12 months, and then yearly after the start of lithium carbonate in 430 patients (Maarbjerg et al. 1987). Mean T_4 levels were decreased and TSH increased at 6 months but returned to baseline at 12 months. Thereafter, mean T_4 increased and mean TSH decreased yearly.

The prevalence of *goiter without hypothyroidism* in four studies ranged from 0% to 61% (mean 6%) (Prakash 1985; Vestergaard 1992). The higher percentage rate was determined with ultrasound, whereas the lower figure was determined by clinical assessment (i.e., palpation). The goiter is usually diffuse and nontender and may spontaneously resolve with continued lithium carbonate treatment. It often goes unnoticed unless the thyroid is examined before and during the course of lithium carbonate therapy. However, in 4 of 45 cases, the enlarged thyroid gland produced difficult swallowing (Berens and Wolff 1975). No relationship has been demonstrated between lithium carbonate treatment and thyroid cancer.

The prevalence of *hypothyroidism* in 16 studies ranged from 0% to 23% (mean 3.4%) (Lazarus 1986). The female:male ratio was 5:1. Age greater than 40 years was associated with a higher incidence of hypothyroidism. Of 41 cases reporting time of onset, 36 (88%) occurred within 4 years of lithium carbonate initiation. Serum lithium levels do not correlate with the incidence and severity of hypothyroidism (Berens and Wolff 1975).

Monitoring should include a baseline free T_4 and TSH. Repeat values should be obtained at 6 months and 1 year. If a mildly elevated TSH (i.e., 8–20 μU/mL) or decreased T_4 are observed during the first 6 months to 1 year of lithium carbonate treatment in patients without signs or symptoms of hypothyroidism, monitoring should be performed every 6 months. Yearly routine monitoring has been recommended for the duration of lithium carbonate treatment (Price and Heninger 1994). However, given that the majority of patients on lithium carbonate who develop hypothyrodism do so within the first 4 years of treatment, routine laboratory monitoring after this period has a low return rate (DasGupta and Jefferson

1990). Because symptoms may develop between routine laboratory assessments, patients should be regularly questioned about signs and symptoms of hypothyroidism. Such monitoring is especially important for women over 40 years of age.

Treatment may not be necessary for early-onset hypothyroidism with mildly abnormal thyroid values, as the majority of cases are transient, without clinical symptoms, and spontaneously resolve (Lazarus 1986; Salata and Klein 1987). However, if the patient develops affective symptoms, has signs and symptoms of hypothyroidism, and/or the values do not normalize, thyroid supplementation should be instituted (DasGupta and Jefferson 1990). Goiter and the hypothyroid state can be reversed with thyroid supplementation (e.g., levothyroxine). Lithium discontinuation also will reverse the thyroid abnormalities, usually within 1 to 2 months. Patients taken off lithium and receiving thyroid supplementation for lithium carbonate–induced hypothyroidism should be gradually tapered off the thyroid over 1 month; in addition, thyroid indices should be monitored monthly until they return to normal. Preexisting hypothyroidism is not an absolute contraindication to lithium carbonate treatment.

Lithium has been shown to reduce iodine uptake by the thyroid gland, inhibit iodine's addition to tyrosine, reduce T_3 and T_4 release, reduce the peripheral metabolism of thyroid hormones, and decrease the thyroid gland's sensitivity to TSH (Salata and Klein 1987). It is unlikely that lithium has a direct effect on the hypothalamic-pituitary axis to reduce TSH release. Seven studies have reported a higher incidence (10%–33%, average 21%) of thyroid autoantibodies in patients receiving lithium carbonate compared with control subjects (10%) (Lazarus 1986). Lithium may accelerate the production of autoantibodies that are present before lithium carbonate initiation. However, autoimmune thyroiditis is not the sole cause of lithium carbonate–induced hypothyroidism, as not all patients have thyroid antibodies. Also, increased levels of antibodies are observed in patients without hypothyroidism. It appears that thyroid failure due to lithium is usually, but not necessarily, dependent on antibody-mediated damage. Although preexisting thyroid dysfunction is not a prerequisite for the development of lithium-induced hypothyroidism, patients with impaired function may be at a higher risk.

▶ **Calcium Metabolism**
Lithium can raise serum calcium, reduce serum phosphorous, and increase parathyroid hormone (PTH) (DasGupta and Jefferson

1990). Slightly elevated calcium and PTH will develop in 10%–15% of patients within less than 4 weeks of lithium carbonate initiation. These values may reverse within 1 week of lithium carbonate discontinuation and should be normal within 2 to 4 weeks. It is unknown whether lithium carbonate unmasks parathyroid pathology. Complications of primary hyperparathyroidism do not occur, although osteopenia has been reported (DasGupta and Jefferson 1990). Lithium may increase the threshold calcium level required to suppress PTH by preventing calcium binding to the parathyroid gland or may increase the release of PTH at therapeutic concentrations (Birnbaum et al. 1988). Hypercalcemic patients receiving lithium carbonate can exhibit dysphoria, apathy, or ataxia. A lithium and calcium level should be performed in patients showing signs of intoxication (DasGupta and Jefferson 1990). Routine monitoring is not recommended, as most changes in serum calcium are without clinical consequence.

Gastrointestinal

Milder GI complaints include epigastric bloating and slight abdominal pain. More severe symptoms such as nausea, vomiting, and anorexia occur most commonly with lithium levels greater than 1.5 mEq/L. Therefore, any assessment of lithium carbonate's role in a patient's GI complaints should include a lithium level. The most serious GI problems are loose stools, diarrhea, and occasional bloody stools (Vacaflor 1975). These adverse effects can produce water and electrolyte disturbances, most significantly loss of sodium, which may result in lithium retention and toxicity (see *Renal* adverse effects [page 249]). Patients are 2–20 times more likely to complain of GI adverse effects during a manic phase than during a euthymic period (Bone et al. 1980).

GI disturbances are usually transient in duration and often subside after the initial treatment period (Prien et al. 1971). Lithium should be administered with food to minimize GI adverse effects (Jeppsson and Sjogren 1975). Readjustment of the dosage schedule by dividing the total daily dose into small divided doses may reduce these disturbances.

Nausea is related to the rate and extent of lithium absorption (Kirkwood et al. 1994). In early studies using European-manufactured products, it was reported that nausea occurred more often after administration of immediate-release dosage forms than of sustained-release products. However, the only U.S. study comparing immediate-release lithium with a sustained-release product (Lithobid®) found no overall difference in the side-effect profiles of the two products (Lyskowski and Nasrallah 1981). Nonetheless, a trial with a sustained-release product is indicated in patients who experience nausea and/or vomiting, as an individual patient might respond to this change. Abdominal pain, diarrhea, and loose stools occur more often with sustained-release than with immediate-release products (Kirkwood et al. 1994), probably because the slow-release formulation releases lithium in the large intestine, which pulls water into the lumen by osmotic pressure (Jeppsson and Sjogren 1975). Switching to an immediate-release product may alleviate the problem.

Hematological
Hematological effects are not related to age, sex, or psychiatric diagnosis (Prakash 1985). Red blood cells are not affected by lithium.

▶ Platelets
In one study, 81% of patients developed thrombocytosis secondary to lithium (Joffe et al. 1984). Platelet counts increased by an average of 13% after 4 weeks of treatment, and 24% of patients had platelet counts above the normal limit. The elevated counts were maintained for 2–4 months after lithium carbonate discontinuation.

▶ White Blood Cells
It is reported that 75%–100% of patients on lithium carbonate demonstrate some degree of leukocytosis (Joffe et al. 1984). All white blood cells, with the exception of basophils, are affected by lithium carbonate (Prakash 1985). The increase in the white blood count (WBC) is usually on the order of 30%–45% and is primarily due to neutrophilia. The maximum reported WBC secondary to lithium carbonate is 24,000/mm^3. There is no left shift to the leukocyte profile. The peak elevation typically occurs within 1 week and is generally maintained. Upon lithium carbonate discontinuation, the effect is reversible within 1 to 2 weeks. It does not appear to be dose related. The exact mechanism of the effect is unknown; however, it may result both from demargination and from increased production of cells. Lithium has not been associated with leukemia in long-term treatment (Volf and Crismon 1991).

Hepatic
Lithium has not been associated with liver-induced disease (Das-Gupta and Jefferson 1990). However, lithium's effect on the liver has not been investigated in patients with liver disease.

Neurological

Cognitive and intellectual problems are frequently reported by patients receiving lithium. Studies investigating these claims have yielded inconclusive results (Vestergaard 1992). If possible, patients complaining of cognitive problems should have their lithium levels reduced during maintenance treatment (see Every-Other-Day Dosing [page 236] under *Dosing Regimens*, above).

Cognitive changes may occur with therapeutic levels of lithium (Sansone and Ziegler 1985). The symptoms often appear insidiously. The electroencephalogram (EEG) may be abnormal, with minor asymmetries of frequency or an increase of 4–6 Hz in theta activity. With higher lithium levels, increasing episodes of intermittent high-amplitude diffuse delta waves (below 4 Hz), with accentuation of previous focal abnormalities, are common findings. Patients with cognitive or psychotic diagnoses may be predisposed to this adverse effect (Shopsin et al. 1970; Tucker et al. 1965). Lithium-induced encephalopathy may be reversed with dosage reduction or may require discontinuation of the drug.

Neurotoxicity has been reported when lithium carbonate is combined with haloperidol, thioridazine, chlorpromazine, or fluphenazine. However, two retrospective reviews of 425 patients (Baastrup et al. 1976) and 55 patients (Juhl et al. 1977), as well as two controlled prospective studies (Biederman et al. 1979; Goldney and Spence 1986) involving a total of 158 patients, found no cases of neurotoxicity. It was hypothesized that cases of neurotoxicity resulting from lithium carbonate in combination with an anti-psychotic might represent antipsychotic-induced neuroleptic malignant syndrome (Kemperman et al. 1989). Although clinical manifestations of neurotoxicity may occur with lithium levels less than or equal to 1.5 mEq/L, patients with levels over 1.5 mEq/L may present with confusion, poor concentration, clouding of consciousness, delirium, and/or coma. Cerebellar disturbances are manifested by dysarthria, nystagmus, and ataxia (Hansen and Amdisen 1978) (see **Lithium** overdose management [pages 519–521] in Chapter 9).

Neuromuscular

▶ Tremor

The reported incidence of lithium-induced tremor is 4%–65% (Carroll et al. 1987; Gelenberg and Jefferson 1995). Lithium-induced tremor may occur both at rest and during movement, although the tremor may be aggravated by the performance of delicate hand movements. The tremor does not often interfere with patients' daily activities (Jarrett et al. 1975). An exacerbation of the tremor or extension of the tremor to other parts of the body may signify rising lithium levels. Emotional stress and caffeine may worsen tremor. However, reducing caffeine intake may increase lithium concentrations and also worsen tremor (Jefferson 1988).

Lithium-induced tremor is reversible with drug discontinuation. If possible, the first management option is to lower the lithium carbonate dose. Tremor is associated with the rate of lithium absorption, the maximum plasma concentration, and the extent of absorption (Kirkwood et al. 1994). Sustained-release lithium carbonate products that slow the rate of absorption and reduce peak concentrations have been suggested to reduce tremor. However, the only study comparing immediate-release and sustained-release (Lithobid®) lithium carbonate found no overall difference in the side-effect profiles of the two formulations (Lyskowski and Nasrallah 1981). Nonetheless, a trial might be attempted, as the tremor may respond to a sustained-release product.

Case reports and a controlled study have reported that propranolol 30–80 mg/day is an effective treatment for tremor (Kirk et al. 1973). Metoprolol, a cardioselective β-blocker, can also improve lithium-induced tremor (Gaby et al. 1983). However, in one case, bronchospasm occurred at the dose required to improve the tremor (Zubenko et al. 1984a). Although the propranolol dose is low, propranolol's depressogenic effect should be considered before institution of this treatment. Likewise, primidone has been reported to be useful (Gelenberg and Jefferson 1995). Lithium tremor is not alleviated by levodopa or anticholinergic agents (Carroll et al. 1987). Direct-comparison studies are needed to determine the best pharmacological treatment for lithium-induced tremor.

▶ **Muscle Weakness**

A transient muscle weakness has been reported in 40% of patients during the first 2 weeks of lithium carbonate treatment (Schou et al. 1970). However, this effect is rarely observed in long-term follow-up studies (Schou et al. 1970; Vestergaard et al. 1980). Muscle weakness appears to be dose related and disappears with reduction or discontinuation of lithium carbonate. Case reports of a severe neuromuscular disorder resembling myasthenia gravis have been described in lithium carbonate–treated patients (Neil et al. 1976). The symptoms improved with drug discontinuation.

Renal

Renal effects reported with lithium carbonate after 10–20 years of treatment include tubular dysfunction (e.g., polyuria, polydipsia), morphological changes, reduction in glomerular filtration rate, renal tubular acidosis, and nephrotic syndrome (Bendz et al. 1994; DasGupta and Jefferson 1990; Vestergaard 1992).

▶ Renal Tubular Acidosis

Renal tubular acidosis (RTA) is a clinically unimportant finding in most patients receiving lithium carbonate (DasGupta and Jefferson 1990). However, patients with preexisting acidosis or urinary acidification defects may be at an increased risk of sustaining renal damage should they develop RTA. In lithium-treated patients with urinary acidification defects, periodic assessment of capillary blood pH, carbon dioxide, and bicarbonate levels is warranted.

▶ Polyuria/Polydipsia

In early studies, urine volumes greater than 2 L/24 hours were reported in more than 70% of the patients treated with lithium carbonate (Schou et al. 1970). Between 2% and 35% of patients may have urine outputs greater than 3 L/24 hours (DasGupta and Jefferson 1990). Most prevalence studies of lithium carbonate–induced polyuria involved patients receiving long-term lithium carbonate maintenance treatment with levels greater than 0.8 mEq/L. In one study, 20% of patients with lithium levels greater than 0.8 mEq/L had a 24-hour urine output of more than 4 L (Vestergaard 1992). However, in the majority of patients with lithium levels less than 0.8 mEq/L, renal concentrating ability was not significantly impaired (Vestergaard 1992). Renal concentrating ability may return completely or only partially to normal, depending on the duration of treatment and the lithium carbonate maintenance levels used (e.g., >0.8 mEq/L) (Bucht and Wahlin 1980).

Polyuria as high as 9 L/24 hours has been reported (Ramsey et al. 1982). In severe cases, polyuria and nocturia may become not only a nuisance but also a hazard, leading to serious fluid and electrolyte disturbances if the patient does not maintain an adequate fluid intake. Also, patient compliance can be adversely affected. Fortunately, most patients with lithium carbonate–induced polyuria have mild symptoms and do not require management, except for maintaining adequate hydration (DasGupta and Jefferson 1990).

Prevention is the key consideration in lithium carbonate–induced polyuria. Maintaining a patient's lithium level between 0.4 and 0.8 mEq/L will minimize this adverse effect (see Maintenance Treatment [page 241] under *Therapeutic Concentrations,* above). Another strategy for preventing polyuria is single daily dosing (DasGupta and Jefferson 1990). Although some studies have reported a reduction in urine output when patients were switched to a once-a-day schedule, this finding has not been confirmed in other reports. However, most studies of single daily dosing have been performed in patients with preexisting polyuria. The utility of once-daily dosing in preventing polyuria has not been rigorously tested. Patients should be placed on the q24h dosing schedule early in the course of treatment to improve compliance and possibly reduce the risk of polyuria.

Management of patients with existing polyuria includes drug discontinuation, dose reduction, dosing regimen adjustment, and pharmacological management (DasGupta and Jefferson 1990). *Drug discontinuation* may lead to reversal of polyuria if the patient has not received lithium carbonate for an extended period of time (i.e., years). In one study of patients treated long-term with lithium carbonate, significant improvement in renal concentrating ability did not occur until up to 4 years after lithium carbonate discontinuation (DasGupta and Jefferson 1990). As previously noted, dosage reduction is an important consideration in reducing polyuria. Attempts should be made to maintain the lowest possible lithium level. Switching a patient to once-daily lithium carbonate dosing may reduce urine output, as noted above (see *Dosing Regimens* [page 235] under "Dosage," above). *Pharmacological management* includes the use of a thiazide or potassium-sparing diuretic (DasGupta and Jefferson 1990). Two separate case studies of chlorothiazide 500 mg/day (Levy et al. 1973) and hydrochlorothiazide 50 mg/day (Juhl et al. 1976) reported reductions in the urine output of 64% and greater than 67%, respectively. However, thiazides may reduce lithium renal clearance, thereby necessitating lithium carbonate dosage adjustment, and may also produce hypokalemia (see **Lithium–*Thiazide Diuretic*** drug interaction [page 473] in Chapter 8). In a 3-week study, amiloride 10–20 mg/day decreased the mean daily urine output by 34%, from 4.7 to 3.1 L/24 hours (Batlle et al. 1985). However, a replication study reported that amiloride decreased the urine output only by about 1 L/24 hours in 33% of patients (Kosten and Forrest 1986). In an unpublished placebo-controlled, single-blind cross-over study, amiloride 20 mg/day and hydrochlorothiazide 50 mg/day were equally effective, both reducing urine output by an average of 1.5 L/ 24 hours (B. Alexander, B.L. Cook, P. Dorenbos, D.E. Smith, "A Placebo-Controlled, Single-Blind, Cross-Over Trial of Hydrochlorothiazide and Amiloride in Lithium-Induced Polyuria" [manuscript in preparation], December 1996). However, some patients preferentially responded to one or the other treatment. Although amiloride may be less likely to increase lithium plasma levels, interactions have been reported in some patients. In addition, elevations in potassium levels have required reductions in amiloride daily dosages.

Polyuria is due to lithium's ability to inhibit the activity of adenylate cyclase in the collecting ducts of the kidney (Price and Heninger 1994). This interference prevents antidiuretic hormone–mediated water reabsorption and results in an inability to concentrate urine.

▶ **Glomerular Filtration Rate**

Most long-term studies (i.e., 5–20 years) have not found a correlation between lithium carbonate use and reduction in glomerular filtration rate (GFR) (DasGupta and Jefferson 1990; Price and Heninger 1994; Vestergaard 1992). Potential risk factors for renal changes include a previous history of lithium intoxication, long-term concurrent treatment with antipsychotics and/or antidepressants, and an affective diagnosis (Bendz et al. 1994). However, conservatively, some authors recommend that a serum creatinine level be obtained at least every 6–12 months (Bendz et al. 1994; Price and Heninger 1994). Although 24-hour urine collection may provide the most accurate assessment of creatinine clearance, a 24-hour urine collection is not very practical. The Cockcroft-Gault equation may be used for estimating creatinine clearance (Cl_{cr}) (Cockcroft and Gault 1976):

$$Cl_{cr} \text{ (mL/minute)} = \frac{(140 - \text{age}) \times \text{weight (kg)}}{72 \times \text{fasting serum creatinine (mg/dL)}}$$

First, calculate the current Cl_{cr} by inserting variables. Second, calculate the expected Cl_{cr} by using normal serum creatinine values as follows: 18–29 years, 1.0 g/100 mL; 30–39 years, 1.1 g/100 mL; 40–49 years, 1.2 g/100 mL; 50–59 years, 1.5 g/100 mL; 60–69 years, 1.4 g/100 mL; and 70–79 years, 1.8 g/100 mL. The following rules apply to this equation: 1) the expected Cl_{cr} should be reduced by 15% in women; 2) a correction to lean or ideal body weight is necessary in excessively obese and/or edematous patients; and 3) the serum creatinine should be obtained after the patient has been in a fasting state for 8 hours.

It is unknown whether patients with preexisting kidney disease are at an increased risk for sustaining additional damage secondary to lithium carbonate (DasGupta and Jefferson 1990). Although lithium carbonate is contraindicated in acute renal failure, it may be used in patients with chronic, stable disease. Lithium has been safely used in renal transplant patients (DasGupta and Jefferson 1990).

❱ Nephrotic Syndrome

Nephrotic syndrome is a rare complication of lithium carbonate treatment. As of 1990, nine cases of nephrotic syndrome from lithium carbonate had been reported (DasGupta and Jefferson 1990). Lithium discontinuation and treatment with diuretics, hemodialysis, or prednisone produced improvement in all cases. Lithium rechallenge may result in recurrence of signs. Alternative treatments should be considered for patients who develop this condition (see **Carbamazepine, Valproate,** and **Verapamil** sections in this chapter). Because nephrotic syndrome occurs so infrequently, routine urinalysis to detect protein excretion is not recommended (DasGupta and Jefferson 1990).

❱ Morphological Changes

A 1977 study reported biopsy evidence of chronic nephropathy in patients who had developed lithium carbonate intoxication or lithium-induced diabetes insipidus (Hestbeck et al. 1977). Biopsy results in unselected patients treated long-term with lithium carbonate indicated that 15% had interstitial fibrosis, tubular atrophy, or glomerular sclerosis (DasGupta and Jefferson 1990; Vestergaard 1992). Interestingly, these changes have also appeared in control patients who have never been treated with lithium carbonate (Kincaid-Smith et al. 1979).

Unique distal-nephron lesions have been associated with long-term lithium carbonate treatment (DasGupta and Jefferson 1990; Vestergaard 1992). These changes may be associated with polyuria. The lesions may or may not be reversible.

Teratogenicity and Excretion Into Breast Milk

❱ Teratogenicity

The International Register of Lithium Babies was established in the 1970s to collect voluntarily reported data on the offspring of mothers who received lithium carbonate treatment during the course of their pregnancies (Weinstein 1980). Of 225 children born to lithium-treated mothers, 25 (11%) had some form of malformation. Eighteen (8%) patients had cardiovascular malformations (e.g., Ebstein's anomaly, atrial septal defect, tricuspid valve malformation). By contrast, the rate of major cardiovascular abnormalities in the general population is 1%–7% (average 3%). The findings of the Registry were questioned because babies with congenital abnormalities were more likely to be reported than were healthy babies. However, epidemiological and case–control studies have reported a risk of 0.056% in lithium-treated patients versus 0.023% in control patients—a non–statistically significant difference (Cohen et al. 1994; Jacobsen et al. 1992; Kallen and Tandberg 1983).

Recommendations regarding lithium use during pregnancy (Cohen et al. 1994; Price and Heninger 1994) are as follows:

1. Appropriate contraceptive practices should be used to minimize unplanned drug exposure.
2. Women who have experienced a single affective episode should gradually taper and discontinue lithium before becoming pregnant and should remain lithium-free throughout the pregnancy.
3. Women at a substantial risk of relapse should discontinue lithium during the first trimester of pregnancy and should consider resuming it only if clinical deterioration occurs.
4. Women at an unacceptable risk of relapse should maintain lithium use throughout pregnancy.
5. Women exposed to lithium during the first trimester should receive reproductive counseling as well as fetal echocardiology and high-resolution ultrasound examinations at gestational weeks 16 through 18 (Cohen et al. 1994).

(See Pregnant Patients [page 230] under *Special Populations.*)

▶ **Neonatal Effects**
Fetal and neonatal lithium toxicity has been reported frequently and is characterized by cyanosis, hypotonia, bradycardia, thyroid depression with goiter, atrial flutter, hepatomegaly, T-wave inversion, cardiomegaly, GI bleeding, diabetes insipidus, polyhydraminos, seizures, and shock. Because lithium's half-life in neonates ranges from 68 to 96 hours, most of the minor effects are self-limited and reverse within 1 to 2 weeks of drug discontinuation (Briggs et al. 1994).

▶ **Dosing in Pregnancy**
See Pregnant Patients (page 230) under *Special Populations.*

▶ **Breast Feeding**
Lithium concentrations in breast milk are about 40%–50% those in maternal serum (Kirksey and Groziak 1984; Schou and Amdisen 1973). Infant serum and milk concentrations are approximately equal (Briggs et al. 1994). Infants may be especially susceptible to lithium toxicity. A breast-fed baby with a serum concentration of 0.6 mEq/L developed cyanosis, poor muscle tone, and T-wave changes on ECG (Tunnessen and Hertz 1972). Because of the risk of lithium toxicity, the American Academy of Pediatrics considers

lithium carbonate to be contraindicated during breast feeding (Committee on Drugs 1994). Conversely, if lithium carbonate is indicated, breast feeding is contraindicated unless it is necessary for the baby's well-being.

■ Rational Prescribing

1. Lithium is the first-line treatment for acute mania and prophylaxis of bipolar illness. Lithium's efficacy is equal to that of antidepressants in the prophylaxis of unipolar affective disorder.
2. Control of a manic episode requires a serum lithium level of between 0.9 and 1.4 mEq/L.
3. Because lithium carbonate usually requires 1–2 weeks to exert its effect, a therapeutic trial in acute mania should last 3 weeks.
4. In manic patients with significant motor activity, the use of antipsychotics and/or benzodiazepines in combination with lithium carbonate may be required to control agitated behavior.
5. Continuation treatment for a period of 4–6 months after resolution of affective symptoms should be considered even if maintenance treatment is not to be initiated. Conservatively, lithium carbonate should be tapered over a 4-week period when it is discontinued.
6. Lithium levels may increase with stable doses when a patient cycles out of mania. Steady-state serum lithium concentrations should be monitored twice weekly in inpatients and every 2 weeks for several months in outpatients.
7. A trial of lithium carbonate for treatment of depression consists of a minimum of 3 weeks at concentrations of 0.9–1.4 mEq/L. However, some depressed patients may require 4–6 weeks to show a response.
8. Lithium should be given as a single dose if the lithium carbonate dose is less than 1,800 mg/day and twice daily if the dose is greater than 1,800 mg/day. It is recommended that lithium carbonate doses be given with food.
9. Maintenance treatment is strongly recommended for patients with recurrent episodes. Patients experiencing a single affective episode may not require maintenance treatment.
10. Maintenance lithium levels in the range of 0.40–0.80 mEq/L on a single-daily-dosing schedule are recommended to reduce long-term adverse effects. However, some patients may require higher maintenance doses.
11. The lithium formulation of choice depends on side effects and cost considerations. Most patients prefer capsules rather than

tablets because of the latter's unpleasant taste. The use of a sustained-release form of lithium may reduce nausea and tremor but increase the incidence of diarrhea and loose stools. Sustained-release products are more expensive than immediate-release ones. It is recommended that patients be initially treated with immediate-release lithium carbonate. Lithium citrate syrup might be used in patients who are suspected or found to be "cheeking" solid dosage forms of the drug.

Carbamazepine

■ Indications

Indications for carbamazepine include treatment of trigeminal neuralgia, pain syndromes, diabetes insipidus, and temporal lobe epilepsy (Ballenger 1988). It has been used clinically to treat aggression.

Carbamazepine has been extensively used in the treatment of affective disorders since 1971. It is not approved by the FDA for the acute and prophylactic treatment of bipolar disorder.

■ Efficacy

Acute Treatment

❱ Mania

Fourteen studies have compared carbamazepine's efficacy in mania with that of placebo, chlorpromazine, or lithium (Keck and McElroy 1996).

It is important to separate study populations into lithium-refractory and lithium-naive (i.e., lithium responsive or potentially lithium responsive) patients to determine whether the rate of response to carbamazepine is greater than, equal to, or less than that to lithium in lithium-naive patients. It is also important to determine the percentage of lithium-refractory patients who will respond to carbamazepine so that the drug can be compared with other suggested treatments such as valproate and verapamil. Unfortunately, many studies 1) do not provide information on the patient's past lithium experience; 2) include lithium-naive and lithium-refractory patients in the same study; and/or 3) do not report results by subjects' previous lithium treatment outcome.

Carbamazepine's onset of action varies from 1 to 2 weeks (Post 1988). A therapeutic trial consists of 3 weeks.

Suggested clinical predictors of carbamazepine response have included lithium nonresponse, rapid-cycling (i.e., more than four episodes per year) or continuous-cycling affective illness, and more-severe mania (Calabrese et al. 1996). In addition, patients with dysphoric mania, schizoaffective or psychotic features, or evidence of organic brain damage, as well as those with primarily manic episodes, no family history of affective illness, and an early onset of bipolar illness, may preferentially respond to carbamazepine (Ballenger 1988). Abnormal EEGs have not been found to consistently predict a positive response to carbamazepine.

Lithium response unknown. *Open reports.* In four reports of 109 patients treated with carbamazepine, 48 (44%) had a moderate to marked response (Stromgren and Boller 1985).

Double-blind design. One study reported that carbamazepine 600 mg/day was as effective as the combination of carbamazepine 600 mg/day and haloperidol 24 mg/day in patients experiencing mania (Chou 1991).

Lithium-naive patients. Studies were included here if it was clear either that subjects were not lithium refractory or that only a few subjects in the study population were lithium refractory.

Carbamazepine versus lithium. In five double-blind studies, the overall response rates for carbamazepine ($n = 164$) and lithium ($n = 120$) were 62% and 67%, respectively (Lenzi et al. 1986; Lerer et al. 1987; Lusznat et al. 1988; Okuma et al. 1990; Placidi et al. 1986).

Carbamazepine versus chlorpromazine. Two studies involving 43 patients receiving carbamazepine 200–1,200 mg/day and 38 patients receiving chlorpromazine 200–800 mg/day reported response rates of 70% and 61%, respectively (Chou 1991).

Carbamazepine versus haloperidol. One study reported that 6 of 8 patients (75%) and 3 of 9 patients (33%) responded to carbamazepine and haloperidol, respectively (Chou 1991).

Lithium-refractory patients. *Open reports.* Two studies involving a total of 35 patients reported that 49% responded to carbamazepine (Fawcett and Kravitz 1985; Stromgren and Boller 1985).

Carbamazepine versus placebo. All six double-blind studies existing in the literature were reported from the National Institute of Mental Health and typically involved patients with rapid-cycling illness (i.e., more than four episodes per year) (Ballenger 1988; Stromgren and Boller 1985). Of 84 patients, 52% responded to a trial of carbamazepine.

Carbamazepine versus lithium.   An 8-week double-blind study involving 48 patients reported a 33% response rate for both carbamazepine and lithium (Small et al. 1991). The average serum levels for carbamazepine and lithium at the end of the study were 9.1 mg/mL and 0.73 mEq/L, respectively. It is unknown whether more patients may have responded to both drugs if higher levels had been achieved (see *Therapeutic Concentrations* under "Pharmacokinetics" of **Lithium** and **Carbamazepine** [pages 240 and 264, respectively]).

Carbamazepine plus haloperidol versus haloperidol alone.   One study reported that carbamazepine plus haloperidol was about equal in efficacy to carbamazepine alone, as approximately 46% and 43% of patients responded, respectively (E. Klein et al. 1984). About 50% of patients in this study were refractory to lithium. However, the authors did not report separate response rates based on previous lithium treatment outcomes.

Carbamazepine plus lithium.   Numerous uncontrolled studies have reported that carbamazepine added to lithium produces a significant response in manic patients who are partially or completely unresponsive to lithium alone (Ballenger 1988). Use of this combination might be considered in a patient who has failed to respond to an individual trial of each drug (see *Neurological* adverse effects [page 248]).

▶ Major Depressive Disorder

The onset of action of carbamazepine varies from 14 to 28 days (Post 1988). A therapeutic trial is considered to be 3–4 weeks.

Clinical predictors of antidepressant response to carbamazepine have included rapid-cycling illness (i.e., more than four episodes per year), more manic and fewer depressive hospitalizations, more bipolar than unipolar depressions, depression of greater severity, and positive response to sleep deprivation.

Carbamazepine alone.   Twelve studies have investigated the efficacy of carbamazepine in the treatment of bipolar and unipolar depression (Ballenger 1988; Janicak et al. 1995; Stromgren and Boller 1985). The authors of three of the studies did not indicate patients' prior treatment response (*n* = 28). The other nine studies included patients who were refractory to lithium and/or standard antidepressants. Overall, carbamazepine's antidepressant response rate was 54%, but only 26% of patients experienced a marked response (see Table 3–3). Interestingly, in two studies involving 13 patients, lithium plus carbamazepine produced a marked response in 8 patients (62%).

Table 3–3. **Summary of carbamazepine's (CBZ's) antidepressant effects**

Study design	Patients (N)	Overall response (%)	Moderate response (%)	Marked response (%)
Lithium + CBZ (open)	13	77	15	62
Open	41	63	27	36
Double-blind	64	44	31	13
Total	118	54	28	26

Source. Ballenger 1988; Stromgren and Boller 1985.

Lithium augmentation.   When lithium was added to carbamazepine in 15 nonresponding depressed patients, 8 (53%) had a moderate response within 2 to 6 days (Ballenger 1988). Of the 8 responders, 6 experienced "clinical remission."

▶ Schizoaffective Disorder

Several open and two controlled trials suggest that carbamazepine alone or in combination with antipsychotics may reduce psychotic and affective symptoms in some patients with schizoaffective disorder (Keck et al. 1996). Double-blind, controlled trials are needed to determine the efficacy of carbamazepine in the acute treatment of schizoaffective disorder.

▶ Aggression

Few double-blind studies have investigated carbamazepine's efficacy in the management of aggression (Pabis and Stanislav 1996). In uncontrolled trials, carbamazepine has shown mild to moderate efficacy in reducing aggressive behavior in schizophrenia, borderline personality disorder, Alzheimer's disease, cognitive disorders, developmental disorders, and impulse dyscontrol syndromes. EEG abnormalities do not predict a response to carbamazepine. Carbamazepine has been reported to reduce impulsivity, irritability, and hostility and to improve mood. Typical carbamazepine serum levels have been 8–12 µg/mL (Pabis and Stanislav 1996). However, in a recent retrospective report, patients were found to respond better to valproate than to carbamazepine (Alam et al. 1995; see *Aggression* [page 273] under "Efficacy" of **Valproate**). More controlled studies are needed to determine carbamazepine's efficacy in controlling aggression.

Continuation Treatment

(General principles for the use of carbamazepine in continuation treatment are the same as those for lithium; see *Continuation Treatment* [page 225] under "Efficacy" of **Lithium**.)

There is no evidence that carbamazepine, like lithium, needs to be tapered to reduce the rate of recurrent manic or depressive episodes. Conservatively, if the drug is to be discontinued in affective disorder patients, it might be tapered by 25% per week.

Maintenance Treatment

(General principles for the use of carbamazepine in maintenance treatment are the same as those for lithium; see *Maintenance Treatment* [page 226] under "Efficacy" of **Lithium**.)

▶ Bipolar Disorder and Unipolar Depression

Open reports.   *Carbamazepine alone.*   Twenty-six reports have investigated carbamazepine's efficacy in the maintenance treatment of primarily bipolar illness, but also recurrent unipolar illness (Ballenger 1988; Solomon and Bauer 1993; Stromgren and Boller 1985). The majority of patients included in these studies did not respond to or tolerate lithium. Overall, carbamazepine was reported to be moderately or markedly effective in preventing recurrences of mania and depression in 60% and 50% of patients, respectively.

Carbamazepine plus lithium.   Several reports have examined the efficacy of combining carbamazepine and lithium in patients who were partially or completely unresponsive to lithium and carbamazepine monotherapy (Ballenger 1988). The combination treatment significantly reduced the number of manic and depressive episodes experienced in most patients. Use of a carbamazepine/lithium combination therapy might be considered in patients unresponsive to individual trials of these drugs (see *Neurological* adverse effects [page 248]).

Double-blind studies.   One placebo-controlled and eight lithium comparison studies have been performed (Janicak et al. 1995; Solomon and Bauer 1993). Although the placebo-controlled trial did not find a difference between carbamazepine and placebo, the numbers in the study may have been too small to detect a difference. The comparison studies involved 133 patients and concluded that carbamazepine was as effective as lithium in preventing affective episodes.

Several reports have suggested that tolerance may develop to carbamazepine's effects in up to 50% of patients receiving maintenance treatment (Frankenburg et al. 1988; Post et al. 1990). However, this finding needs to be confirmed in larger studies. The mechanism for tolerance may be related to pharmacodynamic adaptation.

▶ Schizoaffective Disorder
Several open and two controlled trials suggest that carbamazepine alone or in combination with antipsychotics may reduce relapse of psychotic and affective symptoms in some patients with schizoaffective disorder (Keck et al. 1996). Double-blind, controlled trials are needed to determine the efficacy of carbamazepine in the maintenance treatment of schizoaffective disorder.

▶ Aggression
The efficacy of carbamazepine in the maintenance treatment of aggression has not been extensively studied.

■ Mechanism of Action

The exact mechanism of carbamazepine's effect in affective disorders is unknown (Post 1988). Carbamazepine produces a wide variety of biochemical changes in neurotransmitters, neuromodulators, second messengers, and neuropeptides. The drug's antimanic effect usually begins between 7 and 14 days after treatment initiation and coincides with biochemical changes. Carbamazepine increases acetylcholine in the striatal regions. Unlike typical antipsychotics, carbamazepine decreases dopamine turnover. Carbamazepine also decreases norepinephrine turnover by reducing presynaptic release. Both dopamine and norepinephrine are purported to play a role in mania.

It is also postulated that affective illness may result from a deficiency of γ-aminobutyric acid (GABA). Carbamazepine reduces GABA turnover in the hippocampus and cortex. Lithium and valproate have also been reported to potentiate GABA. Like lithium, carbamazepine acutely inhibits adenylate cyclase activity stimulated by norepinephrine and dopamine.

■ Dosage

Mania and Depression—Acute Treatment
The recommended starting dose for carbamazepine is 200 mg administered twice daily with meals. The daily dose may be increased in 200-mg increments every other day (Ballenger 1988). Initial target doses of 10–15 mg/kg/day are recommended. If necessary, an increase in dose may be made after the patient has received this dose for 1–3 weeks (Bertilsson and Tomson 1986; Kudriakova

et al. 1992). Most patients require doses ranging from 600 to 1,600 mg/day; however, some patients may require between 2,000 and 3,000 mg/day.

If the patient experiences dose-related side effects within the first 3–7 days of treatment initiation, the next dose should be held and the total daily dose reduced by 200 mg/day. After several days, increase of the dose may again be attempted, at a slower rate.

Initially, tid dosing is suggested to minimize peak-related adverse effects. After dose stabilization, bid dosing might be attempted to facilitate compliance.

Maintenance Treatment

There is no evidence that maintenance dosage requirements differ from those for antimanic doses (Janicak 1993).

■ Pharmacokinetics

Carbamazepine-Level Sampling

❱ Acute Mania and Depression

Serum carbamazepine levels should be obtained in the morning 12 hours after the last dose to allow absorption and distribution to be completed (Neppe et al. 1988). A serum level might be obtained after the initial target dose is achieved (see "Dosage," above) and the patient has been on carbamazepine for at least 2 weeks (see Metabolism under *Pharmacokinetic Parameters,* below).

In a nonresponding patient, a linear dose increase to achieve a level of 10–12 mg/mL might be tried (see *Therapeutic Concentrations,* below). A repeat carbamazepine level may be obtained 3 days after the target dose is reached. A serum level measured just before discharge may also be useful for monitoring compliance. Unless drug interactions are involved, it should not be necessary to obtain more than three carbamazepine serum levels during an acute hospitalization.

❱ Maintenance Treatment

There are no guidelines for the frequency at which carbamazepine concentrations should be obtained in a patient stabilized on carbamazepine. Appropriate indications for drug-level measurement might include a change in the patient's clinical condition or anticipation of a drug interaction.

Pharmacokinetic Parameters

❱ Absorption

Absorption of carbamazepine from the GI tract during initial dosing is slow and erratic, as the time required for plasma concentrations to peak varies from 2 to 24 hours (Pugh and Garnett 1991). In general, during chronic therapy, carbamazepine plasma concentrations peak 3–6 hours after the last dose (Pynnonen 1979). The absorption of carbamazepine tablets is approximately 85%–90%. Carbamazepine tablets should be stored in a cool, dry place, as moisture may decrease the potency of the tablets by 30%.

▶ **Distribution**
The volume of distribution of carbamazepine is 1 L/kg (Bertilsson and Tomson 1986). It is estimated that carbamazepine is 70%–80% protein bound.

▶ **Metabolism**
Carbamazepine is extensively metabolized by the liver to the primary active metabolite 10,11-epoxide (CBZE) (Pugh and Garnett 1991). CBZE appears in the plasma at concentrations of 10%–40% of the parent compound.

The half-life of carbamazepine in single-dose studies in patients with epilepsy ranged from 30 to 40 hours (Pynnonen 1979). However, after 3 weeks of exposure, the half-life was reduced to 12–20 hours as the result of enzyme induction. After autoinduction is complete, dosage changes result in steady-state concentrations within 2 to 4 days. CBZE's half-life after autoinduction is estimated to be 6–20 hours (Pynnonen 1979).

In patients with epilepsy, carbamazepine plasma concentrations peak within 3 to 4 days and then fall by approximately 50% over the next 4 weeks if the dosage is not increased. However, a recent study in 77 affectively ill patients reported that maximal enzyme induction occurred within 1 week with carbamazepine doses of 100–1,200 mg/day (Kudriakova et al. 1992).

Dosage Forms
Carbamazepine is available as a 200-mg immediate-release tablet, a 100-mg chewable tablet, and a suspension. The 100- and 200-mg dosage forms have comparable bioavailability and may be exchanged without adjusting the dosage or dosing interval (Pugh and Garnett 1991). The AUC is the same for the suspension and the tablets. However, the suspension produces rapid absorption of the drug, which may lead to peak-related adverse effects. The tablets administered on a bid schedule and the suspension given on a tid schedule yield similar AUCs and minimum and maximum serum concentrations (Pugh and Garnett 1991). The suspension may be administered as an enema if the oral route is unavailable (Pugh and Garnett 1991).

Patients started on a particular generic form of carbamazepine should continue to receive that same product throughout treatment. If a patient is switched from a brand name to a generic product or from one generic product to another, plasma concentrations should be monitored weekly for 2 weeks to determine the effect, if any, of the substitution.

Therapeutic Concentrations

▶ Mania and Depression—Acute Treatment

A correlation between carbamazepine plasma concentrations and affective-symptom response has not been demonstrated (Ballenger 1988). Although one study reported a correlation between the CBZE metabolite and improvement in affective symptoms, this finding has not been replicated (Post et al. 1983). CBZE is not routinely measured by commercial laboratories.

It has been recommended that a nonresponding patient's carbamazepine dosage be increased until initial adverse effects appear (Ballenger 1988). Onset of such effects usually coincides with levels of 10–12 mg/mL (see *Gastrointestinal* and *Neurological* adverse effects [pages 267 and 268, respectively]).

▶ Mania and Depression—Maintenance Treatment

There is no generally accepted therapeutic range for carbamazepine in the maintenance treatment of affective disorders (Ballenger 1988). One maintenance study in bipolar patients reported that a carbamazepine plasma concentration of 4–7 mg/mL (mean 5.7 mg/mL) was effective in most patients (Stuppaeck et al. 1990). In a more recent open trial, 84 patients (52 bipolar, 32 unipolar) with recurrent illness were treated with either "low" or "high" serum carbamazepine levels of 3.5–5.9 µg/L or 6.6–9.4 µg/L, respectively, for 2 years (Simhandl et al. 1993). In the bipolar patients, both low and high serum carbamazepine levels were equally effective in reducing affective episodes. In the unipolar patients, however, the "high" serum-level group had a better outcome than did the "low" serum-level group. More therapeutic-response studies of carbamazepine and its metabolite are needed.

■ Adverse Effects

Adverse-effect frequencies were similar in 255 patients with a convulsive-disorder diagnosis and 24 affectively ill patients treated with carbamazepine (see Table 3–4) (Ballenger and Post 1980; Livingston et al. 1974). A comparison of the primary adverse effects of carbamazepine and valproate is presented in Table 3–5.

Table 3–4. **Carbamazepine's adverse effects**

Reaction	Epileptic patients (N = 255) Number (%)	Number discontinued	Manic-depressive patients (N = 24) Number (%)
Diplopia	44 (17)	0	3 (13)
Drowsiness	28 (11)	0	3 (13)
Leukopenia	16 (6.3)	3	0 (0)
Transient blurred vision	14 (5.5)	0	1 (4)
Rash	7 (2.7)	4	2 (8)
Disequilibirum, dizziness	6 (2.4)	0	7 (29)
Transient paresthesias	5 (2.0)	0	1 (4)
Proteinuria	3 (1.2)	0	0 (0)
Neutropenia	1 (0.4)	1	0 (0)
Systemic lupus erythematosis recurrence	1 (0.4)	1	0 (0)
Ataxia			5 (21)
Clumsiness			4 (17)
Slurred speech			3 (13)
Tremor			2 (8)
Nausea			2 (8)
Poor memory			1 (4)
Confusion			1 (4)
Blurred vision			1 (4)
Cardia arrhythmias (atrial fibrillation)			1 (4)

Source. Ballenger and Post 1980; Livingston et al. 1974.

Cardiac

Carbamazepine can suppress both atrioventricular (AV) conduction and ventricular automaticity. These changes have been reported only in patients with preexisting conduction disturbances. Bradyarrhythmia and AV block occur at therapeutic or mildly elevated serum concentrations and are more commonly observed in elderly women. Thus, like the tricyclic antidepressants, carbamazepine is contraindicated in patients with bundle branch block (Boesen et al. 1983; Kasarskis et al. 1992).

Table 3–5.   **Adverse drug reaction (ADR) comparison between carbamazepine (CBZ) and valproate
(VPA)**

ADR	ADRs reported at any time		ADRs reported at 12-month follow-up	
	CBZ (n = 231) (%)	VPA (n = 240) (%)	CBZ (n = 130) (%)	VPA (n = 136) (%)
Gastrointestinal	29	33	6	2
Rash	11*	1	1	0
Hepatotoxicity	4	3	0	0
Weight gain > 12 pounds	8	20*	3	13*
Hair change or loss	6	12*	1	4
Impotence	7	10	2	1

*$P < .05$.
Source.   Ballenger and Post 1980; Guay 1995; Mattson et al. 1992.

▶ **Dermatological**

Note: It has been suggested that the onset of a rash may be a
harbinger of bone-marrow suppression (Silverstein et al. 1983).
Thus, in patients experiencing dermatological reactions, a complete blood count (CBC) should be obtained.

Dermatological reactions associated with carbamazepine are estimated to occur in 2%–12% of patients (Denicoff et al. 1994;
Livingston et al. 1974). The onset is generally within 2 weeks to
5 months of the start of therapy. A maculopapular rash is the most
common reaction. Usually the rash will resolve with drug discontinuation (Denicoff et al. 1994), but it may also resolve if the drug
is continued without any specific treatment. Nonetheless, oral
antihistamines and prednisone may provide symptomatic relief. In
one series, carbamazepine rechallenge produced recurrence of the
rash in 4 of 7 patients (Livingston et al. 1974).

Other dermatological ADRs include rashes with edema, systemic
lupus erythematosus, dermatomyositis, erythema multiforme, and
Stevens-Johnson syndrome. Stevens-Johnson syndrome requires
drug discontinuation, and the patient should not be rechallenged.

Endocrinological/Metabolic

Carbamazepine is a vasopressin agonist and has been reported
to cause hyponatremia and water intoxication in 5% of patients

(Brewerton and Jackson 1994; Uhde and Post 1983). Serum sodium may decrease to 117 mEq/L. In six patients, demeclocycline 600 mg bid prevented a decrease in serum sodium (Brewerton and Jackson 1994). Hyponatremia has precipitated lithium intoxication (manifested primarily as neurotoxicity) when carbamazepine was combined with lithium. Serum sodium should be measured when patients are treated with this combination (Chaudhry and Waters 1983; Shulka et al. 1984).

Gastrointestinal

Nausea and vomiting are the adverse reactions most commonly experienced during carbamazepine initiation (Mattson et al. 1992). If they appear during dose titration, the next dose may be held and the total daily dosage reduced by 200 mg. Once the signs and/or symptoms resolve, dosage increase may again be attempted, but at a slower rate. Less-frequently reported GI adverse effects are diarrhea and abdominal cramps.

Hematological

Aplastic anemia, agranulocytosis, thrombocytopenia, leukopenia, eosinophilia, leukocytosis, red-cell aplasia, hemolytic anemia, and reticulocytosis have been reported with carbamazepine (Sobotka et al. 1990). With the exception of leukopenia, these dyscrasias are rare occurrences and do not warrant routine hematological monitoring.

Leukopenia (i.e., WBC greater than $4,000/mm^3$) develops in approximately 12% of adults and 7% of children (Sobotka et al. 1990). Its onset is usually within the first 3 months of carbamazepine initiation, with patients at risk having a low or low-normal pretreatment WBC or neutrophil count. Most patients will have a 25% decrease in WBC. However, in nearly all cases, the WBC will return to baseline with carbamazepine continuation. In a few cases, the leukopenia will continue but without adverse hematological or medical consequences. In some patients, a dose-related decline in WBC occurs that reverses with dose maintenance or reduction.

Recommended hematological monitoring for patients receiving carbamazepine is as follows:

1. Obtain a baseline CBC. If all indices are in the middle or upper-normal range, no further laboratory checks are necessary. The patient should be educated to report signs and symptoms of leukopenia (e.g., fever, sore throat, easy bruising, ulcers in the mouth) to the prescriber.
2. Patients with low-normal or below-normal WBCs and neutrophil counts should be monitored every 2 weeks for the first

3 months of treatment. Subsequent monitoring should be individualized based on the previous blood counts.

3. If the WBC falls below 3,000/mm³ or the neutrophil count drops below 1,000/mm³, the dosage should be decreased or, if necessary, the drug discontinued. The risks and benefits of carbamazepine use should be carefully evaluated in patients with dangerously low counts, as alternative treatments are available (see "Efficacy" under **Lithium, Verapamil**, and **Valproate** sections) (Hart and Easton 1982; Silverstein et al. 1983; Sobotka et al. 1990).

Hepatic

▶ Benign Enzyme Elevation
It has been reported that 20% of patients receiving carbamazepine may have elevated liver enzymes (e.g., alkaline phosphatase) (Soffer et al. 1983). Most enzyme levels stabilize and do not continue to rise.

▶ Hepatotoxicity
Rarely, cholestatic jaundice, hepatic necrosis, and granulomatous hepatitis have been associated with carbamazepine (Ballenger 1988; Pugh and Garnett 1991). Twelve cases of hepatotoxicity have been reviewed (Howrie et al. 1983). Ten cases occurred within 4 weeks of treatment initiation and two occurred at 2 and 6 months. Signs and symptoms included fever, jaundice, rash, liver tenderness or enlargement, anorexia, and/or nausea. In one case, bilirubin was increased to 3.4 mg%, and mild elevation in other enzymes were noted. Carbamazepine discontinuation led to rapid improvement in clinical symptoms, although laboratory abnormalities remained elevated for months. Two fatalities occurred. Because hepatotoxicity is believed to be a hypersensitivity reaction, patients who experience this effect should not be rechallenged (Howrie et al. 1983).

Neurological

▶ Sedation/Ataxia
The most common central nervous system (CNS) adverse effects associated with carbamazepine—vertigo, drowsiness, unsteadiness, and dizziness—occur transiently during the first few weeks of therapy (Killian and Fromm 1968; Pugh and Garnett 1991). If these effects occur during initial dose titration, either the dosage can be temporarily reduced until the symptoms subside or the rate of increase can be slowed. Serum carbamazepine CBZE concentra-

tions greater than 2.2 µg/mL are directly correlated with acute CNS carbamazepine toxicity (Patsalos et al. 1985). The CBZE metabolite is not routinely measured in clinical practice.

▶ Dystonic Reactions
Dystonic reactions—possibly caused by carbamazepine's antagonism of dopamine—have been associated with carbamazepine use in children (Crosley and Swender 1979). Unlike dystonia from antipsychotics, these reactions usually occur 2–3 weeks after the drug is started.

▶ Neurotoxicity
Neurotoxic effects generally occur with the combination of carbamazepine and lithium at therapeutic doses. Although most patients tolerate the combination, approximately 12% of patients may experience muscle fasciculation, nystagmus, confusion, disorientation, hyperreflexia, slurred speech, and/or incoordination (Ballenger 1988). (See **Lithium–*Carbamazepine*** drug interaction [page 474] in Chapter 8.)

Ophthalmological
Dose-dependent visual disturbances have been reported to be rare at carbamazepine dosages less than 1,200 mg/day (Livingston et al. 1974).

Psychiatric

▶ Behavioral
Delirium and hallucinations have been reported with carbamazepine use (Silverstein et al. 1983), as have difficulty in sleeping, agitation, irritability, and emotional liability (Pugh and Garnett 1991). If such effects occur, the drug should be stopped and reinitiated at a lower dose, if possible. These reactions are probably the result of carbamazepine's anticholinergic activity.

▶ Cognitive
Although carbamazepine appears to cause minimal cognitive impairment at therapeutic doses (Pugh and Garnett 1991), such impairment may occur at high doses. Psychomotor performance does not correlate with dose or plasma concentration.

Renal
Proteinuria that disappeared on carbamazepine discontinuation has been reported (Livingston et al. 1974).

Teratogenicity and Excretion Into Breast Milk

▶ **Teratogenicity**

Physical effects.   A recent study that used retrospective and prospective data on 35 children born to women treated with carbamazepine alone reported anomaly incidences of 11% for craniofacial defects, 26% for fingernail hypoplasia, 1% for spina bifida, and 20% for developmental delay (Jones et al. 1989; Scolnik et al. 1994). However, other studies have found no adverse fetal effects (Scolnik et al. 1994).

Intellectual effects.   In another recent study, carbamazepine did not adversely effect the global IQs of children born to mothers treated with carbamazepine alone (Scolnik et al. 1994).

▶ **Breast-Milk Excretion**

The milk-to-plasma ratio of carbamazepine ranges from 0.24 to 0.69 (Briggs et al. 1994). Carbamazepine in breast milk produced nontoxic plasma concentrations that averaged 0.4 μ/mL (Inoue and Unno 1984). The drug is considered compatible with breast feeding (Committee on Drugs 1994).

■ Rational Prescribing

1. Carbamazepine is the second-line drug (i.e., after lithium) for the acute treatment of mania and prophylaxis of manic and depressive episodes.
2. As an antidepressant, carbamazepine is less effective than lithium in both unipolar and bipolar depression.
3. Carbamazepine may be more effective than lithium in patients with rapid-cycling illness, a negative family history for affective illness, and/or an early onset of bipolar illness.
4. In highly active manic patients, carbamazepine combined with an antipsychotic and/or a benzodiazepine may produce greater improvement than carbamazepine alone. The antipsychotic and benzodiazepine should be discontinued once manic signs and symptoms resolve.
5. A combination of lithium and carbamazepine may be more effective than either drug alone in the acute treatment of mania and prophylaxis of recurrent affective episodes.
6. The onset of action of carbamazepine requires 1–2 weeks. A therapeutic trial consists of 3 weeks.
7. A carbamazepine therapeutic range has not been conclusively established for the acute treatment or prophylaxis of mania or depression.

8. A baseline CBC should be obtained for each patient.
9. Except for leukopenia, all carbamazepine-associated hematological adverse effects should be monitored, with patients educated about the signs and symptoms of leukopenia (e.g., sore throat, mucosal ulcers, fever, easy bruising) and instructed to report these should they occur. Blood counts should be monitored if the patient has a low or low-normal WBC. If the neutrophil count is less than $1,000/mm^3$ or the WBC is less than $3,000/mm^3$, the carbamazepine dosage should be decreased or the drug discontinued, and the patient should be monitored with serial blood counts.

Valproate

■ Indications

Valproate is indicated alone or in combination with other anticonvulsants in the prophylactic management of simple and complex (petit mal) seizures. It was approved in May 1995 for the acute treatment of mania. Valproate has been used in the management of aggression.

■ Efficacy

Acute Treatment

▶ Mania
Sixteen open and six controlled trials have investigated valproate's efficacy in the treatment of mania (Bowden et al. 1994; Guay 1995; Keck and McElroy 1996; McElroy and Keck 1993). The trials compared valproate with lithium and/or placebo.

It is important to separate study populations into lithium-refractory and lithium-naive (i.e., lithium responsive or potentially lithium responsive) patients to determine whether valproate's response rate is greater than, equal to, or less than lithium's rate in lithium-naive patients. It is also important to determine the percentage of lithium-refractory patients who respond to valproate so that the drug can be compared with other suggested treatments (e.g., carbamazepine, verapamil). Unfortunately, many studies 1) do not provide information on patients' past lithium experience; 2) include both lithium-naive and lithium-refractory patients; and/or 3) may not report results by patients' previous lithium treatment outcomes.

Valproate's onset of action varies from 7 to 14 days (Bowden et al. 1994). A therapeutic trial consists of 3 weeks.

Suggested clinical predictors of response to valproate include rapid-cycling illness (i.e., more than four episodes per year), dysphoric or mixed mania, and neurological abnormalities (e.g., abnormal EEG, mental retardation, history of head trauma or panic attacks) (Calabrese et al. 1996; Freeman et al. 1992; Janicak et al. 1995; McElroy and Keck 1993; Schaff et al. 1993). Conversely, a history of substance abuse predicts a poor outcome. It is important to note that these conclusions are preliminary and need to be replicated in controlled trials.

Lithium-naive patients. *Open reports.* There are no open reports of valproate in the acute treatment of lithium-naive manic patients.

Lithium-refractory patients. *Open reports.* Because in most of the available reports, valproate was added to existing lithium regimens (McElroy and Keck 1993), it is difficult to determine the role of valproate per se. Overall, 198 of 297 patients (67%) experienced a moderate to marked response to valproate.

Valproate versus placebo. Five double-blind studies reported that overall response rates to valproate and placebo were 49% and 16%, respectively (Bowden et al. 1994; McElroy and Keck 1993).

Valproate versus lithium. One double-blind study reported that 12 of 13 patients (92%) and 9 of 14 patients (64%) responded to lithium and valproate, respectively (Freeman et al. 1992). Interestingly, 6 of 13 patients in the lithium group had reportedly failed a previous lithium trial, while 7 of the 14 valproate-treated patients had a history of lithium nonresponse. A larger sample size may have demonstrated a more significant difference between the response rates to the two drugs.

A recent study reported that approximately 50% of valproate- and lithium-treated patients experienced more than a 50% reduction in manic symptoms (Bowden et al. 1994). However, 47% of the patients in the lithium group had failed to respond to a previous trial of lithium. It is important to note that lithium responders in this study improved more with lithium than with valproate.

Valproate versus carbamazepine. One double-blind case study reported that a patient responded to carbamazepine but not valproate (Post et al. 1984).

▶ Schizoaffective Disorder

Lithium-naive patients. No open or double-blind studies of valproate have been performed in this population (Keck and McElroy 1996).

Lithium-refractory patients. *Open reports.* In three reports, 58 of 100 patients (58%) experienced moderate to marked improvement with valproate (Keck et al. 1996; McElroy and Keck 1993).

Double-blind studies. There are no controlled trials of valproate in lithium-refractory patients with schizoaffective disorder (Keck and McElroy 1996).

▶ **Major Depressive Disorder**

Open reports. Of 195 patients with unipolar, bipolar, or schizoaffective depression, only 58 (30%) demonstrated a significant antidepressant response to valproate (McElroy and Keck 1993).

Double-blind studies. There are no controlled trials of valproate in major depressive disorder.

▶ **Aggression**

Uncontrolled trials and case reports in adults and mentally retarded children suggest that valproate has some antiaggressive activity (Pabis and Stanislav 1996). In a large retrospective case series, valproate was more effective than carbamazepine in reducing mechanical-restraint hours in 82 psychiatric inpatients (Alam et al. 1995). Recommended initial doses were 250 mg tid; however, some patients have required dosages up to 60 mg/kg/day. No specific therapeutic range for the management of aggression has been defined.

Continuation Treatment

(General principles for the use of valproate in continuation treatment are the same as those for lithium; see *Continuation Treatment* [page 225] under "Efficacy" of **Lithium.**)

There is no evidence that valproate, like lithium, needs to be tapered to reduce the rate of recurrent manic or depressive episodes. Conservatively, if the drug is to be discontinued in affective disorder patients, it might be tapered by 25% per week.

Maintenance Treatment

(General principles for the use of valproate in maintenance treatment are the same as those for lithium; see *Maintenance Treatment* [page 226] under "Efficacy" of **Lithium.**) All figures noted in this section are from open reports in which observation periods ranged from 6 to 163 months (McElroy and Keck 1993). In most cases, valproate was added to existing regimens of lithium, carbamazepine, antidepressants, and/or antipsychotics.

There are no controlled trials of valproate in the maintenance treatment of affective illness (Keck et al. 1996).

▶ **Bipolar Disorder**

Lithium-naive patients. Two studies reported that 70 of 157 patients (45%) responded to valproate with moderate to marked improvement (McElroy and Keck 1993).

Lithium-refractory patients. Overall, 121 of 138 patients (88%) improved with valproate in six reports (McElroy and Keck 1993; Schaff et al. 1993).

Carbamazepine-refractory patients. Of 29 patients who had failed to respond to a trial of carbamazepine, 20 (69%) responded to valproate (Schaff et al. 1993).

▶ **Schizoaffective Disorder**

Lithium-naive patients. There are no reports of valproate's use in this population.

Lithium-refractory patients. In two reports, valproate produced a moderate to marked response in 14 of 17 patients (83%) (McElroy and Keck 1993; Schaff et al. 1993).

▶ **Unipolar Depression**

Minimal information exists on the efficacy of valproate in the maintenance treatment of unipolar depression. General principles for the use of valproate in maintenance treatment are the same as those for lithium; see *Maintenance Treatment* [page 226] under "Efficacy" of **Lithium.**)

■ Mechanism of Action

The exact cause of bipolar illness and of valproate's efficacy in the disorder is unknown (Post et al. 1992). Overall, valproate enhances the effect of GABA by inhibiting its degradation, stimulating its synthesis and release, and directly enhancing its postsynaptic effects. In addition, valproate reduces dopamine turnover and sodium influx while increasing potassium efflux.

■ Dosage

Most patients can be treated with valproate 1,000–1,500 mg/day (Brown 1989). However, the required dose may range from 750 to 6,000 mg/day. Once a patient's dose is stabilized, the drug may be administered on a twice-daily or once-daily-at-bedtime dosing regimen (Gerner 1993; McElroy and Keck 1993).

The following dosing regimens apply to the treatment of a patient with a bipolar, unipolar, or schizoaffective disorder diagnosis who is either in an acute manic or depressive phase or is not currently experiencing affective symptoms.

Dosage Titration
The patient may be started on valproate 500–1,000 mg/day in two to four divided doses (McElroy and Keck 1993). The dose can be adjusted upward by 250 or 500 mg/day every 2–4 days until a response occurs or adverse effects are experienced (see "Adverse Effects" [page 277]) (Gerner 1993).

Loading Doses
Divalproex sodium 20 mg/kg/day divided into three doses yielded average plasma valproate concentrations of 89 mg/mL ± 19 mg/mL on day 2 of administration (Keck et al. 1993). The calculated dose was administered for 6 consecutive days and was well tolerated by 19 patients, as only 4 patients noted sedation and 1 complained of nausea. The drug was not discontinued in any patient because of adverse effects.

Maintenance Treatment
Maintenance doses of valproate have not been extensively studied. At present, it is recommended that patients continue to receive the same dose that was required for acute treatment (McElroy and Keck 1993; Sachs 1996).

■ Pharmacokinetics

Valproate-Level Sampling
Valproate levels should be obtained at steady state 12 hours after the last dose in the morning (McElroy and Keck 1993). Sampling time should always be at approximately the same time each day, as the drug shows an endogenous circadian elimination. Levels will vary from day to night (Pugh and Garnett 1991).

▶ Acute Treatment
Valproate levels should be obtained 3 days after a patient reaches 20 mg/kg/day of valproate; however, if adverse effects occur, a valproate level might be obtained earlier (Keck et al. 1993; McElroy and Keck 1993).

▶ Maintenance Treatment
Inpatients. Inpatients' valproate levels should be checked on admission and then 1 week later to assess compliance. Thereafter, monitoring should not be necessary unless the clearance of valproate is altered by changes in liver function or the addition/deletion of interacting drugs (see **Valproic Acid** drug interactions [pages 481–482] in Chapter 8).

Outpatients.   A consensus recommendation for the frequency of valproate-level monitoring in stable outpatients is not available. However, once a maintenance dose is achieved, very little change in serum lithium levels would be expected. The addition or deletion of interacting drugs or a change in liver function would indicate the need for a valproate level to be taken within 2 to 4 days (Janicak 1993).

Pharmacokinetic Parameters

▶ Absorption
Valproate is almost completely bioavailable (McElroy and Keck 1993; Pugh and Garnett 1991; Wilder 1992). Food will delay the absorption of all oral formulations except the sprinkle (see *Dosage Forms,* below).

▶ Distribution
Valproate is rapidly distributed within minutes into the CNS (Mc-Elroy and Keck 1993). Cerebrospinal fluid concentrations equal those of free drug in the plasma. When valproate concentrations exceed 100 mg/mL, a disproportionate increase occurs in the free fraction of drug (Pugh and Garnett 1991). This increase may explain some of valproate's dose-related adverse effects (e.g., GI, neurological, hepatic) (see "Adverse Effects" [page 277]).

▶ Metabolism
Valproate is primarily metabolized by oxidation in the liver, producing active and inactive glucuronide metabolites (McElroy and Keck 1993). The plasma elimination half-life ranges from 8 to 17 hours (Janicak 1993). Because the drug follows linear kinetics, proportional increases or decreases in dose should result in equivalent changes in the serum level. Valproate may inhibit the metabolism of many compounds (see **Valproic Acid** drug interactions [pages 481–482] in Chapter 8).

Dosage Forms
Valproate is currently available as a syrup, a soft gelatin capsule, an enteric-coated delayed-release tablet, and a capsule containing coated pellets to be "sprinkled" on food (see Product List [page 291]) (McElroy and Keck 1993; Wilder 1992). Whereas the syrup and soft capsules produce peak concentrations within 0.5 to 1 hour, drug concentrations from the coated tablet and the sprinkle formulations require 4–6 hours to peak. The enteric-coated tablet and sprinkle products contain divalproex sodium, which is a 50/50 combination of sodium valproate and valproate. These two

products reduce the GI adverse effects of valproate by decreasing mucosal contact, slowing the rate of absorption, and lowering the peak valproate concentration (see *Gastrointestinal* adverse effects [page 278]). The enteric-coated tablet's absorption is considerably delayed; complete distribution may require 12 hours or more (Pugh and Garnett 1991). A true trough may not occur until 14–16 hours after the last dose.

The pharmacokinetics of the different dosage forms are similar (Pugh and Garnett 1991); therefore, dosage adjustments typically are not necessary when switching from one product to another. However, a blood level might be obtained 3 days after such a conversion to confirm a stable valproate level.

Therapeutic Concentrations

A therapeutic range for valproate in the acute or maintenance treatment of affective disorders has not been established (Janicak 1993; McElroy and Keck 1993; Sachs 1996). However, many uncontrolled reports have recommended levels between 50 and 150 mg/mL. A recent study reported that serum valproate levels greater than 45 μg/mL were associated with a better therapeutic outcome after 5 days of treatment than were levels less than or equal to 45 μg/mL (Bowden et al. 1994). Unfortunately, dosages were not fixed after the first 5 days of treatment, and an exact therapeutic range cannot be determined from this study. In a blinded study of 14 patients with acute mania, valproate serum levels of 76–125 μg/mL were associated with a better response than valproate serum levels in the range of 25–75 μg/mL (Ellenor et al. 1995). Additional studies need to be performed to assess the relationship between valproate serum levels and therapeutic outcome.

■ Adverse Effects

A comparison of adverse drug reactions (ADRs) associated with valproate and carbamazepine was presented in Table 3–5 (see page 266).

Cardiovascular
Pitting edema has been infrequently reported with valproate (McElroy and Keck 1993; Pugh and Garnett 1991).

Dermatological
Transient alopecia has been reported in 3.6% of patients receiving valproate (Barnes and Bower 1975; Sherard et al. 1980).

Endocrinological

Weight gain and increased appetite not associated with changes in either basal metabolism or thyroid activity occur commonly with valproate. Dietary counseling is recommended, although calorie restriction will not always reverse the weight gain (Penry and Dean 1989).

Idiosyncratic pancreatitis occurring within the first 6 months of treatment has been reported (Wyllie et al. 1984). Abdominal pain associated with an increased amylase level necessitates drug discontinuation.

Gastrointestinal

GI problems are the most commonly reported adverse effects from valproate (Barnes and Bower 1975; Penry and Dean 1989; Sherard et al. 1980). They include anorexia (11.6%); indigestion, heartburn, and nausea (13.8%); vomiting (19.2%); and transient diarrhea (1.7%). These effects can be minimized by administering the drug with food, slowly titrating the dose, and/or switching dosage forms (see *Dosage Forms* [page 276] under "Pharmacokinetics," above, and the Product List [page 291]). In one study, 85% of patients unable to tolerate the soft gelatin formulation of valproate were successfully switched to the enteric-coated tablet (Pugh and Garnett 1991). The addition of a histamine$_2$-blocking agent (e.g., ranitidine) has been reported to reduce GI complaints (McElroy and Keck 1993). It is important to note that the enteric-coated and sprinkle formulations are much more expensive than the soft gelatin capsule (see the Product List [page 291]).

Hematological

Thrombocytopenia and neutropenia are the most common hematological abnormalities associated with valproate. In 45 children followed for more than 1 year, neutropenia and thrombocytopenia were observed in 27% and 33% of the population, respectively (Barr et al. 1982). Both conditions resolved despite drug continuation. No information was presented on the time required for resolution. Prolongation of bleeding time is correlated with both dosage and concentration (Gidal et al. 1994). Thus, dosage reduction or drug discontinuation may be required. A baseline CBC with differential should be obtained for patients starting valproate treatment. One group of authors recommends that patients with affective disorder receive these tests monthly for the first 3 months of drug therapy and every 6–24 months thereafter (McElroy and Keck 1993). Patients should be instructed to contact the prescriber if signs of hematological dysfunction occur (e.g., high fever, extremely sore throat, easy bruising).

Hepatic

▶ Enzyme Elevations

An increase in hepatic transaminases has been reported in 2%–44% of patients receiving valproate (McElroy and Keck 1993). These abnormalities do not necessarily mean that more-serious liver complications will occur (see below). Typically, the enzymes will return to baseline values with drug discontinuation, dosage reduction, or drug continuation. A baseline liver profile is advisable before starting valproate. One group of authors recommends that patients with affective disorder receive these tests monthly for the first 3 months of drug therapy and every 6–24 months thereafter (McElroy and Keck 1993). Patients should be instructed to contact the prescriber if signs or symptoms of hepatic dysfunction occur (e.g., abdominal pain, nausea/vomiting, change in conjunctiva color).

▶ Fatal Hepatotoxicity

The most serious valproate adverse effect is fatal hepatotoxicity (McElroy and Keck 1993; Pugh and Garnett 1991), a rare event that occurs within 6 months of treatment initiation. The onset of the hepatotoxic reaction is preceded by symptoms of vomiting, lethargy, anorexia, and weakness. Risk factors include age less than 2 years, mental retardation, use of multiple anticonvulsants, and refractory seizures (McElroy and Keck 1993; Pugh and Garnett 1991). Although no fatalities from valproate monotherapy have been reported in patients more than 10 years of age, a 13-year-old girl recently died of valproate-induced liver disease when abnormalities in liver function tests were ignored (Clin-Alert 1994).

Neurological

Sedation is the most common CNS effect of valproate. This effect was observed in 4% of adult patients receiving 600–2,400 mg/day (Volzke and Doose 1973). Less commonly experienced ADRs include confusion, fatigue, dizziness, and headache. Minimal or no effects on cognitive skills have been reported with valproate (Gerner 1993; Pugh and Garnett 1991). An essential tremor occurred within 1 month of the start of treatment in 7 of 10 adult patients receiving valproate (Karas et al. 1982). This adverse effect is dose related (Pugh and Garnett 1991).

Teratogenicity and Excretion Into Breast Milk

▶ **Teratogenicity**

There is an increased risk (1%–2%) of neural tube defects in children exposed to valproate during the first trimester of pregnancy (Jeavons 1982). Minor facial defects are also associated with valproate exposure (Briggs et al. 1994). Women taking valproate during days 17 through 30 of gestation should consult their physician about prenatal testing (Briggs et al. 1994).

▶ **Breast Feeding**

No ADRs from valproate exposure in the nursing infant have been reported (Briggs et al. 1994). The drug is considered compatible with breast feeding (Committee on Drugs 1994).

■ Rational Prescribing

1. Valproate is more effective than placebo but probably less effective than lithium in lithium-naive patients.
2. In lithium-refractory patients, valproate produced a 49% response rate in controlled trials (Bowden et al. 1994) and a 67% response rate in open reports (McElroy and Keck 1993).
3. Approximately 70% of patients refractory to carbamazepine may respond to valproate (Schaff et al. 1993).
4. Valproate has not been directly compared with carbamazepine in the management of patients with rapid-cycling illness, organic mania, or mixed/dysphoric mania.
5. In mania, valproate's onset of action ranges from 7 to 14 days. A therapeutic trial consists of 3 weeks.
6. In the treatment of mania, valproate can be combined with antipsychotics and/or benzodiazepines to achieve early control of agitation. The antipsychotic or benzodiazepine should be discontinued after the manic symptoms resolve.
7. Valproate produced an antidepressant response in only 30% of patients with major depressive disorder (McElroy and Keck 1993).
8. Valproate's use in the maintenance treatment of affective disorders has not been studied in controlled trials. In open trials, valproate produced a response rate of 45% and 88% in lithium-naive and -refractory patients, respectively (McElroy and Keck 1993).
9. In open reports of patients with schizoaffective disorder, valproate produced response rates of 58% and 83% in acute treatment and maintenance treatment, respectively (McElroy

and Keck 1993). The relative efficacy of valproate and other treatments needs to be determined in direct-comparison studies.

10. A therapeutic range has not been established for valproate in affective disorders. The dosage should be increased until either therapeutic response or dose-related adverse effects occur.

11. Baseline hepatic and hematological tests should be obtained. Patients should be informed of the signs and symptoms of infection and liver disease and instructed to notify their prescriber should these effects occur.

12. Gastrointestinal adverse effects are dose related and may be relieved by changing to a coated dosage formulation.

13. Valproate is regarded as a third-line treatment for mania (i.e., behind lithium and carbamazepine).

Verapamil

■ Indications

Verapamil, a calcium channel–blocking agent, is indicated for the treatment of supraventricular tachyarrhythmias, angina, and hypertension. It has been found useful in the treatment of acute mania.

■ Efficacy

Although many calcium channel blockers are available on the market, verapamil has been the most widely studied.

Acute Treatment

▶ Mania
It is important to separate study populations into lithium-refractory and lithium-naive (i.e., lithium-responsive or potentially lithium-responsive) patients to determine whether the response rate for verapamil is greater than, equal to, or less than that of lithium in lithium-naive patients. It is also important to determine the percentage of lithium-refractory patients who will respond to verapamil so that verapamil's efficacy can be ranked against that of other suggested treatments (e.g., carbamazepine, valproate).

Verapamil has not been systematically studied either in carbamazepine responders or in valproate responders or nonresponders.

The onset of action of verapamil varies from 7 to 14 days (Garza-Trevino et al. 1992; Giannini et al. 1985; Hoschl and Kozeny 1989). A therapeutic trial is 3 weeks.

Lithium-naive patients. *Open reports.* One patient responded within 4 days of verapamil initiation (Patterson 1987).

Verapamil versus placebo. Three double-blind studies involving a total of 16 patients reported an 81% response rate for verapamil (Dose et al. 1986; Dubovsky et al. 1982, 1986). One study reported that verapamil was more effective than placebo, but did not indicate the patient response rate (Giannini et al. 1984).

Verapamil versus lithium. Three double-blind studies involving a total of 36 patients found that verapamil was as effective as lithium alone or a lithium/antipsychotic combination. However, one of these studies treated patients with an average lithium level of 0.75 mEq/L (Hoschl and Kozeny 1989). The other studies used a lithium-level range of 0.75–1.5 mEq/L and 0.84–1.26 mEq/L, but did not report average or final lithium levels for individual patients (Garza-Trevino et al. 1992; Giannini et al. 1984).

Verapamil combined with an antipsychotic or a benzodiazepine. Verapamil has been successfully combined with haloperidol and/or lorazepam for control of psychomotor agitation (Garza-Trevino et al. 1992).

Lithium-refractory patients. *Open reports.* Only 5 of 13 patients (38%) included in two reports responded to a verapamil trial (Barton and Gitlin 1987; Brotman et al. 1986).

Verapamil versus clonidine. A double-blind study reported that verapamil was significantly more effective than clonidine (Giannini et al. 1985).

Carbamazepine-refractory patients. Only 4 of 14 patients who had failed to respond to a lithium and a carbamazepine trial demonstrated improvement with verapamil (Barton and Gitlin 1987).

▶ **Major Depressive Disorder**

Open report. One report concluded that verapamil was ineffective in two patients with bipolar depression (Barton and Gitlin 1987).

Double-blind study. A study involving 26 patients reported a 38% response rate, which was similar to the placebo response rate of 31% (Hoschl and Kozeny 1989). Ten of the 26 patients had a diagnosis of unipolar depression, while 3 had bipolar depression. The remaining 13 patients had atypical or unspecified depressive disorder.

Continuation Treatment
(General principles for the use of verapamil in continuation treatment are the same as those for lithium; see *Continuation Treatment* [page 225] under "Efficacy" of **Lithium**.)

There is no evidence that verapamil, like lithium, needs to be tapered to reduce the rate of recurrent manic or depressive episodes. Conservatively, if the drug is to be discontinued in affective disorder patients, it might be tapered by 25% per week.

Maintenance Treatment

(General principles for the use of verapamil in maintenance treatment are the same as those for lithium; see *Maintenance Treatment* [page 226] under "Efficacy" of **Lithium**.)

Open reports. One patient unresponsive to lithium responded well to verapamil prophylaxis (Gitlin and Weiss 1984). Two of four patients who had been unresponsive to lithium and probably carbamazepine demonstrated mild improvement in a verapamil trial (Barton and Gitlin 1987).

Double-blind study. In a 6-month crossover study, verapamil was more effective than lithium in 20 lithium-responsive patients (Giannini et al. 1987).

■ Mechanism of Action

Verapamil blocks the influx of calcium into myocardial cells (Giannini et al. 1985). It also inhibits neurosecretory processes, including excitation-secretion coupling at norepinephrine synapses. Verapamil's action on calcium metabolism may be similar to lithium's effect. Both drugs block adenylate cyclase activity in most organs and compete with calcium ions in neuromuscular cells. Interestingly, the onset of mania is associated with transient increases in serum calcium concentrations.

■ Dosage

Antimanic verapamil dosages range from 160 to 480 mg/day, with a median dose of 320 mg/day. Verapamil can be started at 80 mg bid or tid and the dose increased daily or every other day to a dosage of 320 mg/day. Nonresponse after 2 weeks warrants increasing the dosage to 480 mg/day administered on a tid schedule. Dosages greater than 480 mg/day have not been investigated.

■ Pharmacokinetics

Absorption

Approximately 90% of an orally administered verapamil dose is absorbed; however, because of a large first-pass effect in the liver, only 20%–35% reaches the systemic circulation (Kates 1983). The sustained-release formulation has a similar bioavailability profile. Oral bioavailability increases significantly in patients with hepatic dysfunction (e.g., cirrhosis). Peak plasma levels are attained within 1 to 2 hours with the immediate-release formulation and within 4 to 8 hours with the sustained-release formulation. The presence of food in the stomach does not affect the absorption characteristics of the regular tablets, but does affect the rate and extent of absorption of the sustained-release formulation.

Distribution

The volume of distribution ranges from 4.5 to 7 L/kg in healthy adults but increases to approximately 12 L/kg in patients with cirrhosis (Kates 1983). The drug is 90% protein bound, with 6% of verapamil and 4% of norverapamil being present in the cerebrospinal fluid.

Metabolism

Verapamil is extensively metabolized, generating norverapamil as its primary active metabolite (Kates 1983). After 1–2 days of chronic administration, verapamil's elimination half-life increases to 5–12 hours in healthy adults and to 14–16 hours in patients with cirrhosis due to saturation kinetics. Within 4 to 6 hours of administration, norverapamil achieves plasma concentrations similar to those of verapamil.

Therapeutic Range

A therapeutic range for verapamil in the acute or maintenance treatment of affective disorders has not been determined.

■ Adverse Effects

Verapamil is generally well tolerated in affective disorder patients and rarely requires discontinuation because of adverse effects. The incidence data presented in the following sections are based on summed adverse-effect frequencies reported in five studies (Lewis 1986; Madtbo and Hals 1980; Madtbo et al. 1982, 1986; Speders et al. 1989). A total of 43 patients were observed for 6–52 weeks.

Cardiovascular

◗ Conduction Disturbance

Impulse generation may be reduced in the sinoatrial node, conduction in the AV node may be blocked, and a negative inotropic effect can occur as a result of inhibition of calcium influx (Epstein and Rosing 1981). The most commonly reported conduction changes include bradycardia (1.4%), AV block (1.2%), and congestive heart failure or peripheral edema (1.8%) (Calan® Product Information 1993). Verapamil is contraindicated in patients with 1) sick sinus syndrome untreated with a pacemaker if significant second- or third-degree AV junctional disease is present, 2) advanced heart failure, 3) cardiogenic shock, 4) severe hypertension, and/or 5) Wolff-Parkinson-White syndrome with prior atrial fibrillation. The drug should not be used in combination with β-blockers (e.g., propranolol) in patients with congestive heart failure.

▶ Blood Pressure
The most commonly reported vascular reactions associated with orally administered verapamil in patients without affective disorders are hypotension (2.5%) and peripheral edema (1.9%) (Calan® Product Information 1993). Manic patients usually tolerate verapamil's blood pressure–lowering effects very well (Garza-Trevino et al. 1992). Monitoring parameters include lying and orthostatic blood pressure and pulse.

Dermatological
Minor skin reactions occur in 0.55% of patients and include urticaria, itching, and exanthema (Speders et al. 1989). These effects usually do not require drug discontinuation. However, verapamil has also been associated with Stevens-Johnson syndrome, erythema multiforme, exfoliative dermatitis (1 case per million prescriptions), and urticaria (0.85 case per million prescriptions). The most serious dermatological reactions occur within the first 14 days of treatment initiation (Stern and Khalsa 1989).

Gastrointestinal
Mild to moderate constipation secondary to smooth muscle relaxation is reported in 7.3% of patients (Lewis 1986; Madtbo and Hals 1980; Madtbo et al. 1982, 1986; Speders et al. 1989). Constipation may be treated with increased fluid intake, a psyllium derivative, and/or stool softeners. Nausea (2.7%) and vomiting are also associated with oral administration (Calan® Product Information 1993). Nausea may be relieved by taking the medication with food (Speders et al. 1989).

Neurological
Common CNS adverse effects include fatigue (1.1%), headache (1.6%), and dizziness (3.6%) (Madtbo and Hals 1980; Madtbo et al. 1982, 1986; Speders et al. 1989). Generally, the complaints are mild, transient, and rarely require verapamil's discontinuation (see **Lithium–Verapamil** drug interaction [page 476] in Chapter 8).

Teratogenicity and Excretion Into Breast Milk

▶ **Teratogenicity**

A surveillance study of 229,101 Michigan Medicaid recipients reported major birth defects in 76 newborns exposed to verapamil during the first trimester. According to the incidence rate in the general population, only 3 children would have been expected to be so affected (Briggs et al. 1994).

▶ **Breast-Milk Secretion**

Although verapamil is excreted in breast milk, the infant receives less than 0.01% of the mother's dose (Anderson et al. 1987). The American Academy of Pediatrics considers verapamil to be compatible with breast feeding (Committee on Drugs 1994).

■ Rational Prescribing

1. Verapamil is more effective than placebo and equal in efficacy to lithium in lithium-naive patients; however, fewer than 70 patients have been studied.
2. Verapamil produced a 38% response rate in 13 patients with lithium-refractory mania (Barton and Gitlin 1987; Brotman et al. 1986).
3. Approximately one-third of patients refractory to lithium and carbamazepine responded to a verapamil trial (Barton and Gitlin 1987).
4. In mania, verapamil's onset of action varies from 7 to 14 days. A therapeutic trial consists of 3 weeks.
5. Verapamil can be combined with antipsychotics and/or benzodiazepines in the treatment of mania.
6. Verapamil produced an antidepressant response in only one-third of patients with major depressive disorder (Hoschl and Kozeny 1989).
7. Verapamil was more effective than lithium in one 6-month maintenance treatment trial (Giannini et al. 1987).
8. Verapamil has not been directly compared with carbamazepine and valproate in the acute and maintenance treatment of affective disorders.
9. Because of the small number of patients studied, verapamil is considered only a fourth-line treatment for mania. More research is needed to determine this drug's efficacy in comparison with other treatments.

Benzodiazepines

The use of benzodiazepines alone is discussed in this section. (The use of benzodiazepines in combination with lithium is addressed in *Acute Treatment,* Mania [pages 221–223] under "Efficacy" of **Lithium**). The pharmacokinetics and adverse effects of benzodiazepines are covered in Chapter 4.

■ Indications

Benzodiazepines are not approved by the FDA for the acute or prophylactic treatment of unipolar or bipolar disorders.

■ Efficacy

Acute Treatment

Open reports. The successful use of clonazepam or lorazepam has been reported (Aronson et al. 1989; Gerner 1993).

Double-blind studies. In a 10-day study in which 12 manic patients were treated with clonazepam or lithium (Chouinard et al. 1983), clonazepam was significantly superior to lithium in improving symptoms of motor overactivity and logorrhea, but there was no significant difference in the two drugs' effects on elevated mood, pressure of speech, or insight. Nonsignificantly smaller haloperidol dosages were used with clonazepam than with lithium therapy. Because lithium may require more than 10 days to exert an antimanic effect, this study may have been too short in duration to detect a difference between the two treatments.

One study reported that lorazepam was more efficacious than clonazepam in the management of mania (Bradwejn et al. 1990). After 2 weeks of treatment, the response and remission rates for lorazepam were 61% and 39%, respectively, whereas those for clonazepam were 18% and 0%, respectively. Lithium was added during days 14 through 28 of the study. At the end of the study, five lorazepam + lithium patients were discharged, as compared with none of the clonazepam + lithium patients.

Continuation Treatment

(General principles for the use of benzodiazepines in continuation treatment are the same as those for lithium; see *Continuation Treatment* [page 225] under "Efficacy" of **Lithium.**)

There is no evidence that a benzodiazepine, like lithium, needs to be tapered to reduce the rate of recurrent manic or depressive episodes. Conservatively, if the drug is to be discontinued in affective-disorder patients, it might be tapered by 25% per week.

No trials have been conducted of a benzodiazepine alone in the continuation treatment of bipolar illness.

Maintenance Treatment

(General principles for the use of benzodiazepines in maintenance treatment are the same as those for lithium; see *Maintenance Treatment* [page 226] under "Efficacy" of **Lithium**.)

No trials have been conducted of a benzodiazepine alone in the maintenance treatment of bipolar illness.

■ Mechanism of Action

The mechanism of action of the benzodiazepines in mania is unknown. However, benzodiazepines may exert antimanic activity, enhancing the effect of GABA and stimulating serotonin synthesis (Chouinard et al. 1983).

■ Dosage

Lorazepam doses have ranged from 2 to 80 mg/day administered orally or parenterally (Gerner 1993). Typical doses are 2–4 mg po/im every 2 hours. Typical daily doses are less than 36 mg.

Clonazepam doses ranged from 2 to 22 mg/day in controlled trials (Gerner 1993).

■ Rational Prescribing

1. The relative efficacy of benzodiazepines versus lithium, carbamazepine, verapamil, or valproate is unknown.
2. Benzodiazepines can reduce agitation when used in combination with lithium. Benzodiazepines need to be studied in combination with carbamazepine, verapamil, and valproate to determine their relative efficacy.
3. More studies need to be performed to determine the relative efficacy of the benzodiazepines and the antipsychotics in combination with lithium, carbamazepine, verapamil, or valproate.
4. Benzodiazepines may provide an "antipsychotic-dose–sparing" effect when used in combination with scheduled doses of typical antipsychotics.
5. Lorazepam may be more effective than clonazepam in the management of manic agitation. Also, lorazepam has the advantages of being less expensive and being available for parenteral administration.

6. It is unknown whether tolerance develops to the antimanic activity of benzodiazepines.

Miscellaneous Treatments

The following subsections briefly summarize what is known about selected miscellaneous agents studied in the treatment of refractory bipolar illness. Readers wishing to obtain more detailed information on these agents should consult the cited references accompanying each topic. Reviews of treatment options in mania have recently been published (Chou 1991; Gerner 1993; Keck and McElroy 1996; Sachs 1996).

■ Clonidine

Efficacy

▶ Open Reports
Overall, four open reports involving 36 patients suggested that 23 (66%) experienced moderate to marked improvement with clonidine (Hardy et al. 1986; Jouvent et al. 1980; Kontaxakis et al. 1989; Zubenko et al. 1984b).

▶ Controlled Trials
A total of 45 patients have received clonidine in controlled trials. Clonidine reduced manic symptoms in one study, but was equal in efficacy to placebo in another (Giannini et al. 1983; Janicak et al. 1989). In two comparison studies, lithium and verapamil were more effective than clonidine (Giannini et al. 1985, 1986).

Mechanism of Action
The catecholamine theory of affective illness postulates exaggerated noradrenergic activity in mania. Clonidine stimulates presynaptic inhibitory receptors to reduce CNS norepinephrine activity.

Dosage
In the studies cited above, daily doses ranged from 0.2 to 1.2 mg divided into three doses.

Adverse Effects
Primarily dose-related sedation and hypotension have been reported with clonidine. Blood pressure should be monitored during clonidine treatment.

Rational Prescribing

1. Clonidine is less effective than lithium and verapamil in the acute treatment of mania. However, some patients may preferentially respond to clonidine.
2. Clonidine has not been studied in the maintenance treatment of affective disorder, the acute treatment of depression, or the management of schizoaffective disorder.
3. Clonidine's primary adverse effects are sedation and hypotension.

■ Fenfluramine

Efficacy

One uncontrolled study reported that 7 of 7 manic patients responded to fenfluramine (Cookson and Silverstone 1976). Two double-blind studies reported improvement in 5 of 8 patients (Murphy et al. 1978; Pearce 1973).

Mechanism of Action

Fenfluramine is a serotonin agonist (Murphy et al. 1978).

Dosage

Daily dosages reported for fenfluramine ranged from 60 to 180 mg.

■ Thyroid Supplementation

Efficacy

Two studies in which levothyroxine or triiodothyronine were administered at dosages sufficient to produce supranormal thyroid levels reported improvement in 10 of 15 rapid-cycling patients (Bauer and Whybrow 1990; Stancer and Persad 1982).

Adverse Effects

Although thyroid supplementation therapy was well tolerated by patients in the aforementioned studies, a consultation with an endocrinologist is recommended before initiating treatment with these agents (Gerner 1993).

■ Antipsychotics

The use of antipsychotics in the acute treatment of mania and schizoaffective mania as well as their use in maintenance treatment is discussed in the "Efficacy" subsections of **Typical Antipsychotics** and **Clozapine** in Chapter 1.

Product List

Carbamazepine

- Daily dose range: 600–2,000 mg
- Generic cost index: ≈ 0.40 (200 mg); 0.94 (100 mg)

Tablets:	**Tegretol**®
200 mg	[$38] Tegretol/27, pink
Chewable tablets:	**Tegretol**®
100 mg	[$20] Tegretol/52, pink/red speckled
Suspension:	**Tegretol**®
100 mg/5 mL	[$24/450 mL] yellow-orange, citrus/vanilla flavor

Lithium

- Daily dose range: 600–3,000 mg; generically available
- Generic cost index: ≈ 0.29

Tablets:	**Lithotabs**™
300 mg	[$10] Solvay 7516, white
Capsules:	**Eskalith**®
300 mg	[$18] SKF Eskalith, yellow/gray
	Lithonate®
300 mg	[$8] Solvay 7512, peach
Tablets, sustained release:	**Lithobid**®
300 mg	[$24], peach
450 mg	**Eskalith CR**®
	[$38] SKFJ10, buff, scored
Concentrate:	**Lithium citrate**
300 mg/5 mL	[$13/480 mL]

Valproic Acid

- Daily dose range: 1,000–1,500 mg; generically available
- Generic cost index: (valproic acid) ≈ 0.12

Capsules:	**Depakene**® (valproic acid)
250 mg	[$116], orange
	Depakote® **Sprinkle** (divalproex sodium)
125 mg	[$31], orange
Syrup:	**Depakene**® **Syrup** (valproate sodium)
250 mg/5 mL	[$119/480 mL], red, cherry (valproic acid)
Tablets, delayed release:	**Depakote**® (divalproex sodium)
125 mg	[$31], salmon pink
250 mg	[$61], peach
500 mg	[$112], lavender

Verapamil
- Daily dose range: 320–480 mg; generically available
- Generic cost index: ≈ 0.14

Tablets:	**Isoptin**®
40 mg	[$31] Isoptin 40 Knoll, blue
80 mg	[$44] Isoptin 80 Knoll, yellow
120 mg	[$60] Isoptin 120 Knoll, white

Film-coated tablets, extended release:	**Isoptin SR**®
120 mg	[$89] Isoptin SR 120, pink
180 mg	[$113] Isoptin SR 180, salmon
240 mg	[$129] Isoptin SR 240, light green

References

Abou-Saleh MT, Coppen A: The efficacy of low-dose lithium: clinical, psychological, and biological correlates. J Psychiatr Res 23:157–162, 1989

Abou-Saleh MT, Coppen A: Who responds to prophylactic lithium? J Affect Disord 10:115–125, 1986

Alam MY, Klass DB, Luchin DJ, et al: Effectiveness of divalproex sodium, valproic acid, and carbamazepine in aggression (abstract). Psychopharmacol Bull 31:546, 1995

Almy GL, Taylor MA: Lithium retention in mania. Arch Gen Psychiatry 29:232–234, 1973

Amdisen A: Lithium, in Applied Pharmacokinetics: Principles of Therapeutic Drug Monitoring. Edited by Evans WE, Schentag JJ, Jusko WJ. San Francisco, CA, Applied Therapeutics, 1980, pp 586–617

Anderson P, Bondesson U, Mattiasson I, et al: Verapamil and norverapamil in plasma and breast milk during breast feeding. Eur J Pharmacol 31:625–627, 1987

Angst J: Clinical indications for a prophylactic treatment of depression. Adv Biol Psychiatry 7:218–229, 1981

Aronson TA, Shukla S, Hirschowitz J: Clonazepam treatment of five lithium-refractory patients with bipolar disorder. Am J Psychiatry 146:77–80, 1989

Baastrup PC, Hollnagel P, Sorenson R, et al: Adverse reactions in treatment with lithium carbonate and haloperidol. JAMA 236:2645–2646, 1976

Ballenger JC: The clinical use of carbamazepine in affective disorders. J Clin Psychiatry 49 (suppl 4):13–19, 1988

Ballenger JC, Post RM: Carbamazepine in manic-depressive illness: a new treatment. Am J Psychiatry 137:782–790, 1980

Barnes SE, Bower BD: Sodium valproate in the treatment of intractable childhood epilepsy. Dev Med Child Neurol 17:175–181, 1975

Barr RD, Copeland SA, Stockwell ML, et al: Valproic acid and immune thrombocytopenia. Arch Dis Child 57:681–684, 1982

Barton BM, Gitlin MJ: Verapamil in treatment-resistant mania: an open trial. J Clin Psychopharmacol 7:101–103, 1987

Batlle DC, von Riotte AB, Gaviria M, et al: Amelioration of polyuria by amiloride in patients receiving long-term lithium therapy. N Engl J Med 312:408–414, 1985

Bauer MS, Whybrow PC: Rapid-cycling bipolar affective disorder, II: treatment of refractory rapid-cycling with high-dose levothyroxine: a preliminary study. Arch Gen Psychiatry 47:435–440, 1990

Bendz H, Aurell M, Balldin J, et al: Kidney damage in long-term lithium patients: a cross-sectional study of patients with 15 years or more on lithium. Nephrology, Dialysis, Transplantation 9:1250–1254, 1994

Berens SC, Wolff J: The endocrine effects of lithium, in Lithium Research and Therapy. Edited by Johnson FN. London, Academic Press, 1975, pp 443–472

Bertilsson L, Tomson T: Clinical pharmacokinetics and pharmacological effects of carbamazepine and carbamazepine-10,11-epoxide. Clin Pharmacokinet 11:177–198, 1986

Biederman J, Lerner Y, Belmaker RH: Combination of lithium carbonate and haloperidol in schizoaffective disorder. Arch Gen Psychiatry 36:327–333, 1979

Birnbaum J, Klandorf H, Builian A, et al: Lithium stimulates the release of human parathyroid hormone in vitro. J Clin Endocrinol Metab 66:1187–1191, 1988

Boesen F, Andersen EB, Jensen EK, et al: Cardiac conduction disturbances during carbamazepine therapy. Acta Neurol Scand 69:49–52, 1983

Bone S, Roose SP, Dunner DL, et al: Incidence of side effects in patients on long-term lithium. Am J Psychiatry 137:103–104, 1980

Bowden CL, Brugger AM, Swann AC, et al: Efficacy of divalproex vs lithium and placebo in the treatment of mania. JAMA 271:918–924, 1994

Bradwejn J, Shriqui C, Koszycki D, et al: Double-blind comparison of the effects of clonazepam and lorazepam in acute mania. J Clin Psychopharmacol 10:403–408, 1990

Brenner R, Cooper TB, Yablonski ME, et al: Measurement of lithium concentration in human tears. Am J Psychiatry 139:678–679, 1982

Brewerton TD, Jackson CW: Prophylaxis of carbamazepine-induced hyponatremia by demeclocycline in six patients. J Clin Psychiatry 55:249–251, 1994

Briggs GG, Freeman RK, Yaffe SJ: A Reference Guide to Fetal and Neonatal Risk: Drugs in Pregnancy and Lactation, 4th Edition. Baltimore, MD, Williams & Wilkins, 1994

Brotman AW, Farhadi AM, Gelenberg AJ: Verapamil treatment of acute mania. J Clin Psychiatry 47:136–138, 1986

Brown R: U.S. experience with valproate in manic-depressive illness: a multicenter trial. J Clin Psychiatry 50 (suppl 3):13–16, 1989

Bucht G, Wahlin A: Renal concentrating capacity in long-term lithium treatment and after withdrawal of lithium. Acta Med Scand 207:309–314, 1980

Burrows GD: Long-term clinical management of depressive disorders. J Clin Psychiatry 55 (suppl 3):32–35, 1992

Calabrese JR, Mitchell PB, Paggaglia PJ, et al: International Psychopharmacology Algorithm Project report, B: algorithms for the treatment of bipolar, manic-depressive illness. Psychopharmacol Bull 31:469–474, 1995

Calabrese JR, Fatemi SH, Kujawa M, et al: Predictors of response to mood stabilizers. J Clin Psychopharmacol 16 (suppl 1):24S–31S, 1996

Calan® [verapamil] Product Information. Chicago, IL, Searle, 1993

Carroll JA, Jefferson JW, Greist JH: Treating tremor induced by lithium. Hospital and Community Psychiatry 38:1280–1288, 1987

Carson S: Lithium, in Applied Pharmacokinetics: Principles of Therapeutic Drug Monitoring, 3rd Edition. Edited by Evans WE, Schentag JJ, Jusko WJ. Vancouver, BC, Canada, Applied Therapeutics, 1992, p 34–3

Chaudhry RP, Waters BG: Lithium and carbamazepine interaction: possible neurotoxicity. J Clin Psychiatry 44:30–31, 1983

Chou J C: Recent advances in treatment of acute mania. J Clin Psychopharmacol 11:3–21, 1991

Chouinard G, Young SN, Annable L: Antimanic effect of clonazepam. Biol Psychiatry 18:451–466, 1983

Clayton PJ: Bipolar illness, in The Medical Basis of Psychiatry, 2nd Edition. Edited by Winokur G, Clayton PJ. Philadelphia, PA, WB Saunders, 1994, pp 47–68

Clin-Alert: Divalproex sodium: failure to monitor liver function; death; legal action. Clin-Alert 22:291–292, 1994

Cockcroft DW, Gault MH: Prediction of creatinine clearance from serum creatinine. Nephron 16:31–47, 1976

Cohen LS, Friedman JM, Jefferson JW, et al: A reevaluation of risk of in utero exposure to lithium. JAMA 271:146–150, 1994

Committee on Drugs, American Academy of Pediatrics: The transfer of drugs and other chemicals in human milk. Pediatrics 93:137–150, 1994

Cookson J, Silverstone T: 5-Hydroxytryptamine and dopamine pathways in mania: a pilot study of fenfluramine and pimozide. Br J Clin Pharmacol 3:942–947, 1976

Coppen A, Abou-Saleh M, Milln P, et al: Decreasing lithium dosage reduces morbidity and side effects during prophylaxis. J Affect Disord 5:353–362, 1983

Crosley CJ, Swender PT: Dystonia associated with carbamazepine administration: experience in brain-damaged children. Pediatrics 63:612–615, 1979

DasGupta K, Jefferson JW: The use of lithium in the medically ill. Gen Hosp Psychiatry 12:83–97, 1990

Deandrea D, Walker N, Mehmauer M, et al: Dermatological reactions to lithium: critical review. J Clin Psychopharmacol 2:199–204, 1982

Dempsey GM, Dunner DL, Fieve RR, et al: Treatment of excessive weight gain in patients taking lithium. Am J Psychiatry 133:1082–1084, 1976

Denicoff KD, Meglathery SB, Post RM, et al: Efficacy of carbamazepine compared with other agents: a clinical practice survey. J Clin Psychiatry 55:70–76, 1994

Dilsaver SC, Swann AC, Shoaib A, et al: The manic syndrome: factors which may predict a patient's response to lithium, carbamazepine, and valproate. J Psychiatry Neurosci 18:61–66, 1993

Dose M, Emrich HM, Cording-Tommel C, et al: Use of calcium antagonists in mania. Psychoneuroendocrinology 11:241–243, 1986

Dubovsky SL, Franks RD, Lifschitz M, et al: Effectiveness of verapamil in the treatment of a manic patient. Am J Psychiatry 139:502–504, 1982

Dubovsky SL, Franks RD, Allen S, et al: Calcium antagonists in mania: a double-blind study of verapamil. Psychiatry Res 18:309–320, 1986

Edwards R, Stephenson U, Flewett T: Clonazepam in acute mania: a double blind trial. Aust N Z J Psychiatry 25:238–242, 1991

Eggert AE, Crismon ML, Kamp M: Evaluation of potential nonlinear lithium clearance (abstract). Psychopharmacol Bull 31:562, 1995

Ellenor G, Lohr JB, Ito M, et al: The comparative efficacy of divalproex low and high serum level in bipolar disorder and schizophrenia (abstract). Psychopharmacol Bull 31:563, 1995

Epstein SE, Rosing DR: Verapamil: its potential for causing serious complications in patients with hypertropic cardiomyopathy. Circulation 64:437–441, 1981

Faedda GL, Tondo L, Baldessarini RJ, et al: Outcome after rapid versus gradual discontinuation of lithium treatment in bipolar disorders. Arch Gen Psychiatry 50:448–455, 1993

Fawcett J, Kravitz HM: The long-term management of bipolar disorders with lithium, carbamazepine, and antidepressants. J Clin Psychiatry 46:58–60, 1985

Frankenburg FR, Tohen M, Cohen BM, et al: Long-term response to carbamazepine: a retrospective study. J Clin Psychopharmacol 8:130–132, 1988

Freeman TW, Clothier JL, Pazzaglia P, et al: A double-blind comparison of valproate and lithium in the treatment of acute mania. Am J Psychiatry 149:108–111, 1992

Gaby NS, Lefkowitz DS, Israel JR: Treatment of lithium tremor with metoprolol. Am J Psychiatry 140:593–595, 1983

Garland EJ, Remick RA, Zis AP: Weight gain with antidepressants and lithium. J Clin Psychopharmacol 8:323–330, 1988

Garza-Trevino ES, Overall JE, Hollister LE: Verapamil versus lithium in acute mania. Am J Psychiatry 149:121–122, 1992

Gelenberg AJ, Kane JM, Keller MB, et al: Comparison of standard and low serum levels of lithium for maintenance treatment of bipolar disorder. N Engl J Med 321:1489–1493, 1989

Gelenberg AJ, Jefferson JW: Lithium tremor. J Clin Psychiatry 56:283–287, 1995

Gerner RH: Treatment of acute mania. Psychiatric Clin North Am 16:443–460, 1993

Giannini AJ, Extein I, Gold MS, et al: Clonidine in mania. Drug Development Research 3:101–103, 1983

Giannini AJ, Houser WL, Loiselle RII, et al: Antimanic effects of verapamil. Am J Psychiatry 141:1602–1603, 1984

Giannini AJ, Loiselle RH, Price WA, et al: Comparison of antimanic efficacy of clonidine and verapamil. J Clin Pharmacol 25:307–308, 1985

Giannini AJ, Pascarzi GA, Loiselle RH, et al: Comparison of clonidine and lithium in the treatment of mania. Am J Psychiatry 143:1608–1609, 1986

Giannini AJ, Taraszewski R, Loiselle RH: Verapamil and lithium in maintenance therapy of manic patients. J Clin Pharmacol 27:980–982, 1987

Gidal B, Spencer N, Maly M, et al: Valproate-mediated disturbances of hemostasis: relationship to dose and plasma concentration. Neurology 44:1418–1422, 1994

Gitlin MJ, Weiss J: Verapamil as maintenance treatment in bipolar illness: a case report. J Clin Psychopharmacol 4:341–343, 1984

Goldney RD, Spence ND: Safety of the combination of lithium and neuroleptic drugs. Am J Psychiatry 143:882–884, 1986

Goodnick PJ, Meltzer HY: Treatment of schizoaffective disorders. Schizophr Bull 10:30–48, 1984

Goodnick PJ, Meltzer HY, Fieve RR, et al: Differences in lithium kinetics between bipolar and unipolar patients. J Clin Psychopharmacol 2:48–50, 1982

Goodwin FK, Zis AP: Lithium in the treatment of mania: comparison with neuroleptics. Arch Gen Psychiatry 36:840–844, 1979

Grell W, Schmidt ST: Lithium withdrawal reactions, in Lithium: Inorganic Pharmacology and Psychiatric Use. Edited by Birch NJ. Washington, DC, IRL Press, 1988, pp 149–153

Guay DRP: The emerging role of valproate in bipolar disorder and other psychiatric disorders. Pharmacotherapy 15:631–647, 1995

Hammond CM: Single daily dosage of lithium carbonate (letter). Ann Pharmacother 28:472–474, 1994

Hansen HE, Amdisen A: Lithium intoxication (report of 23 cases and review of 100 cases from the literature). Quarterly Journal of Medicine 47:123–144, 1978

Hardy MC, Lecrubier Y, Widlocher D: Efficacy of clonidine in 24 patients with acute mania. Am J Psychiatry 143:1450–1453, 1986

Hart RG, Easton JD: Carbamazepine and hematological monitoring. Ann Neurol 11:309–312, 1982

Hestbeck J, Hansen HE, Amdisen A, et al: Chronic renal lesions following long-term treatment with lithium. Kidney Int 12:305–313, 1977

Hewick DS, Newbury P, Hopwood S, et al: Age as a factor affecting lithium therapy. Br J Clin Pharmac 4:201–205, 1977

Hirschfeld RMA, Clayton PJ, Cohen I, et al: Practice guidelines for the treatment of patients with bipolar disorder. Am J Psychiatry 151 (suppl):1–36, 1994

Hoschl C, Kozeny J: Verapamil in affective disorders: A controlled, double-blind study. Biol Psychiatry 25:128–140, 1989

Howrie DL, Zitelli BJ, Painter MJ: Anticonvulsant-induced hepatotoxicity. Hospital Formulary 18:564–570, 1983

Hullin RP: Minimum effective plasma lithium levels for long-term preventive treatment of recurrent affective disorders, in Lithium: Controversies and Unresolved Issues. Edited by Copper TB, Gershon S, Kline NS, et al. Amsterdam, Excerpta Medica, 1979, pp 333–334

Inoue H, Unno N: Excretion of verapamil in human milk. BMJ 288:644–645, 1984

Jacobsen SJ, Jones K, Johnson K, et al: Prospective multicentre study of pregnancy outcome after lithium exposure during first trimester. Lancet 339:550–553, 1992

Janicak PG: The relevance of clinical pharmacokinetics and therapeutic drug monitoring: anticonvulsant mood stabilizers and antipsychotics. J Clin Psychiatry 54 (suppl 9):35–41, 1993

Janicak PG, Sharma RP, Easton M, et al: A double-blind, placebo-controlled trial of clonidine in the treatment of acute mania. Psychopharmacol Bull 25:243–245, 1989

Janicak PG, Davis JM, Ayd FJ, et al: Advances in the pharmacotherapy of bipolar disorder. Principles and Practice of Psychopharmacotherapy 1(3):1–19, 1995

Jarrett DB, Serry J, Graham DB: Lithium-induced tremor (letter). Med J Aust 62:21, 1975

Jeavons PM: Sodium valproate and neural tube defects. Lancet 2:1282–1283, 1982

Jefferson JW: Lithium tremor and caffeine intake: two cases of drinking less and shaking more. J Clin Psychiatry 49:72–73, 1988

Jefferson JW, Kaufman P, Ackerman D: Tear lithium concentration: a measurement of dubious clinical value. J Clin Psychiatry 45:304–305, 1984

Jensen HV, Plenge P, Mellerup ET, et al: Lithium prophylaxis of manic-depressive disorder: daily lithium dosing schedule versus every second day. Acta Psychiatr Scand 92:69–74, 1995

Jeppsson J, Sjogren J: The influence of food on side effects and absorption of lithium. Acta Psychiatr Scand 51:285–288, 1975

Joffe RT, Kellner CG, Post RM, et al: Lithium increases in platelet count (letter). N Engl J Med 311:674–675, 1984

Jones KL, Lacro RV, Johnson KA, et al: Pattern of malformations in the children of women treated with carbamazepine during pregnancy. N Engl J Med 320:1661–1666, 1989

Jouvent R, Lecrubier Y, Fuech AJ, et al: Antimanic effect of clonidine. Am J Psychiatry 137:1275–1276, 1980

Juhl RP, Kronfol Z, Tsuang MT: Lithium-induced nephrogenic diabetes insipidus. Am J Hosp Pharm 33:843–845, 1976

Juhl RP, Tsuang MT, Perry PJ: Concomitant administration of haloperidol and lithium in acute mania. Diseases of the Nervous System 38:675–680, 1977

Kallen B, Tandberg A: Lithium and pregnancy: a cohort study on manic-depressive women. Acta Psychiatr Scand 68:134–139, 1983

Karas BJ, Wilder BJ, Hammond EJ, et al: Valproate tremors. Neurology 32:428–432, 1982

Kasarskis EJ, Kuo CS, Berger R, et al: Carbamazepine-induced cardiac dysfunction: characterization of two distinct clinical syndromes. Arch Intern Med 152:186–191, 1992

Kates RE: Calcium antagonists: pharmacokinetic properties. Drugs 25:113–124, 1983

Keck PE, McElroy SL: Outcome in the pharmacologic treatment of bipolar disorder. J Clin Psychopharmacol 16 (suppl 1):15S–23S, 1996

Keck PE, McElroy SL, Tugrul KC, et al: Valproate oral loading in the treatment of acute mania. J Clin Psychiatry 54:305–308, 1993

Keck PE, McElroy SL, Strakowski SM: New developments in the pharmacologic management of schizoaffective disorder. J Clin Psychiatry 57 (suppl 9):41–48, 1996

Kemperman CJF, Gerdes JH, DeRooij J, et al: Reversible lithium neurotoxicity at normal serum level may refer to intracranial pathology (letter). J Neurol Neurosurg Psychiatry 52:679–680, 1989

Killian FM, Fromm GH: Carbamazepine in the treatment of neuralgia. Use and side effects. Arch Neurol 19:129–136, 1968

Kincaid-Smith P, Burrows GD, Davies BM, et al: Renal biopsy findings in lithium and pre-lithium patients. Lancet 2:700–701, 1979

Kirk L, Baastrup PC, Schou M: Propranolol treatment of lithium-induced tremor. Lancet 2:1086–1087, 1973

Kirksey A, Groziak SM: Maternal drug use: evaluation of risks to breast-fed infants. World Rev Nutr Diet 43:60–79, 1984

Kirkwood CK, Wilson SK, Hayes PE, et al: Single-dose bioavailability of two extended-release lithium carbonate products. Am J Hosp Pharm 51:486–489, 1994

Klein E, Bental E, Lerer B, et al: Carbamazepine and haloperidol vs. placebo and haloperidol in excited psychoses. Arch Gen Psychiatry 41:165–172, 1984

Klein DF, Gittelman R, Quitkin F, et al: Review of the literature on mood-stabilizing drugs, in Diagnosis and Drug Treatment of Psychiatric Disorders: Adults and Children. Baltimore, MD, Williams & Wilkins, 1980, pp 268–408

Kontaxakis V, Markianos M, Markidis M, et al: Clonidine in mixed bipolar disorder. Acta Psychiatr Scand 79:108–110, 1989

Kook KA, Stimmel GL, Wilkins JN, et al: Accuracy and safety of a priori lithium loading. J Clin Psychiatry 46:49–51, 1985

Kosten TR, Forrest JN: Treatment of severe lithium-induced polyuria with amiloride. Am J Psychiatry 143:1563–1568, 1986

Kudriakova TB, Sirota LA, Rozova GI, et al: Autoinduction and steady-state pharmacokinetics of carbamazepine and its major metabolite. Br J Clin Pharmacol 33:611–615, 1992

Lapensee MA: A review of schizoaffective disorder, II: somatic treatment. Can J Psychiatry 37:347–349, 1992

Lauritsen BJ, Mellerup ET, Plenge P, et al: Serum lithium concentrations around the clock with different treatment regimens and the diurnal variation of the renal lithium clearance. Acta Psychiatr Scand 64:314–319, 1981

Lazarus JH: Endocrine and metabolic effects of lithium. New York, Plenum, 99–124, 1986

Lenox RH, Modell JG, Weinder S: Acute treatment of manic agitation with lorazepam. Psychosomatics 27 (suppl):28–32, 1986

Lenox RH, Newhouse PA, Creelman WL, et al: Adjunctive treatment of manic agitation with lorazepam versus haloperidol: a double-blind study. J Clin Psychiatry 53:47–52, 1992

Lenzi A, Lazzerini F, Grossi E, et al: Use of carbamazepine in acute psychosis: a controlled study. J Int Med Res 14:78–84, 1986

Lerer B, Moore N, Meyendorf E, et al: Carbamazepine versus lithium in mania. J Clin Psychiatry 48:89–93, 1987

Levy ST, Forrest JN, Heninger GR: Lithium-induced diabetes insipidus: manic symptoms, brain and electrolyte correlates, and chlorothiazide treatment. Am J Psychiatry 130:1014–1018, 1973

Lewis GR: Long-term results with verapamil in essential hypertension and its influence on serum lipids. Am J Cardiol 57:35D–38D, 1986

Livingston S, Pauli L, Berman W: Carbamazepine in epilepsy: 9-year follow-up with special emphasis on untoward reactions. Diseases of the Nervous System 35:103–107, 1974

Lobeck F: A review of lithium dosing methods. Pharmacotherapy 8:248–255, 1988

Lusznat RM, Murphy DP, Numm MH: Carbamazepine versus lithium in mania: a double-blind study. Br J Psychiatry 153:198–204, 1988

Lyskowski J, Nasrallah HA: Slow-release lithium: a review and a comparative study. J Clin Psychopharmacol 1:406–408, 1981

Maarbjerg K, Vestergaard P, Schou M: Changes in serum thyroxine (T4) and serum thyroid stimulating hormone (TSH) during prolonged lithium treatment. Acta Psychiatr Scand 75:217–221, 1987

Madtbo KA, Hals O: Verapamil in the treatment of hypertension. Curr Ther Res Clin Exp 27:830–837, 1980

Madtbo KA, Hals O, Van der Meer J: Verapamil compared with nifedipine in the treatment of essential hypertension. J Cardiovasc Pharmacol 4 (suppl 3):S363–S368, 1982

Madtbo KA, Hals O, Lauve O: A new sustained-release formulation of verapamil in the treatment of hypertension. Journal of Clinical Hypertension 3 (suppl):125S–132S, 1986

Maj M, Pirozzi R, Magliano L: Nonresponse to reinstituted lithium prophylaxis in previously responsive bipolar patients: prevalence and predictors. Am J Psychiatry 152:1810–1811, 1995

Marken PA, McCrary KE, Lacombe S, et al: Preliminary comparison of predictive and empiric lithium dosing: impact on patient outcome. Ann Pharmacother 28:1148–1152, 1994

Mattson RH, Cramer JA, Collins JF, et al: A comparison of valproate with carbamazepine for the treatment of complex partial seizures and secondarily generalized tonic-clonic seizures in adults (Department of Veterans Affairs Epilepsy Cooperative Study No. 264 group). N Engl J Med 327:765–771, 1992

McElroy SL, Keck PE: Treatment guidelines for valproate in bipolar and schizoaffective disorders. Can J Psychiatry 38 (suppl 2):S62–S66, 1993

McEvoy GK, Litvak K, Welsh OH Jr, et al (eds): AHFS Drug Information. Bethesda, MD, American Hospital Formulary Service, 1993, pp 1457–1464

Mendels J, Ramsey TA, Dyson WL, et al: Lithium as an antidepressant. Arch Gen Psychiatry 36:845–846, 1979

Mirchandani IC, Young RC: Management of mania in the elderly: an update. Ann Clin Psychiatry 5:67–77, 1993

Mitchell JE, Mackenzie TB: Cardiac effects of lithium in man: a review. J Clin Psychiatry 43:47–51, 1982

Modell JG, Lenox RH, Weiner S: Inpatient clinical trial of lorazepam for the management of manic agitation. J Clin Psychopharmacol 5:109–113, 1985

Murphy DL, Slater S, de la Vega CE, et al: The serotonergic neurotransmitter system in the affective disorders—a preliminary evaluation of the antidepressant and antimanic effects of fenfluramine, in Neuropsychopharmacology. Edited by Deniker P. Oxford, UK, Pergamon, 1978, pp 675–682

Needham TE, Javid P, Brown W: Bioavailability and dissolution parameters of seven lithium carbonate products. J Pharm Sci 68:952–954, 1979

Neil JF, Himmelhoch JM, Licata SM: Emergence of myasthenia gravis during treatment with lithium carbonate. Arch Gen Psychiatry 33:1090–1092, 1976

Neppe VM, Tucker GJ, Wilensky AJ: Introduction: Fundamentals of carbamazepine use in neuropsychiatry. J Clin Psychiatry 49 (suppl 4):4–6, 1988

Okuma T, Yamashita I, Takahashi R, et al: Comparison of the antimanic efficacy of carbamazepine and lithium carbonate by double-blind controlled study. Pharmacopsychiatry 23:143–150, 1990

Pabis DJ, Stanislav SW: Pharmacotherapy of aggressive behavior. Ann Pharmacother 30:278–287, 1996

Patsalos PN, Stephenson TJ, Krishna S, et al: Side effects induced by carbamazepine-10,11-epoxide (letter). Lancet 2:1432, 1985

Patterson JF: Treatment of acute mania with verapamil. J Clin Psychopharmacol 7:206–207, 1987

Pearce JB: Fenfluramine in mania (letter). Lancet 1:427, 1973

Penry JK, Dean JC: The scope and use of valproate in epilepsy. J Clin Psychiatry 50 (suppl):17–22, 1989

Perry PJ, Alexander B, Dunner FJ, et al: Pharmacokinetic protocol for predicting serum lithium levels. J Clin Psychopharmacol 2:114–118, 1982

Perry PJ, Alexander B, Prince RA, et al: A single point dosing protocol for predicting steady state lithium levels. Br J Psychiatry 148:401–405, 1986

Perry PJ, Alexander B: Dosage and serum levels, in Modern Lithium Therapy. Edited by Johnson FN. Lancaster, UK, MTP Press, 1987, pp 67–73

Placidi GF, Lenzi A, Lazzerini F, et al: The comparative efficacy and safety of carbamazepine versus lithium: a randomized, double-blind 3-year trial in 83 patients. J Clin Psychiatry 47:490–494, 1986

Plenge P, Mellerup ET: WHO cross cultural study on lithium every second day. Clin Neuropharmacol 15 (suppl 1):487A–488A, 1992

Post RM, Berrettini W, Uhde TW, et al: Selective response to the anticonvulsant carbamazepine in manic-depressive illness: a case study. J Clin Psychopharmacol 4:178–185, 1984

Post RM, Uhde TW, Ballenger JC, et al: Carbamazepine and its -10, 11 epoxide metabolite in plasma in CSF: relationship to antidepressant response. Arch Gen Psychiatry 40:673–676, 1983

Post RM: Time course of clinical effects of carbamazepine: implications for mechanisms of action. J Clin Psychiatry 49 (suppl 4):35–46, 1988

Post RM, Leverich GS, Rosoff AS, et al: Carbamazepine prophylaxis in refractory affective disorders: a focus on long-term follow-up. J Clin Psychopharmacol 10:318–27, 1990

Post RM, Weiss SRB, De-Maw C: Mechanism of actions of anticonvulsants in affective disorders: comparisons with lithium. J Clin Psychopharmacol 12 (suppl):23S–35S, 1992

Prakash R: A review of the hematologic side effects of lithium. Hospital and Community Psychiatry 36:127–128, 1985

Preskorn SH, Burke MJ, Fast GA: Therapeutic drug monitoring. Psychiatr Clin North Am 16:611–645, 1993

Price LH, Heninger GR: Lithium in the treatment of mood disorders. N Engl J Med 331:591–598, 1994

Prien RF, Caffey EM, Klett CJ: Lithium carbonate: a survey of the history and current status of lithium in treating mood disorders. Diseases of the Nervous System 32:521–531, 1971

Prien RF, Caffey EM, Klett CJ: Relationship between serum lithium level and clinical response in acute mania treated with lithium. Br J Psychiatry 120:409–414, 1972

Pugh CB, Garnett WR: Current issues in the treatment of epilepsy. Clinical Pharmacy 10:335–358, 1991

Pynnonen S: Pharmacokinetics of carbamazepine in man: a review. Ther Drug Monit 1:409–431, 1979

Ramsey TA, Mendels J, Stokes JW, et al: Lithium carbonate and kidney function: a failure in renal concentrating ability. JAMA 219:1446–1449, 1982

Sachs GS: Use of clonazepam for bipolar affective disorders. J Clin Psychiatry 51 (suppl 5):31–34, 1990

Sachs GS: Bipolar mood disorders: Practical strategies for acute and maintenance phase treatment. J Clin Psychopharmacol 16 (suppl 1):32S–47S, 1996

Salata R, Klein I: Effects of lithium on the endocrine system: a review. J Lab Clin Med 110:130–136, 1987

Sansone MEG, Ziegler DK: Lithium toxicity: a review of neurologic complications. Clin Neuropharmacol 8:242–248, 1985

Schaff MR, Fawcett J, Zajecka JM: Divalproex sodium in the treatment of refractory affective disorders. J Clin Psychiatry 54:380–384, 1993

Schou M, Amdisen A: Lithium and pregnancy, III: lithium ingestion by children breast-fed by women on lithium treatment (abstract). BMJ 2:138, 1973

Schou M, Baastrup PC, Grof P, et al: Pharmacological and clinical problems of lithium prophylaxis. Br J Psychiatry 116:615–619, 1970

Scolnik D, Nulman I, Rovet J, et al: Neurodevelopment of children exposed in utero to phenytoin and carbamazepine monotherapy. JAMA 271:767–770, 1994

Sherard ES, Steiman GS, Couri D: Treatment of childhood epilepsy with valproic acid: results of the 100 patients in a 6-month trial. Neurology 31:31–35, 1980

Shopsin B, Johnson G, Gershon S: Neurotoxicity with lithium: differential drug responsiveness. International Pharmacopsychiatry 5:170–182, 1970

Shulka S, Godwin CD, Long LE, et al: Lithium-carbamazepine neurotoxicity and risk factors. Am J Psychiatry 141:1604–1606, 1984

Silverstein FS, Boxer L, Johnston MF: Hematological monitoring during therapy with carbamazepine in children. Ann Neurol 13:685–686, 1983

Simhandl C, Denk E, Thau K: The comparative efficacy of carbamazepine low and high serum level and lithium carbonate in the prophylaxis of affective disorder. J Affect Disord 28:221–231, 1993

Small JC, Klapper MH, Milstein V, et al: Carbamazepine compared with lithium in the treatment of mania. Arch Gen Psychiatry 48:915–921, 1991

Sobotka JL, Alexander B, Cook BL: A review of carbamazepine's hematologic reactions and monitoring recommendations. DICP Ann Pharmacother 24:1214–1219, 1990

Soffer EE, Taylor RJ, Bertram PD, et al: Carbamazepine-induced liver injury. South Med J 76:681–683, 1983

Solomon DA, Bauer MS: Continuation and maintenance pharmacotherapy for unipolar and bipolar mood disorders. Psychiatr Clin North Am 16:515–540, 1993

Souza FGM, Goodwin GM: Lithium treatment and prophylaxis in unipolar depression: a meta-analysis. Br J Psychiatry 158:666–675, 1991

Speders S, Sosma H, Schumacher A, et al: Efficacy and safety of verapamil SR 240 mg in essential hypertension: results of multicentric phase IV study. J Cardiovasc Pharmacol 13 (suppl 4):547–549, 1989

Stancer HC, Persad E: Treatment of intractable rapid-cycling manic-depressive disorder with levothyroxine. Arch Gen Psychiatry 39:311–312, 1982

Stern R, Khalsa JH: Cutaneous adverse reactions associated with calcium channel blockers. Arch Intern Med 149:829–832, 1989

Stromgren LS, Boller S: Carbamazepine in treatment and prophylaxis of manic-depressive disorder. Psychiatric Developments 4:349–367, 1985

Stuppaeck C, Barnas C, Miller C, et al: Carbamazepine in the prophylaxis of mood disorders. J Clin Psychopharmacol 10:39–42, 1990

Suppes T, Baldessarini RJ, Faedda G, et al: Discontinuing maintenance treatment in bipolar manic-depression: risks and implications. Harvard Review of Psychiatry 1:131–144, 1993

Thornhill DP, Field SP: Distribution of lithium elimination rates in a selected population of psychiatric patients. Eur J Clin Pharmacol 21:351–354, 1982

Tucker GJ, Detre T, Harrow M, et al: Behavior and symptoms of psychiatric patients and the EEG. Arch Gen Psychiatry 12:278–286, 1965

Tunnessen WW, Hertz CG: Toxic effects of lithium in newborn infants: a commentary. J Pediatr 81:804–807, 1972

Uhde TW, Post RM: Effect of carbamazepine on serum electrolytes: clinical and theoretical implications. J Clin Psychopharmacol 3:103–106, 1983

Vacaflor L: Lithium side effects and toxicity: the clinical picture, in Lithium Research and Therapy. Edited by Johnson FN. London, Academic Press, 1975, pp 211–225

Vestergaard P: Treatment and prevention of mania: a Scandinavian perspective. Neuropsychopharmacology 7:249–259, 1992

Vestergaard P, Amdisen A, Schou M: Clinically significant side effects of lithium treatment: a survey of 237 patients in long-term treatment. Acta Psychiatr Scand 62:193–200, 1980

Volf N, Crismon ML: Leukemia in bipolar mood disorders: is lithium contraindicated? DICP Ann Pharmacother 25:948–951, 1991

Volzke E, Doose H: Dipropylacetate in the treatment of epilepsy. Epilepsia 14:185–193, 1973

Weinstein MR, Goldfield M: Cardiovascular malformations with lithium use during pregnancy. Am J Psychiatry 132:529–531, 1975

Weinstein MR: Lithium treatment of women during pregnancy and in the post delivery period, in Handbook of Lithium Therapy. Edited by Johnson FN. Lancaster, UK, MTP Press, 1980, pp 421–430

Wilder BJ: Pharmacokinetics of valproate and carbamazepine. J Clin Psychopharmacol 12:64S–68S, 1992

Winokur G: Unipolar depression, in The Medical Basis of Psychiatry, 2nd Edition. Edited by Winokur G, Clayton PJ. Philadelphia, PA, WB Saunders, 1994, pp 69–86

Wyllie E, Wyllie R, Cruse RP, et al: Pancreatitis associated with valproate therapy. American Journal of Diseases of Children 138:912–914, 1984

Zubenko GS, Cohen BM, Lipinski JF: Comparison of metoprolol and propranolol in the treatment of lithium tremor (letter). Psychiatry Res 11:163–164, 1984a

Zubenko GS, Cohen BM, Lipinski JF, et al: Clonidine in the treatment of mania and mixed bipolar disorder. Am J Psychiatry 141:1617–1618, 1984b

4

Antianxiety Agents (Anxiolytics)

Benzodiazepines

All benzodiazepines (BZDs) are Drug Enforcement Administration (DEA) Schedule IV (C-IV) controlled substances. This categorization indicates that these agents have limited dependence liability and less abuse potential than other addictive drugs (e.g., opiates, barbiturates, lysergic acid diethylamide [LSD], marijuana, amphetamines, cocaine). BZD prescriptions may not be dispensed or refilled more than 6 months after the date issued or be refilled more than five times. (See Table 5–2 [page 365] for an explanation of the DEA classification system.)

■ Indications

Pharmacological studies have shown varying degrees of muscle relaxant, sedative, anxiolytic, anticonvulsant, and hypnotic properties for most of the BZDs. The following BZDs have *anxiety* as an approved indication: alprazolam (Xanax®), chlordiazepoxide (Librium®, other names), clorazepate (Tranxene®, other names), diazepam (Valium®, other names), halazepam (Paxipam®), lorazepam (Ativan®, other names), oxazepam (Serax®, other names), and prazepam (Centrax®). Five BZDs are approved for the management of *insomnia:* estazolam (ProSom®), flurazepam (Dalmane®, other names), quazepam (Doral®), temazepam (Restoril®, other names), and triazolam (Halcion®). There is evidence that a given BZD can serve as either a hypnotic or an anxiolytic, depending on whether the dosage is adjusted upward or downward, respectively (Dubovsky 1990). Only those BZDs marketed specifically as antianxiety agents are discussed in this chapter. BZDs marketed specifically as hypnotics are discussed in Chapter 5.

Diazepam and clonazepam (Klonopin®) are approved for treatment of *convulsive disorders,* and diazepam is also approved for adjunctive treatment of *muscle spasm.* Midazolam (Versed®) is approved for use as a *preoperative sedative* and as an agent for *induction of general anesthesia.* The BZD antagonist flumazenil (Romazicon®) reverses the sedative effects of BZDs used in general anesthesia and is used in the management of BZD overdoses.

■ **Efficacy**

Generalized Anxiety Disorder
Epidemiological data indicate that the lifetime prevalence in the United States of DSM-III-R (American Psychiatric Association 1987) generalized anxiety disorder (GAD) is 5.1% (Kessler et al. 1994). In the DSM-III (American Psychiatric Association 1980) classification system, *anxiety neurosis* was divided into panic disorder and GAD (Noyes 1988). The essential characteristics of this condition as it is now defined are persistent, excessive worry accompanied by symptoms suggestive of central nervous system (CNS) arousal (e.g., a "keyed up" feeling, irritability, muscle tension, insomnia, restlessness, sweating).

A 1978 review critiqued the research methodology of 78 double-blind anxiolytic drug studies that had been conducted between 1961 and 1977 (Solomon and Hart 1978). The authors assessed the studies' adequacy with regard to subject selection, study design, assessment of clinical response, data analysis, inclusion/exclusion parameters, and diagnostic criteria. Generally, there was a lack of uniformity in patient populations, making it difficult to determine whether predominant symptoms were anxiety, depression, or phobias. Additionally, anxiety neurosis was so poorly defined that it was difficult to compare the results of more recent drug efficacy studies that used Research Diagnostic Criteria (RDC; Spitzer et al. 1978) or DSM-III or DSM-III-R criteria.

A 1990 review of 17 recent controlled studies noted numerous problems that made it difficult to draw overall conclusions (Perry et al. 1990). Fifty-six percent of the reviewed studies found BZDs much better and 33% slightly better than placebo for the treatment of anxiety. However, 18% found no difference between the two, and 1% (one study) found placebo better than diazepam. About 35% of GAD patients treated with BZD experience marked improvement, 40% are moderately improved but still symptomatic, and 25% are unresponsive (Dubovsky 1990). There is some evidence that BZDs have greater benefit when used to treat patients with moderate to high levels of anxiety (Shapiro et al. 1983) and in anxious patients with concomitant dysphoric mood (Zung 1987).

It is estimated that half of GAD patients seen in primary care experience a return of symptoms after the discontinuation of diazepam treatment lasting 6, 14, or 22 weeks (Rickels et al. 1983). Thus, the BZDs may be tapered and discontinued after an initial 2-month treatment course (Dubovsky 1990). However, because the symptoms of GAD wax and wane in many individuals, chronic long-term treatment may be necessary in some patients. Despite this clinical practice, BZDs and other anxiolytics require further investigation before long-term efficacy can be precisely defined (Murphy et al. 1989; Rickels et al. 1988).

Although most reviews indicate no significant difference in efficacy (Dubovsky 1990) of one BZD compared with another, some authors challenge this conclusion (Baskin and Esdale 1982; Greenblatt et al. 1983a, 1983b). It is important to remember that individual response (determined through trial and error) as well as economic and pharmacokinetic factors should be considered in choosing a BZD.

Panic Disorder/Agoraphobia

Recent epidemiological data indicate that the lifetime prevalence in the United States of DSM-III-R panic disorder is 3.5% and that the prevalence of DSM-III-R agoraphobia without panic disorder is 5.3% (Kessler et al. 1994). Early experience with BZDs suggested that they were only partially effective for the treatment of panic disorder (Ballenger 1986). However, controlled trials have concluded that alprazolam, clonazepam, clorazepate, diazepam, and lorazepam are effective as antipanic and antiphobic agents when taken regularly and in sufficient doses (Andersch et al. 1991; Ballenger et al. 1988; Chouinard et al. 1982; Cross-National Collaborative Panic Study 1992; Dunner et al. 1986; Noyes et al. 1984; Rizley et al. 1986; Sheehan et al. 1984, 1993; Swinson et al. 1987; Tesar et al. 1987; Uhlenhuth et al. 1989). BZDs proved effective on all of the assessment scales used in these various studies and were also ranked high in subjective evaluations. Symptoms responding to them included anxiety, the frequency and severity of panic attacks, and phobic fear and avoidance. With alprazolam, the number of panic attacks per week decreased by an average of 81%, and attacks were often eliminated completely. As many patients experienced moderate to marked improvement with BZDs as with any other class of drugs. Decreases in anticipatory anxiety and disability in work, family life, and social life were observed. Somatic complaints, including cardiovascular, respiratory, gastrointestinal, and muscular, also responded well (Sheehan and Raj 1990). Other factors supporting the effectiveness of BZDs included greater medication compliance with this treatment group, fewer dropouts due to ineffectiveness, a smaller proportion of nonresponders, and the return of symptoms when doses are tapered (Sheehan and Raj 1990).

In comparisons of BZDs and other classes of drugs used for the treatment of panic disorder, buspirone has been found less effective than the BZDs and no more effective than placebo. Propranolol is somewhat more efficacious than placebo but causes the undesirable adverse drug reactions (ADRs) of hypotension, bradycardia, and sedation. Tricyclic antidepressants (TCAs), notably imipramine, are effective but have several disadvantages, including slower onset and more ADRs. Monoamine oxidase inhibitors (MAOIs), despite being effective, have cardiac ADRs, and drug and food interactions make them less than ideal. Selective serotonin reuptake inhibitors (SSRIs) are also effective but in about one-third of patients require a slower dose titration schedule to avoid the CNS ADRs of jitteriness and insomnia (Louie et al. 1993). As is true for these other agents, the BZDs' ADRs limit their usefulness. The addiction potential of the BZDs is usually a problem only in substance abuse patients. Additionally, the most common ADR, daytime sedation, can be a persistent problem in patients whose dosages cannot be decreased.

Response to BZDs may be noted within the first week of treatment. Uncontrolled reports of long-term treatment with clonazepam (1 year) and alprazolam (2½ years) indicate that the drugs maintained their efficacy and were well tolerated (Pollack 1990). Studies of the relative efficacy of BZDs and antidepressants in panic disorder have found no difference between the two classes (Cross-National Collaborative Panic Study 1992; Dunner et al. 1986; Rizley et al. 1986; Uhlenhuth et al. 1989).

Social Phobias

Epidemiological data indicate that the lifetime prevalence in the United States of DSM-III-R social phobia is 13.3% (Kessler et al. 1994). BZDs are reported to be of value in the treatment of social phobia (Jefferson 1995). Two pilot studies found alprazolam dosages up to 10 mg/day (mean 2.9 mg/day) (Reich and Yates 1988) and clonazepam dosages of 1–6 mg/day (mean 2.8 mg/day) (Munjack et al. 1990) beneficial in the treatment of social phobia. In a placebo-controlled trial (Davidson et al. 1993), clonazepam 0.5–3.0 mg/day (mean 2.4 mg/day) demonstrated significant improvement in symptoms of social phobia within 1 week, according to some measures.

Specific (Simple) Phobias

Epidemiological data indicate that the lifetime prevalence in the United States of DSM-III-R simple phobia is 11.3% (Kessler et al.

1994). However, BZDs in the treatment of simple phobia have not been extensively researched (Noyes et al. 1986). BZDs should be used with caution in combination with exposure-based psychotherapy, because BZD blood levels are negatively correlated with extinction rates (Hafner and Marks 1976).

Obsessive-Compulsive Disorder

Epidemiological data indicate that the lifetime prevalence in the United States of DSM-IV (American Psychiatric Association 1994) obsessive-compulsive disorder (OCD) is 2.5%. A 6-week study suggested that the BZD clonazepam may be a useful adjunct in the treatment of OCD (Hewlett et al. 1992). Clonazepam 2–10 mg/day (mean 7 mg/day) was as effective as clomipramine in reducing OCD symptoms. However, only a 25% and a 19% decrease in the Yale-Brown Obsessive-Compulsive Scale (Y-BOCS; Goodman et al. 1989b) for clomipramine and clonazepam, respectively, were observed. More typically, longer efficacy studies demonstrate mean decreases in the Y-BOCS of 40% or more (Pigott et al. 1990). Thus, the effectiveness of BZDs in OCD requires replication before they can be regarded as an alternative treatment in OCD.

Posttraumatic Stress Disorder

The lifetime prevalence in the United States of DSM-IV posttraumatic stress disorder (PTSD) ranges from 1% to 14%. Studies of the population at risk (e.g., combat veterans, victims of volcanic eruption or criminal violence) yield a prevalence rate of 3%–58% (American Psychiatric Association 1994). A placebo-controlled trial of alprazolam 2.5–6 mg/day for 5 weeks demonstrated only minimal benefit in the treatment of PTSD (Braun et al. 1990). Controlled trials suggest that whereas SSRIs are effective in the treatment of PTSD, psychotropic drugs without prominent serotonin-agonist effects, such as the BZDs (γ-aminobutyric acid [GABA] agonists), are not. BZDs may be used as pharmacotherapeutic adjuncts to TCA or SSRI treatment if the latter agents do not control a patient's free-floating anxiety.

Miscellaneous Uses

Psychiatric disorders in which BZDs have been shown to be no more effective than placebo include antisocial personality disorder and the paraphilias. Efficacy has been claimed but not established for the following: allergic disorders, spastic colon, peripheral arterial occlusive disease, asthma, peptic ulcer, acid stomach, spasticity from trauma, and degenerative disease.

■ Mechanism of Action

The limbic system has been postulated as the neurophysiological and anatomical center of emotion. BZDs are thought to affect the limbic system by attenuating the emotional response expressed as anxiety. Several mechanisms have been proposed. Primarily, BZDs directly occupy the BZD receptor, thereby causing increased chloride channel permeability which, in turn, extends and prolongs the inhibitory actions of GABA neurons. Secondarily, BZDs may block the stress-induced increases in central norepinephrine, serotonin, dopamine, and other transmitters whose neurons have GABA receptors (Suranyi-Cadotte et al. 1990).

■ Dosage

Recommended dosage ranges and relative oral potencies for currently available BZDs are provided in the Product List (page 340).

There are two approaches for determining the dose schedule for the BZDs. The first is based on BZD half-life, and the second is based on the lipid solubility of the individual agents. The *half-life theory* suggests that because the long-acting BZDs (e.g., chlordiazepoxide, clorazepate, diazepam, halazepam, and prazepam) have plasma half-lives (including active metabolites) that exceed 24 hours, the entire daily dose can be given at bedtime, when the medication's anxiolytic and hypnotic properties may prove useful. The dosing approach for this theory assumes that BZD anxiolytic action is continuous throughout the day. However, this is not necessarily the case, given that diazepam usually needs to be taken three to four times per day to be effective.

The *lipophilicity theory* hypothesizes that diazepam, a very lipid-soluble BZD, has a shorter clinical duration of action than do the less lipid-soluble BZDs (e.g., clonazepam and oxazepam), because the latter are less extensively distributed into the peripheral compartments, regardless of their half-lives. Alprazolam, chlordiazepoxide, halazepam, and lorazepam have an intermediate degree of lipid solubility. Thus, among the BZDs used to treat panic disorder, the following order of lipophilicity is observed: diazepam > alprazolam, chlordiazepoxide, halazepam, and lorazepam > clonazepam and oxazepam.

The lipophilicity approach seems more rational than the half-life method, because clinicians conclude that whereas clonazepam has a duration of action of 6–8 hours, alprazolam's is 4–6 hours and diazepam's is even shorter. Thus, if a patient taking clonazepam on a q8h schedule becomes symptomatic within 2 to 3 hours after the drug is administered, the dose is probably too low and should be increased. However, if the patient becomes symptomatic 7 hours after the dose is administered, the dose is being scheduled too infrequently. On the basis of lipid solubility, the use of sustained-release diazepam (Valrelease™) is rational (Sheehan and Raj 1990).

Duration of therapy for the initial treatment of panic disorder is recommended by clinicians to be 6–12 months. BZDs can be used alone or as transient adjunctive medication for the treatment of panic disorder. Patients are first treated with a combination of a BZD and an antidepressant to take advantage of the more rapid onset of action of the BZD. However, once the antidepressant has taken effect (after approximately 2 weeks of combined treatment), the BZD is discontinued. The recommended duration of therapy for the initial treatment of GAD is 6–22 weeks. However, because approximately half of GAD patients relapse on discontinuation of the medication, many patients may require considerably longer treatment. The dose and administration schedule is dependent on patient age, presence of liver disease, and the pharmacokinetic profile of the BZD.

Doses should be titrated based on a balance of therapeutic effect and ADRs. The dose and administration schedule for a BZD used in the management of anxiety depends on 1) the patient's clinical presentation (chronic and persistent anxiety, anxiety limited to episodes lasting days to weeks with full recovery between anticipated episodes, or transient anxiety associated with a particular stimulus), 2) the age and sex of the patient, 3) whether the patient has concurrent liver disease, 4) whether the patient smokes, and/or 5) the pharmacokinetic profile of the BZD (Hollister 1986). The interaction of these factors and drug selection are discussed in the "Pharmacokinetics" subsection below.

Interdose anxiety complaints in panic disorder patients is a problem associated with alprazolam use. Patients complain that they feel jittery an hour or so before their next scheduled dose. This is a potential problem with any of the shorter-acting (i.e., highly lipid soluble) BZDs such as diazepam, alprazolam, and lorazepam. It can be alleviated by substituting 1 mg of clonazepam for every 2 mg of alprazolam that the patient is taking. In one study, 82% of patients preferred clonazepam to alprazolam because of decreased interdose anxiety and fewer doses being required per day (e.g., twice-daily dosing versus four-times-daily dosing) (Herman et al. 1987).

Generalized Anxiety Disorder

In 17 controlled trials that evaluated BZD efficacy in the treatment of GAD, the mean or median doses of the BZDs reported were alprazolam (2 mg/day), chlordiazepoxide (55 mg/day), clorazepate (22 mg/day), diazepam (14 mg/day), lorazepam (10 mg/day), and prazepam (28 mg/day) (Perry et al. 1990). Because these doses tend to represent an effort to achieve maximal benefit in a short period of time, they may be somewhat higher than those used in clinical practice.

Panic Disorder

Based on 59 trials of BZDs in the treatment of panic disorder, the mean or median doses of the BZDs reported were alprazolam (6 mg/day), chlordiazepoxide (55 mg/day), clorazepate (29 mg/day), diazepam (30 mg/day), lorazepam (4 mg/day), and clonazepam (3 mg/day) (Sheehan and Raj 1990). As with the GAD study doses, these doses reflect an attempt to achieve maximum benefit in the short run and thus may be higher than those used in clinical practice.

Data suggest that patients receiving treatment continue to improve for up to 6 months. Newly diagnosed patients who respond to BZDs should be treated for at least 1 year before a trial discontinuation is considered to determine continuing pharmacological need (Noyes et al. 1984).

■ Pharmacokinetics

BZDs differ in their lipid and water solubility, protein binding, volume of distribution (V_d), elimination half-life ($t_{1/2}$), absorption rate, and pattern of metabolic transformation.

Absorption

After oral administration, chlordiazepoxide, diazepam, lorazepam, halazepam, and alprazolam are rapidly and completely absorbed, with peak serum levels occurring at about 1–2 hours (Baskin and Esdale 1982). Clorazepate, itself inactive, is rapidly converted to the active metabolite desmethyldiazepam, which reaches peak levels in 1–2 hours. Absorption of oxazepam may require up to 8 hours in some patients, although the average peak is 2.7 hours (Shader and Greenblatt 1981). Prazepam is slowly absorbed, as peak levels of its major metabolite desmethyldiazepam are reached 6 hours after administration of prazepam (Baskin and Esdale 1982). Serum levels of sustained-release diazepam peak at about 3 hours after a dose (Valium® Product Information 1984).

Distribution

All BZDs are highly protein bound (Baskin and Esdale 1982; Greenblatt et al. 1983a). The differences in available BZD lipid and water solubility are used to explain the duration of action after a single dose of the drug. Also, changes in distribution of the drugs as a result of aging and/or liver disease may increase or decrease the drug's therapeutic effects or ADRs, depending on the direction of the change (see Table 4–1).

Metabolism and Elimination

BZDs exhibit first-order (linear) kinetics over the therapeutic dosage range.

BZDs fall into one of two classes, depending on their biotransformation pathways (Table 4–2). One group includes those that are transformed primarily by oxidative pathways (*N*-dealkylation, *N*-demethylation, or aliphatic hydroxylation) to active metabolites and then synthesized to inactive metabolites. The other group consists of BZDs that are metabolized only by conjugation to water-soluble glucuronides that are pharmacologically inactive (e.g., lorazepam and oxazepam). Table 4–2 presents the half-life profiles of the BZDs.

Relationship of Plasma BZD Levels to Therapeutic Response

The relationship between antianxiety effects and serum levels of diazepam, desmethyldiazepam, chlordiazepoxide, and desmethyl-chlordiazepoxide have been investigated in only a few studies (Baskin and Esdale 1982; Bowden and Fisher 1982). These studies reported either no relationship or a slightly positive relationship between BZD serum levels and clinical effects. However, the Cross-National Collaborative Panic Study found that alprazolam plasma concentrations between 20 and 40 ng/mL produced significantly greater decreases in panic attacks than lower concentrations as well as optimum improvement of symptoms of anxiety and dysphoria symptoms (Greenblatt et al. 1993). Finally, sustained-release diazepam (Valrelease™) does not produce serum levels of diazepam significantly different from those produced by regular-release diazepam (Valium® Product Information 1984).

■ Clinical Comparisons

Oral Administration—Single-Dose Kinetics

The duration of action of a single dose of a BZD is determined largely by the drug's V_d and absorption rate rather than by its elimination $t_{1/2}$ (Greenblatt et al. 1983a). BZDs with fast gastroin-

Table 4–1. Cirrhosis and age effects on benzodiazepine pharmacokinetics

Drug	Volume of distribution		Elimination half-life		Plasma clearance	
	Cirrhosis	Age	Cirrhosis	Age	Cirrhosis	Age
Alprazolam	NI	↓	NI	↑	NI	↓
Chlordiazepoxide	↑	↑	↑	↑	↓	↓
Clorazepate (as DD)	NI	↑	NI	↑M	NI	↓M
Diazepam	↑	↑	↑	↑	↓	↔
Lorazepam	↔	↓	↑	↔ or ↑	↔	↓
Oxazepam	↔	↔	↑	↔	↔	↔
Prazepam (as DD)	NI	↑	NI	↑M ↔F	NI	↓M ↔F

Note. DD = desmethyldiazepam; F = female; M = male; ↓ = decrease; ↑ = increase; ↔ = no difference; NI = no information.

Table 4–2.   Benzodiazepine half-lives

Parent drug	Fate	Half-life range (hours)	Time to steady state (days)
Alprazolam[a, b]		6–20	1–4
	α-hydroxyalprazolam benzophone (minor)		
Chlordiazepoxide[c]		7–14	1.5–3
	desmethychloridiazepoxide	8–24	1.5–5
	demoxepam	14–95	3–20
	desmethyldiazepam	30–60	6–13
	oxazepam (minor)		
Clorazepate[c]			
	desmethyldiazepam	30–60	6–13
	oxazepam (minor)		
Diazepam[c]		14–90	3–19
	desmethyldiazepam	30–60	6–13
	temazepam	4–37	1–8
	oxazepam (minor)		
Halazepam[d, e]		14	3
	desmethyldiazepam	30–60	6–13
	3–hydroxyhalazepam (minor)		
Lorazepam[f, g]		10–20	2–4
	inactive glucuronide metabolite		
Oxazepam[g, h]		6–24	1–5
	inactive glucuronide metabolite		
Prazepam[g]	100% biotransformed on first pass through liver		
	desmethyldiazepam	30–60	6–13
	oxazepam (minor)		

Note.   [a] Gall et al. 1978; [b] Greenblatt et al. 1981; [c] Greenblatt and Shader 1974; [d] Baskin and Esdale 1982; [e] Garzone and Kroboth 1989; [f] Breimer 1979; [g] Greenblatt and Shader 1978; [h] Scharf et al. 1988.

testinal (GI) absorption rates (i.e., clorazepate and diazepam) produce a rapid and profound onset of activity after a single dose.
Diazepam is a very lipid-soluble drug and is rapidly and extensively
taken up by fatty tissue. Although its $t_{1/2}$ is quite long, the duration
of action of a single dose is very short because of diazepam's large

V_d. Furthermore, it has been noted that a drug with a short $t_{1/2}$, such as lorazepam, may have longer lasting clinical effects after a single dose than might be expected based on its $t_{1/2}$. This is because lorazepam's tissue distribution is considerably less rapid and extensive than is diazepam's (Greenblatt 1980). As an example, in 10 healthy volunteers, a single dose of lorazepam 2.5 mg po produced significant impairment of psychomotor skills and visual functions related to driving for 24 hours, whereas the impairment in performance after diazepam 10 mg lasted only 5–7 hours. The slow disappearance of lorazepam from the serum (still 50% of peak value at 12 hours) coincided with its longer duration of action (Seppala et al. 1976).

Oral Administration—Multiple-Dose Kinetics
The major distinction to be made for multiple-dose BZD treatment is between drugs with active metabolites and long $t_{1/2}$s and those with no active metabolites and short $t_{1/2}$s. BZDs with active metabolites will accumulate in the body and not reach steady state until days or weeks of continuous dosing have elapsed. However, because of initial tolerance, this accumulation usually has little therapeutic consequence. Notwithstanding, insomnia—a worsening of sleep compared with baseline—has been reported after withdrawal of short-acting BZDs (e.g., triazolam, nitrazepam, flunitrazepam) that were given in nightly doses for short periods (Kales et al. 1979). Diazepam and flurazepam, which have a longer $t_{1/2}$, did not cause rebound insomnia on discontinuation. The rebound insomnia was attributed to the short and intermediate $t_{1/2}$s of certain BZDs.

The onset, severity, and duration of withdrawal signs and symptoms after abrupt discontinuation of BZDs is believed to be related to how rapidly a BZD is eliminated from the body (Browne and Hauge 1986; Busto et al. 1986; Hollister 1980; Perry and Alexander 1986). (See section on anxiolytic-hypnotic withdrawal [page 569] in Chapter 10.)

Intramuscular Administration—Single Dose
Absorption of chlordiazepoxide or diazepam from a gluteal intramuscular injection site is slow and possibly incomplete, presumably leading to unpredictable and unsatisfactory clinical effects. However, the absorption of diazepam and lorazepam from a deltoid intramuscular injection site is rapid and nearly complete. Thus, with nearly 100% bioavailability, intramuscular and intravenous doses are equivalent to oral doses. Lorazepam causes injection-site pain to the same extent as do chlordiazepoxide and diazepam (Greenblatt and Shader 1978).

Intravenous Administration—Single Dose

After an intravenous bolus injection of diazepam, serum concentrations decline very rapidly over a period of several minutes to several hours, owing to rapid and extensive drug distribution. This reduction is generally accompanied by rapid diminution or termination of the desired sedative, anticonvulsant, or amnestic effects. With lorazepam, drug distribution is less rapid and extensive, thereby prolonging the clinical effects. If BZDs are injected too rapidly intravenously, hypotension and/or respiratory depression may occur. Thus, in adults, diazepam should be injected no faster than 5 mg/minute and lorazepam no faster than 2 mg/minute. Anterograde amnesia lasting as long as several hours is consistently reported to follow injection of lorazepam 4 mg, whereas amnesia after diazepam 10 or 20 mg may last only 30 minutes (George and Dundee 1977).

Effects of Liver Disease on Pharmacokinetics

Reduction of plasma clearance and an increase in V_d have been reported with both *diazepam* and *chlordiazepoxide* in patients with liver disease (Baskin and Esdale 1982). Although plasma clearance and V_d appear to be minimally affected by liver disease, $t_{1/2}$ in some patients with alcohol-induced cirrhosis has been reported to increase by 50% and 27% with *lorazepam* and *oxazepam,* respectively (Baskin and Esdale 1982). Acute viral hepatitis has been shown not to affect the pharmacokinetics of lorazepam and oxazepam (Wilkinson 1978) (see Table 4–1). Although drug metabolism declines in patients with liver disease, drugs that are transformed by oxidation and conjugation are affected to a greater extent than those that are only conjugated. Thus, lorazepam is the BZD of choice in patients with liver disease, at dosages one-half those usually prescribed. It is important to remember that because the margin of safety of all BZDs is large, the choice of which particular BZD to use is not as important as are gradual dose titration and close monitoring (Greenblatt 1980).

Effects of Age and Sex on Pharmacokinetics

BZDs can produce greater CNS effects in elderly than in younger patients. This is due partly to increased target-organ sensitivity to BZDs and partly to changes in drug disposition in the elderly (Reidenberg et al. 1978). The effects of aging on a BZD's distribution and elimination kinetics depends on the specific compound. However, as can be discerned from Table 4–1, lorazepam would be the preferred BZD in elderly patients with anxiety disorder diagnoses.

Alprazolam's clearance decreases with age in both sexes. In one study, $t_{1/2}$ increased significantly with age in men but not in women, whereas V_d decreased equally in men and women with increasing age (Moschitto et al. 1981).

Chlordiazepoxide also has a prolonged $t_{1/2}$ in the elderly; it can increase from 7 hours at 20 years to 40 hours at 80 years (Roberts et al. 1978). The mechanism of this prolongation is due both to a reduced hepatic clearance (chlordiazepoxide is cleared by hydroxylation) and to an increased V_d similar to that observed with diazepam (Shader et al. 1977).

Clorazepate and *prazepam* are both *prodrugs* in that they are entirely converted to their common active metabolite, desmethyldiazepam (Allen et al. 1980; Shader et al. 1981). Intrinsic clearance of desmethyldiazepam by the liver depended more on sex than on age in both studies. Clearance was greater in women than in men in both young and elderly groups, whereas it declined with age in men but not in women.

Diazepam has a longer $t_{1/2}$ in the elderly; the $t_{1/2}$ may increase from 20 hours in 20-year-olds to 90 hours in 80-year-olds (Klotz et al. 1975). The V_d of this BZD increases linearly with age over the range of 20–80 years, such that there is a three- to fourfold difference between individuals at the extremes of age studied. Hepatic clearance of diazepam, which is eliminated primarily by demethylation, is independent of age.

The clearance of desmethyldiazepam, the active hydroxylated metabolite of diazepam, is affected by age; it was found to be 40% less in an elderly (65–85 years) than in a younger (29–34 years) population (Klotz and Muller-Seydlitz 1979). Women may clear diazepam more rapidly than men regardless of age (Greenblatt et al. 1980). Half-life is prolonged to a mean of 100 hours in elderly men, whereas the mean in elderly women is about 40–70 hours (Greenblatt et al. 1980).

Lorazepam and *oxazepam* do not have major changes in their pharmacokinetics associated with aging. Neither distribution volume nor hepatic clearance is significantly affected, because these two compounds are metabolized only by glucuronidation, and not by the hepatic mixed-function oxidase system (as are desmethyldiazepam and chlordiazepoxide). The fact that lorazepam and oxazepam have a lower lipid solubility than chlordiazepoxide and diazepam may explain the lack of change in their distribution volume. Gender has no apparent effect on lorazepam clearance (Allen et al. 1980).

All BZDs, given in repeated doses, will accumulate to some

degree and may produce ADRs (Thompson et al. 1983). The extent and severity of the ADRs can be minimized by attention to the drug's $t_{1/2}$, dosage, and frequency of administration. In elderly patients, BZDs with longer $t_{1/2}$s, such as diazepam, chlordiazepoxide, clorazepate, prazepam, and halazepam, should be prescribed in smaller doses (50% or less) and at more widely spaced intervals (once or twice daily rather than two to three times daily) than is recommended for younger patients. BZDs with shorter $t_{1/2}$s, such as oxazepam, lorazepam, and alprazolam, likewise should be administered in smaller doses. However, because the pharmacokinetics of BZDs are not greatly changed in the elderly, the dosage and administration schedule can be similar to that in younger patients.

■ Adverse Effects

Because BZDs have few pharmacological effects outside the CNS, the majority of ADRs are mediated through the CNS. A wide range of non-CNS ADRs have been attributed to BZDs, but their reported incidence is less than 1% (Cole et al. 1981).

Allergic
There have been few documented allergies to the BZDs.

Cardiovascular
The effects of BZDs on blood pressure, heart rate, and cardiac output are minimal. Occasionally, transient episodes of bradycardia and hypotension have been noted after rapid intravenous injection of diazepam (see *Complications of Parenteral Administration* [page 319]).

Dependence
Data indicate that the risk of BZD dependence is small. A survey of physicians with a catchment area of 300,000 identified only 31 BZD-dependent patients (Ladewig and Grossenbacher 1988). Thus, the prevalence rate of benzodiazepine addiction in the general population is 0.01%, or 1 in 10,000. A retrospective analysis of 33,000 consecutive admissions at a German state psychiatric hospital between 1974 and 1983 diagnosed BZD dependence in only 150 (0.45%) patients, whereas substance abuse, primarily alcoholism, was diagnosed in 24% (7,944 of 32,762) of the admissions (Laux and Konig 1987). Dependence is variously defined, and, of course, these studies may have underestimated the prevalence in the general and clinical populations. Nevertheless, the risk of benzodiazepine dependence appears to be low in comparison with the dependency risks of other drugs, especially alcohol. Despite the low prevalence of BZD addiction, however, alcoholic patients are at

greater risk. A study of 1,000 admissions to an alcohol treatment unit found that 35% of the patients used BZDs; however, only 10% were identified as abusers or misusers of the drugs (Ashley et al. 1978). It therefore appears that excessive physician and patient concern about the risk of benzodiazepine abuse, misuse, or dependence is unwarranted, except in alcoholic or polysubstance-abusing individuals. Thus, the data indicate that anxiety disorder patients with coexisting substance abuse who use BZDs for more than 3 months are at a higher risk for BZD addiction, whereas anxiety disorder patients who do not abuse substances are not. Common sense would dictate that it would be preferable to treat such polysubstance abusers with an SSRI or a TCA rather than a benzodiazepine.

Because of the risk of either a withdrawal reaction or a relapse of anxiety symptoms, it is generally recommended that the drug be gradually withdrawn over 1 to several months in patients who have been taking BZDs regularly for more than 1 month.

Patients with chronic anxiety disorders may be an exception to this rule. (For a suggested withdrawal schedule and more information on BZD dependence, see section on anxiolytic-hypnotic withdrawal [page 569] in Chapter 10.)

Hematological and Hepatic

Case reports have attributed reactions involving these systems to BZDs, but a causal factor has not been established.

Neurological

Excessive **CNS depression** (drowsiness, muscle weakness, ataxia, nystagmus, and dysarthria) is the most common side effect attributed to BZDs. It has been reported in 4%–12% of patients taking diazepam or chlordiazepoxide. Elderly individuals and patients with low serum albumin levels are more likely to experience these side effects. Additionally, elderly institutionalized patients are at risk for confusion, falls, and hip fractures as a result of ataxia secondary to BZD sedation (Greenblatt et al. 1991). These ADRs are more likely to occur with the longer half-life BZDs (Greenblatt et al. 1991). Cigarette smokers are less likely to experience CNS depression than are nonsmokers. The interaction between nicotine and BZDs probably occurs in the CNS, given that BZD metabolism is not affected by smoking (Klotz et al. 1975). The subjective incidence of sedation is not significantly different for sustained-release diazepam and regular-release diazepam (Valium® Product Information 1984). This is also the case with a soon-to-be-released sustained-release formulation of alprazolam (Ferguson 1993). These ADRs are dose dependent and disappear when the dose is lowered or the drug discontinued. Central depressant effects of BZDs tend to decline as the duration of exposure increases, thereby reducing the sedative effects (Cole et al. 1981). Thus, patients should be counseled to expect morning sedation and daytime drowsiness or fatigue for the first week or two of treatment.

The BZDs have been demonstrated in the laboratory to impair reaction time, motor coordination, and intellectual functioning in a dose-related fashion. However, studies of long-term BZD users suggest that tolerance develops to these effects (Lucki et al. 1985; Scharf et al. 1988; Valium® Product Information 1984). In patients requiring BZDs, diazepam 15–30 mg/day or placebo was adminis-tered for 2 weeks. The differences between the diazepam and pla-cebo groups decreased over the 2-week period even though blood levels of diazepam were continually rising. Apparently, familiarity with the test and decreased drug-depressant effects improved per-formance (Dubovsky 1990). Because BZDs may impair driving performance in some patients, all patients should be cautioned about driving and operating machinery, especially during the first 2 weeks of treatment. Additionally, patients should be cautioned that the risk of being involved in a traffic accident is increased fivefold in drivers taking BZDs. This finding suggests that the intermittent or prn use of BZDs may be particularly hazardous in patients needing to drive a car.

Anterograde amnesia (memory loss after drug ingestion) may occur with all BZDs (Garzone and Kroboth 1989; Gelenberg 1985; Scharf et al. 1988). Although in the past this effect was most often associated with parenteral administration, it is now commonly reported with oral use. BZDs exert their primary effect on the consolidation (recent) phase without impairment at the acquisition (immediate) or retention (short-term) phases of memory. Thus, although patients taking BZDs will appear to be functioning nor-mally in day-to-day situations, they may later have difficulty recall-ing information communicated to them while they were on the drug (Salzman 1992). Patients should avoid taking BZDs shortly before doing schoolwork, making important decisions, or perform-ing other tasks dependent on an intact memory (Lister 1985).

Complications of Parenteral Administration
Intramuscular chlordiazepoxide, diazepam, and lorazepam injec-tions are painful because of precipitated particles or the propylene glycol solvent, and cause elevations in serum creatine phosphoki-nase (Cole et al. 1981).

Diazepam causes local pain in about 5%–7% of patients receiving it intravenously. This rate is similar for chlordiazepoxide and lorazepam (Greenblatt and Shader 1978). To avoid these problems, 1) the rate of injection should not exceed 5 mg (1 mL) per minute, 2) large veins should be used, 3) injection sites should be alternated, and 4) the veins should be flushed well after each injection (Katcher 1978).

Psychiatric

BZDs, like ethanol and barbiturates, have been reported to produce disinhibition, intoxication, paradoxical excitement, hostility, rage, and even violent, destructive behavior. It is suggested that such reactions are more likely if the BZDs are taken in a setting of interpersonal frustration. This type of ADR occurs infrequently, and some clinicians question whether such reactions actually represent drug effects (Salzman 1992). Triazolam has been associated with an ADR symptom cluster of severe anxiety, agitation, paranoia, hyperacusis, altered smell and taste, irritability, and anger. This reaction is dose dependent, occurring more commonly at doses of 0.5 mg or greater (Salzman 1992).

Respiratory

Compared with other anxiolytic/hypnotics, BZDs are relatively benign in their effects on respiration. Even though overdoses with BZDs are frequent, serious sequelae are rare because of minimal pulmonary function effects. However, in patients with compromised pulmonary function, BZDs may produce clinically significant respiratory effects. All anxiolytic/hypnotics should be used with caution in patients with reduced pulmonary function (Katcher 1978). It has been suggested anecdotally that pulmonarily compromised patients should be treated with lorazepam or oxazepam, short–$t_{1/2}$ BZDs that do not undergo metabolism to any active metabolites.

Teratogenicity and Excretion Into Breast Milk

Studies indicate that diazepam and its metabolites are excreted in breast milk in levels sufficient to produce pharmacological effects (e.g., sedation) in newborns. Milk levels have been reported to be 8%–50% of serum levels. Infant serum levels have been noted to be initially high; the fact that they fall by 6 days is probably due to increased hepatic conjugation, an elimination pathway necessary for all BZDs. Accumulation of BZDs may occur in the infant.

Although some studies have suggested an association between ingestion of BZDs and increased risk of congenital anomalies, this has not been a consistent finding (Calabrese and Gulledge 1985; "Teratogenicity of Minor Tranquilizers" 1975; Gelenberg 1987; St. Clair and Schirmer 1992). When malformations were reported, they consisted of cleft lip and palate and involved women who ingested BZDs during the first trimester of pregnancy. Although the data do not conclusively indicate an association between BZDs and teratogenicity, risk-benefit considerations are such that BZD use during pregnancy, at least during the first trimester, should be avoided, since such use is rarely uncircumventable (Altshuler and Szuba 1994).

Reports indicate that a neonate may experience a BZD withdrawal syndrome if the mother has taken a BZD during pregnancy (Katcher 1978). This observation has led to the recommendation that BZDs should be gradually tapered during the last month of pregnancy.

■ Rational Prescribing

1. With the exception of clonazepam, halazepam, and midazolam, all BZDs are now generically available and relatively inexpensive.
2. There is no evidence that one BZD is clinically superior to another.
3. Antianxiety agents are useful in the short-term management of anxiety but should not be regarded as the mainstay of or sole treatment. Initial treatment for GAD should last for 2 months; that for panic disorder should last for 6–12 months and conclude with a 2- to 4-month drug tapering and discontinuation period.
4. See "Rational Prescribing" (page 328) under **Antidepressants** for a discussion of the long-term treatment of panic disorder.

Antidepressants

■ Indications

For a complete discussion of antidepressant indications, see Chapter 2.

■ Efficacy

Generalized Anxiety Disorder
Although antidepressants have not been extensively studied in the treatment of GAD, there is support for their consideration. Con-

trolled studies have reported that imipramine (Hoehn-Saric et al. 1988; Kahn et al. 1986; McLeod et al. 1990; Rickels et al. 1993) was as effective as chlordiazepoxide and alprazolam, and that doxepin (Haskell et al. 1978) was as effective as diazepam. When the two drug classes, TCAs and BZDs, were directly compared, alprazolam was found to be primarily effective in lowering the somatic component of GAD, whereas imipramine predominantly affected the psychic component (Hoehn-Saric et al. 1988).

Panic Disorder/Agoraphobia
MAOIs and TCAs were first investigated in the pharmacological management of panic disorder and agoraphobia with panic attacks in the early 1960s (Ballenger 1986; Jann and Kurtz 1987; Noyes et al. 1989).

TCAs. A total of 11 controlled trials have investigated the efficacy of TCAs in the treatment of panic disorder and/or agoraphobia (Charney et al. 1986; Cross-National Collaborative Panic Study 1992; Deltito et al. 1991; Gloger et al. 1981; Mavissakalian and Perel 1985; Modigh et al. 1992; Munjack et al. 1985; Rosenberg et al. 1991; Sheehan et al. 1980; Uhlenhuth et al. 1989; Zitrin et al. 1983). The TCAs imipramine and clomipramine were effective in the treatment of panic attacks with or without agoraphobia. The mean percentage of patients who responded to TCA treatment was approximately 67%. (Response was defined as either the complete remission of panic attacks or an 80% reduction in the number of attacks.) Only 1 of the 11 studies (Uhlenhuth et al. 1989) did not find the TCAs to be significantly more effective than placebo in reducing the severity of agoraphobia on the patients' self-rated scale of severity. It has been suggested that antidepressants were found to be effective in panic disorder only because the studies included a large proportion of dysphoric patients, in whose absence the drugs would not have produced their antipanic and antiphobic effects (Marks and O'Sullivan 1988). However, an analysis of more than 1,000 panic disorder patients found that the antipanic/antiphobic effect of alprazolam and imipramine was independent of the presence of depression or dysphoria (Deltito et al. 1991).

The question of efficacy of pharmacological versus behavioral treatment remains unanswered because of research limitations. One controlled study has reported that imipramine is an effective antipanic and antiphobic agent when used alone (Mavissakalian and Perel 1989). A literature review revealed an additional three studies that reported that TCAs were effective alone (Mavissakalian and Perel 1989). Another study reported that the combination of imipramine and behavior therapy provided the greatest response rate (Mavissakalian and Michelson 1986). The other available TCAs have not been as widely studied as imipramine; however, clinical experience suggests that amitriptyline, clomipramine, desipramine, doxepin, and nortriptyline are also effective (Ballenger 1986; Den Boer and Westenberg 1988; Gloger et al. 1989; Hollister 1986; Liebowitz 1985; Muskin and Fyer 1981). Clomipramine may be effective, as might other sedating TCAs such as imipramine, amitriptyline, and doxepin in low doses (e.g., 50–100 mg/day). Comparison studies with TCAs are needed to determine their relative efficacy.

MAOIs. Six placebo-controlled trials (five using phenelzine) reported that MAOIs were effective in 65%–70% of patients (Ballenger et al. 1977; Mountjoy et al. 1977; Sheehan et al. 1980; L. Solyom et al. 1971, 1973; Tyrer et al. 1973). Although the overall response rate with MAOIs was slightly less than that for the TCAs, this may be attributable to the smaller sample sizes, mixed groups of patients, and low doses of drugs used in the studies. An open trial using average phenelzine doses of 55 mg/day reported that panic attacks were blocked in 95% of patients (Buigues and Vallejo 1987). Avoidant behavior improved in 74% of subjects, although this improvement was not statistically significant.

SSRIs and trazodone. Nine studies—three open, one single-blind, one double-blind, and four double-blind and placebo-controlled—have examined the efficacy of trazodone (Charney et al. 1986; Mavissakalian et al. 1987) and the SSRIs fluoxetine (Gorman et al. 1987; Schneier et al. 1990), fluvoxamine (Black et al. 1993; Den Boer and Westenberg 1988, 1990; Hoehn-Saric et al. 1993), and paroxetine (Oehrberg et al. 1995). Response to the treatments was judged by decrease in 1) the number of panic attacks experienced, 2) avoidance of agoraphobic situations, and 3) score on the Hamilton Rating Scale for Anxiety (HAM-A; Hamilton 1959). The studies reported approximately a 60% overall mean decrease of panic attack severity and about a 30% decrease in the phobic avoidance subscale score on the Fear Questionnaire (Mavissakalian et al. 1986) with the SSRIs. When reported, the decreases in HAM-A scores averaged about 50% with the SSRIs.

Bupropion. In a single-blind, placebo-controlled trial, bupropion was shown to be ineffective in treating panic disorder (Sheehan et al. 1983).

Maprotiline.   Maprotiline has been reported to be effective in open trials. One double-blind trial found maprotiline to be ineffective in preventing panic attacks (Den Boer and Westenberg 1988).

Social Phobia

TCAs.   The only TCA that has been studied in the treatment of social phobia is clomipramine. Three of four uncontrolled trials found clomipramine, in doses ranging from 25 to 225 mg/day, to be effective in the treatment of social phobia (Allsopp et al. 1984; Beaumont 1977; Gringras 1977). The fourth study found clomipramine ineffective in a series of social phobia patients who eventually responded to the MAOI tranylcypromine (Versiani et al. 1988).

MAOIs.   A controlled trial involving 74 social phobia patients found phenelzine 45–90 mg/day (mean 76 mg/day) to be effective in 64% of the patients, in contrast to only 30% for atenolol and 23% for placebo (Liebowitz et al. 1992). Another controlled trial involving 78 patients found the MAOIs phenelzine (mean 68 mg/day) and moclobemide (mean 581 mg/day) more effective than placebo, with response rates of 91%, 82%, and 43%, respectively (Versiani et al. 1992).

SSRIs.   Two controlled trials involving a total of 42 social phobia patients found fluvoxamine 150 mg/day for 12 weeks (van Vliet et al. 1994) and sertraline (mean 134 mg/day) (Katzelnick et al. 1995) more effective than placebo in treating this disorder.

Obsessive-Compulsive Disorder

Drugs effective in the treatment of OCD are thought to have one common mechanism of action. The antiobsessional effect seems to be mediated by serotonin agonist activity, because the effective drugs have serotonergic effects. In general, 40%–60% of OCD patients who receive a 10-week course of drug treatment experience approximately a 20%–35% reduction in their obsessions and compulsions, as measured by the Y-BOCS (Goodman et al. 1993). Although both clomipramine and the SSRIs are effective in the short-term treatment of OCD, clomipramine produces a greater increase in the improvement rate over placebo than do the SSRIs. Direct-comparison efficacy studies of clomipramine and the SSRIs have found no difference between the two. Clomipramine and fluvoxamine have been found to be more effective than antidepressants with no serotonergic activity. Finally, the presence or absence of depressive symptoms does not confound the effectiveness of clomipramine and the SSRIs in the treatment of OCD (Piccinelli et al. 1995).

TCAs. The potent serotonin agonist clomipramine is effective in the treatment of OCD, whereas the less-potent serotonin agonists nortriptyline, amitriptyline, and imipramine are not (McDougle et al. 1993a). Twenty-three trials have documented the effectiveness of clomipramine in the treatment of OCD in both adults and children (Piccinelli et al. 1995).

MAOIs. Three reports have suggested that MAOIs may be effective in the treatment of OCD (Annesley 1969; Jain et al. 1970; Jenike 1981). However, no controlled trials exist to support these reports.

SSRIs. Twenty-one controlled trials have demonstrated the effectiveness of fluoxetine, fluvoxamine, sertraline, and paroxetine (Jenike et al. 1990b; Piccinelli et al. 1995; Wheadon et al. 1993) in OCD.

Posttraumatic Stress Disorder

TCAs. Two of three controlled trials have found the TCAs amitriptyline (Davidson et al. 1990) and imipramine (Frank et al. 1988) effective in treating PTSD in World War II and Vietnam War veterans. A 4-week trial of desipramine 200 mg/day or less was not effective (Reist et al. 1989).

MAOIs. Two controlled trials have evaluated the effectiveness of phenelzine in the treatment of PTSD (Frank et al. 1988; Shestatzky et al. 1988). Phenelzine (75 mg/day or less) was effective (Frank et al. 1988) in the 8-week study but not the 4-week study (30–90 mg/day) (Shestatzky et al. 1988).

SSRIs. A controlled 5-week trial found fluoxetine 20–60 mg/day effective in the treatment of PTSD (Van der Kolk et al. 1994). The trauma patients (e.g., rape victims) experienced greater benefit from the fluoxetine treatment than did the soldiers.

■ Mechanism of Action

The mechanism by which TCAs and MAOIs exert their antipanic effects is unclear (Ballenger 1986). Although antidepressants do not directly bind with the BZD receptor, they may exert their anxiolytic effect by interacting with components of the BZD–GABA receptor complex. This system then enhances GABAergic neurotransmission at the level of the chloride channel (Suranyi-Cadotte et al. 1990). The mechanism by which SSRIs exert anxiolytic effects is unclear but obviously related to their effects on serotonin (Suranyi-Cadotte et al. 1990).

■ Dosage

Generalized Anxiety Disorder

TCAs.   The effective mean doses of imipramine in the treatment of GAD ranged from 91 to 135 mg/day.

Panic Disorder

TCAs.   Although some patients respond to imipramine doses of 25 mg/day, most patients require 150 mg/day to achieve a response, and a few require 200–400 mg/day. Imipramine doses should be initiated at 10–25 mg/day, which can be increased in increments of 10–25 mg every 3 days to 150–200 mg/day. If a response is not seen in 4–6 weeks, the dosage may be increased to 400 mg/day (Sheehan and Raj 1990). Antipanic doses of antidepressants other than imipramine are typically in the antidepressant range. In one study, a dose-response pattern emerged for imipramine's antiphobic efficacy (Mavissakalian and Perel 1985). Patients were more likely to respond to imipramine doses of ≥150 mg/day than to lower doses of ≤125 mg/day. The same investigators found that the antipanic effect of imipramine was achieved with 1.5 mg/kg/day, whereas the antiphobic effect required a higher dose of 3.0 mg/kg/day (Mavissakalian and Perel 1989). These researchers recently concluded that a total imipramine (imipramine + desipramine) plasma concentration of 110–140 ng/mL and a target imipramine dose of 2.25 mg/kg/day are optimal in the acute treatment of patients with panic disorder with agoraphobia (Mavissakalian and Perel 1995). Regarding prophylactic drug treatment, panic disorder patients experienced better outcomes at 3-month follow-up if their imipramine dosages were halved rather than completely discontinued (Mavissakalian and Perel 1992).

MAOIs.   MAOI treatment is usually initiated at 15 mg/day and increased to 15 mg/day every 3–4 days until 90 mg/day is reached. Tranylcypromine is started at 10 mg in the morning. The dose may be raised by 10 mg every 3–4 days to a maximum dosage of 80 mg/day (Sheehan and Raj 1990).

SSRIs.   In retrospect, the fluoxetine studies (Gorman et al. 1987; Schneier et al. 1990) were compromised in that the dosages administered were excessive. Most panic disorder patients will respond to doses of 20 mg/day or less. This dosage will minimize the number of patients who discontinue the medication because of adverse effects. The optimum titration rate for fluoxetine is 5 mg/day for week 1, 10 mg/day for week 2, and 15–20 mg/day for week 3 (Sheehan and Raj 1990). For paroxetine, the initially recommended dosages are 10 mg/day for week 1 and 20 mg/day for week 2 (Oehr-berg et al. 1995).

Social Phobia

Clomipramine doses ranging from 25 to 225 mg/day are effective in the treatment of social phobia. Effective phenelzine doses range from 45 to 90 mg/day, whereas fluoxetine doses range from 20 to 80 mg/day.

Obsessive-Compulsive Disorder

TCAs.   An adequate trial of clomipramine consists of 10–12 weeks at a minimum mean daily dose of 150 mg for at least the first 6 weeks (Goodman et al. 1993).

SSRIs.   Daily doses of SSRIs for the treatment of OCD were 250–300 mg/day for fluvoxamine (Goodman et al. 1989a; Jenike et al. 1990a; Perse et al. 1988), 75 mg/day (mean) for fluoxetine (Pigott et al. 1990), 180 mg/day (mean) for sertraline (Chouinard et al. 1990), and 40–60 mg/day for paroxetine (Wheadon et al. 1993).

Posttraumatic Stress Disorder

Controlled treatment trials with amitriptyline (Davidson et al. 1993), imipramine (Frank et al. 1988; Kosten et al. 1991), desipramine (Reist et al. 1989), phenelzine (Shestatzky et al. 1988), and fluoxetine (Van der Kolk et al. 1994) have concluded that for antidepressants to be effective in the treatment of PTSD, they 1) must possess a serotonin agonist effect, 2) must be administered in high doses, and 3) must be administered for a minimum of 8 weeks. Because of the risk of "jitteriness syndrome" (see "Adverse Effects," below), it is recommend that upward dosage titration be done slowly. In chronic PTSD patients, it may be necessary to continue treatment for up to 1 year (Vargas and Davidson 1993).

■ Pharmacokinetics

For a complete discussion of antidepressant pharmacokinetics, see Chapter 2.

■ Adverse Effects

For a complete discussion of antidepressant adverse effects, see Chapter 2.

TCAs in panic patients have been associated with adverse effects severe enough to result in treatment discontinuation in 35% of patients (Noyes et al. 1989).

A reaction that appears almost exclusively in anxiety disorder patients is the *jitteriness syndrome,* or "hypersensitivity" reaction

(Pohl et al. 1988). Forty-nine of 158 patients (30%) with panic disorder developed this reaction in one retrospective study. Symptoms included jitteriness, shakiness, increased anxiety, and insomnia. Although TCA doses were most often started at 10 mg/day, symptoms still occurred. The syndrome appears with initial doses and tolerance develops over 7–10 days (Pohl et al. 1988; Zitrin et al. 1983). However, if tolerance does not develop within this time period, it is unlikely to occur. Desipramine was reported to be more likely to produce this reaction than imipramine, based on retrospective data (Pohl et al. 1988). If slow upward dose titration or dose reduction are ineffective, a 1-month course of low-dose propranolol (20–40 mg/day) or benzodiazepine is a useful treatment option (Lipinski et al. 1989).

■ Rational Prescribing

1. Studies indicate that TCAs are as efficacious as BZDs in the treatment of GAD.
2. Overall, antidepressants and BZDs are superior to β-blockers in prevention of panic attacks.
3. For the treatment of panic disorder, the data suggest that BZDs and antidepressants are approximately equivalent in efficacy and ADRs.
4. Antidepressants rather than BZDs are the preferred treatment in panic disorder patients who are significantly depressed or who have a history of major depressive disorder. Because of the dietary restrictions needed with MAOIs, TCAs are usually the antidepressant class of choice, followed by the less adequately researched SSRIs.
5. BZDs may be used in patients to achieve rapid control of anxiety symptoms while antidepressant treatment is being initiated.
6. If an adequate trial with one treatment fails, monotherapy with another pharmacological class should be tried. Although not well studied, combination treatment with various agents has been reported to succeed when monotherapy fails (Jann and Kurtz 1987).
7. For all of the anxiety disorders, evidence exists from controlled trials that patients continue to improve for up to 6–12 months with pharmacological management.
8. As a general rule for panic disorder or GAD, regardless of whether the patient has been successfully treated with an antidepressant or a benzodiazepine, most patients will eventu-

ally experience a recurrence of symptoms (Coryell et al. 1983; Rickels et al. 1983; Wheeler et al. 1953). An undetermined proportion of patients can remain off medications during the second year of treatment, but many will require long-term treatment. Therefore, after 6–12 months of successful treatment, it is reasonable to consider discontinuing medications to determine whether the patient is among the minority that can do without medication (Pecknold et al. 1988). However, overall, the data suggest that treatment-responsive panic disorder patients whose medication is completely discontinued do worse than patients whose medication is simply reduced to a 50% maintenance dose (Mavissakalian and Perel 1992).

9. Clomipramine, phenelzine, and fluoxetine are effective in the treatment of social phobia.

10. High-dose SSRIs or clomipramine for 10–12 weeks is regarded as the first-line treatment for OCD.

11. As in the treatment of OCD, high doses of SSRIs are required for the treatment of social phobia.

12. Therapeutic doses of the serotonergic TCAs amitriptyline and imipramine, the MAOI phenelzine, and the SSRI fluoxetine for a minimum of 8 weeks are beneficial for the treatment of PTSD.

13. It is recommended that BZDs, TCAs, MAOIs, and SSRIs be tapered gradually over a 2- to 4-month period to allow early detection of relapse. Alprazolam's tapering should be done very slowly to avoid significant withdrawal symptoms, especially if higher doses are being used (Pecknold et al. 1988) (see section on anxiolytic-hypnotic withdrawal [page 569] in Chapter 10). If the patient relapses after the first taper, reinstitution of treatment often achieves clinical control. It is recommended that tapering be reattempted in 3–6 months.

β-Adrenergic–Blocking Drugs

■ Indications

Of the β-adrenergic receptor–blocking agents available in the United States, propranolol is the most extensively studied in the management of anxiety. It was first introduced into medicine in 1964 and is used in the treatment of angina, hypertension, specific tremors, and certain cardiac arrhythmias. At present, it is not approved by the U.S. Food and Drug Administration (FDA) for use as an anxiolytic. β-blockers may be useful in the treatment of performance or situational anxiety, and they have potential value in the treatment of PTSD. Their anxiolytic activity is relatively weak, and they are of little value in panic disorder with or without agoraphobia.

■ **Efficacy**

Generalized Anxiety Disorder
The anxiolytic effect of propranolol was first examined in 1966. Approximately half of the β-blocker anxiolytic efficacy studies were conducted before the DSM-III GAD diagnosis was introduced. Only one study (Peet and Ali 1986) exists in which subjects met the criteria for GAD. Both propranolol 160 mg/day and atenolol 100 mg/day were more effective than placebo in that study. No efficacy studies are available that used only GAD patients. Despite these limitations, 19 trials have documented the β-blockers' effectiveness versus placebo in the treatment of "anxiety." Of these trials, 12 reported positive results for β-blockers, 4 yielded equivocal findings, and 3 found no difference in effectiveness (Birkett and Tyrer 1990). No studies are available that used DSM-III-R criteria. Eight studies have compared β-blockers with diazepam and chlordiazepoxide. Five of these studies (Burrows et al. 1976; McMillin 1973; Meibach et al. 1987a, 1987b; Wheatley 1969) found no difference between the β-blockers and the BZD, and three (Hallstrom et al. 1981; Johnson et al. 1976; Tyrer and Lader 1974) found the BZDs clearly superior to the β-blockers. Overall, the β-blockers are inferior to the BZDs, although the difference in efficacy is less marked after 1 or 2 weeks of treatment.

Panic Disorder/Agoraphobia
A placebo comparison trial suggested that propranolol 160 mg/day might be more effective than placebo in the treatment of panic disorder with or without agoraphobia. However, a 2-week study comparing propranolol 240 mg/day with diazepam 30 mg/day found propranolol less effective than diazepam (Noyes et al. 1984). Likewise, another study found propranolol (mean dosage 185 mg/day) less effective than alprazolam (mean dosage 4 mg/day) and only as effective as placebo in preventing panic attacks (Munjack et al. 1989). However, one trial found propranolol 160 mg/day as effective as imipramine 150–300 mg/day in 23 patients with panic disorder (Munjack et al. 1985). Thus, β-blockers appear to be less effective than BZDs in the treatment of panic disorder.

Social Phobias

An open trial of atenolol 50–100 mg/day (Gorman et al. 1985) reported the drug to be beneficial in the treatment of social phobia. However, propranolol was no more effective than placebo in the treatment of social phobia (Falloon et al. 1981). Likewise, atenolol, when compared with phenelzine, was less effective than the MAOI and not superior to placebo (Liebowitz et al. 1992). β-blockers do not appear to be useful as antiphobic agents.

β-blockers have not been investigated in the treatment of simple (specific) phobia (Noyes et al. 1986).

Acute Situational Anxiety (Performance Anxiety)

β-blockers are effective in the treatment of acute situational, or performance, anxiety (Lader 1988). The drugs appear to be most effective when somatic symptoms predominate (Hollister 1986; Schuckit 1981). β-blockers have improved performance in students taking examinations, decreased tachycardia and lessened stress responses in race car drivers, decreased stress-induced somatic symptoms experienced during public speaking, reduced tremor in string instrument players, and alleviated symptoms of anxiety related to stress in anxious outpatients (Lader 1988).

Obsessive-Compulsive Disorder

β-blockers are of no value in the treatment of OCD.

Posttraumatic Stress Disorder

According to anecdotal reports and open trials, propranolol is effective in the treatment of PTSD among Vietnam veterans (Kolb et al. 1984) and physically and/or sexually abused children (Famularo et al. 1988).

■ Mechanism of Action

The mechanism by which propranolol and other β-blockers exert their antianxiety effects is not known. Some authors believe the main action is primarily peripherally mediated, given that lower doses have been shown to decrease tremor without entering the CNS and because non-CNS–acting β-blockers have been used with success (Tyrer 1992). It has been hypothesized that propranolol, which crosses the blood-brain barrier, acts peripherally and centrally to reduce symptoms mediated by overactive or hypersensitive β-adrenergic receptors (Kathol et al. 1980). Whether the proposed anxiolytic effects of β-blockers are mediated through a central or a peripheral site of action has not been resolved. The drugs may also reduce somatic symptoms by interrupting the negative feedback loop associated with anxiety disorders (Tyrer 1992).

■ Dosage

For the treatment of GAD and PTSD, a propranolol dose of 80–160 mg/day is most commonly associated with a beneficial effect (Birkett and Tyrer 1990; Kolb et al. 1984). Single doses of propranolol 40–60 mg have been successfully used in acute situational anxiety and for social phobia (Liebowitz et al. 1985). The dose should be administered 1–2 hours before the stressful event.

■ Pharmacokinetics

Propranolol is well absorbed after oral administration. A saturable, high-affinity binding mechanism exists in the liver, and, hence, the drug undergoes a significant first-pass effect. It is extensively metabolized in the liver to 4-hydroxypropranolol, which is pharmacologically active. Propranolol is more than 90% bound to plasma proteins. During chronic dosing, the $t_{1/2}$ varies from 3.5 to 6 hours, but may be as high as 24 hours in patients with chronic liver disease (Young and Riddiough 1978).

■ Adverse Effects

The reported incidence of ADRs with propranolol in patients with anxiety is 25%–40% (Kathol et al. 1980). This is higher than the 9%–17% ADR incidence reported in disorders other than anxiety. The explanation may be that the common ADRs of propranolol (i.e., dizziness, fatigue, insomnia) resemble symptoms of anxiety.

Cardiovascular

At the doses used in antianxiety studies, propranolol has been reported to produce cardiac failure in patients with and without preexisting impairment of myocardial function, arrhythmias such as bradycardia and heart block, and hypotension.

Nearly 9% of 268 patients treated with propranolol experienced significant ADRs, one-third of which were life-threatening: bradycardia, impaired atrioventricular conduction, acute pulmonary edema, hypotension, and bronchospasm (in asthmatic patients) (Young and Riddiough 1978). These reactions occurred more frequently in the elderly. Long-term use of propranolol at doses of 160–400 mg/day resulted in a 9% incidence of left-ventricular failure (Young and Riddiough 1978). These effects are a result of propranolol's β-blocking effects. All are reversible upon discontinuation of the drug. Because of reports of myocardial infarction associated with rapid withdrawal (Kathol et al. 1980; Young and Riddiough 1978), it is recommended that propranolol be discontinued gradually in patients receiving the drug for angina.

Dermatological
Erythemas, maculopapular rashes, and erythema multiforme have been reported, albeit only rarely (Robinson 1975).

Gastrointestinal
The percentage of patients experiencing GI symptoms has varied widely among studies. Nausea occurs occasionally but can be avoided if doses are given with meals. Vomiting is rare, but diarrhea accompanied by abdominal cramps occurs frequently. These GI side effects are not generally severe enough to require discontinuation of treatment (Robinson 1975; Young and Riddiough 1978).

Hematological
Eosinophilia, usually transient, has been reported frequently in patients receiving propranolol. This effect appears to be a direct result of β-blockade, given that propranolol blocks the eosinophil-decreasing action of epinephrine (Robinson 1975).

Metabolic
Propranolol-induced hypoglycemia due to β-blockade of hepatic glycogenolysis has been reported but appears to be infrequent. In addition, β-blockade may make clinical detection of hypoglycemia more difficult, as it attenuates certain autonomic manifestations of this condition (Young and Riddiough 1978).

Neuropsychiatric
Reactions such as fatigue and lethargy are frequently reported. Effects such as vivid dreams and nightmares are also common. Hallucinations, almost always visual and often of a hypnagogic nature, have been reported, although rarely. Toxic psychosis may occur and responds to stopping the drug temporarily and restarting it at a lower dose (Erman and Guggenheim 1981; Robinson 1975).

Depression has been reported as a complication of β-blocker therapy; however, the true incidence of this effect is difficult to determine. The possibility of depression should be considered in patients treated with propranolol who have a history of depression (Erman and Guggenheim 1981). The incidence of depression is more often associated with the more-lipophilic β-blocking drugs such as propranolol than with the less-lipophilic β-blockers such as atenolol (Westerlund 1985).

Respiratory

Respiratory complications of propranolol are related to increased airway resistance that may become symptomatic in asthmatic patients or those with chronic obstructive pulmonary disease. Approximately 0.5%–2% of patients have developed dyspnea and wheezing after initiation of propranolol (Young and Riddiough 1978). Although cardioselective β-blockers are thought to cause fewer respiratory complications, higher doses may overcome the cardioselectivity of the drug, resulting in respiratory symptoms (Fisher 1985).

Teratogenicity and Excretion Into Breast Milk

Use of propranolol during pregnancy has been reported to cause decreased placental size, fetal growth retardation, and neonatal bradycardia and hypoglycemia.

Studies in breast-feeding women receiving propranolol found drug levels in the milk to be 50%–100% of the plasma levels in the mothers. Adverse effects on the infant are unknown (Young and Riddiough 1978).

■ Rational Prescribing

1. β-blockers are considered second-line drugs in the treatment of generalized anxiety disorder. However, in some patients, they may prove to be beneficial adjunctive treatments in combination with the antidepressants and BZDs.
2. Propranolol and other β-blockers are not as effective as antidepressants or BZDs for panic disorder or agoraphobia.
3. Propranolol may be effective in acute situational anxiety (performance anxiety) but is probably not useful in social phobia.

Buspirone

Buspirone, a member of a new class of agents known as azaspirodecanediones, is the first nonbenzodiazepine anxiolytic to be introduced in the United States in 25 years. It is not a controlled substance.

■ Indications

Buspirone is indicated for the short-term treatment of GAD when symptoms are mild to moderate in severity (Dommisse and De Vane 1985; Goldberg 1984).

■ Efficacy

Generalized Anxiety Disorder

Seven controlled trials have compared the anxiolytic activity of buspirone with that of diazepam in the treatment of GAD (Feighner et al. 1982; Goldberg and Finnerty 1979; Jacobson et al. 1985; Olajide and Lader 1987; Pecknold et al. 1985; Rickels et al. 1982; Wheatley 1982). Three of the studies (Jacobson et al. 1985; Olajide and Lader 1987; Pecknold et al. 1985) found diazepam more effective than buspirone during either the first 2 weeks or the entire study. Buspirone's anxiolytic effectiveness compared favorably with other BZDs, including clorazepate (Cohn et al. 1986; Goldberg and Finnerty 1982), alprazolam (Cohn and Wilcox 1986), and lorazepam (Cohn and Wilcox 1986). Interestingly, according to the physician global ratings in all three studies, a greater percentage of patients responded to the BZDs than to buspirone, although this finding never reached statistical significance. Buspirone appears to have a slower onset of action than the BZDs. Patients who have been exposed to BZDs are less likely to respond to buspirone than are those who have never taken a BZD (Schweizer et al. 1986). Additionally, the maximum therapeutic benefit from buspirone may not occur until 4–6 weeks of treatment have elapsed, and women may respond better than men. Buspirone's delayed onset prevents its prn use.

Panic Disorder

One controlled trial comparing buspirone, imipramine, and placebo found buspirone to be less effective than imipramine and equal to placebo in treating panic disorder (Sheehan et al. 1990). A second study showed that imipramine and buspirone were no better than placebo in a double-blind trial (Pohl et al. 1989). The studies were criticized by the manufacturer because the maximal drug dosage, 60 mg/day, was not used. The most recent study (Sheehan et al. 1993) used a 60-mg/day dose in comparing the drug's efficacy with that of alprazolam and placebo. Once again, buspirone was less effective than alprazolam and no more effective than placebo in the treatment of panic disorder.

Social Phobia

Buspirone's efficacy in the treatment of DSM-III-R social phobia was evaluated in 21 patients (Schneier et al. 1993). Eight of the patients randomized to treatment were rated as very much improved. Although buspirone may be effective in the treatment of social phobia, this remains to be conclusively shown in a controlled trial.

Obsessive-Compulsive Disorder

An open-design, 8-week trial found buspirone ineffective in the treatment of OCD (Jenike and Baer 1988). However, a controlled trial comparing clomipramine with buspirone in 18 OCD patients found both drugs equally effective, as determined by the improvement observed in Y-BOCS scores (Pato et al. 1991). Buspirone augmentation of clomipramine (Pigott et al. 1992) or fluoxetine (Jenike et al. 1991) has been suggested; however, two controlled trials found such augmentation ineffective (McDougle et al. 1993b; Pigott et al. 1992).

Posttraumatic Stress Disorder

Anecdotal reports suggest that buspirone 30–60 mg/day may be useful in the treatment of PTSD (La Porta and Ware 1992; Wells et al. 1991).

Schizophrenia

Because buspirone has dopamine antagonistic activity, its effectiveness in the treatment of psychotic patients was evaluated. In an early open trial, schizophrenic patients treated with buspirone 600–2,400 mg/day showed no improvement in psychopathology (Goldberg 1984).

■ Mechanism of Action

In contrast to standard anxiolytic agents, buspirone does not appear to have significant sedative, muscle relaxant, or anticonvulsant actions. It has also been demonstrated that buspirone does not directly interact with the GABA-BZD receptor (Riblet et al. 1984).

Buspirone interacts with dopaminergic pathways as both an agonist and an antagonist. Like classical dopamine-blocking agents (i.e., antipsychotics), it increases prolactin levels in rats and human volunteers and also increases the rate of dopamine synthesis. However, buspirone cannot be classified as a typical antipsychotic because it does not inhibit dopamine-stimulated adenylate cyclase or alter the density of [^{3}H]spiroperidol-binding sites after long-term treatment. The latter two effects are found in drugs that cause tardive dyskinesia.

Buspirone appears to be a serotonin antagonist. It acts on the noradrenergic system to increase the firing of the locus coeruleus (LC). Typically, drugs that stimulate the LC produce a syndrome resembling anxiety, and drugs that suppress the LC have anxiolytic actions. It appears that buspirone has actions that override its activating effects in the LC. With regard to serotonin, buspirone has been shown to decrease the firing of serotonergic neurons in the dorsal raphe nucleus (presynaptic) and to antagonize serotonin's effects in the hippocampal (postsynaptic) region (Yocca 1990).

■ Dosage

The usual anxiolytic dose of buspirone is 15–45 mg/day (Riblet et al. 1984). The initial starting dose is 15 mg/day given on a bid or tid dosage schedule. The dose may be increased by 5 mg/day, and the maximum recommended daily dose is 60 mg.

■ Pharmacokinetics

Absorption
Buspirone is rapidly absorbed in humans, with peak plasma concentrations occurring 1 hour after oral administration. Peak plasma concentrations of buspirone were 1.0–3.9 ng/mL after a single 20-mg dose (Dommisse and De Vane 1985; Goldberg 1984).

Although the clinical significance of this finding is not known, food may increase the amount of buspirone entering the systemic circulation.

Distribution
Buspirone is approximately 95% protein bound (Dommisse and De Vane 1985).

Metabolism
Buspirone is extensively metabolized by the liver, as less than 1% appears in the urine as unchanged drug. Its elimination half-life has been calculated to be 2.5 ± 0.5 hours. The 5-hydroxy derivative of buspirone is pharmacologically active and exists in plasma in greater concentrations than the parent compound. It has a half-life of 4.8 ± 1.0 hours and is excreted after conjugation in the urine. Oxidative dealkylation of buspirone produces pyrimidinylpiperazine (1-PP), which may contribute pharmacologically to buspirone's effect. Buspirone may undergo dose-dependent metabolism (Dommisse and De Vane 1985; Goldberg 1984).

Elimination was markedly impaired in patients with cirrhosis and, to a lesser extent, in patients with renal disease, compared with that in healthy subjects. Although the clinical implications of these findings are not known, buspirone should be used cautiously in patients with liver and kidney disease (Dommisse and De Vane 1985; Goldberg 1984).

■ Adverse Effects

All reviews of the overall side-effect profile of buspirone have concluded that the drug (45%) has more ADRs than placebo (33%) but fewer than the BZDs (45%–60%) (Newton et al. 1982).

Central Nervous System

Dizziness, drowsiness, and headache occurred in 12%, 10%, and 6% of buspirone-treated patients, respectively. These side effects are more common with doses higher than 20 mg/day. Dizziness was reported 30–60 minutes after buspirone was administered, especially when subjects were walking or standing.

Dysphoria has been reported, primarily with doses less than 30 mg/day.

Initial studies indicate that buspirone at or below 20 mg/day produces less psychomotor impairment than do BZDs. The effects of buspirone in combination with ethanol were compared with those of lorazepam plus ethanol (two studies) or diazepam plus ethanol (one study) (Matilla et al. 1982; Moskorvitz and Smiley 1982; Seppala et al. 1982). All three studies demonstrated that in healthy subjects receiving buspirone plus ethanol, objective performance was impaired significantly less than it was in subjects receiving lorazepam or diazepam. Interestingly, the healthy subjects reported some drowsiness, weakness, and faintness after ingesting buspirone plus ethanol, although their objective performance was not impaired. However, after taking lorazepam plus ethanol, the subjects did not perceive ADRs associated with psychomotor impairment.

Dependence

Studies of the abuse potential of buspirone in animals and recreational sedative users have demonstrated no overt sedative or euphoric effects (Bolster and Woolverton 1982; Cole et al. 1982; Taylor et al. 1984).

It is important to note that buspirone is not cross-tolerant with standard anxiolytics/hypnotics (i.e., BZDs, barbiturates). Therefore, buspirone will not prevent withdrawal signs and symptoms that may occur if a patient is abruptly changed from one of these drugs to buspirone (see section on anxiolytic-hypnotic withdrawal [page 569] in Chapter 10).

Gastrointestinal

Nausea was the most common GI adverse effect, occurring in 8% of patients.

Neurological

In a series of six stable patients with Parkinson's disease on anti-parkinsonian medication who were treated with buspirone dosages of less than 100 mg/day, four experienced a mild worsening of their parkinsonian symptoms and four were clinically unchanged (Sussman 1986). In a study designed to investigate the antipsychotic activity of buspirone 600–2,400 mg/day, one patient developed extrapyramidal symptoms of akathisia, tremor, and rigidity (Dommisse and De Vane 1985).

Teratogenicity and Excretion Into Breast Milk

Use of buspirone during pregnancy or while breast-feeding is not recommended, as it has not been adequately investigated.

■ Rational Prescribing

1. Overall, clinical studies with buspirone suggest that it is more effective than placebo in treating GAD and perhaps equal in efficacy to the BZDs. The drug does has no antipanic activity and only mild antiphobic activity. Its utility in OCD is questionable, and its value in the treatment of PTSD remains to be proven.

2. Buspirone may be useful in treating GAD patients who are unable to take BZDs (i.e., disinhibition), those with a history of anxiolytic/hypnotic abuse, and pulmonary disease patients who cannot to take BZDs.

3. Buspirone is by far the most expensive anxiolytic treatment currently available (Modell 1995).

Miscellaneous Agents

■ Indications

The following drugs are not approved by the FDA for the treatment of anxiety disorders.

■ Efficacy

Panic Disorder

Baclofen 30 mg/day in a double-blind trial was significantly more effective than placebo (Breslow et al. 1989).

    Carbamazepine produced a marked improvement in only in 1 of 14 patients with panic disorder (Uhde et al. 1988).

    Valproic acid 2,250 mg/day in an open trial produced moderate improvement in 6 of 10 panic disorder patients treated for 7 weeks.

Adverse effects included nausea and dizziness ($n = 4$), drowsiness, tremor, diarrhea ($n = 3$) and constipation, dry mouth, and headaches ($n = 2$) (Primeau et al. 1990).

In a double-blind, placebo-controlled, 5-week crossover-design trial, **verapamil** 480 mg/day produced a significant reduction in panic attacks but not in symptoms of agoraphobia in 11 patients. Overall, in self-ratings, patients considered themselves markedly improved ($n = 4$), marginally improved ($n = 3$), and unimproved ($n = 4$) (Klein and Uhde 1990).

Obsessive-Compulsive Disorder

Because 40%–60% of OCD patients may not respond to either clomipramine or one of the SSRIs, a number of serotonin augmentation treatments have been tried with varying success that has been documented anecdotally. Augmentation of clomipramine or an SSRI with L-tryptophan, lithium, fenfluramine, or *buspirone* may be of benefit in treatment-refractory OCD patients (McDougle et al. 1993b).

Posttraumatic Stress Disorder

Anecdotal reports have supported the use of lithium, carbamazepine, clonidine, or valproic acid as adjunctive agents to stabilize the mood of agitated PTSD patients (Sutherland and Davidson 1994).

Product List

(For the antidepressant product list, see Chapter 2.)

Alprazolam (benzodiazepine)
- Relative oral potency: 1 mg
- Daily dose range: 0.75–10 mg; generically available
- Generic cost index: ≈ 0.10

Tablets:	**Xanax**®
0.25 mg	[$62] Xanax 0.25, white
0.5 mg	[$77] Xanax 0.5, peach
1.0 mg	[$103] Xanax 1, blue
2.0 mg	[$175] Xanax 2, white

Buspirone (azaspirodecanedione)
- Daily dose range: 15–60 mg

Tablets:	**BuSpar**®
5 mg	[$60] BuSpar MJ 5, white
10 mg	[$104] BuSpar MJ 10, white

Chlordiazepoxide (benzodiazepine)
- Relative oral potency: 25 mg
- Oral daily dose range: 5–100 mg; generically available
- Generic cost index: ≈ 0.10

Capsules:	**Librium**®
5 mg	[$37] Roche Librium 5, green/yellow
10 mg	[$54] Roche Librium 10, green/black
25 mg	[$92] Roche Librium 25, green/white

Tablets:	**Libritabs**®
5 mg	[$35] Libritabs 5, green
25 mg	[$87] Libritabs 25, green

Injection:	**Librium**®
100 mg/mL	[$8/1-mL ampule]

Clonazepam (benzodiazepine)
- Relative oral potency: 1 mg
- Daily dose range: 1–10 mg

Tablets:	**Klonopin**®
0.5 mg	[$76] Roche Klonopin 0.5, orange
1 mg	[$87] Roche Klonopin 1, blue
2 mg	[$121] Roche Klonopin 2, white

Clorazepate (benzodiazepine)
- Relative oral potency: 15 mg
- Daily dose range: 15–60 mg; generically available
- Generic cost index: ≈ 0.04

Tablets:	**Tranxene**®
3.75 mg	[$116] aTL, blue
7.5 mg	[$144] aTM, peach
15.0 mg	[$196] aTN, lavender

Tablets:	**Tranxene SD**®
11.25 mg	[$307] aTX, blue
22.5 mg	[$394] aTY, tan

Diazepam (benzodiazepine)
- Relative oral potency: 10 mg
- Daily dose range: 4–40 mg; generically available
- Generic cost index: ≈ 0.05

Tablets:	**Valium**®
2 mg	[$42] Roche 2 Valium, white
5 mg	[$65] Roche 5 Valium, yellow
10 mg	[$109] Roche 10 Valium, blue

Injection:	**Valium**®
5 mg/mL	[$6/2-mL ampule]
5 mg/mL	[$19/10-mL vial]
5 mg/mL	[$4/2-mL unit dose syringe]
Capsules:	**Valrelease**™
15 mg	[$173] Roche Valrelease 15, yellow/blue

Halazepam (benzodiazepine)
- Relative oral potency: 40 mg
- Daily dose range: 60–160 mg

Tablets:	**Paxipam**®
20 mg	[$47] Schering 251, orange
40 mg	[$66] Schering 538, white

Lorazepam (benzodiazepine)
- Relative oral potency: 1 mg
- Daily dose range: 1–10 mg; generically available
- Generic cost index: ≈ 0.03

Tablets:	**Ativan**®
0.5 mg	[$63] Wyeth 81, white
1 mg	[$83] Wyeth 64, white
2 mg	[$120] Wyeth 65, white
Injection:	**Ativan**®
2 mg/mL	[$107/10-mL vial]
4 mg/mL	[$134/10-mL vial]
2 mg/mL	[$13/0.5-mL unit dose syringe]
2 mg/mL	[$13/1.0-mL unit dose syringe]
4 mg/mL	[$13/1.0-mL unit dose syringe]

Oxazepam (benzodiazepine)
- Relative oral potency: 10 mg
- Daily dose range: 30–120 mg; generically available
- Generic cost index: ≈ 0.09

Capsules:	**Serax**®
10 mg	[$70] Serax 10 Wyeth-Ayerst, pink/white
15 mg	[$89] Serax 15 Wyeth-Ayerst, red/white
30 mg	[$128] Serax 30 Wyeth-Ayerst, maroon/white
Tablets:	**Serax**®
15 mg	[$85] S Wyeth 317, yellow

Propranolol (β-blocker)
- Oral daily dose range: 80–320 mg; generically available
- Generic cost index: ≈ 0.04

Tablets:	**Inderal**®
10 mg	[$33] Inderal 10, peach
20 mg	[$46] Inderal 20, blue
40 mg	[$60] Inderal 40, green
60 mg	[$83] Inderal 60, pink
80 mg	[$92] Inderal 80, yellow

Capsules:	**Inderal**® LA
60 mg	[$80] Inderal LA 60, blue/white
80 mg	[$94] Inderal LA 80, light blue
120 mg	[$117] Inderal LA 120, two-tone blue
160 mg	[$153] Inderal LA 160, royal blue

Injection:	**Inderal**®
1 mg/mL	[$4/1-mL ampule]

References

Allen MD, Greenblatt DJ, Harmatz JS, et al: Desmethyldiazepam kinetics in the elderly after oral prazepam. Clin Pharmacol Ther 28:196–202, 1980

Allsopp LF, Cooper GL, Poole PH: Clomipramine and diazepam in the treatment of agoraphobia and social phobia in general practice. Curr Med Res Opin 9:64–70, 1984

Altshuler LL, Szuba MP: Course of psychiatric disorders in pregnancy: dilemmas in pharmacologic management. Neurol Clin 12:613–635, 1994

American Psychiatric Association: Diagnostic and Statistical Manual of Mental Disorders, 3rd Edition. Washington, DC, American Psychiatric Association, 1980

American Psychiatric Association: Diagnostic and Statistical Manual of Mental Disorders, 3rd Edition, Revised. Washington, DC, American Psychiatric Association, 1987

American Psychiatric Association: Diagnostic and Statistical Manual of Mental Disorders, 4th Edition. Washington, DC, American Psychiatric Association, 1994

Andersch S, Rosenber NK, Kullingsjo H, et al: Efficacy and safety of alprazolam, imipramine and placebo in treating panic disorder: a Scandinavian multicenter study. Acta Psychiatr Scand 365 (suppl):18–27, 1991

Annesley PT: Nardil response in a chronic obsessive compulsive. Br J Psychiatry 115:748, 1969

Ashley MJ, LeRiche WH, Olin GS, et al: "Mixed" (drug abusing) and "pure" alcoholics: a socio-medical comparison. British Journal of Addiction 73:19–34, 1978

Ballenger JC: Pharmacotherapy of the panic disorders. J Clin Psychiatry 6 (suppl):27–32, 1986

Ballenger JC, Sheehan DV, Jacobsen G: Antidepressant treatment of severe phobic anxiety (174), in Abstracts of the Scientific Proceedings of the 130th Annual Meeting of the American Psychiatric Association, Toronto, Canada, May 1977, pp 103–104

Ballenger JC, Burrows GD, DuPont RL Jr, et al: Alprazolam in panic disorder and agoraphobia: results from a multicenter trial, I: efficacy in short-term treatment. Arch Gen Psychiatry 45:413–422, 1988

Baskin SI, Esdale A: Is chlordiazepoxide the rational choice among benzo-diazepines? Pharmacotherapy 2:110–119, 1982

Beaumont G: A large open multicenter trial of clomipramine in the man-agement of phobic disorders. J Int Med Res 5 (suppl 5):116–123, 1977

Birkett P, Tyrer P: β-blocking drugs for the treatment of generalized anxiety disorder, in Handbook of Anxiety, Vol 4. Edited by Noyes R, Roth M, Burrows GD. Amsterdam, Elsevier, 1990, pp 147–168

Black DW, Wesner R, Bowers W, et al: A comparison of fluvoxamine, cognitive therapy and placebo in the treatment of panic disorder. Arch Gen Psychiatry 50:44–50, 1993

Bolster RL, Woolverton WL: Intravenous buspirone self-administration in rhesus monkeys. J Clin Psychiatry 43:34–37, 1982

Bowden CL, Fisher JG: Relationship of diazepam serum level to antianxiety effects. J Clin Psychopharmacol 2:110–114, 1982

Braun P, Greenberg D, Dasberg H, et al: Core symptoms of post-traumatic stress disorder unimproved by alprazolam treatment. J Clin Psychiatry 51:236–238, 1990

Breimer DD: Pharmacokinetics and metabolism of various benzodiazepines used as hypnotics. Br J Clin Pharmacol 8 (suppl):75–135, 1979

Breslow MF, Fankhauser MP, Potter RL, et al: Role of gamma-aminobutyric acid in antipanic drug efficacy. Am J Psychiatry 146:353–356, 1989

Browne JL, Hauge KJ: A review of alprazolam withdrawal. Drug Intelligence and Clinical Pharmacy 20:837–841, 1986

Buigues J, Vallejo J: Therapeutic response to phenelzine in patients with panic disorder and agoraphobia with panic attacks. J Clin Psychiatry 48:55–59, 1987

Burrows GD, Davies B, Fail L, et al: A placebo controlled trial of diazepam and oxprenolol for anxiety. Psychopharmacology 50:177–179, 1976

Busto U, Sellers EM, Naranjo CA, et al: Withdrawal reactions after long-term therapeutic use of benzodiazepines. N Engl J Med 315:854–859, 1986

Calabrese JR, Gulledge AD: Psychotropics during pregnancy and lactation: a review. Psychosomatics 26:413–426, 1985

Charney DS, Woods SW, Goodman WK, et al: Drug treatment of panic disorder: the comparative efficacy of imipramine, alprazolam, and tra-zodone. J Clin Psychiatry 47:580–586, 1986

Chouinard G, Annable L, Fontaine R, et al: Alprazolam in the treatment of generalized anxiety and panic disorders: a double-blind, placebo-controlled study. Psychopharmacology 77:229–233, 1982

Chouinard G, Goodman W, Greist J, et al: Results of a double-blind placebo-controlled trial of a new SSRI, sertraline, in the treatment of obsessive-compulsive disorder. Psychopharmacol Bull 26:279–284, 1990

Cohn JB, Wilcox CS: Low-sedation potential of buspirone compared with alprazolam and lorazepam in the treatment of anxious patients: a double-blind study. J Clin Psychiatry 47:409–412, 1986

Cohn JB, Bowden CL, Fisher JG, et al: Double-blind comparison of buspirone and clorazepate in anxious outpatients. Am J Med 80 (suppl 3B):10–16, 1986

Cole JO, Haskell DS, Orzack MH: Problems with benzodiazepines: an assessment of the available evidence. McLean Hospital Journal 6:46–74, 1981

Cole JO, Orzack MH, Beake B, et al: Assessment of the abuse liability of buspirone in recreational sedative users. J Clin Psychiatry 43:69–74, 1982

Coryell W, Noyes R, Clancy J: Panic disorder and primary unipolar depression: a comparison of background and outcome. J Affect Disord 5:311–317, 1983

Cross-National Collaborative Panic Study, Second Phase Investigators: Drug treatment of panic disorder: comparative efficacy of alprazolam, imipramine, and placebo. Br J Psychiatry 160:191–202, 1992

Davidson JRT, Kudler HS, Smith RD, et al: Treatment of post-traumatic stress disorder with amitriptyline and placebo. Arch Gen Psychiatry 4:259–269, 1990

Davidson JR, Potts N, Richichi E, et al: Treatment of social phobia with clonazepam and placebo. J Clin Psychopharmacol 13:423–428, 1993

Deltito JA, Argyle N, Klerman GL: Patients with panic disorder unaccompanied by depression improve with alprazolam and imipramine treatment. J Clin Psychiatry 52:121–127, 1991

Den Boer JA, Westenberg HGM: Effect of a serotonin and noradrenaline uptake inhibitor in panic disorder: a double-blind comparative study with fluvoxamine and maprotiline. Int Clin Psychopharmacol 3:59–74, 1988

Den Boer JA, Westenberg HGM: Serotonin function in panic disorder: a double-blind, placebo-controlled study with fluvoxamine and ritanserin. Psychopharmacology 102:85–94, 1990

Dommisse CS, De Vane CL: Buspirone: a new type of anxiolytic. Drug Intelligence and Clinical Pharmacy 19:624–628, 1985

Dubovsky SL: Generalized anxiety disorder: new concepts and psychopharmacologic therapies. J Clin Psychiatry 51 (suppl):3–10, 1990

Dunner DL, Ishiki D, Avery DH, et al: Effect of alprazolam and diazepam on anxiety and panic attacks in panic disorder: a controlled study. J Clin Psychiatry 47:458–460, 1986

Erman MK, Guggenheim FG: Psychiatric side effects of commonly used drugs. Drug Ther 11:117–126, 1981

Falloon IRH, Lloyd GG, Harpin RE: The treatment of social phobia: real-life rehearsal with non-professional therapists. J Nerv Ment Dis 169:180–184, 1981

Famularo R, Kinscherff R, Fenton T: Propranolol treatment for childhood post-traumatic stress disorder. J Clin Psychiatry 46:385–388, 1988

Feighner JP, Meredith CH, Hendrickson GH: A double-blind comparison of buspirone and diazepam in outpatients with generalized anxiety disorder. J Clin Psychiatry 43 (12 pt 2):102–107, 1982

Ferguson JM: Alprazolam-XR: patient acceptability, safety, and tolerability. Psychiatr Ann 23 (10, suppl):20–24, 1993

Fisher HK: Drug-induced asthma syndromes, in Bronchial Asthma: Mechanisms and Therapeutics. Edited by Weiss EB, Segal MS, Stein M. Boston, MA, Little, Brown, 1985, pp 938–949

Frank JB, Giller EL, Kosten T, et al: A randomized clinical trial of phenelzine and imipramine for post-traumatic stress disorder. Am J Psychiatry 145:1289–1291, 1988

Gall M, Kamdar BV, Collins RJ: Pharmacology of some metabolites of triazolam, alprazolam, and diazepam prepared by a simple, one-step oxidation of benzodiazepines. Journal of Medicinal Chemistry 21:1290–1294, 1978

Garzone PD, Kroboth PD: Pharmacokinetics of the newer benzodiazepines. Clin Pharmacokinet 16:337–364, 1989

Gelenberg AJ: Amnesia and benzodiazepines. Biological Therapies in Psychiatry 8:27, 1985

Gelenberg AJ: Benzodiazepines in pregnancy. Biological Therapies in Psychiatry 10:18–19, 1987

George KA, Dundee JW: Relative amnesic actions of diazepam, flunitrazepam, and lorazepam in man. Br J Clin Pharmacol 4:45–50, 1977

Gloger S, Grunhaus L, Birmacher B, et al: Treatment of spontaneous panic attacks with clomipramine. Am J Psychiatry 138:1215–1217, 1981

Gloger S, Brunhaus L, Gladic D, et al: Panic attacks and agoraphobia: low dose clomipramine treatment. J Clin Psychopharmacol 9:28–32, 1989

Goldberg HL: Buspirone hydrochloride: a unique new anxiolytic agent. Pharmacotherapy 4:314–324, 1984

Goldberg HL, Finnerty RJ: Comparative efficacy of buspirone and diazepam in the treatment of anxiety. Am J Psychiatry 136:1184–1187, 1979

Goldberg HL, Finnerty RJ: Comparison of buspirone in two separate studies. J Clin Psychiatry 43 (12 pt 2):87–91, 1982

Goodman WK, Price LH, Rasmussen SA, et al: Efficacy of fluvoxamine in obsessive-compulsive disorder: a double-blind comparison with placebo. Arch Gen Psychiatry 46:36–43, 1989a

Goodman WK, Price LH, Rasmussen SA, et al: The Yale-Brown Obsessive-Compulsive Scale, I: development, use, and reliability. Arch Gen Psychiatry 46:1006–1011, 1989b

Goodman WK, McDougle CJ, Barr LC, et al: Biological approaches to treatment-resistant obsessive compulsive disorder. J Clin Psychiatry 54 (suppl 6):16–26, 1993

Gorman JM, Liebowitz MR, Fyer AJ, et al: Treatment of social phobia with atenolol. J Clin Psychopharmacol 5:298–301, 1985

Gorman JM, Liebowitz MR, Fyer AJ, et al: An open trial of fluoxetine in the treatment of panic attacks. J Clin Psychopharmacol 7:258–260, 1987

Greenblatt DJ: Pharmacokinetic comparisons. Psychosomatics 21 (suppl):9–14, 28, 1980

Greenblatt DJ, Shader RI: Detection and quantification, in Benzodiazepines in Clinical Practice. New York, Raven, 1974, pp 17–19

Greenblatt DJ, Shader RI: Prazepam and lorazepam, two new benzodiazepines. N Engl J Med 299:1342–1344, 1978

Greenblatt DJ, Allen MD, Hormatz JS, et al: Diazepam disposition determinants. Clin Pharmacol Ther 27:301–312, 1980

Greenblatt DJ, Shader RI, Divoll M, et al: Benzodiazepines: a summary of pharmacokinetic properties. Br J Clin Pharmacol 11 (suppl):115–165, 1981

Greenblatt DJ, Shader RI, Abernathy DR: Current status of benzodiazepines, part I. N Engl J Med 309:354–358, 1983a

Greenblatt DJ, Shader RI, Abernathy DR: Current status of benzodiazepines, part II. N Engl J Med 309:410–416, 1983b

Greenblatt DJ, Harmatz JS, Shader RI: Clinical pharmacokinetics of anxiolytics and hypnotics in the elderly. Clin Pharmacokinet 21:165–177, 1991

Greenblatt DJ, Harmatz JS, Shader RI: Plasma alprazolam concentrations: relation to efficacy and side effects in the treatment of panic disorder. Arch Gen Psychiatry 50:715–722, 1993

Gringras M: An uncontrolled trial of clomipramine in the treatment of phobic and obsessional states in general practice. J Int Med Res 5 (suppl 5):111–115, 1977

Hafner RJ, Marks IM: Exposure in vivo of agoraphobics: contribution of diazepam, group exposure, and anxiety evocation. Psychol Med 6:71–88, 1976

Hallstrom C, Treasaden J, Edwards G: Diazepam, propranolol and their combination in the management of chronic anxiety. Br J Psychiatry 139:417–421, 1981

Hamilton M: The assessment of anxiety states by rating. Br J Med Psychol 32:50–55, 1959

Haskell DS, Gambill JD, Gardos G, et al: Doxepin or diazepam for anxious and anxious-depressed outpatients. J Clin Psychiatry 39:135–139, 1978

Herman JB, Rosenbaum JR, Brotman AW: The alprazolam to clonazepam switch for the treatment of panic disorder. J Clin Psychopharmacol 7:175–178, 1987

Hewlett WA, Vinogradov S, Agras WS: Clomipramine, clonazepam, and clonidine treatment of obsessive-compulsive disorder. J Clin Psychopharmacol 12:420–430, 1992

Hoehn-Saric R, McLeod DR, Zimmerli WD: Differential effects of alprazolam and imipramine in generalized anxiety disorder: somatic versus psychic symptoms. J Clin Psychiatry 49:293–301, 1988

Hoehn-Saric R, McLeod DR, Hipsley PA: Effect of fluvoxamine on panic disorder. J Clin Psychopharmacol 13:321–326, 1993

Hollister LE: Benzodiazepines 1980—current update: a look at the issues. Psychosomatics 21 (suppl):4–8, 1980

Hollister LE: Pharmacotherapeutic considerations in anxiety disorders. J Clin Psychiatry 47 (suppl):33–36, 1986

Jacobson AF, Dominguez RA, Goldstein BJ, et al: Comparison of buspirone and diazepam in generalized anxiety disorder. Pharmacotherapy 5:290–296, 1985

Jain VK, Swinson RP, Thoms JG: Phenelzine in obsessional neurosis. Br J Psychiatry 117:237–238, 1970

Jann MW, Kurtz NM: Treatment of panic and phobic disorders. Clinical Pharmacy 6:647–662, 1987

Jefferson JW: Social phobia: a pharmacologic treatment overview. J Clin Psychiatry 56 (suppl 5):18–24, 1995

Jenike MA: Rapid response of severe obsessive-compulsive disorder to tranylcypromine. Am J Psychiatry 138:1249–1250, 1981

Jenike MA, Baer L: An open trial of buspirone in obsessive-compulsive disorder. Am J Psychiatry 145:1285–1286, 1988

Jenike MA, Hyman S, Baer L, et al: A controlled trial of fluvoxamine in obsessive-compulsive disorder: implications for a serotonergic theory. Am J Psychiatry 147:1209–1215, 1990a

Jenike MA, Baer L, Summergrad P, et al: Sertraline in obsessive-compulsive disorder: a double-blind comparison with placebo. Am J Psychiatry 147:923–928, 1990b

Jenike MA, Baer L, Buttolph L: Buspirone augmentation of fluoxetine in patients with obsessive-compulsive disorder. J Clin Psychiatry 52:13–14, 1991

Johnson G, Singh B, Leeman M: Controlled evaluation of the β-adrenoceptor–blocking drug oxprenolol in anxiety. Med J Aust 1:909–912, 1976

Kahn RJ, McNair DM, Lipman RS, et al: Imipramine and chlordiazepoxide in depressive and anxiety disorders, II: efficacy in anxious outpatients. Arch Gen Psychiatry 43:79–85, 1986

Kales A, Schard MB, Kales JD, et al: Rebound insomnia: a potential hazard following withdrawal of certain benzodiazepines. JAMA 241:1692–1695, 1979

Katcher BS: General care: anxiety and insomnia, in Applied Therapeutics for Clinical Pharmacists, 2nd Edition. Edited by Koda-Kimble MA, Katcher BS, Young LY. San Francisco, CA, Applied Therapeutics, 1978, pp 71–85

Kathol RG, Noyes R, Slymen DJ, et al: Propranolol in chronic anxiety disorders. Arch Gen Psychiatry 37:1361–1365, 1980

Katzelnick DJ, Kobak KA, Greist JH, et al: Sertraline for social phobia: a double-blind, placebo-controlled crossover study. Am J Psychiatry 152:1368–1371, 1995

Kessler RC, McGonagle KA, Zhao S, et al: Lifetime and 12-month prevalence of DSM-III-R psychiatric disorders in the United States: results from the National Comorbidity Survey. Arch Gen Psychiatry 51:8–19, 1994

Klein E, Uhde TW: Controlled study of verapamil for treatment of panic disorder. Am J Psychiatry 145:431–434, 1990

Klotz U, Muller-Seydlitz P: Altered elimination of desmethyldiazepam in the elderly. Br J Clin Pharmacol 7:119–120, 1979

Klotz U, Avant GR, Hoyumpa A, et al: The effects of age and liver disease on the disposition and elimination of diazepam in adult man. J Clin Invest 55:347–359, 1975

Kolb LC, Burris BC, Griffiths S: Propranolol and clonidine in the treatment of PTSD of war, in Post-Traumatic Stress Disorder: Psychological and Biological Sequelae. Edited by Van der Kolk BA. Washington, DC, American Psychiatric Press, 1984, pp 98–105

Kosten TR, Frank JB, Dan E, et al: Pharmacotherapy for posttraumatic stress disorder using phenelzine or imipramine. J Nerv Ment Dis 179:366–370, 1991

La Porta LD, Ware MR: Buspirone in the treatment of posttraumatic stress disorder (letter). J Clin Psychopharmacol 12:133–134, 1992

Lader M: β-adrenoceptor antagonists in neuropsychiatry: an update. J Clin Psychiatry 49:213–223, 1988

Ladewig D, Grossenbacher H: Benzodiazepine abuse in patients of doctors in domiciliary practice in the Basle area. Pharmacopsychiatry 21:104–108, 1988

Laux G, Konig W: Long-term use of benzodiazepines in psychiatric patients. Acta Psychiatr Scand 76:64–70, 1987

Liebowitz MR: Imipramine in the treatment of panic disorder and its complications. Psychiatr Clin North Am 8:37–47, 1985

Liebowitz MR, Gorman JM, Fyer AJ, et al: Social phobia: review of a neglected disorder. Arch Gen Psychiatry 42:729–736, 1985

Liebowitz MR, Schneier F, Campeas R, et al: Phenelzine versus atenolol in social phobia: a placebo-controlled comparison. Arch Gen Psychiatry 49:290–300, 1992

Lipinski JF, Mallya G, Zimmerman P, et al: Fluoxetine-induced akathisia: clinical and theoretical implications. J Clin Psychiatry 50:339–342, 1989

Lister RG: The amnesic action of benzodiazepines in man. Neurosci Biobehav Rev 9:87–94, 1985

Louie AK, Lewis TB, Lannon RA: Use of low-dose fluoxetine in major depression and panic disorder. J Clin Psychiatry 54:435–438, 1993

Lucki I, Rickels K, Geller AM: Psychomotor performance following the long-term use of benzodiazepines. Psychopharmacol Bull 21:93–96, 1985

Marks I, O'Sullivan G: Drugs and psychological treatments for agoraphobia/panic and obsessive-compulsive disorders: a review. Br J Psychiatry 153:650–658, 1988

Matilla MJ, Aranko K, Seppala T: Acute effects of buspirone and alcohol on psychomotor skills. J Clin Psychiatry 43:56–60, 1982

Mavissakalian M, Michelson L: Agoraphobia: relative and combined effectiveness of therapist-assisted in vivo exposure and imipramine. J Clin Psychiatry 47:117–122, 1986

Mavissakalian M, Perel J: Imipramine in the treatment of agoraphobia: dose-response relationships. Am J Psychiatry 142:1032–1036, 1985

Mavissakalian MR, Perel JM: Imipramine dose-response relationship in panic disorder with agoraphobia: preliminary findings. Arch Gen Psychiatry 46:127–131, 1989

Mavissakalian MR, Perel JM: Protective effects of imipramine maintenance treatment in panic disorder with agoraphobia. Am J Psychiatry 149:1053–1057, 1992

Mavissakalian MR, Perel JM: Imipramine treatment of panic disorder with agoraphobia: dose ranging and plasma level–response relationships. Am J Psychiatry 152:673–682, 1995

Mavissakalian M, Perel J, Michelson L: The Fear Questionnaire: a validity study. Behav Res Ther 24:83–85, 1986

Mavissakalian M, Perel J, Bowler K, et al: Trazodone in the treatment of panic disorder and agoraphobia with panic attacks. Am J Psychiatry 144:785–787, 1987

McDougle CJ, Goodman WK, Leckman JF, et al: The psychopharmacology of obsessive compulsive disorder: implications for treatment and pathogenesis. Psychiatr Clin North Am 16:749–766, 1993a

McDougle CJ, Goodman WK, Leckman JF, et al: Limited therapeutic effect of addition of buspirone in fluvoxamine-refractory obsessive-compulsive disorder. Am J Psychiatry 150:647–649, 1993b

McLeod DR, Hoehn Saric R, Zimmerli WD, et al: Treatment effects of alprazolam and imipramine: physiological versus subjective changes in patients with generalized anxiety disorder. Biol Psychiatry 28:849–861, 1990

McMillin WP: Oxprenolol in anxiety. Lancet 1:1193, 1973

Meibach RC, Mullane JF, Binstok G: A placebo-controlled multicenter trial of propranolol and chlordiazepoxide in the treatment of anxiety. Current Therapeutic Research 41:65–70, 1987a

Meibach RC, Dunner D, Wilson LG, et al: Comparative efficacy of propranolol, chlordiazepoxide, and placebo in the treatment of anxiety: a double-blind trial. J Clin Psychiatry 48:355–358, 1987b

Modell JG: The high cost of buspirone (letter). J Clin Psychiatry 56:375, 1995

Modigh K, Westberg P, Eriksson E: Superiority of clomipramine over imipramine in the treatment of panic disorder: a placebo-controlled trial. J Clin Psychopharmacol 12:251–259, 1992

Moschitto L, Greenblatt DJ, Divoll M, et al: Alprazolam kinetics in the elderly: relation to antipyrine disposition (abstract). Clin Pharmacol Ther 29:267, 1981

Moskorvitz H, Smiley A: Effects of chronically administered buspirone and diazepam on driving-related skills performance. J Clin Psychiatry 43:45–56, 1982

Mountjoy CQ, Roth M, Garside RF, et al: A clinical trial of phenelzine in anxiety depressive and phobic neuroses. Br J Psychiatry 131:486–492, 1977

Munjack DJ, Rebal R, Shaner R, et al: Imipramine versus propranolol for the treatment of panic attacks: a pilot study. Compr Psychiatry 26:80–89, 1985

Munjack DJ, Crocker B, Cabe D, et al: Alprazolam, propranolol, and placebo in the treatment of panic disorder and agoraphobia with panic attacks. J Clin Psychopharmacol 9:22–27, 1989

Munjack DJ, Baltazar PL, Bohn PB, et al: Clonazepam in the treatment of social phobia: a pilot study. J Clin Psychiatry 51 (suppl):35–40, 1990

Murphy SM, Owen R, Tyrer P: Comparative assessment of efficacy and withdrawal symptoms after 6 and 12 weeks' treatment with diazepam or buspirone. Br J Psychiatry 154:529–534, 1989

Muskin PR, Fyer AJ: Treatment of panic disorder. J Clin Psychopharmacol 1:81–90, 1981

Newton RE, Casten GP, Alms DR, et al: The side effect profile of buspirone in comparison to active controls and placebo. J Clin Psychiatry 43:100–102, 1982

Noyes R: History of the treatment of anxiety, in Handbook of Anxiety: Biological, Clinical and Cultural Perspectives, Vol 1. Edited by Roth M, Noyes R Jr, Burrows GD. Amsterdam, Elsevier, 1988, pp 3–25

Noyes R, Anderson D, Clancy J: Diazepam and propranolol in panic disorder and agoraphobia. Arch Gen Psychiatry 41:287–292, 1984

Noyes R, Chaudry DR, Domingo DV: Pharmacologic treatment of phobic disorders. J Clin Psychiatry 47:445–452, 1986

Noyes R, Garvey MJ, Cook BL, et al: Problems with tricyclic antidepressant use in patients with panic disorder or agoraphobia: results of a naturalistic follow-up study. J Clin Psychiatry 50:163–169, 1989

Oehrberg S, Christiansen PE, Behnke K, et al: Paroxetine in the treatment of panic disorder: a randomized, double-blind, placebo-controlled study. Br J Psychiatry 167:374–379, 1995

Olajide D, Lader MH: A comparison of buspirone, diazepam and placebo in patients with chronic anxiety states. J Clin Psychopharmacol 7:148–152, 1987

Pato MT, Pigott TA, Hill JL, et al: Controlled comparison of buspirone and clomipramine in obsessive-compulsive disorder. Am J Psychiatry 148:127–129, 1991

Pecknold JC, Familamiri P, Chang H, et al: Buspirone: anxiolytic? Prog Neuropsychopharmacol Biol Psychiatry 9:639–642, 1985

Pecknold JC, Swinson RP, Kuch K, et al: Alprazolam in panic disorder and agoraphobia: results from a multicenter trial. Arch Gen Psychiatry 45:429–436, 1988

Peet M, Ali S: Propranolol and atenolol in the treatment of anxiety. International Clinical Psychopharmacology 1:314–320, 1986

Perry PJ, Alexander B: Sedative/hypnotic dependence: patient stabilization, tolerance testing, and withdrawal. Drug Intelligence and Clinical Pharmacy 20:532–537, 1986

Perry PJ, Garvey M, Noyes R: Benzodiazepine treatment of generalized anxiety disorder, in Handbook of Anxiety, Vol 4. Edited by Noyes R, Roth M, Burrows GD. Amsterdam, Elsevier, 1990, pp 111–124

Perse TL, Greist JH, Jefferson JW, et al: Fluvoxamine treatment of obsessive-compulsive disorder. Am J Psychiatry 144:1543–1548, 1988

Piccinelli M, Pini S, Bellantuono C, et al: Efficacy of drug treatment in obsessive-compulsive disorder: a meta-analytic review. Br J Psychiatry 166:424–443, 1995

Pigott TA, Pato MR, Berenstein SE, et al: Controlled comparison of clomipramine and fluoxetine in the treatment of obsessive-compulsive disorder. Arch Gen Psychiatry 47:926–932, 1990

Pigott TA, Pato MT, L'Heureux F, et al: A double-blind study of adjuvant buspirone hydrochloride in clomipramine-treated patients with obsessive-compulsive disorder. J Clin Psychopharmacol 12:11–18, 1992

Pohl R, Yeragani VK, Balon R, et al: The jitteriness syndrome in panic disorder patients treated with antidepressants. J Clin Psychiatry 49:100–104, 1988

Pohl R, Balon R, Yeragani VK, et al: Serotonergic anxiolytics in the treatment of panic disorder: a controlled study with buspirone. Psychopathology 22 (suppl):S60–S67, 1989

Pollack MH: Long-term management of panic disorder. J Clin Psychiatry 51 (suppl):11–13, 1990

Primeau F, Fontaine R, Beauclair L: Valproic acid and panic disorder. Can J Psychiatry 35:248–250, 1990

Reich J, Yates W: A pilot study of treatment of social phobia with alprazolam. Am J Psychiatry 145:733–736, 1988

Reidenberg MM, Levy M, Warner H, et al: Relationship between diazepam dose, plasma level, age, and central nervous system depression. Clin Pharmacol Ther 23:371–374, 1978

Reist C, Kauffman CD, Haier RJ: A controlled trial of desipramine in 18 men with post-traumatic stress disorder. Am J Psychiatry 146:513–516, 1989

Riblet LA, Eison AS, Eison MS, et al: Neuropharmacology of buspirone. Psychopathology (suppl 3):69–78, 1984

Rickels K, Weisman K, Norstad N, et al: Buspirone and diazepam in anxiety: a controlled study. J Clin Psychiatry 43:81–86, 1982

Rickels K, Case G, Downing RW, et al: Long-term diazepam therapy and clinical outcome. JAMA 250:767–771, 1983

Rickels K, Schweizer E, Csanalosi I, et al: Long-term treatment of anxiety and risk of withdrawal: prospective comparison of clorazepate and buspirone. Arch Gen Psychiatry 45:444–450, 1988

Rickels K, Downing R, Schweizer E, et al: Antidepressants for the treatment of generalized anxiety disorder: a placebo-controlled comparison of imipramine, trazodone, and diazepam. Arch Gen Psychiatry 50:884–895, 1993

Rizley R, Kahn RJ, McNair DM, et al: A comparison of alprazolam and imipramine in the treatment of agoraphobia and panic disorder. Psychopharmacol Bull 22:167–172, 1986

Roberts RK, Wilkinson GR, Branch RA, et al: Effects of age and parenchymal liver disease on the disposition and elimination of chlordiazepoxide (Librium). Gastroenterology 75:479–485, 1978

Robinson BF: Drugs acting on the cardiovascular system, in Meyler's Side Effects of Drugs, Vol 8. Edited by Dukes MNG. New York, Excerpta Medica, 1975, pp 442–445

Rosenberg AS, Kullingsjo NK, Bruun-Hansen BP, et al: Efficacy and safety of alprazolam, imipramine, and placebo in treating panic disorder: a Scandinavian multicenter study. Acta Psychiatr Scand 365:18–27, 1991

Salzman C: Behavioral side effects of benzodiazepines, in Adverse Effects of Psychotropic Drugs. Edited by Kane J, Lieberman JA. New York, Guilford, 1992, pp 139–152

Scharf MB, Jennings SW, Graham JP: Therapeutic substitution: clinical differences among benzodiazepine compounds. U.S. Pharmacist (Dec):1–12, 1988

Schneier FR, Liebowitz MR, Davies SO, et al: Fluoxetine in panic disorder. J Clin Psychopharmacol 10:119–121, 1990

Schneier FR, Saoud JB, Campeas R, et al: Buspirone in social phobia. J Clin Psychopharmacol 13:251–256, 1993

Schuckit MA: Current therapeutic options in the management of typical anxiety. J Clin Psychiatry 42 (sec 2):15–26, 1981

Schweizer E, Rickels K, Lucki I: Resistance to the anti-anxiety effect of buspirone in patients with a history of benzodiazepine use (letter). N Engl J Med 314:719–720, 1986

Seppala T, Korttila K, Hakkinen S, et al: Residual effects and skills related to driving after a single oral administration of diazepam, medazepam or lorazepam. Br J Clin Pharmacol 3:831–841, 1976

Seppala T, Aranko K, Matilla MJ, et al: Effects of alcohol on buspirone and lorazepam actions. Clin Pharmacol Ther 32:201–207, 1982

Shader RI, Greenblatt DJ: The use of benzodiazepines in clinical practice. Br J Clin Pharmacol 11:55–89, 1981

Shader RI, Greenblatt DJ, Harmatz JS, et al: Absorption and distribution of chlordiazepoxide in young and elderly male volunteers. J Clin Pharmacol 17:709–718, 1977

Shader RI, Greenblatt DJ, Ciraulo DA, et al: Effect of age and sex on disposition of desmethyldiazepam formed from its precursor clorazepate. Psychopharmacology 75:193–197, 1981

Shapiro AK, Stuening EL, Shapiro E, et al: Diazepam: How much better than placebo? J Psychiatr Res 17:51–73, 1983

Sheehan DV, Raj BA: Benzodiazepine treatment of panic disorder, in Handbook of Anxiety, Vol 4. Edited by Noyes R, Roth M, Burrows GD. Amsterdam, Elsevier, 1990, pp 169–206

Sheehan DV, Ballenger JC, Jacobsen G: Treatment of endogenous anxiety with phobic, hysterical, and hypochrondriacal symptoms. Arch Gen Psychiatry 37:511–519, 1980

Sheehan DV, Davidson J, Manschreck T, et al: Lack of efficacy of a new antidepressant (bupropion) in the treatment of panic disorder with phobias. J Clin Psychopharmacol 3:28–31, 1983

Sheehan DV, Coleman JH, Greenblatt DJ, et al: Some biochemical correlates of panic attacks with agoraphobia and their response to a new treatment. J Clin Psychopharmacol 4:66–75, 1984

Sheehan DV, Raj AB, Sheehan KH, et al: Is buspirone effective for panic disorder? J Clin Psychopharmacol 10:3–11, 1990

Sheehan DV, Raj AB, Harnett-Sheehan K, et al: The relative efficacy of high-dose buspirone and alprazolam in the treatment of panic disorder: a double-blind-controlled study. Acta Psychiatr Scand 88:1–11, 1993

Shestatzky M, Greenberg D, Lerer B: A controlled trial of phenelzine in posttraumatic stress disorder. Psychiatry Res 24:149–155, 1988

Solomon K, Hart R: Pitfalls and prospects in clinical research on antianxiety drugs: benzodiazepines and placebo—a review. J Clin Psychiatry 39:823–831, 1978

Solyom L, Heseltine GFD, Ledwidge B, et al: A comparative study of aversion relief and systematic desensitization in the treatment of phobias. Br J Psychiatry 119:299–303, 1971

Solyom L, Heseltine GFD, McClure DJ, et al: Behavior therapy versus drug therapy in the treatment of phobic neurosis. Canadian Psychiatric Association Journal 18:25–32, 1973

Spitzer RL, Endicott J, Robins E: Research Diagnostic Criteria: rationale and reliability. Arch Gen Psychiatry 35:773–782, 1978

St. Clair SM, Schirmer RG: First-trimester exposure to alprazolam. Obstet Gynecol 80:843–846, 1992

Suranyi-Cadotte BE, Bodnoff SR, Welner SA, et al: Antidepressant–anxiolytic interactions: involvement of the benzodiazepine–GABA and serotonin systems. Prog Neuropsychopharmacol Biol Psychiatry 14:633–654, 1990

Sussman N: Diazepam, alprazolam, and buspirone: review of comparative pharmacology, efficacy, and safety. Hospital Formulary 21:110–127, 1986

Sutherland SM, Davidson JRT: Pharmacotherapy for post-traumatic stress disorder. Psychiatr Clin North Am 17:409–423, 1994

Swinson RP, Pecknold JC, Kuch K: Psychopharmacological treatment of panic disorder and related states: a placebo controlled study of alprazolam. Prog Neuropsychopharmacol Biol Psychiatry 11:105–113, 1987

Taylor DP, Allen LE, Becker JA, et al: Changing concepts of the biochemical action of the anxioselective drug buspirone. Drug Development and Research 4:95–105, 1984

Teratogenicity of minor tranquilizers. FDA Drug Bulletin 5:14–15, 1975

Tesar GE, Rosenbaum JF, Pollack MH, et al: Clonazepam versus alprazolam in the treatment of panic disorder: interim analysis of data from a prospective, double-blind, placebo-controlled trial. J Clin Psychiatry 48 (suppl):S16–S19, 1987

Thompson TL, Moran MG, Nies AS: Drug therapy: psychotropic drug use in the elderly, part I. N Engl J Med 308:134–138, 1983

Tyrer P: Anxiolytics not acting at the benzodiazepine receptor: β-blockers. Prog Neuropsychopharmacol Biol Psychiatry 16:17–26, 1992

Tyrer PJ, Lader MH: Response to propranolol and diazepam in somatic and psychic anxiety. BMJ 2:14–16, 1974

Tyrer P, Candy J, Kelly D: A study of the clinical effects of phenelzine and placebo in the treatment of phobic anxiety. Psychopharmacologia 32:237–254, 1973

Uhde TW, Stein MB, Post RM: Lack of efficacy of carbamazepine in the treatment of panic disorder. Am J Psychiatry 145:1104–1109, 1988

Uhlenhuth EH, Matuzas W, Glass RM, et al: Response of panic disorder to fixed doses of alprazolam or imipramine. J Affect Disord 17:261–270, 1989

Valium® [diazepam] Product Information. Nutley, NJ, Roche Laboratories, 1984

Van der Kolk BA, Dreyfuss D, Michaels M, et al: Fluoxetine in posttraumatic stress disorder. J Clin Psychiatry 55:517–522, 1994

van Vliet IM, Den Boer JA, Westenberg HGM: Psychopharmacological treatment of social phobia: a double-blind placebo-controlled study with fluvoxamine. Psychopharmacology 115:128–134, 1994

Vargas MV, Davidson J: Post-traumatic stress disorder. Pediatr Clin North Am 16:737–748, 1993

Versiani M, Mundim FD, Nardi AE, et al: Tranylcypromine in social phobia. J Clin Psychopharmacol 8:279–283, 1988

Versiani M, Nardi AE, Mundim FD, et al: Pharmacotherapy of social phobia: a controlled study with moclobemide and phenelzine. Br J Psychiatry 161:353–360, 1992

Wells BG, Chu GC, Johnson R, et al: Buspirone in the treatment of posttraumatic stress disorder. Pharmacotherapy 11:340–343, 1991

Westerlund A: Central nervous system side-effects with hydrophilic and lipophilic β-blockers. Eur J Clin Pharmacol 28 (suppl):73–76, 1985

Wheadon DE, Bushnell W, Steiner M: A fixed-dose comparison of 20, 40, and 60 mg paroxetine to placebo in the treatment of obsessive-compulsive disorder. Paper presented at the Annual Meeting of the American College of Neuropharmacology, San Juan, PR, December 1993

Wheatley D: Comparative effects of propranolol and chlordiazepoxide in anxiety states. Br J Psychiatry 115:1411–1412, 1969

Wheatley D: Buspirone: multicenter efficacy study. J Clin Psychiatry 43 (12 pt 2):92–94, 1982

Wheeler EO, White PD, Reed EW, et al: Neurocirculatory asthenia: a 20-year follow-up study of 173 patients. JAMA 142:878–889, 1953

Wilkinson GR: The effects of liver disease and aging on the disposition of diazepam, chlordiazepoxide, oxazepam, and lorazepam in man. Acta Psychiatr Scand 274 (suppl):56–74, 1978

Yocca FD: Neurochemistry and neurophysiology of buspirone and gepirone: interactions at presynaptic and postsynaptic 5-HT$_{1A}$ receptors. J Clin Psychopharmacol 10 (suppl 3):6S–12S, 1990

Young LY, Riddiough MA: Essential hypertension, in Applied Therapeutics for Clinical Pharmacists, 2nd Edition. Edited by Koda-Kimble MA, Katcher BS, Young LY. San Francisco, CA, Applied Therapeutics, 1978, pp 146–147, 240–242

Zitrin CM, Klein DF, Woerner MG, et al: Treatment of phobia, I: comparison of imipramine hydrochloride and placebo. Arch Gen Psychiatry 40:125–138, 1983

Zung WW: Effect of clorazepate on depressed mood in anxious patients. J Clin Psychiatry 48:13–14, 1987

5

Hypnotics

Insomnia

Insomnia is defined as a nocturnal disturbance of the normal sleep cycle that produces adverse daytime consequences (Rosekind 1992). Before the indications for a hypnotic can be delineated, an understanding of the etiology of insomnia is necessary.

Sleep disturbances affect approximately 33% of the population annually. Only about 17% of patients consider the problem serious enough to seek help from a physician, and an even smaller group actually have insomnia (Rosekind 1992). Elderly patients over 65 years of age experience insomnia far more commonly than younger patients. The prevalence rate for insomnia is estimated to be 9% in the 20- to 30-year-old population versus 35%–50% in the population 65 years or older (Miles and Dement 1980). Insomnia can arise from a variety of underlying causes, which may be classified into five general areas.

Situational insomnia stems from circadian rhythm disturbances caused by shift work, jet lag, delayed sleep phase syndrome, and advanced sleep phase syndrome; poor sleep habits resulting from extended time in bed naps or an irregular sleep schedule; or a poor sleep environment secondary to noise, temperature, light, sleeping surface, or bed partner. Situational insomnia is usually a short-term problem that resolves once the psychological or physical stressor is removed (Gillin and Byerley 1990).

The most common diagnoses associated with *medical insomnia* are heart diseases, endocrinopathies, and neurological disorders (Moran and Stoudemire 1992). Cardiac diseases commonly associated with insomnia include coronary artery disease, angina, hypertension, and congestive heart failure. Endocrine disorders associated with insomnia include hyperthyroidism, diabetic neuropathies, acromegaly, Cushing's syndrome, premenstrual syndrome, and pregnancy. Neurological conditions associated with insomnia include Parkinson's disease, seizure disorders, Alzheimer's disease, and cerebral injuries (e.g., birth trauma, brain tumors, thalamotomy, Down's syndrome, mental retardation). Proper pharmacotherapy of the medical condition normally will result in attenuation or reversal of the insomnia. Other medical disorders also commonly associated with insomnia are hiatal hernia and esophagitis, chronic renal failure, chronic liver failure, urinary tract infections, prostatitis, sleep apnea, and chronic obstructive pulmonary disease (COPD). Narcolepsy and nocturnal myoclonus account for about 15% of patients with medical insomnia (Coleman et al. 1982).

It is estimated that between one-third and two-thirds of patients with *psychiatric illness* have chronic insomnia. Diagnoses commonly associated with psychiatric insomnia include panic disorder, generalized anxiety disorder, depression, borderline personality disorder, posttraumatic stress syndrome, bulimia, anorexia, obsessive-compulsive disorders, alcohol abuse, and drug abuse (Gillin and Byerley 1990). Again, as in medical insomnia, treatment consists of ameliorating the primary illness rather than prescribing sedative-hypnotic drugs for symptomatic relief of insomnia. About 35% of insomniac patients have psychiatric diagnoses (Coleman et al. 1982).

Drug-intake insomnia is associated with alcohol, caffeine, nicotine, and sympathomimetic ingestion. Dopamine-blocking drugs (e.g., phenothiazines, haloperidol, metoclopramide) may cause akathisia, which can result in insomnia. Other prescription drugs reported to disrupt sleep include methyldopa, propranolol, theophylline, β-adrenergic agonists (e.g., isoproterenol), antiarrhythmics, oral contraceptives, thyroid hormone, and stimulating antidepressants such as the selective serotonin reuptake inhibitors (SSRIs), bupropion, and protriptyline (Moran and Stoudemire 1992). Polysubstance abusers who experience insomnia are predisposed to drug abuse problems and for them use of sedative-hypnotics is not appropriate. Use of low-dose antidepressants such as amitriptyline or trazodone is indicated in such patients if medication is necessary.

Drug withdrawal insomnia is associated with the abrupt withdrawal of alcohol, anxiolytics, hypnotics, and all other rapid eye movement (REM)–suppressant drugs. The lengthy duration of REM rebound demands that *patients abusing central nervous system (CNS) depressants* be slowly titrated off the offending agent by substituting a long-acting benzodiazepine (BZD) such as diazepam over at least a 7- to 10-day period. It is estimated that 12% of patients with chronic insomnia have drug and alcohol dependency problems (Coleman et al. 1982). Primary or idiopathic insomnia is the most difficult to treat because the vagueness of the presentation makes it difficult to identify an obvious source of the complaint (Consensus Development Conference 1984). Patients with insomnia who suffer from sleep apnea, restless legs syndrome, or nocturnal myoclonus, or whose insomnia is treatment resistant, should be referred to a sleep-disorder specialist.

Patients' insomnia complaints can be characterized as either *sleep latency problems* or *sleep maintenance problems* (Rosekind 1992). Younger patients are more likely to have sleep latency problems, whereas older patients complain of sleep maintenance difficulties. Sleep problems increase with age and are more common among women (Rosekind 1992). Insomnia can also be classified according to its course. *Transient insomnia* and *short-term insomnia* usually develop in response to an acute stressor or to environmental changes associated with time zone and altitude changes. Stressors include drug use, examinations, bereavement reactions, hospitalization, recovery after surgery, and pain of more than 3 weeks' duration. Normally, transient or short-term insomnia improves with the passage of time as the patient adapts to the stress. If this does not occur, the physician should help the patient to identify and implement adaptive coping mechanisms (J. D. Kales et al. 1982).

Air travel across time zones also is commonly associated with insomnia (Gillin and Byerley 1990). Ordinarily a person requires 1 day to adjust to each eastward time zone crossed and slightly less than that for each westward time zone crossed. If an individual is traveling from Chicago to London (a 6-hour time change) and plans to stay for only a few days, there is obviously a problem. To minimize the effects of the time change in this situation, it is recommended that the individual sleep during his or her conventional nocturnal bedtime and avoid all substances such as alcohol and caffeine that interfere with sleep. The person may adjust more rapidly to the new environment if exposed to the "bright light" of morning on eastward trips and the "bright light" of evening on westward trips. Ideally, frequent airline fliers ought to schedule their flights so that their normal sleep cycle is not altered.

Insomnia can be induced in those living at **high altitudes** (>2,800 meters [9,300 feet]), a disturbance referred to as acute mountain sickness (AMS). This benign condition results from increased sympathetic nervous system activity. Other symptoms of AMS include headache, nausea, vomiting, irritability, dizziness, lethargy, and peripheral edema. Because of their respiratory-depressant properties, hypnotics should be avoided; acetazolamide, however, has been found effective (Gillin and Byerley 1990).

Chronic insomnia, by definition greater than 3 weeks in duration, is often multifaceted in its origin. Therefore, effective treatment frequently requires both nonpharmacological and pharmacological measures. Nonpharmacological treatments include the use of general measures (discussed in the following section), supportive counseling, and behavioral treatment. Pharmacological treatment primarily consists of the adjunctive use of hypnotic medication in patients with primary or idiopathic insomnia (A. Kales and J. D. Kales 1983).

Nonpharmacological Treatment of Insomnia

General *nonpharmacological treatment* measures should be recommended as the initial mode of therapy for patients experiencing insomnia. A meta-analysis involving more than 2,100 subjects from 59 controlled trials found that behavioral treatment of insomnia resulted in improvement in sleep induction and sleep maintenance. Sleep latency and sleep maintenance were 84% and 74% better, respectively, in the treated patients than in the untreated ones (Morin et al. 1994). General principles for nonpharmacological treatment of insomnia are presented in Table 5–1.

Sleep hygiene information.   The sleeping environment should be comfortable, familiar, and used specifically for sleep. Comfort can be maximized by the appropriate choice of mattress (not too hard), proper hygiene, temperature ($<75°F$), and humidity (Berlin 1984; A. Kales and J. D. Kales 1984). Familiarity includes the actual bedroom setting, amount of noise, and whether the patient normally sleeps alone or with a partner. Additionally, the patient should be informed to refrain from taking daytime naps, lounging in bed, keeping irregular sleep/wake schedules, using drugs that affect sleep (e.g., caffeine, alcohol, cigarettes [nicotine], sympathomimetics [appetite suppressants and decongestants], REM suppres-

---

Table 5–1.   Principles for nonpharmacological treatment of insomnia

Restrict bedroom use to sleep
Restrict time in bed
Avoid napping and daytime inactivity
Establish bedtime and wakeup time
Use outdoor light exposure
Discontinue use of alcohol, tobacco, caffeine, and REM-
    suppressant drugs

Note.   REM = rapid eye movement.

sants), exercising close to bedtime, and exposing him- or herself to stressful situations just before bedtime (Bootzin and Perlis 1992).

Sleep restriction.   Sleep restriction therapy is a simple maneuver that may be helpful. Because insomniac individuals often underestimate the amount of time they spend sleeping, their time in bed sleeping is restricted to their estimate. This underestimate results in mild sleep deprivation, which hastens the onset and improves the efficiency of sleep. As sleep improves, patients are gradually allowed to increase the amount of time spent in bed (Gillin and Byerley 1990). Sleeping schedules should be developed to provide not only for approximately 7 hours of sleep per night but also for a relaxation time before going to bed. This relaxation time should not take place in the bedroom.

Stimulus control.   Excessive sleeping, reading in bed, watching television in bed, or lounging in bed are not allowed. This form of stimulus control requires that if patients are unable to fall asleep within 15 to 20 minutes, they should leave the bedroom and not return until they feel sleepy. The bedtime schedule should be flexible, however, to allow for slight variations without causing undue anxiety to the patient. Sleep scheduling for patients should not only consider their sleeping habits but also include other daily activities. It is estimated that 26% of men and 18% of women work swing shifts. Daily activities should be synchronized around the work schedule. Thus, after work, regardless of the time of day, these individuals should eat dinner, relax, sleep, eat breakfast, and then return to work. External factors, such as lighting and temperature, should simulate those experienced during the normal evening sleep cycle (Gillin and Byerley 1990; A. Kales and J. D. Kales 1984). It is also known that, when rotating work shifts, employee productivity and morale are improved if the change is in a clockwise direction (Gillin and Byerley 1990).

Nutrition.   Good nutritional habits appear to be more important than using specific diets to induce sleep (Crisp 1980; Philips et al. 1975). Increases in body weight are associated with increases in total sleep time and other sleeping parameters, whereas abnormally low weight produces the opposite effect (A. Kales and J. D. Kales 1984). No foods have been found to have exceptional sleep-inducing properties, but a snack at bedtime consisting of either warm milk or cheese with cookies or crackers may be helpful, because the carbohydrate in the latter helps facilitate the transport of the dairy product's L-tryptophan into the brain.

Exercise. Moderate exercise appears to be most beneficial for improving sleep when practiced on a regular basis. However, it has less effect if performed during the late evening or in the morning. The data tentatively suggest that exercise may initially aggravate insomnia, but when conducted on a regular basis, it may help attenuate the problem (A. Kales and J. D. Kales 1984).

Relaxation therapy, meditation, and biofeedback. Probably the most important nonpharmacological strategy for treating insomnia has been the development of methods for managing the associated stress. The primary thrust of supportive counseling is to teach the insomniac person to externalize emotions during the day so that his or her thinking is not overwhelmed by daytime conflicts at bedtime. To accomplish this goal, the patient may find it useful to discuss problems on a regular basis with his or her spouse, friends, relatives, or a trusted professional (Bootzin and Perlis 1992). Behavioral treatments that have been helpful include relaxation therapy, meditation, yoga, hypnosis, and electromyogram biofeedback. These techniques help patients divert their attention away from the unpleasant ruminations that lead to insomnia (Bootzin and Perlis 1992). In transient insomnia, patients often do not associate their insomnia with daily stresses. Too often these stresses get taken to bed and may compound the problem. Therefore, patients should be instructed on how to recognize stressful situations and should be told to work through their stress before bedtime. In cases of chronic insomnia, the stress is often self-generated and may be an extension of smaller daily stressful situations that have not been dealt with properly. In these circumstances it is usually not sufficient to simply instruct the patient to take time each day to relax. Thus, insomniac patients may benefit from more formal stress management techniques. Biofeedback, progressive muscle relaxation, autogenic training, hypnosis, guided imagery–meditation training, and systematic desensitization have been used with success, although data substantiating their efficacy still are required (Gillin and Byerley 1990).

Bright-light therapy. Exposure to bright light from a light box (7,000–12,000 lux) for 2–3 days can shift the phase of the sleep cycle. To advance the sleep cycle, bright-light exposure in the morning will cause the patient to become sleepy earlier in the evening. Delaying the sleep cycle (i.e., a phase delay) is accomplished with light exposure in the evening. As an example, night-shift workers exposed to bright light will have their daytime sleep increase and be more alert on the job (Bootzin and Perlis 1992).

Benzodiazepines and Nonbenzodiazepines

■ Indications

Although limited, circumstances exist in which a hypnotic may be indicated. Pharmacological treatment of insomnia is advocated for transient insomnia. An individual facing a clearly identified external stress (e.g., grief reaction) may become acutely anxious and have difficulty sleeping. In such instances, the prn use of hypnotics for up to 3 weeks may be justified. However, the use of hypnotics should be considered only as an adjunct to primary nonpharmacological or medical therapeutic measures directed toward reversing the underlying cause of the insomnia. Additionally, it is incumbent on the physician to monitor closely the patient's use and need for hypnotics, because the patient is being exposed to a potentially addictive drug. Additionally, hypnotics may be used as adjunctive treatments or on an as-needed basis for the treatment of chronic insomnia (Consensus Development Conference 1984). These drugs should never be used for convenience, and should only be prescribed after a careful evaluation of the patient. Most hypnotics suppress REM sleep, and their effects may be seen the next day. These effects may include confusion, disorientation, and impairment of motor functions in the elderly (Goldson 1981).

Diagnosis and effective treatment of the primary cause can usually eliminate the need for hypnotic drugs to treat insomnia. Treating just the symptom, insomnia, not only can lead to difficulty in recognizing and treating the underlying illness but also subjects the patient to potential habituation and/or physical dependence on hypnotic drugs. Although seemingly obvious, these principles are often neglected, to the extent that insomnia has become one of the most common indications for therapy in the United States, and treatment of insomnia is usually with hypnotic agents rather than with nonpharmacological measures.

■ Efficacy

A survey by the National Academy of Sciences estimated that about one-third of Americans over 18 years of age have trouble sleeping within a given year, but that only 2% characterize this problem as insomnia (Solomon et al. 1979). About 17% of patients with sleeping problems, or about 6% of Americans, seek the help of a physician. Of these patients, it is estimated that 2.6%–3.1% of the adult population in the United States receive prescriptions for sleeping pills (Dement 1992). However, the use of sedative-hypnotic drugs has decreased dramatically in the last 20 years. Retail pharmacies dispensed approximately 62.5 million prescriptions for these drugs in 1970. That number declined to 31.6 million by 1978, and by 1989 it was 20.8 million (Wysowski and Baum 1991). The passage of the Controlled Substances Act of 1970 and the classification of hypnotics based on their potential for abuse and for physical and psychological dependence were probably the primary precipitants of this decline. Table 5–2 presents the Drug Enforcement Administration (DEA) categories of hypnotic drugs and their respective prescribing restrictions.

Because insomnia is a symptom in numerous diseases (Consensus Development Conference 1984), it must be remembered that hypnotics relieve the symptom only for a relatively short period and will have no effect, or possibly a detrimental effect, on the underlying disorder (Dement 1983). The criteria traditionally used to judge the effectiveness of hypnotic drugs are 1) degree of decrease in the sleep latency period, 2) reduction of nocturnal awakenings, 3) increase in total sleep time, and 4) subjective evaluations of the quality of sleep the patient experiences (Consensus Development Conference 1984). All hypnotics, as expected, reduce sleep latency, increase sleep time, and decrease nocturnal awakenings when first administered to insomniac individuals. However, these medications lose their efficacy as hypnotics after only 1–2 weeks of continuous use. Thus, sleeping pills are indicated only for the treatment of transient or short-term insomnia. There is now general agreement in the literature that BZDs should not be used for long periods of time to treat idiopathic chronic insomnia (Vogel 1992). REM sleep is reduced by all hypnotics and is accompanied by REM rebound after drug discontinuation. This phenomenon occurs with all hypnotic agents, although it may be less severe with chloral hydrate and the BZDs (Consensus Development Conference 1984). The absence of secondary daytime sedation from a particular dose of a hypnotic agent is as important an efficacy parameter as the four traditional criteria for evaluating efficacy noted above. The most common adverse drug reaction (ADR) in patients using hypnotics is a reduced ability to function on the morning after taking the medication. Coupling this ADR with the fact that insomniac patients report that their poor sleep impairs their daytime activities 2–3 days per week underscores the need to use hypnotics judiciously on a prn basis. The ultimate goal is better sleep *and* improved daytime functioning. Therefore, it is recommended that the clinician monitor and evaluate the insomniac

Table 5–2. **Drug Enforcement Administration (DEA) schedules of controlled hypnotics**

DEA Schedule	Drugs	Prescribing restriction
II: High abuse potential with severe dependence liability	amobarbital glutethimide pentobarbital phencyclidine secobarbital mixtures of the above (e.g., Tuinal®)	No telephoned prescriptions, no refills
III: Less abuse potential than Schedule II drugs and moderate dependence liability	Schedule II barbiturates combined with non- controlled drugs or in suppository form aprobarbital butabarbital methyprylon talbutal thiopental	Prescriptions must be re-written after 6 months or five refills
IV: Less abuse potential than Schedule III drugs and limited dependence liability	all benzodiazepines barbital chloral betaine chloral hydrate ethchlorvynol ethinamate mebutamate mephobarbital meprobamate methohexital paraldehyde petrichloral phenobarbital	Prescriptions must be re-written after 6 months or five refills; differs from Schedule III in the penalties for illegal possession

Source. Iowa Pharmacists Association 1992.

patient for a full 24-hour period to determine a hypnotic's effectiveness (Dement 1983).

The pharmacological criteria the clinician should use in selecting a hypnotic are as follows:

1. The agent must have low addiction and low suicide potential (i.e., a high therapeutic index).
2. The agent must alter the normal electroencephalogram (EEG) sleep pattern minimally and, therefore, not depress REM or non-REM sleep.

3. The agent must have minimal interactions with other drugs.
4. The agent must have a rapid rate of absorption, a high degree of lipophilicity to penetrate as well as exit the blood-brain barrier quickly, and a moderately rapid clearance rate, such that most of the drug is cleared from the patient's body once he or she wakes up.

The physician should also remember that because of the various underlying causes of insomnia, there is no one hypnotic that is useful for all patients (Dement 1983).

These criteria suggest that the **BZDs** marketed as hypnotics (e.g., *flurazepam, temazepam, quazepam, estazolam,* and *triazolam*) and *lorazepam* are the most useful hypnotics available to the clinician. Nonbenzodiazepines requiring consideration include *chloral hydrate, zolpidem, trazodone,* the sedating tricyclic *amitriptyline,* and the over-the-counter antihistamines *diphenhydramine* and *doxylamine.* The very favorable therapeutic index of the BZDs may be the single most important reason that there has been such a large shift away from barbiturates and related sleeping medications. More than 90% of the prescriptions currently written for hypnotics are for BZDs (Mendelson 1987). Because BZDs may be effectively used at doses far below toxic levels, fatalities due to overdoses with this class of drugs are extremely rare. Of 1,122 deaths reported to the American Association of Poison Control Centers over a 4-year period, only 66 (5.9%) involved BZDs. Only in five (0.4%) of these cases (three using alprazolam, one triazolam, and one temazepam) was the BZD the only agent ingested (Litovitz 1987). The obvious exception to minimal BZD mortality is the concomitant ingestion of these agents with alcohol or other interacting drugs and the use of these agents in patients with compromised respiratory function.

Benzodiazepines

Estazolam.   Estazolam was consistently more effective than placebo in seven inpatient and outpatient blinded studies of geriatric and nongeriatric populations treated for less than 7 days (Pierce and Shu 1990). Long-term-use (6 weeks) studies of geriatric and nongeriatric outpatient insomniac patients demonstrated the efficacy of estazolam 2 mg in decreasing sleep latency and nocturnal awakenings (Pierce and Shu 1990). Based on patients' daily assessments and the investigators' global evaluations, estazolam 2 mg and flurazepam 30 mg were more effective than placebo in treating outpatient insomniac patients for 7 consecutive nights (Scharf et al. 1990).

Flurazepam. In 16 studies, flurazepam 15–30 mg/night was more effective than chloral hydrate 500 mg, glutethimide 500 mg, diazepam 5 mg, or placebo (Rickels et al. 1983). However, the chloral hydrate and diazepam doses were quite probably subtherapeutic. A hypnotic dose of diazepam is generally considered to be 20 mg. Sustained efficacy was reported at 2–4 weeks for flurazepam 30 mg (some studies reported tolerance within 2 to 3 weeks) and at 1 week for flurazepam 15 mg (Gillin and Byerley 1990). In placebo-controlled studies, significant improvement in the flurazepam 15- and 30-mg groups occurred initially but there were no differences after 2–3 weeks (Gillin and Byerley 1990). In some subjects, decreased sleep latency was not observed until the second night of administration, which is consistent with the long $t_{1/2}$ of flurazepam and the carryover effect of the desalkylflurazepam metabolite (A. Kales et al. 1976). Although effective for up to 4 weeks, flurazepam was associated with some evidence of mild REM suppression in the longer studies. Nightly administration of flurazepam consistently decreased sleep latency, increased total sleep time, and decreased nocturnal awakenings and delta sleep.

Lorazepam. A weeklong trial of lorazepam 2 mg was as effective as temazepam 20 mg in the treatment of insomnia in elderly geriatric patients (Linnoila et al. 1980). Even more intriguing, however, was the 3-week sleep laboratory study that found lorazepam 2 mg more effective on most sleep parameters than flurazepam 30 mg (McClure et al. 1988). These efficacy findings, coupled with the drug's short half-life and lack of active metabolites, make lorazepam an ideal hypnotic for use in the geriatric population.

Quazepam. Four sleep-laboratory studies demonstrated the effectiveness of the short-term use (1–4 days) of quazepam 7.5 mg, 15 mg, and 30 mg in insomniac patients (A. Kales 1990). Another five sleep-laboratory studies documented the continued effectiveness of quazepam after 14 and 28 consecutive days of use, although the drug's effectiveness begins to fade between 14 and 28 days of consecutive use (A. Kales 1990).

Triazolam. Triazolam 0.25–0.5 mg hs (i.e., taken at bedtime) for 1 day to 3 months decreased latency, increased total sleep time, decreased awakenings, and subjectively improved the quality of sleep significantly more than did placebo, chloral hydrate 500 mg, methyprylon 300 mg, or secobarbital 100 mg (Rickels et al. 1983). In placebo-controlled studies, significant improvement in the triazolam 0.5-mg group occurred initially, but there were no differences after 2–3 weeks (Gillin and Byerley 1990). The short-term efficacy of triazolam is documented for doses of 0.125 mg/day in elderly (Bayer et al. 1989; Woo et al. 1991) and of 0.25 mg/day in non-elderly adults (Bonnet et al. 1988; Nicholson et al. 1982). However, a 1-week trial of triazolam 0.25 mg found the drug effective initially but not at the end of the week (Roth et al. 1977). In 1-day crossover studies, it appears that triazolam is preferable to flurazepam, but this difference disappears after several days of chronic use. However, both rebound insomnia and anxiety are more likely when this short-acting BZD is abruptly withdrawn. Additionally, anterograde amnesia occurs at dosages of 0.25 mg or greater. In contrast, it should be noted that the longer-acting BZDs are more likely to cause daytime sedation and morning hangover.

Temazepam.   The original U.S.–marketed formulation of temazepam, a hard gelatin capsule, had a much slower rate of absorption than the European-marketed product, a liquid-filled gelatin capsule, with peak plasma concentrations occurring 2–3 hours after ingestion (Greenblatt 1992). The slow absorption from the gastrointestinal (GI) tract rendered this product ineffective for inducing sleep in patients with initial insomnia (Bixler et al. 1978; Mitler et al. 1979). However, the dosage form was reformulated such that peak plasma concentrations occur at 1.5 hours, which is similar to the absorption rates of other U.S.–marketed BZD hypnotics (Locniskar and Greenblatt 1990). One temazepam 20-mg capsule (liquid-filled gelatin capsule) has been demonstrated to be as effective as flurazepam 30 mg (De Jonghe et al. 1984). Regardless of which pharmaceutical formulation is used, there is general agreement that temazepam improves sleep maintenance in insomniac patients, as evidenced by significant decreases in the number and duration of nocturnal awakenings and an increase in total sleep time (Bixler et al. 1978; Mitler et al. 1979; Nicholson and Stone 1979).

Nonbenzodiazepines

Amitriptyline.   Amitriptyline at low doses has been used for years as a sedative. Amitriptyline 50 mg for 28 consecutive nights increased total sleep time and deep (stages III and IV) sleep and decreased sleep latency and REM sleep compared with placebo. REM rebound occurred upon abrupt discontinuation of the drug (Hartmann and Cravens 1973). In a study in healthy volunteers, the sedative effects of amitriptyline 37.5 mg hs and 75 mg hs persisted for the full 14 days of the study (Sakulsripong et al. 1991). However, because of the CNS anticholinergic effects of the drug, subjects experienced significant cognitive memory deficits as a result of using the amitriptyline as a sedative. Thus, use of sedating tricyclics that have potent CNS anticholinergic activity is not recommended.

Chloral hydrate. A review of seven chloral hydrate sleep-laboratory studies considered only three studies definitive (Kay et al. 1976). These three studies used 500–1,000 mg/night given for 3–28 consecutive nights to healthy subjects. Consistent findings included an increase in total sleep time (primarily spindle—or stage II—sleep), a decrease in wakefulness, and a decrease in sleep latency. No effect was noted on delta or REM (dream) sleep. After drug discontinuation, REM rebound was not noted. The beneficial effects reportedly disappear within 2 weeks (Rall 1990).

Diphenhydramine. This antihistamine is used to treat insomniac patients. Diphenhydramine 50 mg at bedtime for 2 weeks was more effective than placebo in decreasing sleep latency and having patients wake feeling rested (Rickels et al. 1983). A 5-day crossover-design study of diphenhydramine 50 mg versus temazepam 15 mg and placebo found diphenhydramine more effective than placebo in decreasing sleep latency and, by the fifth night, more effective than temazepam in increasing total sleep time (Meuleman et al. 1987). Diphenhydramine 12.5 mg, 25 mg, and 50 mg were effective in improving sleep in 60%–70% of psychiatric patients with insomnia (Kudo and Kurihara 1990). A dose-dependent increase in the "hypnotic" effect was observed in the insomnia treatment–naive patients. Although the drug is effective in the treatment of insomnia, the appropriate dosage will depend on previous medical treatment of insomnia. One important caveat regarding diphenhydramine dosing is that doses greater than 50 mg (e.g., 150 mg) do not increase the effect on sleep but do increase the risk of CNS anticholinergic-induced delirium (Teutsch et al. 1975).

Doxylamine. Single 25- and 50-mg doses of doxylamine, an antihistamine, were equally effective in treating chronically ill hospitalized patients who were accustomed to taking nightly hypnotics (Sjoqvist and Lasagna 1967). The antihistamine was equal in effectiveness to secobarbital 100 mg but less effective than secobarbital 200 mg.

Trazodone. Trazodone 50 mg hs is commonly prescribed as a sleeping medication. Thus, it is important to determine whether the data support this practice. Using noninsomniac subjects, a 4-day sleep-laboratory study compared trazodone 50 mg, 100 mg, 150 mg, and 200 mg with placebo and with the sedating tricyclic trimipramine 25 mg, 50 mg, 100 mg, and 200 mg, respectively, on consecutive nights. The only difference observed among the three treatments was that trazodone significantly increased stage IV—or deep—sleep (Ware and Pittard 1990). In another study in healthy volunteers, the sedative effects of trazodone 100 mg hs and 200 mg hs persisted for the full 14 days of the study (Sakulsripong et al. 1991). In a controlled trial, six patients with chronic insomnia and associated dysthymia were treated with trazodone titrated from 50 to 150 mg/day over 6 weeks (Parrino et al. 1994). By day 4 of treatment, patients receiving trazodone 50 mg/day showed significantly increased stage 2 sleep and slow-wave sleep, although sleep latency and sleep maintenance never benefited from treatment. Higher doses did not produce an additive effect on the affected sleep parameters. A double-blind crossover trial comparing the sleep-inducing effectiveness of trazodone and placebo in 17 depressed patients found trazodone to be an effective hypnotic for antidepressant (i.e., fluoxetine or bupropion)–induced insomnia (Nierenberg et al. 1994).

Zolpidem.   Ten placebo-controlled trials concluded that zolpidem 10 mg and 20 mg are effective in decreasing sleep latency and increasing total sleep duration. The drug's effect on nocturnal awakenings was somewhat equivocal. In the 8 trials in which zolpidem was compared with a BZD (triazolam, oxazepam, flurazepam, or flunitrazepam), zolpidem was found to be as effective as the BZD in inducing and maintaining sleep. Additionally, abrupt discontinuation of zolpidem did not result in rebound insomnia or withdrawal effects, as occurs with the BZDs, probably because zolpidem does not suppress REM sleep (Hoehns and Perry 1993).

■ Mechanism of Action

Despite 70 years of research, the neurochemical basis of sleep and wakefulness and the mechanism of action of hypnotics have not been established. The mechanism of action may be related to the interactions of the drugs with the monoamine neurotransmitters (norepinephrine, dopamine, and serotonin) and acetylcholine. There is some evidence that non-REM sleep is precipitated by the synaptic release of serotonin from neurons originating in the rostral raphe nuclei in the brain stem, whereas REM sleep is initiated by the release of serotonin from neurons originating in the caudal raphe nuclei. Wakefulness and cortical arousal depend on norepinephrine-containing neurons of the anterior locus coeruleus, dopamine-containing neurons in the mesencephalic reticular formation, and acetylcholine-containing neurons in the cortex (Rall 1990).

Most, if not all, of the actions of the BZDs are the result of potentiation of γ-aminobutyric acid (GABA)–mediated neuronal inhibition. Effects of BZDs are decreased by GABA antagonists such as bicuculline or GABA synthesis inhibitors such as thiosemicarbazide. Thus, the BZDs' ability to produce sedation is attributed to their ability to potentiate GABAergic pathways that regulate the firing of neurons containing excitatory monoamine compounds that promote behavioral arousal while they inhibit the behavioral effects of fear and punishment. This dual activity is believed to occur via two pharmacologically distinct BZD receptors: high-affinity (type I) sites and low-affinity (type II) sites (Gershon and Eison 1987). It has been proposed that the anxiolytic effects of BZDs are mediated by type I receptors, whereas sedation effects are mediated by type II receptors (Manfredi and Kales 1987). The high therapeutic index of the BZDs is a result of the self-limited neuronal depression they produce because their action requires the release of the endogenous neurotransmitter GABA at higher doses. The barbiturates, despite having a similar effect on GABA, have a low therapeutic index. Although barbiturates inhibit the release of excitatory neurotransmitters at low doses, at higher doses they mimic the inhibitory action of GABA, thereby producing CNS depression (Rall 1990).

The barbiturates produce their CNS-depressant effects unevenly but diffusely throughout the CNS. The mesencephalic reticular activating system is especially sensitive to the suppression of polysynaptic responses produced by these agents. Inhibition of the responses is most obvious at the synapses, where neuronal inhibition is mediated by GABA, glycine, or the monoamine neurotransmitters. The site of the inhibition is either postsynaptic at the cortical and cerebellar pyramidal cells, cuneate nucleus, substantia nigra, and thalamic relay neurons, or presynaptic in the spinal cord. At low doses, the barbiturates potentiate the GABAergic-induced increase in chloride ion conductance. In high doses, they depress the calcium-dependent action potentials, decrease calcium-dependent release of neurotransmitters, and increase chloride ion conductance in the absence of GABA. It is clinically relevant that the barbiturates do not displace BZDs from binding sites. Instead, they enhance this binding by increasing the binding site's affinity for the BZD. Additionally, the barbiturates also enhance the binding of GABA and its agonist analogs (Rall 1990). Other drugs believed to have mechanisms of actions similar to the barbiturates' include chloral hydrate, glutethimide, and methyprylon (Rall 1990).

Zolpidem, a nonbenzodiazepine sedative-hypnotic, binds to the same GABA–chloride ion channel to which BZDs bind and is believed to act in the same manner as BZDs at these receptors. Its main difference from BZDs is its high affinity for the BZ_1 receptors, which are located in the cerebellum and cerebral cortex. No BZ_1 receptors are found in the spinal cord or the peripheral tissues. Although the relative significance of selective BZ_1 binding is not known, zolpidem's ability to selectively affect sleep suggests that this mechanism is possibly involved in inducing sleep. Unlike the BZDs, zolpidem lacks anticonvulsant and myorelaxant properties, and its anxiolytic activity is not clinically observable because of its overlapping sedative activity (Hoehns and Perry 1993).

Diphenhydramine, doxylamine, and the sedating tricyclic antidepressant amitriptyline are other agents often employed as sedative-hypnotics. Pharmacologically, they are histamine$_1$ blockers (Rall 1990).

■ Dosage

The proper and successful clinical dosing of hypnotic drugs requires that the patient be made aware of the limitations of these agents. First, the drugs should be taken on a *prn* basis rather than a continuous nightly schedule. This practice will decrease the risk of habituation and increase the duration of effectiveness of the drug. The use of short-half-life hypnotics is imperative because accumulation will result with any doses at intervals shorter than five times the drug's half-life. This means that any drug and its metabolites with half-life values of greater than 5 hours will result in accumulation if the drug is administered chronically rather than on a prn basis. Physicians often find it useful to write their hypnotic drug orders so that a patient can have only three hypnotic doses per week. This practice requires patients to be more thoughtful when assessing their needs for a sleeping pill. Thrice-weekly dosing also decreases problems with hangover or daytime sedation, especially from hypnotics with a long $t_{1/2}$. Second, the patient should be aware that occasional insomnia does not constitute a serious health problem. As a result of *intrinsic sleep deprivation*, a night of poor sleep is usually compensated by good sleep on the following night without any drug intervention. Third, the patient should be given the *smallest recommended dose*, to be increased only if there is objective and subjective evidence that the initial dose is ineffective. Interestingly, the short-half-life (mean 5.5 hours) BZD hypnotic brotizolam improved daytime performance at a dose of 0.25 mg and worsened daytime performance at 0.5 mg (Roehrs et al. 1983). Thus, the consequences of increasing the dose of a hypnotic must be carefully monitored. The importance of adhering to the smallest-recommended-dose axiom cannot be overstated, given that this strategy attenuates or prevents the most common ADRs associated with these compounds—namely, daytime sedation and performance decrements, anterograde amnesia, and rebound insomnia.

In November 1991, the U.S. Food and Drug Administration (FDA) approved new labeling for triazolam in which it emphasized that the drug is indicated for the **short-term** (7–10 days) treatment of insomnia ("New Halcion Labeling" 1992): "Treatment lasting longer than 2–3 weeks requires a complete reevaluation." As can be concluded from the preceding paragraph, our dosing recommendations are more conservative than the FDA's. Additionally, the FDA suggests 0.25 mg as an initial dose of triazolam. However, because of possible memory dysfunction associated with the BZDs, it is strongly recommended that the initial dose of triazolam and of flurazepam not exceed 0.125 mg and 15 mg, respectively (Perry and Smith 1991).

When selecting a hypnotic for a geriatric patient, clinicians must take special care to select either a drug with a short $t_{1/2}$ or one with a metabolic pathway that is not affected by age. Aging is associated with an increase in sensitivity to psychotropic drugs and a prolongation of their activity. A good clinical rule to follow is that a standard dose of a drug will result in greater sensitivity and a longer duration of activity in an elderly patient than in a younger patient (Lader 1986). Generally, metabolism of drugs in the elderly is slower. This is particularly true for BZDs that are metabolized by phase I pathways (hydroxylation and demethylation). However, the effect of advancing age on the clearance of BZDs that are metabolized by phase II conjugation pathways (e.g., lorazepam and oxazepam) is negligible (Greenblatt et al. 1982). Although not commonly used as a hypnotic, lorazepam 2 mg can be employed in treating insomnia in the elderly population because its $t_{1/2}$ is relatively short (12–18 hours) and it has no active metabolites (Linnoila et al. 1980). Higher doses (4 mg) are not recommended because they are associated with anterograde amnesia.

■ Pharmacokinetics

In insomnia treatment, drug action is preferably restricted to the evening hours so that no residual sedative effects are discernible to the patient during the day. Thus, a hypnotic with a rapid rate of elimination or a short $t_{1/2}$ is ideal. Patients receiving hypnotics expect a rapid onset of action, which requires that the drug be quickly absorbed after oral administration and rapidly distributed into the CNS. Thus, rapid absorption, distribution, and elimination are desirable for hypnotics (Breimer 1977).

Most barbiturates have long elimination $t_{1/2}$s (i.e., >24 hours). Exceptions include the highly fat-soluble barbiturates used for general anesthesia, methohexital, hexobarbital, and heptabarbital. Barbiturate salts are rapidly absorbed. The presence of liver disease increases the $t_{1/2}$, and the presence of renal disease results in the accumulation of pharmacologically active polar metabolites (Breimer 1977).

Flurazepam and its two active metabolites exhibit characteristics of both short- and long-acting hypnotics. Flurazepam and its hydroxyethyl metabolite are very short acting and are primarily responsible for sleep induction. The elimination $t_{1/2}$ of flurazepam's long-acting metabolite desalkylflurazepam is influenced by aging in males, by liver disease, and by enzyme-inducing and -inhibiting drugs (Greenblatt et al. 1983). Desalkylflurazepam's elimination $t_{1/2}$ ranges from 40 to 103 hours (average 72 hours), whereas that of flurazepam's other metabolite, hydroxyethylflurazepam, is short ranging, from 0.9 to 1.1 hour (mean 1.1 hour) (Eckert et al. 1983). Only 5% of orally administered flurazepam is metabolized to desalkylflurazepam (Amrein et al. 1983). It has been found that the free fraction of the hydroxyethyl metabolite is seven times greater than the desalkyl metabolite, which suggests that the former metabolite is primarily responsible for the hypnotic action for the first few days until the longer-acting desalkyl metabolite begins to accumulate (Cooper and Drolet 1982). Flurazepam has an intermediate rate of absorption, followed by that of triazolam, and then temazepam (Manfredi and Kales 1987).

Peak levels of **estazolam** occur usually within 2 hours (mean 1.9 hour). The drug is extensively metabolized by the liver, with an elimination $t_{1/2}$ of 10–24 hours (mean 14 hours). Estazolam is 93% protein bound, and less than 5% of a dose is excreted in the urine unchanged. Although two active metabolites are generated, they are present in insufficient quantities to contribute significantly to the pharmacological activity of the drug (A. Kales 1990).

Peak levels of **quazepam** usually occur within 2 hours (mean 1.5 hour) of ingestion. The drug is extensively metabolized by the liver, with an elimination $t_{1/2}$ of 25–41 hours (mean 40 hours) for both the parent drug and the 2-oxoquazepam metabolite, whereas the $t_{1/2}$ for the N-desalkylflurazepam metabolite is 70–75 hours. Quazepam and its metabolites are more than 95% protein bound, and 31% of a dose is excreted in the urine unchanged. Although two active metabolites are generated, they are present in insufficient quantities to contribute significantly to the drug's pharmacological activity (Gustavson and Carrigan 1990).

Temazepam, a hydroxylated diazepam metabolite, is slowly absorbed, with peak levels occurring approximately 2.5 hours after ingestion (i.e., hard-gelatin capsule). Thus, this drug is of little benefit for inducing sleep unless ingested approximately 2 hours before bedtime (Rall 1990). The elimination $t_{1/2}$ ranges between 8 and 24 hours (average 13 hours) in healthy subjects. This $t_{1/2}$ is not drastically changed in the elderly, because the drug is metabolized by conjugation (Lader 1986). Temazepam is biotransformed to an inactive glucuronide metabolite (Manfredi and Kales 1987).

Triazolam is metabolized by hepatic oxidation. However, the elimination $t_{1/2}$ is quite short, ranging from 1.5 to 5 hours, so that accumulation of the drug normally will not occur. The drug reaches peak blood concentrations within 1 to 2 hours after ingestion and has a higher hepatic clearance rate than other BZDs. Thus, if a patient's hepatic blood flow is reduced as a result of aging or microsomal enzyme-inhibiting drugs, one would expect to see accumulation of the drug. It appears that the $t_{1/2}$ is not significantly altered in such situations. However, the amount of drug distributed is significantly increased because of a reduced first-pass effect through the liver secondary to a decrease in hepatic blood flow or hepatic enzyme inhibition (Greenblatt et al. 1982).

Chloral hydrate is an inactive drug that is reduced by alcohol dehydrogenase in the liver to its active metabolite trichloroethanol as well as oxidized to its inactive metabolite trichloroacetic acid and conjugated to trichloroethanol glucuronide. Peak concentrations of trichloroethanol occur within 20 to 60 minutes after oral administration, and the elimination $t_{1/2}$ ranges between 4 and 12 hours. Trichloroacetic acid's $t_{1/2}$ is approximately 4 days. The drug is capable of displacing drugs such as tolbutamide, phenytoin, and warfarin from albumin binding sites (see **Chloral Hydrate** drug interactions [page 488] under **Anxiolytic-Hypnotics** in Chapter 8) (Breimer 1977).

Zolpidem is both rapidly and well absorbed on an empty stomach in healthy subjects, with peak levels occurring at approximately 1 hour. The mean terminal elimination $t_{1/2}$ is 1.7 hour. The unbound fraction of zolpidem in plasma was 8.1% in healthy volunteers, 10.8% in renal failure patients (14.9% before and 9.8% after hemodialysis), and 11.3% in cirrhotic patients. Hemodialysis produced a significant reduction of the unbound fraction. Cirrhotic patients had only 60% of the albumin concentration of the healthy volunteers. The hypoalbuminemic state was the cause of decreased protein binding in cirrhotic patients. Zolpidem's pharmacokinetics have also been characterized in the elderly (70–85 years). Zolpidem 20 mg resulted in a 55% increase in C_{max}, a 68% increase in the area under the curve (AUC), and 16% increase in the $t_{1/2}$. The drug is extensively metabolized to three major inactive metabolites. Only trace amounts of the parent drug appear in the urine (Hoehns and Perry 1993).

Table 5–3 summarizes the pharmacokinetic parameters for barbiturates, BZDs, and other hypnotics.

■ Adverse Effects

The Boston Collaborative Drug Surveillance Program (BCDSP) reported efficacy data and adverse reaction rates for hypnotics (Miller and Greenblatt 1976). Its findings are somewhat surprising in that pentobarbital had the lowest failure rate and the lowest adverse reaction rate. These data are presented and summarized in Table 5–4.

Barbiturates

Pentobarbital had ADR rates similar to those of chloral hydrate and diphenhydramine, whereas secobarbital's rate was similar to those of chloral hydrate, diphenhydramine, and flurazepam. The high rate observed for phenobarbital reflects the drug's long $t_{1/2}$, which produces the highest hangover rate of any of these drugs. Tuinal, a combination of secobarbital and amobarbital, probably acquired its high hangover rate of 5.4% because of the higher total dose (200 mg) used in 40% of its recipients. The barbiturates are potent inducers of microsomal enzymes and may antagonize the pharmacological effects of drugs such as monoamine oxidase inhibitors, tricyclic antidepressants, phenytoin, and coumarin oral anticoagulants. However, none of these interactions were observed by the BCDSP despite more than 5,000 patients having received barbiturate doses while hospitalized (Miller and Greenblatt 1976). An increased sensitivity and paradoxical response (including agitation, restlessness, and psychosis) to barbiturates occurs in the elderly (Lader 1986). Because of this, the World Health Organization (1981) recommended that barbiturates not be used in elderly individuals. Additionally, impaired renal and liver function contribute to altered elimination of these drugs and increased toxicity (Lader 1986).

Chloral Hydrate

Although the symptoms of CNS depression (i.e., hangover) were the most common ADRs of chloral hydrate, the incidence of

Table 5–3. Hypnotic pharmacokinetic parameters

Drug	Half-life (hours)	Volume of distribution (L/kg)	Protein binding (%)	Active metabolite(s)
Amobarbital	12–27	0.5–1.2	61	—
Chloral hydrate	7–10	0.6	70–80	trichloroethanol
Ethchlorvynol	19–32	2.4–3.2	—	—
Flurazepam	72	—	—	desalkylflurazepam
Estazolam	10–24	—	93	1-oxoestazolam, 4-hydroxyestazolam
Glutethimide	75–22	2.7	54	—
Hexobarbital	3–7	1.1	—	—
Midazolam	2–5	0.8–1.2	94–97	hydroxymidazolam
Nitrazepam	18–34	2.1	90	—
Oxazepam	76–25	1.6	90	2-oxoquazepam
Paraldehyde	3.4–9.8	—	—	—
Pentobarbital	23–30	0.9–1.0	60–70	—
Phenobarbital	748–144	0.5–0.6	50–60	—
Quazepam	25–41	5–8.6	> 95%	2-oxoquazeapm, N-desalkylflurazepam
Secobarbital	20–28	1.5	46–70	—
Temazepam	78–24	1.3–1.5	96–98	—
Triazolam	1.5–5.0	1.0	80–90	—
Zolpidem	1.7	0.54	92%	—

Source. Breimer 1977; Dundee et al.1984; Greenblatt et al. 1983; Heel and Avery 1980; Hoehns and Perry 1993.

Table 5–4.   Boston Collaborative Drug Surveillance Program efficacy data and adverse reaction rates

Drug	N	Failure rate (%)	Adverse reactions n	%
Chloral hydrate	4,849	14	108	2.2
Diphenhydramine	2,102	16	49	2.3
Ethchlorvynol	150	17	7	4.7
Flurazepam	1,966	10	71	3.6
Glutethimide	222	18	17	7.7
Pentobarbital	1,988	6	34	1.7
Phenobarbital	1,349	10	114	8.5
Secobarbital	1,520	11	40	2.6
Secobarbital/amobarbital	184	14	16	8.7

Source.   Miller and Greenblatt 1976.

hangover (1.1%) with chloral hydrate is lower than with any other hypnotic. It is commonly reported that chloral hydrate causes excessive GI irritation. However, the incidence figure of 0.3%, which was nearly identical to that of secobarbital and lower than that of glutethimide, does not support this allegation. Apparently, chloral hydrate is quite irritating to the GI lining if not taken with a large glass of fluid. Approximately 25% of patients receiving warfarin experience a significant but transient potentiation of the hypoprothrombinemic effect of warfarin after chloral hydrate administration (Miller and Greenblatt 1976). This interaction, a result of the displacement of warfarin from its albumin binding sites by chloral hydrate's inactive metabolite trichloroacetic acid, can occur as early as 12 hours after a 1,000-mg chloral hydrate dose (see *Chloral Hydrate* drug interactions [page 488] under **Anxiolytic-Hypnotics** in Chapter 8) (Sellers and Koch-Weser 1970). Although chloral hydrate is a useful hypnotic, a high rate of paradoxical reactions (including confusion, agitation, and disorientation) is associated with use of this drug in the elderly (Hollaway 1974).

Diphenhydramine
This agent, an antihistamine/anticholinergic, is often used as a sedative. Hangover, occurring in only 1.7% of the recipients, was the most common adverse effect (Miller and Greenblatt 1976). The CNS anticholinergic action of the drug makes it a less-than-ideal agent for sedating geriatric patients. Doses of greater than 50 mg hs

are no more effective than a 50-mg dose and do increase the risk of an anticholinergic delirium.

Estazolam

ADR rates of estazolam 2 mg, flurazepam 30 mg, and placebo have been compared. The ADRs that occurred more often with estazolam in contrast with placebo were somnolence (43% versus 20%), hypokinesia (7% versus 2%), dizziness (7% versus 2%), and abnormal coordination (3% versus <1%). The only ADR that occurred more frequently with flurazepam 30 mg than with estazolam 2 mg was a peculiar taste (11% versus 0%). Estazolam 1 mg and 2 mg at bedtime had no effect on memory and daytime psychomotor performance (Pierce et al. 1990).

Ethchlorvynol

Oversedation, occurring in 3.3% of recipients, was the most common ADR with ethchlorvynol. However, the high failure rate (17%) suggested that inadequate dosages were being used in many of the patients (95% were receiving a dose of 500 mg). Therefore, it was difficult to adequately assess the potential hazards of the drug (Miller and Greenblatt 1976). Excretion of ethchlorvynol is slowed by renal insufficiency (Dawborn et al. 1972).

Flurazepam

According to the BCDSP, adverse reactions are slightly more common with flurazepam 30 mg than with 15 mg (4.1% versus 3.1%, respectively). Hangover and confusion occurred in 3% of patients; all other reactions accounted for only 0.6% of ADRs (Miller and Greenblatt 1976). For subjects less than 70 years old, the total reactions decreased to 1.9% for a 3-mg dose and to 1.3% if 15 mg was used (Greenblatt et al. 1977). Table 5–5 compares the incidence of adverse reactions observed for flurazepam and for placebo in a separate study (Rickels et al. 1983). Daytime sedation may be related more to daily dose than to a drug's elimination $t_{1/2}$ (Johnson and Chernik 1982). However, because accumulation of flurazepam's desalkyl metabolite occurs after daily administration (due to a long elimination $t_{1/2}$), this drug is more likely to produce excessive daytime sedation than either temazepam or triazolam (Johnson and Chernik 1982; A. Kales et al. 1976). Flurazepam is metabolized by age-dependent pathways (hydroxylation and demethylation). Thus, the incidence of CNS depression is age and dose related. One study observed a 1.9% incidence of toxicity in patients under 60 years of age and a 7.1% incidence in patients over 80 years of age. There was a 2% rate of toxicity in patients over

Table 5–5.   Incidence of adverse effects—flurazepam versus placebo

Adverse effect	Flurazepam (%) (n = 2,397)	Placebo (%) (n = 2,101)
Drowsiness	11.4	4.2
Dizziness	2.5	1.3
Lethargy	0.3	0.2
Confusion	0.6	0.3
Euphoria	0.04	0.0
Weakness	2.4	3.0
Anorexia	0.04	0.0
Diarrhea	0.1	0.2
Tremor	0.04	0.04
Ataxia	0.8	0.1
Falling	0.7	0.05
Palpitations	0.2	0.2
Hallucinations	0.04	0.04
Paradoxical reactions	0.4	0.2

Source.   Rickels et al. 1983.

70 years of age who were taking 15 mg of flurazepam per day, and a 39% incidence of toxicity in patients of the same age group who were taking 30 mg or more per day (Greenblatt et al. 1977).

Glutethimide

Hangover was the most common (4.5%) complaint with glutethimide, followed by GI disturbances (Miller and Greenblatt 1976). The drug induces hepatic microsomal enzymes and thereby enhances the metabolism of oral anticoagulants (MacDonald et al. 1969). Warfarin antagonism was observed in one patient. Glutethimide has a very narrow therapeutic index as well as pronounced anticholinergic activity, and therefore should be used very cautiously (if ever) in elderly patients (Hollaway 1974).

Quazepam

The overall frequency of daytime sedation with quazepam is 12%. Another ADR that occurs more frequently with quazepam 15 mg than with placebo is headache (5% versus 2%). Other ADRs that occur at more than a 1% frequency are fatigue (1.9%), dizziness (1.5%), dry mouth (1.5%), and dyspepsia (1.1%). Rebound insomnia and anterograde amnesia have not yet been reported (Roth and Roehrs 1991).

Temazepam

In 795 patients receiving temazepam in clinical studies, the most common ADRs were drowsiness (17%), dizziness (7%), and confusion (5%). A large postmarketing surveillance report, which included more than 12,000 patients treated with doses of temazepam up to 30 mg at night for 2 weeks as well as more than 3,000 patients treated for 3 months, showed that approximately 10% of these patients experienced ADRs. In addition to the usual CNS depressant–related adverse effects, the most common ADRs were headaches, GI complaints, and sleep disturbances (Roth and Roehrs 1991).

Triazolam

As with other BZDs, the types of ADRs reported by patients after taking triazolam were dose dependent and could be characterized as an extension of the CNS-depressant effects of the drug. As presented in Table 5–6, the most common ADRs reported after single-night administration of triazolam were hangover, headache, dizziness, nervousness, and dry mouth (Pakes et al. 1981). ADR frequencies are usually higher in 1-night studies than in those conducted over several weeks.

Because of the short elimination $t_{1/2}$ of triazolam, there is minimal drug accumulation and less potential for daytime sedation (Johnson and Chernik 1982). Triazolam produced significantly less impairment of daytime performance 10 hours after bedtime administration than did flurazepam 15 and 30 mg, secobarbital 100 mg, or nitrazepam 10 mg (Hindmarch and Clyde 1980; Roth et al. 1977;

Table 5–6. **Frequency (%) of ADRs during 1-night studies comparing triazolam, flurazepam, and placebo**

Adverse effect	Placebo	Triazolam (mg)			Flurazepam (mg)	
		0.25	0.5	1.0	15	30
Hangover	6	6	8	22	5	11
Headache	4	1	3	2	3	2
Dizziness	1	1	2	3	1	1
Dry mouth	1	1	1	10	1	1
Nervousness	1	1	1	2	1	2

Note. ADR = adverse drug reaction.
Source. Pakes et al. 1981.

Veldkamp et al. 1974). However, because triazolam is rapidly eliminated, it has a higher likelihood of producing early-morning insomnia and daytime anxiety (Johnson and Chernik 1982). REM rebound (Roth et al. 1977), rebound anxiety (Morgan and Oswald 1982), rebound insomnia (Roehrs et al. 1986), and anterograde amnesia (Schneider and Perry 1990) have been reported if too large a dose of triazolam is used in an individual patient. Rebound insomnia occurs only at doses beyond which there is no further increase in hypnotic efficacy (Roehrs et al. 1986). Regarding the effects of BZDs on memory, immediate recall (acquisition memory) at 1.5 hours after ingestion, the time of the peak BZD plasma concentration, was affected only slightly by triazolam 0.25 mg and not at all by 0.125 mg. However, 24-hour recall was reduced by 41% by triazolam 0.125 mg and by 80% by the 0.25-mg dose (Greenblatt 1992). BZDs exert their primary effect in impairing the consolidation phase without impairing the acquisition or retention phase. Thus, 0.125 mg is the preferred initial dose. Additionally, abrupt withdrawal from triazolam (short $t_{1/2}$) is associated with a greater potential for rebound insomnia and rebound anxiety than is withdrawal from flurazepam. These adverse effects may reinforce habitual use of this drug by patients to suppress anxiety, and may lead to dependence (Manfredi and Kales 1987).

The use of triazolam has been associated with CNS ADRs that can be separated into four general categories: 1) delirium in psychiatric patients, 2) delirium in geriatric patients, 3) withdrawal reactions, and 4) anterograde amnesia (Schneider and Perry 1990). Agents with a greater affinity for BZD receptors such as triazolam, alprazolam, and lorazepam appear most likely to induce the amnestic effects (Scharf et al. 1988), although all BZDs are capable of producing amnesia. Thus, severity of the effect is a function of BZD dose, plasma concentration, and time after BZD administration at which the new information was presented.

Zolpidem

ADR rates in 23 clinical studies involving more than 1,028 insomniac patients have been analyzed. CNS depression symptoms (dysphoria, confusion, ataxia, fatigue, and drowsiness), CNS disinhibition, and nightmares occurred more frequently with zolpidem 20 mg than with either placebo or zolpidem 10 mg. ADRs that occur in 2%–4% of patients and with equal frequency for zolpidem 10 mg and 20 mg include somnolence, anterograde amnesia, headache, nausea, vertigo/dizziness, and falls (Hoehns and Perry 1993).

■ Rational Prescribing

1. Generally hypnotics are best administered an hour before bedtime. Triazolam, an exception to this rule, is best administered 30 minutes or less before bedtime.

2. The preferred hypnotics are BZDs, primarily because of their somewhat longer duration of effectiveness and lower risk of fatal overdose.

3. Pentobarbital and secobarbital may be considered in rare instances in which drug cost is an issue. However, cost is no longer an advantage, given that most of the BZDs are now available as generics (e.g., flurazepam, lorazepam, temazepam, triazolam). The barbiturates' potential for drug interactions, drug abuse, and use in suicide attempts renders these agents obsolete as routine medications for the treatment of insomnia.

4. BZDs should never be combined with ethanol to enhance their hypnotic effect.

5. Difficulties in treating overdoses and the abuse potential of hypnotics such as ethchlorvynol and glutethimide limit their utility.

6. The sedative antihistamine diphenhydramine in a 50-mg dose has been shown to be as effective as a 200-mg dose of pentobarbital. If prescribing diphenhydramine, no more than 50 mg/night need be given, because the sedative effects of the drug do not demonstrate a positive dose-response relationship (i.e., 150 mg is no more sedating than 50 mg) (Teutsch et al. 1975).

7. It is appropriate to require that patients use a hypnotic only a limited number of times each week. It is a good practice to restrict use to a 4- to 6-week period.

8. Patients with chronic insomnia who are being seen by a physician for the first time require sleep, drug, medical, and psychiatric histories as part of their evaluation.

9. In the elderly, pharmacokinetics and ADR considerations conclude that it is best to restrict hypnotic use to lorazepam, triazolam, or chloral hydrate.

10. The clinical effect of the new BZD hypnotic, quazepam, is largely attributable to its primary active metabolite, desalkylflurazepam. Thus, quazepam's profile of clinical efficacy and adverse effects should be identical or very similar to that of flurazepam.

11. Estazolam 1 and 2 mg has been compared only with flurazepam 30 mg in the treatment of insomnia, and was found to be equally effective. The lack of comparison studies with other

similar-acting BZDs and with flurazepam 15 mg suggests that estazolam be restricted at this time to a second-line drug in the treatment of insomnia.

12. The advantages of zolpidem over the BZDs are that its use does not lead to tolerance, withdrawal reactions, or REM rebound. However, if the BZDs are used only on a short-term, as-needed basis, none of zolpidem's advantages are clinically relevant.

Tryptophan

■ Indications

Tryptophan is an essential amino acid contained in high concentrations in meat, milk, and fish. Its efficacy has been investigated as a hypnotic and in the treatment of depression, mania, and schizophrenia (Pakes 1979).

■ Efficacy

A number of studies have examined the efficacy of tryptophan in treating insomnia. One study demonstrated significant increases in total sleep and non-REM sleep (Wyatt et al. 1970), whereas another study demonstrated that doses of 4–5 g significantly increased sleep time while reducing sleep latency and nocturnal awakenings (Hartmann et al. 1971). A long-term study found that 4 weeks of 1- or 4-g nightly doses of tryptophan, unlike other hypnotics, produced no disturbance of REM or non-REM sleep either during treatment or after discontinuation (Hartmann 1977). Tryptophan 3 g was compared with chloral hydrate 500 mg and placebo in a group of nonpsychotic inpatients with dementia, with each treatment lasting 7 days. Only chloral hydrate was more effective in inducing and maintaining sleep than placebo, although it did produce rebound insomnia, whereas tryptophan did not (Linnoila et al. 1980). Eight severely insomniac patients with initial, middle, or terminal insomnia were treated with tryptophan 2 g followed by 4 nights of placebo. This "interval therapy" was based on the observation that the maximal effects on abnormal sleep cycles occurred during the drug-free interval after short-term administration. Results of the study showed that sleep was improved in all patients (Schneider-Helmert 1981).

This observation was replicated in a study in which tryptophan 1 g, secobarbital 100 mg, flurazepam 30 mg, and placebo were compared in 96 insomniac patients for a 7-day treatment trial combined with a 7-day follow-up. During the treatment week, flurazepam produced significant improvement in sleep parameters compared with placebo; tryptophan and secobarbital did not. In addition, sleep latency in the tryptophan patients did not improve during the treatment week but had improved significantly by the end of the follow-up week, while the flurazepam and secobarbital patients were experiencing withdrawal symptoms (Hartmann et al. 1983). A delayed improvement in sleep latency also occurred in a group of 20 patients with chronic sleep-onset insomnia. Subjects were given either tryptophan 3 g or placebo for 6 nights. There was no improvement in sleep latency during the first 3 nights, but on nights 4 through 6, sleep latency improved significantly in the tryptophan group (Spinweber 1986). Finally, a controlled trial of 25 patients with severe insomnia of greater than 2 years' duration (mean 20 years) produced an impressive finding (Demisch et al. 1987): The effect of tryptophan 2 g plus sleep deprivation therapy for 4 weeks was compared with 4 weeks of sleep deprivation only. Nineteen of the 25 patients (76%) experienced an improvement in their sleep while receiving tryptophan.

A review of controlled studies involving tryptophan and its effect on sleep disorders indicates that 1 g of the drug increases subjective sleepiness and reduces sleep latency. The effect of tryptophan on total wakefulness and sleep time is less well documented. Tryptophan seems most beneficial in individuals with mild insomnia (1 g). However, in patients with severe insomnia, a larger dose of tryptophan (2 g), when combined with sleep deprivation therapy, is also effective. Those with chronic sleep-onset insomnia may show improvement after repeated low-dose administration (Hartmann 1982–1983; Schneider-Helmert and Spinweber 1986).

■ Mechanism of Action

The administration of tryptophan produces an increase in serotonin in the serotonin-specific neurons that contain the enzyme tryptophan hydroxylase. This enzyme catalyzes the conversion of tryptophan to 5-hydroxytryptophan (5-HT), which is then catalyzed by a decarboxylase enzyme to serotonin. The administration of 5-HT rather than tryptophan leads to the synthesis of serotonin in many neurons rather than just the serotonin neurons, because the decarboxylase enzyme is found in catecholamine- as well as serotonin-producing neurons. Brain serotonin levels may be directly dependent on circulating plasma tryptophan concentrations. These brain and serum concentrations are very sensitive to the intake of dietary protein and tryptophan. Thus, dietary tryptophan

or exogenously administered tryptophan may influence endogenous serotonin concentrations quickly enough to significantly affect sleep (Hartmann 1977).

■ Dosage

The tryptophan sleep studies in humans have used doses ranging
from 0.25 to 15 g (Hartmann and Spinweber 1979). The lowest
effective dose of tryptophan is 1 g, with no obvious dose-response
relationship existing between 1 and 15 g. Response is more likely
related to the severity of the insomnia. Thus, to maximize tryptophan's sleep latency–reducing effect in acute or short-term insomnia, the effective dose is 1–5 g. Individuals with chronic insomnia
appear to respond to low doses only after repeated administration
of the drug—for example, 2 g at bedtime for 4 weeks (Demisch et
al. 1987).

A diurnal variation in total and free tryptophan concentrations
exists. At midnight the plasma concentration is 45% higher than at
noon (Tagliamonte et al. 1974). Maximum concentrations of free
tryptophan are found between 2 and 5 P.M., and between 4 and
7 P.M. for total tryptophan. The minimum concentrations are found
between midnight and 8 A.M. for both free and total tryptophan
(Eynard et al. 1993). Thus, doses usually effective at night may be
ineffective during the day. Other factors causing fluctuations in
free and total tryptophan concentrations include environmental
temperature and seasonal changes (Eynard et al. 1993).

Tryptophan responders typically have a complaint of multiple
nocturnal awakenings. Nonresponders to tryptophan usually complain of either a single nocturnal awakening or dozing at night
rather than experiencing deep, sound sleep (Lindsley et al. 1983).

■ Pharmacokinetics

Tryptophan is rapidly metabolized. Its mean plasma $t_{1/2}$ varies between 2.7 and 2.9 hours. The drug is 65%–78% bound to albumin.
It is metabolized by tryptophan hydroxylase and excreted in the
urine as 5-hydroxyindoleacetic acid (5-HIAA). This enzyme is
increased either by cortisol or by increases in tryptophan's serum
concentration (Pakes 1979). Tryptophan's conversion to serotonin
is a minor metabolic pathway. One of the major degradative pathways involves the enzymes tryptophan oxygenase or pyrrolase,
which form the immediate precursor formylkeneurenine. This new
precursor is then metabolized to quinolinic acid, which is an agonist
of excitatory amino acid receptors at low concentrations and an

excitotoxin at high concentrations (Fuller 1991). Tryptophan's effects on EEG sleep recordings last only a few hours (Hartmann 1977), although the drug has been effective in patients with terminal insomnia (Schneider-Helmert 1981).

■ Adverse Effects

Because tryptophan is normally present in the diet at the doses required to reduce sleep latency, it would seem reasonable to conclude that a similar nondietary dose would produce no adverse effects. However, nondietary amino acids can produce different effects than a similar mixture contained in food. The long-term use of high doses of tryptophan could present certain potential dangers. A highly abnormal mixture and intake of amino acids could reduce or alter protein synthesis in the growing organism. Additionally, certain tryptophan metabolites have been implicated as possible bladder carcinogens in animals (Dunning et al. 1950). Drug abuse and drug withdrawal problems have not occurred with tryptophan. ADRs noted to occur with the higher doses of L-tryptophan when the agent was being used for treating depression include ataxia, blurred vision, dry mouth, muscle stiffness, palpitations, sweating, tremor, and urticaria (Coppen et al. 1972).

Eosinophilia Myalgia Syndrome

An ADR that has been associated with tryptophan is eosinophilia-myalgia syndrome (EMS). In 1989, the Centers for Disease Control (CDC) found an unequivocal link between the consumption of manufactured tryptophan products and EMS. More than 1,500 patients have been reported to the CDC as being affected by this syndrome. Of these cases, 36 confirmed deaths were related to EMS. Passive surveillance systems, such as those used by the CDC for the detection of EMS, may exclude many patients who do not meet the surveillance case definition. Because of this and other problems, it is estimated that more than 6,000 persons may be affected by this syndrome (Kaufman and Philen 1993). Of these estimated 6,000 patients, only 1,333 have had complete case information reported. In this population of 1,333, the majority of those affected by EMS are white non-Hispanic females with a median age of 48 (range 3–86 years) (Kaufman and Philen 1993). Extensive laboratory tests have been able to identify a specific biochemical by-product known as 1-1' ethylidene bis (EBT) that is thought to be responsible for EMS. This by-product is associated with a single source of tryptophan manufactured by the Japanese company Showa Denko KK. Analysis by high-performance liquid chromatography

(HPLC) has shown that the manufacturer's lot numbers believed to be associated to EMS were positive for EBT (also referred to as "peak E" or "peak 97"). It is not known whether the presence of EBT serves a marker for the causative agent associated with EMS, or whether EBT is the causative agent (Kaufman and Philen 1993).

In the surveillance database, the amount of daily tryptophan ingestion averaged approximately 1,500 mg/day (range 10 mg– 35 g/day). Symptoms usually developed over 1–2 weeks, although there have been reports of a delayed onset occurring after the agent was discontinued. Myalgia and fatigue are the most characteristic symptoms; others include low-grade fever; weakness; weight loss; shortness of breath; a maculopapular, vesicular, or urticarial rash; and peripheral edema. Numerous significant cognitive deficits have been associated with EMS. They include difficulty concentrating (63%), difficulty remembering words or names of persons (52%), difficulty thinking logically (52%), difficulty conversing (43%, and impairment of short-term memory (42%) (CDC 1991). Physical signs include congestive heart failure and skin changes consistent with scleroderma. Laboratory findings include a significant eosinophilia (absolute count $>1,000/mm^3$) and only occasional increases in the creatine phosphokinase, aldolase, and PO_2 levels. Some patients do not show a significant eosinophilia at the time of medical evaluation, thus leading to delays in diagnosis and treatment. In a significant number of patients, the disease has progressed to either a scleroderma-like syndrome or an ascending polymyopathy usually developing 3–6 months after the original manifestations of the syndrome. Common long-term complaints from patients include severe incapacitating muscle cramps and spasms. These generally involve the hands, feet, and subcostal regions of the chest and abdomen. Ascending polyneuropathy with resultant paralysis and respiratory failure is the major cause of EMS-related deaths, in addition to a severe cardioneuropathy leading to arrhythmias and sudden death. Tryptophan has been recalled by the FDA (Kaufman and Philen 1993; Milburn and Myers 1991).

As of October 1996, tryptophan was still not legally on the market and was available only though an investigational drug use permit. This permit is issued by the FDA on a case-by-case basis. The CDC reports that "black market" tryptophan is still in circulation, but strongly cautions against use of this supply because cases of EMS from this black-market supply have been reported. The CDC also reports that for the present, there are no plans to reintroduce tryptophan back into the market for public use (A. M. Wasley, CDC personal communication, October 1996).

■ Rational Prescribing

1. The pharmacokinetic profile of tryptophan suggests that the drug would be most effective in patients with initial insomnia, although it has also been effective in patients with terminal insomnia.
2. Some patients may respond better to tryptophan if the "interval therapy" is used. This therapy consists of a drug-free interval after short-term use of the amino acid.
3. Before the current recall of tryptophan, the drug could be purchased in either pharmacies or health-food stores and did not require a prescription.
4. Because of the lack of evidence that patients develop tolerance to the sleep effects of tryptophan, the agent might be useful in individuals in whom long-term use of traditional hypnotics is not feasible.
5. Unlike other hypnotics, tryptophan does not appear to cause a withdrawal reaction or rebound insomnia upon discontinuation, and some patients may actually show an improvement in the weeks that follow discontinuation.
6. EMS is a potentially fatal adverse effect that has been linked to a contaminant in the tryptophan manufacturing process.
7. EMS is associated with cognitive deficits that include difficulty in thinking, concentrating, remembering, and conversing.

Melatonin

Melatonin (MLT) is a natural substance secreted by the pineal gland in the brain. It has been suggested that MLT improves the sleep-wake cycle and eases jet lag. Melatonin is now being produced synthetically. Because it has been classified as a dietary supplement, MLT is not regulated by the FDA with regard to purity, efficacy, or safety, and no approved labeling or recommended dosages exist.

■ Efficacy

Six controlled trials have examined the effectiveness of MLT as a sleeping aid in insomniac patients and control subjects. In one trial, prerecorded traffic noise (68–90 dB) was used to disrupt the sleep of 20 healthy volunteers receiving MLT 80 mg/day or placebo (Waldhauser et al. 1990). Time awake before sleep onset, sleep latency, and the number of awakenings during a total sleep period decreased significantly in the MLT-treated group. Another trial, in which 10 insomniac patients received MLT 1 mg, MLT 5 mg, or placebo at bedtime for 1 week each, found that changes in sleep latency and sleep efficiency were insignificant, although REM latency was decreased at the 1-mg dosage (James et al. 1990). In eight subjects with delayed sleep-phase syndrome, a 4-week course of MLT 5 mg advanced the sleep phase, advanced sleep onset time, and decreased wake time versus placebo (Dahlitz et al. 1991). A 7-day sleep-laboratory study comparing MLT 100 mg, triazolam 0.125 mg, MLT 100 mg + triazolam 0.0625 mg, and placebo in six patients identified a trend toward reduction of stage 1 non-REM (NREM) sleep and increase of stage 3–4 NREM sleep with the MLT–triazolam combination. However, REM sleep percentage and latency were unchanged by MLT, triazolam, or MLT plus triazolam (Ferini-Strambi et al. 1993). In another study, MLT 0.3 mg and 1 mg decreased sleep-onset latency and stage 2 latency compared with placebo. The higher dosage did not produce an enhanced hypnotic effect (Zhdanova et al. 1995). A 2-mg controlled-release dose of MLT was compared with placebo in a group of chronic-insomnia patients with numerous medical problems. After 3 weeks, sleep efficiency was improved and nocturnal awakenings significantly reduced in the MLT group as compared with the placebo group (Garfinkel et al. 1995).

■ **Mechanism of Action**

Melatonin may play an important role in the induction of sleep. MLT is produced in the pinealocytes which are the cells of the pineal gland, a structure in the midbrain (Cavallo 1993). MLT secretion is controlled by an endogenous rhythm-generating system in the brain which is synchronized by the light-dark cycle; high MLT levels are produced in darkness, low levels produced in light (Cavallo 1993: Jan and Espeze 1994). Stimuli from the suprachiasmatic nuclei of the hypothalamus are carried to the superior cervical ganglion through a complex neuronal network that includes the paraventricular nucleus, the midbrain, and the spinal cord (Cavallo 1993, Stankov 1991). During dark periods (nighttime), the suprachiasmatic nuclei send stimulatory messages to the pineal gland, which results in the secretion of MLT (Cavallo 1993). This activity is suppressed during light.

■ **Pharmacokinetics**

MLT 80 mg as a single oral dose produced relatively stable serum MLT concentrations for approximately 1.5 hours after administration. Serum MLT concentrations returned to the physiological nocturnal range within 8 to 19 hours after taking MLT (Waldhauser et al. 1984).

The daytime concentrations of MLT range between 4 and 10 pg/mL in persons of all ages (Cavallo 1993). MLT secretion changes with age. Plasma concentrations are highest at night, and average 250 pg/mL in children 1–3 years of age (Utiger 1992). MLT concentrations decrease to approximately 120 pg/mL in children and adolescents 8–15 years of age (Utiger 1992). Concentrations continue to decline gradually to about 20 pg/mL in adults 50–70 years of age (Utiger 1992).

In one study, the presence of liver disease was associated with a fivefold decrease in MLT clearance (Iguchi et al. 1982). MLT's high hepatic extraction ratio suggests a prominent first-pass hepatic metabolism and reduced bioavailability for orally administered MLT (Iguchi et al. 1982).

■ Adverse Effects

Few ADR data for MLT are available. No long-term toxicity trials have been conducted. Reported ADRs are headache, pruritis, and an increase in alkaline phosphatase after 20 weeks of continued treatment (Dahlitz et al. 1991).

■ Rational Prescribing

1. Limited information is available about MLT. In addition, because much of the trial data involved noninsomiac subjects, this information may not be applicable to patients with insomnia. Due to the small number of subjects studied, it is difficult to find clinically significant differences between treatment groups.
2. Longer trials are needed to assess MLT's safety and potential side effects (the longest study conducted to date involved only 3 weeks of continuous dosing).
3. The optimal MLT dosage has not yet been determined, given that the trials used doses ranging from 0.3 to 100 mg. These trials also did not record patients' weights (needed to adequately determine a dose/kg) or assess clinical benefit and desired outcomes.
4. Melatonin has been classified as a dietary supplement and therefore is not regulated by the FDA; there are no standards in place for MLT's purity, efficacy, and safety and no approved

labeling or recommended dosages. Manufacturers are not required to demonstrate that MLT is in fact present in the product being sold to consumers. According to *The Medical Letter,* chemical analyses found that four of six MLT products from health-food stores contained impurities that could not be characterized ("Melatonin" 1995).
5. All patients taking MLT should be warned that it is not an FDA-approved medication.

Product List

Chloral Hydrate (nonbarbiturate/nonbenzodiazepine)
- Daily dose range: 0.5–2.0 g; only generically available

Capsules:	generic (Rugby)
500 mg	[$10]
Syrup:	generic
500 mg/5 mL	[$11/480 mL] orange flavor

Diphenhydramine (antihistamine)
- Daily dose range: 25–50 mg; over the counter
- Generic cost index: ≈ 0.08

Capsules:	Benadryl®
25 mg	[$22/48] P-D 471, pink/white
50 mg	[$30] P-D 373, pink/white
Elixir:	generic
12.5 mg/5 mL	[$7/240 mL]
Injection:	generic
50 mg/mL	[$2/1-mL vial; $10/10-mL vial]

Estazolam (benzodiazepine)
- Daily dose range: 1–2 mg

Tablets:	ProSom®
1 mg	[$89], white
2 mg	[$99], coral

Ethchlorvynol (nonbarbiturate/nonbenzodiazepine)
- Daily dose range: 0.5–1.0 g; generically available
- Generic cost index: ≈ 0.42

Capsules:	Placidyl®
200 mg	[$105] red
500 mg	[$129] Placidyl 500, red
750 mg	[$172] Placidyl 750, green

Flurazepam (benzodiazepine)
- Daily dose range: 15–30 mg; generically available
- Generic cost index: ≈ 0.09

Capsules:	**Dalmane**®
15 mg	[$55] Dalmane 15 Roche, orange/ivory
30 mg	[$60] Dalmane 30 Roche, red/ivory

Glutethimide (nonbarbiturate/nonbenzodiazepine)
- Daily dose range: 0.5–1.0 g; only generically available

Tablets:	**generic**
500 mg	[$18]

Lorazepam (benzodiazepine)
- Daily dose range: 1–10 mg; generically available
- Generic cost index: ≈ 0.03

Tablets:	**Ativan**®
0.5 mg	[$63] Wyeth 81, white
1 mg	[$83] Wyeth 64, white
2 mg	[$120] Wyeth 65, white

Injection:	**Ativan**®
2 mg/mL	[$107/10-mL vial]
4 mg/mL	[$134/10-mL vial]
2 mg/mL	[$13/0.5-mL unit dose syringe]
2 mg/mL	[$13/1.0-mL unit dose syringe]
4 mg/mL	[$13/1.0-mL unit dose syringe]

Melatonin (hormone)
- Daily dose range: 0.3–100 mg

Tablets:*	
3 mg	[$12/60], white

Pentobarbital (barbiturate)
- Daily dose range: 50–200 mg po; generically available
- Generic cost index: ≈ 0.14

Capsules:	**Nembutal**®
50 mg	[$33] CF, orange/white
100 mg	[$52] CH, yellow

Injection:	**Nembutal**®
50 mg/mL	[$60/25 2-mL ampule; $2/1 unit]
50 mg/mL	[$12/20-mL vial]
50 mg/mL	[$23/50-mL vial]

---

* Contain 1 mg of vitamin B6.

Suppositories:	**Nembutal**®
30 mg	[$41/12]
60 mg	[$49/12]
120 mg	[$54/12]
200 mg	[$67/12]
Elixir:	**Nembutal**®
18.2 mg/5 mL	[$65/480 mL]

Quazepam (benzodiazepine)

- Daily dose range: 7.5–15 mg

Tablets:	**Doral**®
7.5 mg	[$125] Doral 7.5, light orange with white speckles
15.0 mg	[$137] Doral 15, light orange with white speckles

Secobarbital (barbiturate)

- Daily dose range: 50–200 mg; generically available
- Generic cost index: ≈ 0.31

Capsules:	**Seconal**®
100 mg	[$22] F40 Lilly, orange

Secobarbital/amobarbital (barbiturates)

- Daily dose range: 50–200 mg, total drug

Capsules:	**Tuinal**®
100 mg (50/50)	[$25] F65 Lilly, orange/blue
200 mg (100/100)	[$33] F66 Lilly, orange/blue

Temazepam (benzodiazepine)

- Daily dose range: 15–30 mg; generically available
- Generic cost index: ≈ 0.06

Capsules:	**Restoril**®
7.5 mg	[$60] Restoril 7.5 mg for sleep, blue/pink
15 mg	[$68] Restoril 15 mg for sleep, maroon/pink
30 mg	[$76] Restoril 30 mg for sleep, maroon/blue

Triazolam (benzodiazepine)

- Daily dose range: 0.25–0.5 mg; generically available
- Generic cost index: ≈ 0.68

Tablets:	**Halcion**®
0.125 mg	[$71] Halcion 0.125, white
0.25 mg	[$77] Halcion 0.25, powder blue

Tryptophan (essential amino acid)

- Generically available; recalled by the FDA in November 1989

References

Amrein R, Bovey F, Cano JP, et al: Pharmacokinetics and pharmacodynamics of flurazepam in man, II: investigation of the relative efficacy of flurazepam, desalkylflurazepam and placebo under steady-state conditions. Drugs Exp Clin Res 9:85–99, 1983

Bayer AJ, Bayer EM, Pathy MSJ, et al: A double-blind controlled study of chlormethiazole and triazolam as hypnotics in the elderly. Acta Psychiatr Scand 73 (suppl 329):104–111, 1989

Berlin RM: Management of insomnia in hospitalized patients. Ann Intern Med 100:398–404, 1984

Bixler EO, Kales A, Soldatos CR, et al: Effectiveness of temazepam with short-, intermediate-, and long-term use: sleep laboratory evaluation. J Clin Pharmacol 18:110–118, 1978

Bonnet MH, Dexter JR, Gillin JC, et al: The use of triazolam in the phase-advanced sleep. Neuropsychopharmacology 1:225–134, 1988

Bootzin RR, Perlis ML: Nonpharmacologic treatments of insomnia. J Clin Psychiatry 53 (suppl 6):37–41, 1992

Breimer D: Clinical pharmacokinetics of hypnotics. Clin Pharmacokinet 2:93–109, 1977

Cavallo A: The pineal gland in human beings; relevance to pediatrics. Pediatr 123:843–851, 1993

Centers for Disease Control: Eosinophilia Myalgia Syndrome: follow-up survey of patients—New York, 1990–1991. MMWR Morb Mortal Wkly Rep 401–403, 1991

Coleman RM, Roffwarg HP, Kennedy SJ, et al: Sleep-wake disorders based on a polysomnographic diagnosis: a national cooperative study. JAMA 247:997–1003, 1982

Consensus Development Conference: Drugs and insomnia: the use of medication to promote sleep. JAMA 251:2410–2414, 1984

Cooper SF, Drolet D: Protein binding of flurazepam and its major metabolites in plasma. Curr Ther Res Clin Exp 32:757–760, 1982

Coppen A, Whybrow PC, Noguera R: The comparative antidepressant value of L-tryptophan and imipramine with and without attempted potentiation by liothyronine. Arch Gen Psychiatry 26:234–241, 1972

Crisp AH: Sleep, activity, nutrition and mood. Br J Psychiatry 137:1–7, 1980

Dahlitz M, Alvarez B, Vignau J, et al: Delayed sleep phase syndrome response to melatonin. Lancet 337:1121–1124, 1991

Dawborn JK, Turner A, Pattison G: Ethchlorvynol as a sedative in patients with renal failure. Med J Aust 2:702–704, 1972

De Jonghe F, Ameling EH, Folkers C, et al: Flurazepam and temazepam in the treatment of insomnia in a general hospital population. Pharmacopsychiatry 17:133–135, 1984

Dement WC: Rational basis for the use of sleeping pills. Pharmacology 2 (suppl):3–38, 1983

Dement WC: The proper use of sleeping pills in the primary care setting. J Clin Psychiatry 53 (suppl 6):50–56, 1992

Demisch K, Bauer J, Georgi K: Treatment of severe chronic insomnia with L-tryptophan and varying sleeping times. Pharmacopsychiatry 20:245–248, 1987

Dundee JW, Halliday NJ, Harper KW, et al: Midazolam: a review of its pharmacological properties and therapeutic use. Drugs 28:519–543, 1984

Dunning WF, Curtis MR, Maun MB: The effect of added dietary tryptophan on the occurrence of 2-acetylamino-fluorene–induced liver and bladder cancer in rats. Cancer Res 10:454–459, 1950

Eckert M, Zeigler WH, Cano JP, et al: Pharmacokinetics and pharmacodynamics of flurazepam in man, I: pharmacokinetics of desalkylflurazepam and hydroxyethyl-flurazepam after a single iv injection in comparison with orally administered flurazepam. Drugs Exp Clin Res 9:77–84, 1983

Eynard N, Flachaire E, Lestra C, et al: Platelet serotonin content in free and total plasma tryptophan in healthy volunteers during 24 hours. Clinical Chemistry 39:237–240, 1993

Ferini-Strambi L, Zuccone M, Biella G, et al: Effect of melatonin on sleep microstructure: preliminary results in healthy subjects. Sleep 16:744–747, 1993

Fuller RW: Role of serotonin in therapy of depression and related disorders. J Clin Psychiatry 52 (suppl 5):52–57, 1991

Garfinkel D, Laudon M, Nof D, et al: Improvement of sleep quality in elderly people by controlled-release melatonin. Lancet 346:541–544, 1995

Gershon S, Eison AS: The ideal anxiolytic. Psychiatr Ann 17:156–170, 1987

Gillin JC, Byerley WF: The diagnosis and management of insomnia. N Engl J Med 322:239–248, 1990

Goldson RL: Management of sleep disorders in the elderly. Drugs 21:390–396, 1981

Greenblatt DJ: Pharmacology of benzodiazepine hypnotics. J Clin Psychiatry 53 (suppl 6):7–13, 1992

Greenblatt DJ, Allen MD, Shader RI: Toxicity of high dose flurazepam in the elderly. Clin Pharmacol Ther 21:355–361, 1977

Greenblatt DJ, Sellers EM, Shader RI: Drug disposition in old age. N Engl J Med 306:1081–1088, 1982

Greenblatt DJ, Abernathy DR, Divoll M, et al: Pharmacokinetic properties of benzodiazepine hypnotics. J Clin Psychopharmacol 3:129–132, 1983

Gustavson LE, Carrigan PJ: The clinical pharmacokinetics of single doses of estazolam. Am J Med 88 (suppl 3A):12S, 1990

Hartmann E: L-tryptophan: a rational hypnotic with clinical potential. Am J Psychiatry 134:366–370, 1977

Hartmann E: Effects of L-tryptophan on sleepiness and on sleep. J Psychiatr Res 17:107–113, 1982–1983

Hartmann E, Cravens J: The effects of long term administration of psychotropic drugs on human sleep, III: the effects of amitriptyline. Psychopharmacologia 33:185–202, 1973

Hartmann E, Spinweber CL: Sleep induced by L-tryptophan: effects of dosages within the normal dietary intake. J Nerv Ment Dis 167:497–499, 1979

Hartmann E, Chung R, Chien CP: L-tryptophan and sleep. Psychopharmacologia (Berl) 19:114–127, 1971

Hartmann E, Lindsley JG, Spinweber C: Chronic insomnia: effects of L-tryptophan, flurazepam, secobarbital and placebo. Psychopharmacology (Berl) 80:138–142, 1983

Heel RC, Avery GS: Drug data information, in Drug Treatment: Principles and Practice of Clinical Pharmacology and Therapeutics. Edited by Avery GS. New York, Australian Drug Information Service (ADIS)/ Williams & Wilkins, 1980, pp 1211–1222

Hindmarch I, Clyde CA: The effects of triazolam and nitrazepam on sleep quality, morning vigilance and psychomotor performance. Arzneimit-telforschung 30:1163–1166, 1980

Hoehns JD, Perry PJ: Zolpidem: a nonbenzodiazepine hypnotic for the treatment of insomnia. Clinical Pharmacy 12:814–828, 1993

Hollaway P: Drug problems in the geriatric patients. Drug Intelligence and Clinical Pharmacy 8:632–642, 1974

Iguchi H, Kato KI, Ibayashi H: Melatonin serum levels and metabolic clearance rate in patients with liver cirrhosis. J Clin Endocrinol Metab 54:1025–1027, 1982

Iowa Pharmacists Association: Iowa Pharmacy Law and Information Manual, 2nd Edition. Des Moines, IA, Iowa Pharmacists Association, 1992

James SP, Sack DA, Rosenthal NE, et al: Melatonin administration in insomnia. Neuropsychopharmacol 3:19–23, 1990

Jan JE, Espeze H, Appleton RE: The treatment of sleep disorders with melatonin. Dev Med Child Neurol 36:97–107, 1994

Johnson LC, Chernik DA: Sedative-hypnotics and human performance. Psychopharmacology 76:101–113, 1982

Kales A: Quazepam: hypnotic efficacy and side effects. Pharmacotherapy 10:1–12, 1990

Kales A, Kales JD: Sleep laboratory studies of hypnotic drug: efficacy and withdrawal effects. J Clin Psychopharmacol 3:140–150, 1983

Kales A, Kales JD: General measures for treating insomnia, in Evaluation and Treatment of Insomnia. New York, Oxford University Press, 1984, pp 186–240

Kales A, Bixler EO, Scharf M, et al: Sleep laboratory studies of flurazepam: a model for evaluating hypnotic drugs. Clin Pharmacol Ther 19:576–583, 1976

Kales JD, Soldatos CR, Kales A: Diagnosis and treatment of sleep disorders, in Treatment of Mental Disorders. Edited by Greist JH, Jefferson JW, Spitzer RL. New York, Oxford University Press, 1982, pp 473–500

Kaufman LD, Philen RM: Tryptophan: current status and future trends for oral administration. Drug Saf 8:89–98, 1993

Kay DC, Blackburn AB, Buckingham AB, et al: Human pharmacology of sleep, in Pharmacology of Sleep. Edited by Williams RL, Karacan I. New York, Wiley Medical, 1976, pp 83–210

Kudo Y, Kurihara M: Clinical evaluation of diphenhydramine hydrochloride for the treatment of insomnia in psychiatric patients: a double-blind study. J Clin Pharmacol 30:1041–1048, 1990

Lader M: The use of hypnotics and anxiolytics in the elderly. International Clinical Psychopharmacology 1:273–283, 1986

Lindsley JG, Hartmann EL, Mitchell W: Selectivity in response to L-tryptophan among insomniac subjects: a preliminary report. Sleep 6:247–256, 1983

Linnoila M, Viukari M, Numminen A, et al: Efficacy and side effects of chloral hydrate and tryptophan as sleeping aids in psychogeriatric patients. International Pharmacopsychiatry 15:124–128, 1980

Litovitz T: Fatal benzodiazepine toxicity? the author replies (letter). Am J Emerg Med 5:472–473, 1987

Locniskar A, Greenblatt DJ: Oxidative versus conjugative biotransformation of temazepam. Biopharm Drug Dispos 11:499–506, 1990

MacDonald MG, Robinson DS, Sylvester D, et al: The effects of phenobarbital, chloral betaine, and glutethimide administration on warfarin plasma levels and hypoprothrombinemia responses in man. Clin Pharmacol Ther 10:80–84, 1969

Manfredi RL, Kales A: Clinical neuropharmacology of sleep disorders. Semin Neurol 7:286–295, 1987

McClure DJ, Walsh J, Chang H, et al: Comparison of lorazepam and flurazepam as hypnotic agents in chronic insomniacs. J Clin Pharmacol 28:52–63, 1988

Melatonin. Medical Letter 37:111–112, November 24, 1995

Mendelson WB: Pharmacotherapy of insomnia. Psychiatr Clin North Am 10:555–563, 1987

Meuleman JR, Nelson RC, Clark RL Jr: Evaluation of temazepam and diphenhydramine as hypnotics in a nursing-home population. Drug Intelligence and Clinical Pharmacy 21:716–720, 1987

Milburn DS, Myers CW: L-tryptophan toxicity: a pharmacoepidemiologic review of eosinophilia-myalgia syndrome. DICP Ann Pharmacother 25:1259–1262, 1991

Miles LE, Dement WC: Sleep and aging. Sleep 3:1–220, 1980

Miller RR, Greenblatt DJ: Hypnotics, in Drug Effects in Hospitalized Patients. Edited by Miller RR, Greenblatt DJ. New York, Wiley, 1976, pp 171–191

Mitler MM, Carskadon MA, Phillips RL: Hypnotic efficacy of temazepam: a long-term sleep laboratory evaluation. Br J Clin Pharmacol 8 (suppl):63S–68S, 1979

Moran MG, Stoudemire A: Sleep disorders in the medically ill patient. J Clin Psychiatry 53 (suppl 6):29–36, 1992

Morgan K, Oswald I: Anxiety caused by a short-life hypnotic (abstract). BMJ 284:942, 1982

Morin CM, Culbert JP, Schwartz SM: Nonpharmacological interventions for insomnia: a meta-analysis of treatment efficacy. Am J Psychiatry. 151:1172–1180, 1994

New Halcion labeling. FDA Medical Bulletin 22:7–8, 1992

Nicholson AN, Stone BM: Diazepam and 3-hydroxydiazepam (temazepam) and sleep of middle age. Br J Clin Pharmacol 7:463–468, 1979

Nicholson AN, Stone BM, Pascoe PA: Hypnotic efficacy in middle age. J Clin Psychopharmacol 2:118–121, 1982

Nierenberg AA, Adler LA, Peselow E, et al: Trazodone for antidepressant-associated insomnia. Am J Psychiatry 151:1069–1072, 1994

Pakes GE: L-tryptophan in psychiatry practice. Drug Intelligence and Clinical Pharmacy 13:391–396, 1979

Pakes GE, Brogden RN, Heel RC, et al: Triazolam: a review of its pharmacological properties and therapeutic efficacy in patients with insomnia. Drugs 22:81–110, 1981

Parrino L, Spaggiari MC, Boselli M, et al: Clinical and polysomnographic effects of trazodone CR in chronic insomnia associated with dysthymia. Psychopharmacology 116:389–395, 1994

Perry PJ, Smith DA: Triazolam—the never-ending story (editorial). DICP Ann Pharmacother 25:163–164, 1991

Philips F, Chen CN, Crisp AH, et al: Isocaloric diet changes and electroencephalographic sleep. Lancet 2:723–723, 1975

Pierce MW, Shu VS: Efficacy of estazolam. Am J Med 88 (suppl 3A):12S, 1990

Pierce MW, Shu VS, Groves LJ: Safety of estazolam. Am J Med 88 (suppl 3A):12S, 1990

Rall TW: Hypnotics and sedatives; ethanol, in Goodman and Gilman's The Pharmacological Basis of Therapeutics, 8th Edition. Edited by Gilman AG, Rall TW, Nies AS, et al. New York, Macmillan, 1990, pp 345–382

Rickels K, Morris RJ, Newman H, et al: Clinical trials of hypnotics. J Clin Pharmacol 23:234–242, 1983

Roehrs TA, Zorick F, Koshorek GL, et al: Effects of acute administration brotizolam in subjects with disturbed sleep. Br J Clin Pharmacol 16:371S–376S, 1983

Roehrs TA, Zorick FJ, Wittig RM, et al: Dose determinants of rebound insomnia. Br J Clin Pharmacol 22:143–147, 1986

Rosekind MR: The epidemiology and occurrence of insomnia. J Clin Psychiatry 53 (suppl 6):4–6, 1992

Roth T, Kramer M, Lutz T: The effects of triazolam (0.25 mg) on the sleep of insomnia subjects. Drugs Exp Clin Res 1:279–285, 1977

Roth T, Roehrs TA: A review of the safety profiles of benzodiazepine hypnotics. J Clin Psychiatry 52 (suppl 9):38–41, 1991

Sakulsripong M, Curran HV, Lader M: Does tolerance develop to the sedative and amnestic effects of antidepressants? a comparison of amitriptyline, trazodone, and placebo. Eur J Clin Pharmacol 40:43–48, 1991

Scharf MB, Fletcher K, Graham JP: Comparative amnestic effects of benzodiazepine hypnotic agents. J Clin Psychiatry 49:134–137, 1988

Scharf MB, Roth PR, Dominguez RA, et al: Estazolam and flurazepam: a multicenter, placebo-controlled comparative study in outpatients with insomnia. J Clin Pharmacol 30:461–467, 1990

Schneider PJ, Perry PJ: Triazolam: an "abused drug" by the lay press? DICP Ann Pharmacother 24:389–392, 1990

Schneider-Helmert D: Interval therapy with L-tryptophan in severe chronic insomniacs: a predictive laboratory study. International Pharmacopsychiatry 16:162–173, 1981

Schneider-Helmert D, Spinweber CL: Evaluation of L-tryptophan for treatment of insomnia: a review. Psychopharmacology 89:1–7, 1986

Sellers EM, Koch-Weser J: Potentiation of warfarin-induced hypoprothrombinemia by chloral hydrate. N Engl J Med 283:827–831, 1970

Sjoqvist F, Lasagna L: The hypnotic efficacy of doxylamine. Clin Pharmacol Ther 8:48–54, 1967

Solomon F, White CC, Parron DL, et al: Sleeping pills, insomnia and medical practice. N Engl J Med 300:803–808, 1979

Spinweber CL: L-tryptophan administered to chronic sleep-onset insomniacs: late-appearing reduction of sleep latency. Psychopharmacology (Berl) 90:151–155, 1986

Stankov B, Fraschini F, Reiter RJ: Melatonin binding sites in the central nervous system. Brain Res 16:245–256, 1991

Tagliamonte A, Gessa R, Biggio G, et al: Daily changes of free serum L-tryptophan in humans. Life Sci 14:349–354, 1974

Teutsch G, Mahler DL, Brown CR, et al: Hypnotic efficacy of diphenhydramine, methapyrilene, and pentobarbital. Clin Pharmacol Ther 17:195–201, 1975

Utiger RD: Melatonin—the hormone of darkness. N Engl J Med 327:1377–1379, 1992

Veldkamp W, Straw RN, Metzler CM, et al: Efficacy and residual effect of evaluation of a new hypnotic, triazolam. J Clin Pharmacol 14:102–111, 1974

Vogel G: Clinical use and advantages of low doses of benzodiazepine hypnotics. J Clin Psychiatry 53 (suppl 6):19–22, 1992

Waldhauser F, Waldhauser M, Lieberman H, et al: Bioavailability of oral melatonin in humans. Neuroendocrinol 39:307–313, 1984

Waldhauser F, Saletu B, Trinchard-Lugan I: Sleep laboratory investigations on hypnotic properties of melatonin. Psychopharmacol 100:222–226, 1990

Ware JC, Pittard JT: Increased deep sleep after trazodone use: a double-blind placebo-controlled study in healthy young adults. J Clin Psychiatry 51 (suppl 9):18–22, 1990

Woo E, Proulx SM, Greenblatt DJ: Differential side effect profile of triazolam versus flurazepam in elderly patients undergoing rehabilitation therapy. J Clin Pharmacol 31:168–173, 1991

World Health Organization: Health care in the elderly: report of the technical group on use of medicaments of the elderly. Drugs 22:279–294, 1981

Wyatt RJ, Kupfer DJ, Sjoersma A, et al: Effects of L-tryptophan (a natural sedative) on human sleep. Lancet 2:842–846, 1970

Wysowski DK, Baum C: Outpatient use of prescription sedative-hypnotic drugs in the United States, 1970 through 1989. Arch Intern Med 151:1779–1783, 1991

Zhdanova IV, Wurtman RJ, Lynch HJ, et al: Sleep-inducing effects of low doses of melatonin ingested in the evening. Clin Pharmacol Ther 57:552–558, 1995

Agents for Treating Early-Onset Extrapyramidal Side Effects

This chapter discusses the treatment of dystonia, akathisia, and drug-induced parkinsonism with anticholinergics, amantadine, benzodiazepines, β-adrenergic–blocking drugs, levodopa, and clonidine. (For a discussion of early-onset extrapyramidal side effects, neuroleptic malignant syndrome, and tardive dyskinesia, see *Neurological* adverse effects [page 45] under **Typical Antipsychotics** in Chapter 1.)

Note: A significant benefit in preventing or reducing antipsychotic-induced extrapyramidal side effects (EPS) can be achieved by initiating and maintaining antipsychotic dosages in the low therapeutic range, as all early-onset EPS are dose related (Bezchlibnyk-Butler and Remington 1994; Casey 1993, 1994; Fleischhacker et al. 1990; Tonda and Guthrie 1994). Many studies have demonstrated that EPS are not directly related to therapeutic response (Casey 1994; Tonda and Guthrie 1994). (See "Dosage" [page 12] under **Typical Antipsychotics** in Chapter 1.) These side effects can be quite uncomfortable for the patient and disturbing to family and friends. Recognizing them and instituting appropriate management are an important part of patient care.

The use of clozapine, olanzapine, risperidone, and sertindole, which have a lower rate of EPS, is discussed under these drug headings in Chapter 1.

Anticholinergics

■ Indications

Although numerous anticholinergics are available for management of antipsychotic-induced EPS, no significant clinical differences among agents have been demonstrated (Bezchlibnyk-Butler and Remington 1994).

■ Efficacy

Dystonia

Acute treatment. Dystonias disappear without treatment within 7 to 10 days even if the antipsychotic is continued. However, because of discomfort to the patient and the potential for a rare, serious reaction (e.g., laryngeal spasm), dystonic reactions should be treated as soon after their appearance as possible (Donlon and Stenson 1976; Gelenberg 1983; Tonda and Guthrie 1994). Diphenhydramine (Benadryl®, generic) 50 mg or benztropine (Cogentin®) 2 mg iv or im, for example, reverse dystonia in 100% of cases after a single injection or, rarely, a repeated dose within 5 minutes if the iv route is used (Gagrat et al. 1978; Lee 1979). If more than two injections are required, other possible causes of the dystonia should be considered (Casey 1993).

The preferred route of administration is intravenous. If this is not feasible, intramuscular drug administration can be used. In a study comparing benztropine and diphenhydramine in both routes, iv administration reversed dystonia in 2–3 minutes, whereas im administration produced improvement only after 30–40 minutes, regardless of the drug (Lee 1979). Oral treatment with anticholinergics is not recommended because of the slower onset of action and because some patients may have difficulty in swallowing during acute dystonic reactions.

Because dystonia is usually self-limiting, the antipsychotic need not be discontinued or changed nor the dosage lowered. However, if recurrences are frequent and/or severe, lowering the antipsychotic dose or switching the patient to a lower-potency agent is recommended (Donlon and Stenson 1976; Gelenberg 1983). Finally, the drug-induced nature of the syndrome and its benign course should be explained to the patient and the family.

Prophylactic treatment. There is evidence that prophylactic treatment with antipsychotics is successful in lowering the incidence of acute dystonic reactions (Arana et al. 1988; Gelenberg 1983). In nine open and controlled trials ($n = 1,366$), the risk of a dystonic reaction in patients receiving versus not receiving prophylaxis was 7.7% and 14.8%, respectively (Arana et al. 1988). Patients in these studies were receiving a variety of low- and high-potency antipsychotics. Five of the studies involved 330 patients receiving only high-potency antipsychotics (primarily haloperidol); in these studies, the incidence of dystonic reactions was 51.2% in patients receiving and 9.5% in patients not receiving prophylaxis. Typically, in patients 45 years of age or older, no difference was demonstrated between those receiving versus not receiving prophylaxis, because the rate of dystonia is low above this age. Also, patients receiving low-potency antipsychotics (e.g., chlorpromazine) rarely experienced dystonic reactions. (See "Dosage" [page 12] under **Typical Antipsychotics** in Chapter 1.) It has been suggested that, regardless of patient age, high-dose intravenous haloperidol may be less likely to produce dystonic reactions than standard oral doses. (See *Extrapyramidal side effects* [page 45] under *Neurological* adverse effects of **Typical Antipsychotics** in Chapter 1.)

Prophylaxis would be appropriate in a patient with a high risk of developing dystonia (e.g., a man less than 45 years of age with a history of dystonia who is receiving a piperazine phenothiazine or butyrophenone; a patient likely to develop a reaction for whom medical treatment is not readily accessible) (Bezchlibnyk-Butler and Remington 1994; Casey 1993; Tonda and Guthrie 1994). Recommended prophylactic oral doses of benztropine are 2–4 mg/day (Sramek et al. 1986).

Duration of treatment.   After acute treatment of dystonia, the reaction may recur. Inpatients can be treated with repeat parenteral anticholinergics if the condition reappears. Five days of oral therapy might be prescribed to prevent recurrence of the syndrome in an outpatient unable to obtain prompt medical care.

Duration of prophylactic treatment should cover the risk period of 5–7 days, although a period of 7–10 days has been recommended (Casey 1993).

Akathisia

Acute treatment.   When akathisia develops, it is appropriate in some clinical situations to change to an antipsychotic less likely to produce EPS (i.e., thioridazine, chlorpromazine, risperidone) or to lower the dose of the antipsychotic causing the reaction (Bezchlibnyk-Butler and Remington 1994; Casey 1993; Tonda and Guthrie 1994). These drugs should be considered for patients at a high risk of developing specific types of acute-onset EPS. (See *Neurological* adverse effects [page 45] under **Typical Antipsychotics** in Chapter 1.)

The use of anticholinergics in the treatment of akathisia has been reviewed (Fleischhacker et al. 1990). Of nine studies, four were double-blind in design. Five reports indicated that anticholinergics were effective in akathisia, two had negative findings, and two had equivocal results. In studies that reported results by percentage response, the range was 30%–100% (average 62%). However, not all patients in the positive studies had complete resolution of their akathisia. The time required for akathisia to respond to anticholinergics is usually 3–7 days. Most studies reported that anticholinergics were effective for akathisia in patients who had concomitant drug-induced parkinsonism. Therefore, anticholinergics might be considered the first-line treatment for patients with akathisia with concurrent drug-induced parkinsonism (Fleischhacker et al. 1990).

Two studies have directly compared the effects of benztropine and propranolol in alleviating antipsychotic-induced akathisia. One study of 6 patients compared intravenous benztropine 2 mg, propranolol 1 mg, and saline placebo in a double-blind, crossover investigation (Sachdev and Loneragan 1993). In subjective and objective ratings, benztropine was significantly more effective than propranolol in effecting clinical improvement. However, equivalent doses of benztropine and propranolol have not been determined. In another placebo-controlled, blinded study involving 28 patients, propranolol 80 mg/day and benztropine 6 mg/day produced equal and significantly greater improvement in akathisia symptoms compared with placebo (Adler et al. 1993). Maximal effect with drug treatment occurred between days 3 and 5. Three patients on benztropine developed confusion or forgetfulness by day 3; however, these effects cleared upon drug discontinuation.

Upon discontinuation of the antipsychotic, akathisia symptoms generally resolve within 7 to 10 days but may take several weeks, depending on the drug, the dosage, and the patient.

Prophylactic treatment.   The prophylactic management of akathisia is addressed in the section on drug-induced parkinsonism (see *Prophylactic treatment* under *Parkinsonism*, below).

Duration of treatment.   (See *Duration of treatment* under *Parkinsonism*, below.)

Parkinsonism

Acute treatment.   When drug-induced parkinsonism develops, it is appropriate in some clinical situations to change to an antipsychotic less likely to produce EPS (i.e., thioridazine, chlorpromazine, olanzapine, risperidone, sertindole) or to lower the dosage of the antipsychotic causing the reaction (Bezchlibnyk-Butler and Remington 1994; Casey 1993). Thioridazine, chlorpromazine, olanzapine, risperidone, or sertindole should likewise be considered for patients at a high risk of developing specific types of early-onset EPS. (See *Neurological* adverse effects [page 45] under **Typical Antipsychotics** in Chapter 1.)

Typically, anticholinergics have been used as the first-line treatment for antipsychotic-induced parkinsonism (Bezchlibnyk-Butler and Remington 1994; Chouinard et al. 1987; Friis et al. 1983). There is no consistently reported percentage of patients that responds to anticholinergics. Study results vary because of differences in study design and difficulties in diagnosing and assessing extrapyramidal reactions both objectively and subjectively.

The use of an initial parenteral dose may produce an immediate response, although it is not unusual for drug-induced parkinsonism to be resistant to maximal doses of anticholinergic medication, whether administered orally or parenterally (Tarsy 1983). The time required for drug-induced parkinsonism to respond to anticholinergics is usually 3–7 days; however, this depends on the patient and the dose of anticholinergic. No information exists to suggest that one anticholinergic agent is more efficacious than another (Bezchlibnyk-Butler and Remington 1994).

Upon discontinuation of the antipsychotic, parkinsonism symptoms generally resolve within 7 to 10 days but may take several weeks to months for complete resolution, depending on the drug, the dose, and the patient.

Prophylactic treatment. The efficacy of instituting anticholinergic drugs at the same time antipsychotics are initiated to prevent the onset of drug-induced parkinsonism and akathisia has been reviewed (Tonda and Guthrie 1994). Three of six retrospective studies reported benefit from the prophylactic treatments, whereas three reported no benefit. Of eight prospective studies, six reported prophylactic treatment to be beneficial and two did not. However, in one of the six positive studies, the no-treatment group received higher doses of the antipsychotic.

Opponents of the use of prophylactic and continuous anticholinergics cite the following in support of their view: 1) prophylactic treatment lacks demonstrated efficacy; 2) not all patients treated with antipsychotics develop EPS; 3) anticholinergic drugs have the potential to produce side effects (e.g., memory impairment, anticholinergic effects); 4) anticholinergic drugs can increase patients' susceptibility to tardive dyskinesia; and 5) studies have demonstrated that in the majority of patients, EPS do not recur when anticholinergic drug therapy is discontinued after 3 months of administration.

Those who favor the use of prophylactic and continuous anticholinergics contend that even though some patients will receive these agents unnecessarily, the expense and potential toxicity of anticholinergics are balanced by the benefits of reducing the risk of misdiagnosing EPS (primarily akathisia) that mimic psychopathology. In addition, prophylactic treatment might minimize discouragement in patients who are not highly motivated to take antipsychotics and who would probably stop taking them if EPS emerged (Manos et al. 1981; McEvoy 1983).

Studies indicate that if high-potency antipsychotics (e.g., haloperidol, piperazine phenothiazines) are prescribed, prophylactic anticholinergics can significantly reduce the reported incidence of early-onset EPS as compared with no treatment or placebo (Tonda and Guthrie 1994). Patients with a history of antipsychotic-induced EPS who are taking high-potency antipsychotics at higher doses should receive preventive pharmacological treatment. If a patient receiving an antipsychotic for the first time develops akathisia or drug-induced parkinsonism, treatment should be initiated immediately. For many patients, the onset of EPS is gradual, and if such symptoms occur, they can be treated with anticholinergic medication.

Duration of treatment.   The percentage of patients that will require long-term maintenance anti-EPS medication is controversial; studies report EPS relapse rates varying from 4% to 72% in patients whose anticholinergics are discontinued (Lavin and Rifkin 1991; Manos et al. 1986; Sramek et al. 1986; World Health Organization 1990; Winslow et al. 1986). However, a more recent controlled study reported a relapse rate of only 14% when anti-EPS medication was discontinued in patients who had received long-term treatment with the agent (Double et al. 1993).

In patients with drug-induced akathisia and parkinsonism, the duration of anticholinergic administration should be individually determined (Bezchlibnyk-Butler and Remington 1994; Casey 1993; Tonda and Guthrie 1994). Some patients may require only several months of concomitant anticholinergic drug treatment, because antipsychotic doses are generally decreased when the patient is being managed as an outpatient. Therefore, dose-related EPS may disappear with lower doses. A general recommendation is to manage akathisia and drug-induced parkinsonism as described above, continue the anticholinergic drug for 2–3 months, and then, if the patient has no symptoms of EPS, attempt to taper and discontinue the anticholinergic. If EPS recur, a reasonable approach would be to reinstitute the anticholinergic drug for 3 more months and then reattempt discontinuation (Tonda and Guthrie 1994). If the anticholinergic still cannot be discontinued, a 6-month period of treatment is recommended. At least once a year, the drug should be tapered to determine the lowest effective dose.

■ Mechanism of Action

The dopaminergic-cholinergic balance hypothesis is the foremost theory regarding the etiology of antipsychotic-induced EPS. An equilibrium of dopaminergic (inhibitory) and cholinergic (excitatory) neuronal activity in the corpus striatum is required for normal motor functioning. The interneuronal dopaminergic-blocking action of antipsychotics leads to a functional decrease of dopamine and, hence, a relative increase in interneuronal acetylcholine, resulting in signs and symptoms of EPS (Marsden and Jenner 1980). Of all the EPS, drug-induced akinesia, parkinsonism, and dystonia best fit the dopaminergic-cholinergic equilibrium theory. At this time, little evidence exists for concluding that akathisia is the result of disruption of this equilibrium (Fleischhacker et al. 1990; Marsden and Jenner 1980).

Historically, anticholinergics were believed to act in diminishing or eliminating EPS by reestablishing the dopamine-acetylcholine equilibrium through blockage of acetylcholine in the corpus striatum (Marsden and Jenner 1980). However, recent evidence suggests that these drugs may exert an indirect dopaminergic effect by blocking the presynaptic reuptake and causing the release of dopamine (Bezchlibnyk-Butler and Remington 1994; Modell et al. 1989). In addition, anticholinergics may have agonistic effects on the noradrenergic and serotonin systems and antagonistic effects on glutamate (Tonda and Guthrie 1994). (For a complete discussion of antipsychotic-induced EPS, see *Neurological* adverse effects [page 45] under **Typical Antipsychotics** in Chapter 1.)

■ Dosage

Anticholinergic dosages should be initiated with benztropine 1–2 mg/day or its equivalent (see Product List [page 419]). Smaller initial doses should be used with geriatric patients. Equivalent doses and dosage ranges of anticholinergics are listed under the individual products at the end of this chapter (Bezchlibnyk-Butler and Remington 1994). (For recommended dosing schedules for anticholinergics, see "Pharmacokinetics," below.)

■ Pharmacokinetics

Benztropine has a $t_{1/2}$ of more than 24 hours. Benztropine 6 mg has been successfully and safely administered once daily in a young population (Bezchlibnyk-Butler and Remington 1994). Once-daily dosing of benztropine has not been studied in elderly patients.

Biperiden can be administered once daily, as its $t_{1/2}$ varies from 18 to 24 hours (Bezchlibnyk-Butler and Remington 1994).

Diphenhydramine's availability from an oral dose varies from 65% to 83%. The oral solution and intramuscular injection are 100% absorbed. Diphenhydramine is extensively metabolized in the liver, with more than 4% excreted unchanged in the urine. It has a reported $t_{1/2}$ of 4–15 hours and, therefore, steady state is attained within 2 to 3 days (Alberg et al. 1975; Berlinger et al. 1982; Bezchlibnyk-Butler and Remington 1994).

Orphenadrine has an average $t_{1/2}$ of 12 hours (range 5.5–20.1 hours) and is dosed two to three times a day, as is procyclidine, which also has a $t_{1/2}$ of 12 hours (Bezchlibnyk-Butler and Remington 1994).

Trihexyphenidyl has a relatively short $t_{1/2}$ of 3–10 hours and is dosed three times a day (Bezchlibnyk-Butler and Remington 1994; Gelenberg 1983).

■ Adverse Effects

Adverse effects of anticholinergics are related to their ability to block acetylcholine at muscarinic receptors and, possibly, to their dopamine agonist activity. All anticholinergics will produce these effects in varying degrees, depending on the patient and the drug dosage. In this section, individual differences among these agents are noted, and guidelines are provided for managing their adverse effects (Bezchlibnyk-Butler and Remington 1994).

Allergic
Diphenhydramine is a strong allergen and may cause rash, urticaria, contact dermatitis, and anaphylaxis (Lauderdale et al. 1964; Peters 1989).

Cardiovascular
At recommended anticholinergic doses, the heart rate may increase to 120 beats/minute. Caution should be exercised in patients with angina and/or arrhythmias (Parkes 1981; Peters 1989; Weimer 1980). Dosage reduction should be considered if the patient is symptomatic.

Gastrointestinal

Constipation frequently occurs and should be managed with exercise, a high-bulk diet, and, if necessary, a bulk laxative (e.g., psyllium). Lowering the anticholinergic dosage may be helpful. Adynamic ileus, which presents as abdominal pain, nausea, tenderness in the epigastrium, and reduced bowel sounds, requires discontinuation of the drug and medical management (Parkes 1981; Peters 1989; Weimer 1980).

Dry mouth and/or throat are common complaints of patients who receive anticholinergics. This side effect may or may not be transient. If it persists, the patient is at risk of developing dental caries, gum diseases (e.g., gingivitis, periodontitis), and yeast infections (Gelenberg 1984; Peters 1989).

Dry mouth may be helped symptomatically by agents that stimulate salivation, such as sugarless gum or candy (Gelenberg 1984; Parkes 1981; Weimer 1980). Although not formally studied, commercial artificial saliva preparations or pilocarpine 4% ophthalmic solution 1–2 drops po tid have been clinically reported to afford symptomatic relief (Gelenberg 1984).

Nausea and vomiting have been reported during initial treatment with anticholinergics. Taking doses with food may alleviate this problem, as might reducing the dose.

Genitourinary

Bladder tone and speed of micturition are decreased as a result of anticholinergic effects. Acute urinary retention is a risk, especially in elderly men with enlarged prostate. This condition requires discontinuation of the drug and, possibly, treatment with bethanechol 10–25 mg tid (Peters 1989; Weimer 1980).

Metabolic/Endocrinological/Exocrinological

Hyperpyrexia (i.e., rectal temperatures up to 42°C) has been reported in association with other signs and symptoms of toxicity. This effect is the result of blocking of exocrine sweating and requires discontinuation of the anticholinergic and institution of cooling measures. To prevent hyperpyrexia, patients should avoid excessive heat exposure (Peters 1989; Weimer 1980).

Neurological

Memory impairment may occur acutely with anticholinergics at usual doses, especially in elderly patients (Peters 1989; Tonda and Guthrie 1994). The drug should be discontinued if memory is adversely affected. The acute delirium usually resolves within 36 to 48 hours (Bezchlibnyk-Butler and Remington 1994).

It is unclear whether anticholinergic use increases the risk of tardive dyskinesia, as study results in the literature are conflicting (Casey 1993). (For a complete discussion of this syndrome, see *Tardive dyskinesia* [page 50] under *Neurological* adverse effects of **Typical Antipsychotics** in Chapter 1.)

Ophthalmological

Blurred vision is the result of ciliary muscle paresis. It is rarely serious and generally lasts about 1 week after initiation of treatment. Dose reduction may be helpful, and if the condition persists, it can be treated with topical pilocarpine 0.5%–1% drops. Patients should be cautioned against operating a motor vehicle if the problem is marked and should be instructed to wear sunglasses for photophobia (Parkes 1981; Peters 1989; Weimer 1980). Over time, this effect usually subsides (Bezchlibnyk-Butler and Remington 1994).

Anticholinergics increase intraocular pressure in narrow-angle glaucoma as a result of pupillary dilatation. There is little danger from this effect in a patient with narrow-angle glaucoma if miotic ophthalmic drops are used concurrently with the oral anticholinergic. In wide-angle glaucoma, a significant rise in pressure is unusual, and the drugs can generally be used safely (Parkes 1981; Peters 1989; Reid and Rakes 1983; Weimer 1980).

Psychiatric

A toxic psychosis that develops with usual therapeutic doses of anticholinergics is commonly reported. Often, patients in whom this reaction occurs are also receiving other psychotropic medication with anticholinergic effects (e.g., tricyclic antidepressants, antipsychotics). Geriatric patients may be particularly sensitive to "anticholinergic psychosis"—a condition characterized by visual hallucinations, confusion, disorientation, speech difficulties, emotional liability, and psychotic symptoms. These psychiatric signs are usually accompanied by the physical signs described in this section. Discontinuation of the drug(s) responsible for the reaction usually results in rapid improvement in signs and symptoms within 24 to 36 hours (Bezchlibnyk-Butler and Remington 1994; Peters 1989; Shader and Greenblatt 1980).

Abuse of anticholinergics has been reported (Bezchlibnyk-Butler and Remington 1994; Fleischhacker et al. 1990). Reasons cited for such overuse have included euphoria, reduced anxiety, hallucinations, delusion, memory impairment, and a disturbance of time. However, some patients labeled as anticholinergic abusers may have been appropriately treating their EPS with self-titrated higher doses. Notwithstanding, anticholinergic consumption, especially in polysubstance abusers, should be carefully monitored.

Teratogenicity and Excretion Into Breast Milk

One study reported that the use of diphenhydramine in pregnant women was associated with cleft palate in infants (Saxen 1974). No information is available on breast feeding (Bezchlibnyk-Butler and Remington 1994).

■ Rational Prescribing

1. Anticholinergics should be prescribed only if lowering the dose of the antipsychotic (in an acutely psychotic patient) is not possible and an antipsychotic with lower EPS incidence (e.g., thioridazine, chlorpromazine, olanzapine, risperidone, sertindole) cannot be prescribed (Tonda and Guthrie 1994).
2. Except in special cases, anticholinergics should not routinely be prescribed prophylactically in anticipation of EPS. Not all patients develop EPS and, therefore, some would be receiving these drugs unnecessarily. At regular intervals, all patients receiving antipsychotics should be carefully examined for EPS so that treatment, if necessary, can be promptly instituted.
3. Patients using anticholinergics should be reassessed at least every 3 months for the presence of EPS. Studies indicate that not all patients require long-term anticholinergics, even when the antipsychotic is continued.
4. If a patient does not respond to one anticholinergic at maximal doses, a trial with another may be done empirically.
5. No support exists for the combination use of anticholinergics.

Amantadine

■ Indications

Amantadine was introduced in 1966 for prophylaxis of A2 (Asian) influenza. A patient receiving the drug for this indication noted improvement in her parkinsonian symptomatology. In 1970, an uncontrolled study of amantadine suggested that it was effective in alleviating antipsychotic-induced parkinsonism (Kelly and Abuzzahab 1971).

■ Efficacy

Dystonia
One study reported that amantadine 200–400 mg/day po was more effective than benztropine 4–6 mg/day po in 19 patients with recurrent dystonias who were receiving haloperidol 8–20 mg/day (Borison 1983).

Akathisia
Amantadine has been used as an alternative to anticholinergics and β-blockers in the treatment of akathisia. Three studies, involving a total of 42 patients, have investigated amantadine's utility in managing this symptom (Fleischhacker et al. 1990). One study reported that amantadine was very effective, whereas another reported minimal effect in a group of patients with anticholinergic-refractory akathisia. The third report indicated that tolerance develops to the antiakathistic effect of amantadine within 1 week of treatment initiation (Zubenko et al. 1984a). Thus, the efficacy of amantadine in the treatment of antipsychotic-induced akathisia remains to be demonstrated.

Drug-Induced Parkinsonism
Most studies of drug-induced parkinsonism have found amantadine to be an effective therapy (DiMascio et al. 1976; Fann and Lake 1976; Kelly et al. 1974; Merrick and Schmitt 1973; Silver et al. 1995). Side effects were reported more commonly with anticholinergics (e.g., memory) than with amantadine, and the onset of action of amantadine was within 7 days of initiation of treatment. Few studies have evaluated amantadine's long-term efficacy; however, the development of tolerance to amantadine's effects after 6–12 months has been reported (Bezchlibnyk-Butler and Remington 1994). Amantadine is considered a second-line treatment in drug-induced parkinsonism.

■ Mechanism of Action

Amantadine is a compound with little anticholinergic effects that presumably acts to increase central nervous system (CNS) concentrations of dopamine by blocking dopamine reuptake or by increasing dopamine release from presynaptic fibers (Bezchlibnyk-Butler and Remington 1994). It is theorized that amantadine restores the dopamine-acetylcholine balance in the striatum by enhancing striatal dopamine activity rather than acetylcholine blockade (Fann and Lake 1976).

■ Dosage

Amantadine treatment is initiated at 100 mg/day and increased to 200 mg/day at 1 week. Doses of 300 mg/day may produce further improvement, and 400 mg/day has been tried. Dosing may be once or twice daily (Kelly et al. 1974).

■ Pharmacokinetics

An oral 200-mg dose of amantadine is completely absorbed, and 50%–90% of the drug is excreted unchanged by the kidneys. Half-life varies between 10 and 31 hours in young adults and between 23 and 45 hours in the elderly. Steady-state blood levels are usually achieved within 4 to 7 days. Therapeutic and toxic blood levels have not been established for amantadine, but toxicity has been reported at serum levels of 2.5–5.5 g/mL. Because the kidneys play an important role in elimination of amantadine, lower dosages are used in patients with reduced renal function or congestive heart failure (Gelenberg 1983).

■ Adverse Effects

Cardiovascular

Orthostatic hypotension occurs early in treatment; it may be asymptomatic or cause dizziness and, in some patients, syncope (Parkes 1981). Patients should be monitored with lying and standing blood pressures and warned of possible dizziness and falls.

Approximately 10% of patients treated with amantadine develop ankle edema accompanying livedo (see *Dermatological* adverse effects, below). Edema is usually mild and appears within 6 to 8 weeks of starting treatment. Edema may result from changes in vascular permeability in skin blood vessels, and it is usually unaccompanied by signs of heart, liver, or kidney disease. Although this effect responds to diuretic therapy, amantadine dosage reduction or withdrawal occasionally is required (Parkes 1981).

Dermatological

Livedo reticularis, a reddish-purplish venous marbleization of the skin, occurs in 50%–80% of patients on amantadine. Lesions on the legs are most pronounced, but other parts of the body are involved as well. The lesions may be associated with ankle edema. This reaction occurs at usual dosages, and onset is usually within 2 to 4 months of initiation of treatment. With chronic amantadine use, the livedo reticularis and peripheral edema may subside. The lesions disappear within 2 to 4 weeks after discontinuation of the drug. The mechanism of this effect is not known but may be related to catecholamine depletion in peripheral nerve endings rather than to a pathological change in blood vessels. Although the rash is unsightly and may itch, it is otherwise not troublesome (Parkes 1981).

Gastrointestinal
Nausea, vomiting, constipation, and anorexia occur infrequently with amantadine use. Dosage reduction is recommended to alleviate these adverse effects (Parkes 1981).

Psychiatric

Psychosis. Patients without preexisting psychosis and with a clear sensorium have been reported to experience visual hallucinations within days of starting amantadine 200 mg/day. Hallucinations resolved within 36 to 48 hours after discontinuation of the drug (Parkes 1981). Exacerbation of psychosis has been reported in three patients being treated with an antipsychotic when amantadine was added for treatment of EPS (Nestelbaum et al. 1986).

Delirium. Delirium, or toxic psychosis, is characterized by confusion with auditory and/or visual hallucinations and unpleasant dreams. After drug discontinuation, symptoms generally abate within 2 to 7 days. This adverse reaction is more common with amantadine dosages at the upper therapeutic range and often occurs with overdoses of the drug (Parkes 1981).

Up to 10% of people taking 200 mg/day develop these psychoses. When such symptoms occur, they normally do so within the first 48 hours of treatment (Parkes 1981). They are usually transitory and subside with continued treatment.

The psychiatric adverse effects of amantadine are hypothesized to be the result of the drug's ability to increase dopamine levels in the CNS. It has been suggested that amantadine's CNS adverse effects are more common in patients concurrently receiving anticholinergics (Parkes 1981).

Irritability/hostility. Symptoms of CNS stimulation, with restlessness, nervousness, and irritability, occur in as many as 20% of patients with Parkinson's disease who receive amantadine 100–300 mg/day (Parkes 1981). These symptoms usually occur within 2 to 3 weeks of initiation of amantadine. Depending on the severity of these side effects, the dose should be reduced or the drug discontinued.

Teratogenicity and Excretion Into Breast Milk
Little information is available to draw conclusions about use of amantadine during pregnancy and while nursing. The drug should be avoided during pregnancy, and nursing is not recommended for women receiving amantadine.

■ Rational Prescribing

1. Amantadine is considered a second-line treatment for drug-induced parkinsonism and a fourth-line treatment for antipsychotic-induced akathisia.
2. General guidelines that apply to anticholinergics (see "Rational Prescribing" [page 411] under **Anticholinergics**) should be followed when prescribing amantadine.

Benzodiazepines

Only limited information is available on the use of benzodiazepines (BZDs) to treat antipsychotic-induced EPS. None of the BZDs are approved by the U.S. Food and Drug Administration (FDA) for this purpose. (For a complete discussion of BZD indications, mechanism of action, dosages, pharmacokinetics, and adverse effects, see Chapter 4.)

■ Efficacy

Dystonia
In a single-dose study, diazepam 5 mg iv was as effective as diphenhydramine 50 mg iv in reversing dystonia (Gagrat et al. 1978).

Akathisia
The use of BZDs in the management of antipsychotic-induced akathisia has been reviewed (Fleischhacker et al. 1990). Of eight studies, four used diazepam and two each investigated lorazepam and clonazepam (Fleischhacker et al. 1990; Kutcher et al. 1989). Typical dosages were diazepam 40 mg/day or its equivalent (see Table 10–3 [page 570]). The six studies that reported positive results noted that improvement occurred within 3 to 7 days. It is unknown whether tolerance develops to akathisia, as most cases reported are of short duration (i.e., <1 week). At present there is no evidence to indicate that one BZD is more effective than another in treating this symptom.

■ **Rational Prescribing**

1. Until further investigations are performed, BZDs are considered a second-line treatment of dystonia and akathisia.
2. The same general guidelines that apply to anticholinergics (see "Rational Prescribing" [page 411] under **Anticholinergics**) should be followed when prescribing a BZD for antipsychotic-induced akathisia.

β-Adrenergic–Blocking Drugs

None of the β-blocking drugs are approved by the FDA for treating antipsychotic-induced EPS. (For a complete discussion of BZD indications, pharmacokinetics, and adverse effects, see Chapter 4.)

■ **Efficacy**

The efficacy of β-adrenergic–blocking agents in akathisia has been reviewed (Fleischhacker et al. 1990). Of 14 studies, 13 examined propranolol alone or in comparison with another agent. Other β-adrenergic–blocking agents examined included atenolol, metoprolol, pindolol, nadolol, stadol, and betaxolol. Only 6 of the 14 investigations were performed blind, most were of short duration (i.e., <1 week), and patients typically received anticholinergic agents in addition to the β-blockers.

In summary, studies with propranolol indicate a 50%–65% response rate at doses of 20–80 mg/day. Onset of action varied from 36 hours to 5 days, with minimal side effects. In comparison studies, propranolol has been shown to be equal in efficacy to betaxolol but more effective than atenolol, pindolol, metoprolol, and stadol. One open study reported nadolol to be effective. If a patient fails to respond to a propranolol trial or cannot tolerate the drug, use of pindolol might be considered (Fleischhacker et al. 1990).

Discontinuation of propranolol will result in return of symptoms within 3 to 5 days (Zubenko et al. 1984b). One report indicated that tolerance did not develop to propranolol over a 6-month treatment period.

■ **Mechanism of Action**

The exact mechanism by which β-blockers may reduce akathisia is unknown. The effect may depend predominately on the blockade of CNS β-adrenergic receptors (Fleischhacker et al. 1990).

■ Dosage

See "Efficacy," above.

■ Adverse Effects

In one study, propranolol 30–80 mg/day produced no signs of peripheral β_1 blockade, such as reduction in pulse rate or blood pressure (Adler et al. 1986; Lipinski et al. 1984; Zubenko et al. 1984b). However, metoprolol 300–400 mg/day produced significant β_1 and β_2 blockade, with patients experiencing significant decreases in pulse and blood pressure (Zubenko et al. 1984b). Thus, patients receiving β-blockers should have their blood pressure and pulse routinely monitored until maximum dosages are reached. Two patients, one receiving propranolol and the other receiving metoprolol, were reported to develop bronchospasm (a β_2 effect) while being treated for antipsychotic-induced akathisia.

■ Rational Prescribing

1. β-blockers are an effective treatment for antipsychotic-induced akathisia. Based on preliminary reports, propranolol is the first-line β-blocker.
2. General guidelines that apply to anticholinergics (see "Rational Prescribing" [page 411] under **Anticholinergics**) should be followed when prescribing β-blockers for akathisia.

Clonidine

■ Indications

Clonidine is not approved by the FDA for treating antipsychotic-induced akathisia.

■ Efficacy

Clonidine's efficacy in treating akathisia has been investigated in an open, on-drug/off-drug trial (Zubenko et al. 1984c). Of six patients, four experienced complete remission of their symptoms; the other two demonstrated substantial improvement. Dosages ranged from 0.2 to 0.8 mg/day, and maximal response was achieved within 24 to 48 hours. Symptomatic orthostatic hypotension occurred in two patients. The authors recommended that clonidine be instituted at 0.1 mg twice daily and that the daily dose be increased by a maximum of 0.1 mg twice daily every other day until akathisia remits, hypotension or sedation develops, or the maximum daily dose of 2.4 mg is reached.

This initial report was followed by a single-blind rater trial (Adler et al. 1987). Six patients with antipsychotic-induced akathisia who were receiving clonidine 0.15–0.4 mg/day improved significantly on both objective and subjective ratings. However, increases in clonidine dosages were limited by the onset of sedative and hypotensive effects in four and five patients, respectively.

■ Mechanism of Action

The exact mechanism of clonidine's effect on antipsychotic-induced akathisia is unknown (Adler et al. 1986).

■ Dosage

See "Efficacy," above.

■ Rational Prescribing

1. Current evidence suggests that propranolol is better tolerated than clonidine in patients with antipsychotic-induced akathisia. These preliminary results need to be replicated in double-blind, controlled trials. However, in patients with akathisia who are unresponsive to primary treatments, use of clonidine might be considered.
2. General guidelines applicable to anticholinergics (see "Rational Prescribing" [page 411] under **Anticholinergics**) should be followed when prescribing clonidine for akathisia.

Levodopa

■ Indications

Levodopa (L-dopa) is not approved by the FDA for treating antipsychotic-induced parkinsonism.

■ Efficacy

One study concluded that L-dopa at dosages up to 600 mg/day was slightly but nonsignificantly more effective than placebo, although some patients experienced significant improvement at these doses (Chouinard et al. 1987). The authors of the study suggested that higher doses might improve the response rate.

■ Mechanism of Action

It is theorized that L-dopa restores the dopamine-acetylcholine balance in the striatum by enhancing the activity of striatal dopamine (Chouinard et al. 1987; Fann and Lake 1976).

■ Dosage

See "Efficacy," above.

■ Adverse Effects

L-dopa had previously not been widely studied because of concerns that it might produce or exacerbate psychosis (see "Mechanism of Action" [page 12] under **Typical Antipsychotics** in Chapter 1) (Chouinard et al. 1987).

■ Rational Prescribing

1. L-dopa is considered a third-line treatment for antipsychotic-induced parkinsonism because studies examining its efficacy and safety for this indication are lacking. Patients receiving the drug should be closely monitored for exacerbation of psychosis.
2. The same general guidelines that apply to anticholinergics (see "Rational Prescribing" [page 411] under **Anticholinergics**) should be followed when prescribing L-dopa.

Product List

(See Chapter 4 for the benzodiazepine and β-blocker product lists.)

Amantadine (dopaminergic)
- Daily dose range: 100–400 mg
- Generic cost index: ≈ 0.22

    Capsules: **Symmetrel**®
    100 mg   [$17/20] Endo 105, red

    Syrup: **Symmetrel**®
    50 mg/5 mL   [$81/480 mL]

Benztropine (anticholinergic)
- Relative oral potency: 2 mg
- Daily dose range: 1–12 mg; 1–2 mg iv, im dystonia
- Generic cost index: ≈ 0.13

Tablets:	**Cogentin**®
0.5 mg	[$18] MSD 21, white
1 mg	[$21] MSD 635, white
2 mg	[$26] MSD 60, white

Injection:	**Cogentin**®
1 mg/mL	[$7/2-mL ampule]

Biperiden (anticholinergic)
- Relative oral potency: 2 mg
- Daily dose range: 2–40 mg

Tablets:	**Akineton**®
2 mg	[$26] scored

Injection:	**Akineton**®
5 mg/mL	[$3/1-mL ampule]

Diphenhydramine (anticholinergic)
- Relative oral potency: 25 mg
- Daily dose range: 25–200 mg, 50 mg iv, im dystonia
- Generic cost index: ≈ 0.07

Capsules:	**Benadryl**®
25 mg	[$22] PD 471, pink/white
50 mg	[$30] PD 373, pink/white

Injection:	**Benadryl**®
50 mg/mL	[$17/10-mL vial]
50 mg/mL	[$2/1-mL unit dose syringe]
50 mg/mL	[$2/1-mL ampule]

Elixir:	**Benadryl**®
12.5 mg/5 mL	[$4/120 mL] 14% ethanol
12.5 mg/5 mL	[$7/240 mL] 14% ethanol

Orphenadrine (anticholinergic)
- Relative oral potency: 50 mg
- Daily dose range: 50–400 mg
- Generic cost index: ≈ 0.16

Tablets:	**Norflex**®
100 mg	[$143]
30 mg/mL	[$10/2-mL ampule]

Procyclidine (anticholinergic)
- Relative oral potency: 5 mg
- Daily dose range: 2.5–30 mg

Tablets:	**Kemadrin**®
5 mg	[$42] Kemadrin S3A

Trihexyphenidyl (anticholinergic)
- Relative oral potency: 5 mg
- Daily dose range: 2–30 mg
- Generic cost index: ≈ 0.4

Tablets:	**Artane**®
2 mg	[$16], white
5 mg	[$32], white

| Elixir: | **Artane**® |
| 2 mg/5 mL | [$32/480 mL] 5% ethanol |

References

Adler L, Angrist B, Peselow E, et al: A controlled assessment of propranolol in the treatment of neuroleptic-induced akathisia. Br J Psychiatry 149:42–45, 1986

Adler LA, Angrist B, Peselow E, et al: Clonidine in neuroleptic-induced akathisia. Am J Psychiatry 144:235–236, 1987

Adler LA, Peselow E, Rosenthal M, et al: A controlled comparison of the effects of propranolol, benztropine, and placebo on akathisia: an interim analysis. Psychopharmacol Bull 29:283–286, 1993

Alberg KS, Hallmark MR, Sakmar E, et al: Pharmacokinetics of diphenhydramine in man. Journal of Pharmacokinetics and Biopharmaceutics 3:159–170, 1975

Arana GW, Goff DC, Baldessarini FJ, et al: Efficacy of anticholinergic prophylaxis for neuroleptic-induced acute dystonia. Am J Psychiatry 145:993–996, 1988

Berlinger WG, Goldberg MJ, Spector R, et al: Diphenhydramine: kinetics and psychomotor effects in elderly women. Clin Pharmacol Ther 32:387–391, 1982

Bezchlibnyk-Butler KZ, Remington GJ: Antiparkinsonian drugs in the treatment of neuroleptic-induced extrapyramidal symptoms. Can J Psychiatry 39:74–84, 1994

Borison RL: Amantadine in the management of extrapyramidal side effects. Clin Neuropharmacol 6 (suppl):S57–S63, 1983

Casey DE: Neuroleptic-induced acute extrapyramidal syndromes and tardive dyskinesia. Psychiatr Clin North Am 16:589–610, 1993

Casey DE: Motor and mental aspects of acute extrapyramidal syndromes. Acta Psychiatr Scand 89 (suppl 380):14–20, 1994

Chouinard G, Annable L, Mercier P, et al: Long-term effects of L-dopa and procyclidine on neuroleptic-induced extrapyramidal and schizophrenic symptoms. Psychopharmacol Bull 23:221–226, 1987

DiMascio A, Bernardo DL, Greenblatt DJ, et al: A controlled trial of amantadine in drug-induced extrapyramidal disorders. Arch Gen Psychiatry 33:599–602, 1976

Donlon PT, Stenson RL: Neuroleptic induced extrapyramidal symptoms. Diseases of the Nervous System 37:629–635, 1976

Double DB, Warren GC, Evans M, et al: Efficacy of maintenance use of anticholinergic agents. Acta Psychiatr Scand 88:381–384, 1993

Fann WE, Lake CR: Amantadine versus trihexyphenidyl in the treatment of neuroleptic-induced parkinsonism. Am J Psychiatry 133:940–943, 1976

Fleischhacker WW, Roth SD, Kane JM: The pharmacologic treatment of neuroleptic-induced akathisia. J Clin Psychopharmacol 10:12–21, 1990

Friis T, Christensen TR, Gerlach J: Sodium valproate and biperiden in neuroleptic-induced akathisia, parkinsonism and hyperkinesia. Acta Psychiatr Scand 67:178–187, 1983

Gagrat D, Hamilton J, Belmaker RH: Intravenous diazepam in the treatment of neuroleptic-induced acute dystonia and akathisia. Am J Psychiatry 135:1232–1233, 1978

Gelenberg AJ: Treating extrapyramidal reactions. Biological Therapies in Psychiatry 6:13–16, 1983

Gelenberg AJ: Dry mouth. Biological Therapies in Psychiatry 7:18–19, 1984

Kelly JT, Abuzzahab FS: The antiparkinson properties of amantadine hydrochloride in drug-induced parkinsonism. Journal of Clinical Pharmacology and New Drugs 11:211–214, 1971

Kelly JT, Zimmerman RL, Abuzzahab FS, et al: A double-blind study of amantadine hydrochloride versus benztropine mesylate in drug-induced parkinsonism. Pharmacology 12:65–73, 1974

Kutcher S, Williamson P, MacKenzie S, et al: Successful clonazepam treatment of neuroleptic-induced akathisia in older adolescents and young adults: a double-blind, placebo-controlled study. J Clin Psychopharmacol 9:403–406, 1989

Lauderdale WH, Fred HL, Graber CD: Anaphylactoid reaction to diphenhydramine hydrochloride. Arch Intern Med 114:693–695, 1964

Lavin MR, Rifkin A: Prophylactic antiparkinson drug use, II: withdrawal after long-term maintenance therapy. J Clin Pharmacol 31:769–777, 1991

Lee AS: Treatment of drug-induced dystonic reactions. JACEP 8:453–457, 1979

Lipinski JF, Zubenko GS, Cohen BM, et al: Propranolol in the treatment of neuroleptic-induced akathisia. Am J Psychiatry 141:412–415, 1984

Manos N, Gkiouzepas J, Logothetic J: The need for continuous use of antiparkinsonian medication with chronic schizophrenic patients receiving long-term neuroleptic therapy. Am J Psychiatry 138:184–188, 1981

Manos N, Lavrentiadis G, Gkiouzepas J: Evaluation of the need for prophylactic antiparkinson medication in psychotic patients treated with neuroleptics. J Clin Psychiatry 47:114–116, 1986

Marsden CD, Jenner P: The pathophysiology of extrapyramidal side effects of neuroleptic drugs. Psychol Med 10:55–72, 1980

McEvoy JP: The clinical use of anticholinergic drugs as treatment for extrapyramidal side effects of neuroleptic drugs. J Clin Psychopharmacol 3:288–302, 1983

Merrick EM, Schmitt PP: A controlled study of the clinical effects of amantadine hydrochloride (Symmetrel). Current Therapeutic Research, Clinical and Experimental 15:552–558, 1973

Modell JG, Tandon R, Beresford TP: Dopaminergic activity of the antimuscarinic antiparkinsonian agents. J Clin Psychopharmacol 9:347–351, 1989

Nestelbaum Z, Siris SG, Rifkin A, et al: Exacerbation of schizophrenia associated with amantadine. Am J Psychiatry 143:1170–1171, 1986

Parkes JD: Adverse effects of antiparkinsonian drugs. Drugs 21:341–353, 1981

Peters NL: Snipping the thread of life: antimuscarinic side effects of medications in the elderly. Arch Intern Med 149:2414–2420, 1989

Reid WH, Rakes S: Intraocular pressure in patients receiving psychotropic medications. Psychosomatics 24:665–667, 1983

Sachdev P, Loneragan C: Intravenous benztropine and propranolol challenges in acute neuroleptic-induced akathisia. Clin Neuropharmacol 16:324–331, 1993

Saxen I: Cleft palate and maternal diphenhydramine intake (letter). Lancet 1:407–408, 1974

Shader RI, Greenblatt DJ: Belladonna alkaloids and synthetic anticholinergics: uses and toxicity, in Psychiatric Complications of Medical Drugs. Edited by Shader RI. New York, Macmillan, 1980, pp 120–137

Silver H, Geraisy N, Schwartz M: No difference in the effect of biperiden and amantadine on parkinsonian- and tardive dyskinesia-type involuntary movements: a double-blind crossover, placebo-controlled study in medicated chronic schizophrenic patients. J Clin Psychiatry 56:167–170, 1995

Sramek JJ, Simpson GM, Morrison RL, et al: Anticholinergic agents for prophylaxis of neuroleptic-induced dystonic reactions: a prospective study. J Clin Psychiatry 47:305–309, 1986

Tarsy D: Neuroleptic-induced extrapyramidal reactions: classification, description, and diagnosis. Clin Neuropharmacol 6:9–26, 1983

Tonda ME, Guthrie SK: Treatment of acute neuroleptic-induced movement disorders. Pharmacotherapy 14:543–560, 1994

Weimer N: Atropine, scopolamine, and related antimuscarinic drugs, in The Pharmacological Basis of Therapeutics, 6th Edition. Edited by Gilman AL, Goodman LS, Gilman A. New York, Macmillan, 1980, pp 120–137

Winslow RS, Stillner V, Coons DJ, et al: Prevention of acute dystonic reactions in patients beginning high-potency neuroleptics. Am J Psychiatry 143:706–710, 1986

World Health Organization (heads of centres collaborating in WHO-coordinated studies on biological aspects of mental illness): Prophylactic use of anticholinergics in patients on long-term neuroleptic treatment (editorial). Br J Psychiatry 156:412, 1990

Zubenko GS, Barreira P, Lipinski JF: Development of tolerance to the therapeutic effect of amantadine on akathisia. J Clin Psychopharmacol 4:128–130, 1984a

Zubenko GS, Lipinski JF, Cohen BM, et al: Comparison of metoprolol and propranolol in the treatment of akathisia. Psychiatry Res 11:143–149, 1984b

Zubenko GS, Cohen BM, Lipinski JF, et al: Use of clonidine in treating neuroleptic-induced akathisia. Psychiatry Res 13:253–259, 1984c

6

7

Psychotropic Drug Treatment of Alcohol and Drug Dependence

Three medications—methadone, L-alpha-acetyl methadol (LAAM), and naltrexone—have received U.S. Food and Drug Administration (FDA) approval for treatment of opiate dependence. Many medications are under active investigation for use in the treatment of alcohol and cocaine dependence. However, no medication has received FDA approval for use in the treatment of cocaine dependence, and only two have received approval for use in the treatment of alcohol dependence. These two drugs, disulfiram and naltrexone, are very different in their mechanisms for achieving reduced alcohol consumption in patients.

Disulfiram

■ Indications

A number of substances, when taken with ethanol, produce an adverse or toxic reaction (Table 7–1). Only one of these substances, disulfiram (Antabuse), is used therapeutically in the United States for the treatment of alcohol dependence.

Disulfiram's effect with alcohol was first noted in 1937, and its use as a prophylactic agent in the treatment of alcoholism was first reported in 1948 (Hald and Jacobsen 1948; Wright and Moore 1990). It has been used extensively since that time in the behavioral treatment of alcohol dependence. Alcohol-dependent individuals are usually given disulfiram daily (or, on occasion, two to three times per week) and are informed that if they drink within 7 to 14 days of taking disulfiram, they can suffer a serious and potentially fatal reaction.

Theoretically, therefore, individuals are able to concentrate their daily decision whether to drink to one point in time. Once they have taken the drug, they know they cannot drink for 1–2 weeks without possibly suffering a serious toxic reaction.

425

Table 7-1.   Drugs and chemicals producing effects similar to those of disulfiram when used with ethanol

Antimicrobial agents
  Cephalosporins (cefoperazone, moxalactam, cefotetan)
  Chloramphenicol
  Diethylthiocarbamate (Imuthiol®)
  Furazolidone
  Griseofulvin
  Metronidazole (Flagyl®)
  Quinacrine
  Nitrofurantoin
Oral hypoglycemic agents
  Acetohexamide (Dymelor®)
  Chlorpropamide (Diabenese®)
  Glipizide (Glucotrol®)
  Glyburide (DiaBeta®, Micronase®)
  Tolazamide (Tolinase®)
  Tolbutamide (Orinase®)
Industrial agents
  4-Bromopyrazole
  Carbon disulfide
  Hydrogen sulfide
  Tetraethyl lead
  Pyrogallol
Miscellaneous
  Animal charcoal (amorphous carbon)
  Butanol oxime
  Calcium carbimide (Temposil®; used in Canada as antialcohol
    agent)
  Mushrooms *(Corprinus atramentarius, Clitocybe clavipes)*
  Nitrefazole
  Pargyline
  Phentolamine
  Procarbazine
  Tolazoline

Source.   Goldfrank et al. 1990; Peachey et al. 1981; Sellers et al. 1981.

■ Efficacy

Multiple studies have attested to the effectiveness of disulfiram in the treatment of alcoholism. Unfortunately, most of these studies had significant design flaws (Kwentus and Major 1981; Larson et al. 1992). An exception was the well-designed multicenter Veterans Administration (VA) collaborative study (Fuller et al. 1986), which compared regular-dose disulfiram (250 mg), inactive-dose disulfiram (1 mg), and placebo in 605 alcoholic patients, each of whom was randomly assigned to one of these treatment groups and followed for 1 year in terms of abstinence, drinking days, working days, family stability, and number of attended scheduled visits. No statistical differences in these parameters among the three groups were found. However, when a subgroup of only those patients who were available for all seven scheduled follow-up interviews were assessed, those patients in that subgroup who received disulfiram 250 mg reported fewer drinking days than those who received disulfiram 1 mg or placebo. Even in this subgroup, however, the medication groups differed on no other outcome measures.

The VA study also found that patients compliant with their medication regimen (regardless of which medication group they were in) did better in terms of abstinence than those who were noncompliant.

These findings are compatible with other studies that found that only certain types of patients do well on disulfiram—namely, those who are compliant, older, socially stable, well motivated, not depressed, and not sociopathic (Lundwall and Baekland 1971; Schuckit 1985). The VA study's findings are also compatible with other studies that have reported that patients with such characteristics do well regardless of whether they are taking disulfiram (Kwentus and Major 1981).

There is a general consensus, despite lack of hard data, that disulfiram is a useful adjunctive drug when used in conjunction with other behavioral and psychosocial therapies. Emphasis is usually placed on the ineffectiveness of disulfiram when it is the only form of therapy (Allen and Litten 1992; Sellers et al. 1981; Wright and Moore 1990).

In agreement with this emphasis, a number of studies have reported that the manner of disulfiram's administration may determine its efficacy. These findings indicate that having a spouse or significant other observe and/or supervise the patient taking disulfiram and reporting lapses to a therapist significantly increases compliance and enhances abstinence (Allen and Litten 1992; Azrin et al. 1982; Brewer 1992; Chick et al. 1992; Gerrein et al. 1973; O'Farrell and Bayog 1986). Other studies (Duckert and Johnsen 1987; Duckert et al. 1981) have reported enhanced abstinence rates among disulfiram users when they were instructed to take disulfiram only when they felt a need for it—for example, before entering a situation with a high risk for drinking, to end a bout of drinking, or to maintain a period of sobriety during stressful times.

■ Mechanism of Action

Normally, ethanol is metabolized in the liver first to acetaldehyde by alcohol dehydrogenase and then to acetate by aldehyde dehydrogenase (ALDH). Disulfiram inhibits aldehyde dehydrogenase and, hence, when used in the presence of alcohol, causes an increase in blood acetaldehyde levels. It is postulated that these increased acetaldehyde levels cause the toxic disulfiram–ethanol reaction (DER). This postulate has been questioned, because acetaldehyde poisoning causes hypertension, not hypotension as usually occurs during a DER. It is generally concluded, however, that acetaldehyde is involved in the reaction, perhaps through the release of mediators such as histamine (Kwentus and Major 1981; Petersen 1992).

ALDH inhibition by disulfiram develops slowly over 12–24 hours and is irreversible, with recovery of ALDH activity requiring de novo synthesis of the enzyme, which takes 6 days or more (Peachey and Sellers 1981; Petersen 1992). Disulfiram's alcohol-sensitizing properties follow the time course of the ALDH inhibition. The intensity and duration of the reaction is directly related to the dosage of the drug and the dosage of alcohol ingested. However, there are significant interindividual differences in blood acetaldehyde levels and intensity of response to any given acetaldehyde level, and great variability in these responses in any given individual on different drinking occasions (Brien et al. 1980; Larson et al. 1992).

■ Dosage

Doses of disulfiram higher than 500 mg/day are likely to produce medically serious disulfiram-ethanol reactions (Peachey et al. 1981). In addition, disulfiram doses higher than 500 mg/day are associated with a high incidence of non–alcohol-related adverse effects. For these reasons, disulfiram is generally given at a dose of 500 mg/day for only 5 days and reduced to 250 mg/day thereafter. The DER will not occur at a disulfiram dose of 250 mg until 12 or more hours after initial dosing. This time period can be shortened somewhat with higher doses of disulfiram, and it is for this reason that loading doses of 500 mg are usually prescribed for the first 5 days of use. When used in an inpatient setting, where speed of onset of the drug's effects is not usually crucial, disulfiram can be initiated at a dose of 250 mg/day. Although 250 mg/day is the dose generally given in the United States, in approximately 50% of patients this dose does not reliably cause a DER (Wright and Moore 1990). Thus, if patients report drinking while taking the 250-mg dose without experiencing a DER, the dose is raised to 500 mg.

Only one type of tablet formulation of disulfiram is available in the United States. In Denmark, an effervescent tablet is available that has been demonstrated to have two to three times the bioavailability of the noneffervescent tablet (Andersen 1992).

It has also been demonstrated that a light meal 15 minutes before disulfiram ingestion increases the bioavailability of disulfiram by a factor of 2 to 3, compared with taking disulfiram on an empty stomach (Andersen 1992).

The dose is taken once per day, usually at night, because disulfiram frequently (at least initially) causes drowsiness.

Surgical implantation of disulfiram tablets (800–1,600 mg) under the skin to achieve long-term therapeutic effects is not practiced in the United States but has been used in Canada and England. Studies to date have found active tablets no better than placebo tablets in ameliorating the signs and symptoms of alcoholism. In addition, neither measurable disulfiram blood levels nor reactions to an alcohol challenge have been found in patients receiving active tablets (Bergstrom et al. 1982; Morland et al. 1984; Wilson et al. 1980, 1984).

The failure of implanted disulfiram tablets to have a clinical or therapeutic effect has led to efforts to develop an injectable sustained-release depot form of disulfiram. Testing in humans of the initial formulations has demonstrated mild reactions to alcohol challenges for 14 days and detectable breath acetaldehyde concentrations for 28 days after injection (Johnsen and Morland 1992; Phillips and Greenberg 1992).

Investigations of the metabolism of disulfiram have led to the finding that diethylthiocarbamic acid methyl ester sulfoxide (DETC-MeSo) may be the active metabolite of disulfiram responsible for the inhibition of aldehyde dehydrogenase. The development of this metabolite as a separate pharmacological agent that would have greater potency and perhaps fewer side effects than disulfiram is anticipated (Hart and Faiman 1994; Petersen 1992).

Investigators are also developing an assay of ALDH activity in the leukocytes of peripheral blood. This activity appears to be quite similar to the ALDH activity in the liver, and thus the possibility exists of developing a clinically feasible lab test done on peripheral blood that can be used to determine if an individual has been given a sufficient amount of disulfiram to cause a DER (Petersen 1992).

■ Pharmacokinetics

Disulfiram is 80% absorbed from the gastrointestinal tract, with peak blood levels reached 1 hour after ingestion. The parent compound is metabolized to diethyldithiocarbamate (DDC), which is further metabolized to diethylamine, carbon disulfide, diethyldithiocarbamic glucuronide (DDC glucuronide), sulfate, and methyl ester, and to diethylthiocarbamic acid methyl ester (DETC-Me) and DETC-MeSo (Hart and Faiman 1994; Petersen 1992). Recent work has indicated that DETC-MeSo may be the active metabolite in inhibiting ALDH. Approximately 5%–20% of disulfiram is excreted unchanged in the feces; 30%–80% is excreted via the kidney as diethylamine, DDC glucuronide, and sulfate; and 12%–50% is excreted via the lung as carbon disulfide (Faiman 1979). Excretion is slow, with about 20% of a disulfiram dose detectable 1 week after ingestion (Goldfrank 1994).

Because inhibition of ALDH is irreversible and requires the synthesis of new ALDH, there is no correlation between blood levels of disulfiram or its metabolites and ALDH inhibition or DER intensity (Petersen 1992).

■ Disulfiram-Ethanol Reaction

The DER occurs 10–20 minutes after the ingestion of alcohol and lasts 1–2 hours (Banys 1988; Liskow et al. 1990). The severity of the reaction correlates with the dose of disulfiram and the amount of alcohol ingested; however, because the reaction can occur with even small amounts of alcohol, patients must be warned to avoid ingestion of *any* alcohol, including preparations (e.g., over-the-counter cough medicines and mouthwashes) that contain alcohol (Goldfrank et al. 1990).

The DER consists of flushing, diaphoresis, tachycardia, palpitations, dyspnea, hyperventilation, anxiety, nausea, vomiting, headaches, vertigo, and abdominal pain. Severe reactions can include severe hypotension (shock), loss of consciousness, and death. Treatment is supportive. Hypotension is treated with intravenous saline or lactated Ringer's solution and by placing the patient in the Trendelenburg position. If these actions do not restore blood pressure, a direct-acting sympathomimetic such as norepinephrine may be used (Goldfrank 1994). For refractory vomiting, prochlorperazine may be used.

Although 4-methylpyrazol, which inhibits alcohol dehydrogenase and thus prevents the formation of acetaldehyde, has shown some promise as an antidote for the DER (Lindros et al. 1981), it has not been studied for this purpose to a significant degree.

■ Adverse Effects

The adverse effects discussed below refer to the effects of disulfiram alone and not to those of its combination with alcohol.

Cardiovascular

Concern regarding the cardiovascular effects of disulfiram has arisen from the finding that viscose rayon workers who were exposed to carbon disulfide have a higher rate of cardiovascular disease than a comparable control group (Hernberg et al. 1970). Carbon disulfide is a major metabolite of disulfiram, and it is unknown whether chronic disulfiram users will eventually have an increased incidence of cardiovascular disease. In addition, patients receiving disulfiram 500 mg/day for 6 weeks were noted to have an increase in serum cholesterol, although such an increase did not occur at drug doses of 250 mg/day (Major and Goyer 1978).

Central Nervous System

In the early years of its use, disulfiram was reported to cause psychosis and delusions in up to 16% of users (Bennett et al. 1951). At that time, the maintenance dose of disulfiram was 1.5–2.0 g/day. In recent years, the usual dose of disulfiram has been 250–500 mg/day, and the incidence of psychosis has dropped to occasional case reports related to intentional or accidental overdoses. These psychotic reactions, which include hallucinations, delusions, and bizarre behavior, are often accompanied by disorientation, anxiety, sleep disorders, depression, memory impairment, and disordered intellectual functioning. Electroencephalogram (EEG) correlates of the psychosis consist of a slowing of the basic pattern and the appearance of distinct delta waves. Withdrawal of disulfiram usually results in clearance of psychotic symptoms in 1–4 weeks (Rainey 1977).

Delirium and psychosis have also been postulated to be caused by carbon disulfide, although this explanation has been seriously questioned by studies that indicate that not enough carbon disulfide is produced in the metabolism of disulfiram to account for the degree of neurotoxicity observed (Faiman 1979; Rainey 1977).

There are reports that disulfiram exacerbates underlying schizophrenia, and this effect, as well as the tendency to cause psychosis de novo at high doses, has been attributed to disulfiram's known property of inhibiting dopamine β-hydroxylase (which catalyzes the conversion of dopamine to norepinephrine), leading to an accumulation of dopamine (Goldstein and Nakajima 1967; Heath et al. 1965). A recent review, however, concluded that at its usual dose of 250 mg/ day, disulfiram does not significantly increase the risk of psychiatric complications or of psychiatric drug interactions and can thus be used safely in alcoholic persons with co-occurring psychiatric disorders (Larson et al. 1992).

This conclusion is strengthened by a recent double-blind study that compared the effects of disulfiram 250 mg, disulfiram 1 mg, and placebo in 605 alcoholic patients followed for 1 year. No differences were found in the incidence of psychiatric complications among the three groups (Branchey et al. 1987).

Disulfiram initially induces drowsiness and lethargy in approximately 50% of patients. This side effect generally abates within 2 weeks and usually can be managed by giving the daily dose at bedtime (Gerrein et al. 1973).

Hypersensitivity and Toxic Reactions

One percent to 5% of patients develop a drug-related rash, usually consisting of pruritic erythematous vesicular eruptions on the face and extremities. The peak incidence for occurrence is within 7 to 10 days of beginning disulfiram, but the rash may occur at any time, including after years of use. This rash generally improves with routine symptomatic treatment whether or not the drug is discontinued (Enghusen-Poulsen et al. 1992; Fox 1968).

Reviews of the literature by Kristensen (1981) and Wright et al. (1988) indicate that 53 cases of disulfiram-induced hepatitis have been reported, of which 5 were confirmed by rechallenge testing. Eleven patients died; in those patients who survived, the hepatic damage was reversible. Most patients developed hepatotoxicity within 2 weeks to 2 months of being placed on disulfiram. Based on their review, Wright and colleagues (1988) recommended that liver-function tests be obtained before treatment, at 2-week intervals for 2 months, and at 3- to 6-month intervals thereafter. In a later report, Wright et al. (1993) suggested that alanine aminotransferase (ALT), aspartate aminotransferase (AST), λ-glutamyl transpeptidase (GGTP), and alkaline phosphatase be measured 2–4 weeks after starting therapy and that therapy be discontinued if ALT is three times above the upper limit of normal. However, only 1 in 500 patients with an elevated ALT is estimated to be at risk of developing severe hepatitis. In addition, after 4 weeks on disulfiram, approximately 30% of patients develop one or more elevations above the upper limit of normal for ALT, AST, GGTP, or alkaline phosphatase (Wright et al. 1993). For the vast majority of patients, these elevated values are of no clinical significance and return to normal with continued use of disulfiram. Because of this large number of elevated liver-function test values without clinical consequence, not all authorities recommend that routine liver-function tests be done (Enghusen-Poulsen et al. 1992; Phillips 1990). The low utility of routine testing is supported by one study in which 453 patients assigned to either disulfiram or placebo were followed for 1 year with repeated liver-function tests. Elevated liver-function test values were found to be significantly associated with continued drinking but not with use of disulfiram (Iber et al. 1987).

One putative problem that frequently causes concern among clinicians is the interaction of topically applied alcohol (e.g., aftershave lotion) and disulfiram. Patients taking disulfiram are frequently advised to avoid such topical products. A controlled study (Haddock and Wilkin 1982) has demonstrated, however, that alcoholic persons reacted no differently to topically applied alcohols (ethanol, n-propyl, isopropyl) and acetaldehyde before and 14 days after disulfiram therapy, and reacted no differently than nonalcoholic control subjects on no medication.

Peripheral Nervous System

Thirty-seven cases of peripheral neuropathy induced by disulfiram have been reported. The neuropathy is sensorimotor, affecting all sensory modalities, acting upon autonomic nerve fibers, bilateral, greater in the legs than in the arms, and more prominent distally. Generalized weakness, paresthesias, and vasomotor instability are prominent clinical symptoms (Enghusen-Poulsen et al. 1992). Electron microscopic studies indicate that the primary pathological processes are axonal degeneration, loss of myelinated fibers, and neurofilament accumulation in enlarged axons (Frisoni and Di Monda 1989). Although in one investigation, changes in motor conduction velocity and motor latency were found in the electromyelograms (EMGs) of patients on 250 mg of disulfiram and 10% (3 of 33) of these patients developed frankly abnormal EMGs, none developed symptoms of peripheral neuropathy over the 6-month period of the study. Hence, electrophysiological studies appear to be of no value in predicting clinical neuropathy (Palliyat and Schwartz 1988; Palliyat et al. 1990).

The incidence of neuropathy is probably higher in women, the onset of symptoms is later at lower doses, most cases occur within 2 to 3 months of starting disulfiram, and the severity is dose dependent, with few patients developing neuropathy who are receiving less than 250 mg/day and most receiving 500 or more mg/day (Enghusen-Poulsen et al. 1992; Frisoni and DiMonda 1989). Improvement follows discontinuation of the drug, but it is unclear whether reversibility always occurs (Enghusen-Poulsen et al. 1992; Mokri et al. 1981).

It is postulated that this neuropathy is due to carbon disulfide accumulation based on the fact that a similar neuropathy occurs during carbon disulfide intoxication and disulfiram is known to metabolize to carbon disulfide (Ansbacher et al. 1982). Another postulate is based on the fact that one of disulfiram's metabolites (DDC) chelates copper-containing enzymes (which are necessary for synthesis of catecholamines), and it has been suggested this property of disulfiram may be involved in the pathophysiology of axonal degeneration (Enghusen-Poulsen et al. 1992).

Disulfiram has been implicated in several cases of bilateral optic neuritis; symptoms reversed upon discontinuation of the drug (Norton and Walsh 1972).

Teratogenicity
Although disulfiram is not considered to be teratogenic based on animal studies (Petersen 1992), fetal limb-reduction abnormalities have been reported in the children of women who have taken disulfiram during pregnancy (Nora et al. 1977). These results need to be considered when one is evaluating whether to place alcohol-dependent women of reproductive age on disulfiram.

Sexual Function
Anecdotal reports and research findings exist that associate disulfiram with impotence. One study found that alcoholic men on disulfiram, compared with those on placebo, had a decreased number and duration of full nocturnal erections as measured by all-night penile tumescence recordings (Snyder et al. 1981). Another study (Jensen 1984) reported that more than 60% of alcoholic individuals complained of sexual dysfunction (compared with 10% of a matched control group) and that half of the symptomatic persons in the alcoholic group attributed their dysfunction to disulfiram. In contrast, in a large double-blind, randomized study (Christensen et al. 1984) of the side effects of disulfiram, no significant differences—other than a higher number of sexual complaints in the placebo group—were found in the side effects reported by the disulfiram and placebo groups.

■ Rational Prescribing

1. The patient must be given clear and detailed information (see disulfiram monograph [page 667] in Chapter 13 for patient information on the disulfiram–ethanol interaction), with emphasis on the potential for a serious and potentially fatal reaction up to 14 days after the last dose of disulfiram has been taken.

2. The patient must have abstained from alcohol for at least 24 hours and from paraldehyde, which is also metabolized to acetaldehyde, for 48 hours before the administration of disulfiram.

3. Test reactions in which patients are given disulfiram and then alcohol under controlled conditions, so that the patient experiences the effects of the disulfiram-ethanol interaction, are no longer recommended. The test is unpredictable, severe reactions sometimes occur, and there is no evidence that such a test increases drug compliance or decreases the incidence of relapse (Wright and Moore 1990).

4. Although some authorities insist that patients must be motivated before receiving disulfiram, it is generally recognized that motivation is an extremely complex phenomenon to evaluate. Disulfiram should, therefore, be prescribed for alcohol-dependent patients who have no medical or psychiatric contraindications to the use of the drug, who understand the reason for its use and its dangers, and who state, after such an education, that they desire to take disulfiram. It is worth noting that experiencing a DER or an adverse reaction with disulfiram does not usually deter patients from taking disulfiram again if it is offered (Liskow et al. 1990).

5. Prescribe the daily dose to be taken at bedtime because of the medication's soporific effects, and instruct the patient to take the dose with food, as this increases disulfiram's bioavailability.

6. If a patient receiving 250 mg/day of disulfiram drinks and does not have a reaction, the dosage may be increased to 500 mg/day with the patient's knowledge and consent.

7. Serious consideration should be given to enlisting the patient's spouse or significant other to observe and/or supervise the daily administration of disulfiram. However, such a strategy should be employed only if both parties concur and agree to call the therapist if difficulties arise in adhering to the agreement. In certain circumstances, the therapist may be the supervisor/ observer with the patient's consent.

8.   Although there are no firm guidelines regarding the duration
     of disulfiram treatment, generally the drug is recommended for
     a minimum of 1 year beyond the patient's full social recovery,
     with much longer periods reported necessary and successful in
     selected cases (Brewer 1993; Kristenson 1992).

Naltrexone

■ Indications

A great deal of recent research activity has been devoted to searching for medications that attenuate the neurochemical processes
leading to craving for alcohol. Drugs affecting the dopamine, serotonin, γ-aminobutyric acid (GABA), and opiate systems have all
been clinically evaluated (Chick and Erickson 1996; O'Brien
1994). The only drug thus far to emerge from this research and to
gain FDA approval as effective and safe in the treatment of alcohol
dependence has been the orally active pure opiate-receptor antagonist naltrexone. Although this agent has been in use as a treatment
for opiate dependence since the late 1970s, the two controlled
studies that led to its approval by the FDA for alcohol dependence
were not published until 1992 (O'Malley et al. 1992; Volpicelli et
al. 1992). Hence, an extensive database on the clinical utility of
naltrexone in alcoholism, both short-term and long-term, has yet
to be established. Current data, however, suggest that naltrexone,
like disulfiram, is of greatest benefit when combined with psychosocial treatments and when used in medication-compliant alcoholic individuals (O'Brien et al. 1996). There are also indications
that naltrexone may be especially useful for alcoholic persons with
high levels of craving and somatic symptoms (Volpicelli et al.
1995).

Although naltrexone is used in the treatment of opiate dependence, its impact has been limited because of low compliance, except in highly motivated patient populations or those in whom the
medication can be closely monitored (National Research Council
Committee 1978; Washton et al. 1984).

■ Efficacy

Two separate double-blind placebo-controlled studies have established the value of naltrexone in treating alcohol dependence. In
the first (Volpicelli et al. 1992), 70 alcohol-dependent subjects
were detoxified, entered into an outpatient rehabilitation program,
and randomly assigned to receive either placebo or naltrexone

50 mg/day for 12 weeks. Compared with patients receiving placebo, naltrexone-treated patients relapsed to problem drinking at a lower rate, reported fewer days of alcohol use, and experienced less subjective craving. Also of note was that among patients receiving placebo who had a "slip" (i.e., who drank any alcohol at all), 95% then began to drink heavily, whereas only 50% of naltrexone-treated patients who slipped went on to drink heavily.

In the second study (O'Malley et al. 1992), 97 alcohol-dependent patients were randomly assigned to placebo or naltrexone 50 mg/day and to one of two psychosocial treatments, either coping skills/relapse prevention or supportive therapy. All groups were then followed for 12 weeks. Naltrexone-treated patients, regardless of psychosocial treatment assigned, had fewer drinking days, consumed less alcohol, experienced reduced subjective craving, and had a lower relapse to heavy drinking compared with placebo-treated patients. Also of note, patients receiving supportive therapy and naltrexone had the highest abstinence rate among the four groups, and naltrexone patients receiving coping skills/relapse prevention treatment were the group least likely to relapse to heavy drinking after a slip.

O'Malley and colleagues followed the patients in this second study for 6 months after the study ended and found that up to month 4 of the follow-up period, those who had received naltrexone were less likely to relapse to heavy drinking than were patients who had been treated with placebo (O'Malley et al. 1996). In addition, naltrexone-treated patients were less likely than placebo-treated ones to meet criteria for a current diagnosis of alcohol abuse or dependence at the end of the 6-month follow-up period. The implication of this study is that some of the benefits of naltrexone continue for several months after the termination of treatment, although these effects do eventually dissipate. Studies of the effects of longer-term treatment with naltrexone are in progress, and more are anticipated.

Although naltrexone would seem to be an ideal treatment for opiate dependence, given its absence of agonist effects, minimal side effects, and oral administration, in practice its use is very limited because it is unpopular with patients (Fram et al. 1989). Even when patients agree to take naltrexone, less than 10% remain on the medication for 6 months (Greenstein et al. 1981). Special populations such as physicians and prisoners on probation do demonstrate much better compliance and opiate abstinence when receiving naltrexone (Brahen et al. 1984; Metzger et al. 1990; Washton et al. 1984), as do both patients in meaningful relationships with nonaddicted mates and those who are employed or attending school full-time (Resnick et al. 1979).

■ Mechanism of Action

Animal studies have provided evidence linking the endogenous opioid system with alcohol drinking. Rats and mice that have been bred to prefer alcohol solutions to plain-water solutions have been noted to have increased β-endorphin and met-enkephalin levels in various areas of their brains, compared with non–alcohol-preferring rodents (O'Brien 1994). Other studies in alcohol-preferring rodents (Froehlich et al. 1990) and in monkeys (Altschuler et al. 1980; Myers et al. 1986) have established that opiate antagonists reduce alcohol consumption in these animals.

In human studies, subjects with a family history of alcoholism had lower baseline plasma levels of β-endorphins than did subjects without such a history (Gianoulakis et al. 1996a). In addition, family-history–positive subjects exhibited dose-dependent increases in plasma β-endorphin levels with increasing doses of ethanol, whereas family-history–negative subjects did not demonstrate such increases (Gianoulakis et al. 1996b). β-endorphins have also been found to be reduced in alcoholic persons shortly after heavy alcohol use and to return to normal after 6 weeks of abstinence (Vescovi et al. 1992). These studies have led to the hypothesis that alcohol ingestion causes the release of endogenous opioids, which are reinforcing and hence elicit additional drinking. Naltrexone is postulated to work by blocking the action of endogenous opioids, thereby preventing the reinforcing effects of alcohol. This hypothesis suggests that although naltrexone-treated patients might be just as likely as nontreated alcoholic patients to drink, they would receive fewer reinforcing effects from the alcohol and would thus be less likely to continue to drink. The results of the two placebo-controlled clinical studies described earlier (O'Malley et al. 1992; Volpicelli et al. 1992), with their reports of lower relapse to abusive drinking and lower craving in naltrexone-treated patients, are consistent with this hypothesis.

Naltrexone's mechanism of action in the treatment of opiate dependence rests on its pharmacological activity as a pure opiate-receptor blocker (O'Brien et al. 1978). It thus blocks the effects of opiates, such as heroin, at the cellular level. Dependent patients who attempt to use an opiate will receive no effect from it and will thus discontinue its use.

■ Dosage

The usual dose of naltrexone for treatment of alcohol dependence is 50 mg given once per day. Opiate-dependent patients should be opiate free for 7–10 days before receiving naltrexone. Alternative dosing regimens, such as 100 mg every other day or 150 mg every third day, have been suggested for use in treating opiate dependence, but such regimens have not been used in managing alcohol dependence.

■ Pharmacokinetics

Naltrexone is almost completely absorbed from the gastrointestinal tract and reaches peak plasma concentrations within 1 hour of ingestion. Its major metabolite, β-naltrexol, peaks in the plasma 2 hours after ingestion. This metabolite is a weaker opiate antagonist than the parent compound but reaches plasma levels 2–10 times higher than naltrexone and probably contributes to the drug's long duration of action (Bullingham et al. 1983; Verebely et al. 1976; Wall et al. 1981a).

Naltrexone is approximately 20% bound to plasma protein; its volume of distribution after intravenous injection is 1,350 L/kg (Bullingham et al. 1983).

Naltrexone undergoes extensive first-pass hepatic metabolism, with 95% conversion of the parent drug to conjugated naltrexone, conjugated and unconjugated β-naltrexol, and small amounts of 2-hydroxy-3-0-methyl-β-naltrexol (Bullingham et al. 1983; Wall et al. 1981b). Most of the drug is excreted in the urine as β-naltrexol, although a small amount (2%–3%) is eliminated in the feces (Crabtree 1984; Verebely et al. 1976; Wall et al. 1981b).

The half-life of naltrexone is biphasic, with an initial phase of approximately 10 hours. The second phase occurs after 24 hours and exhibits a slow decline in plasma concentrations, with a half-life of about 96 hours, indicating probable sequestration of the drug in tissue and slow release to the circulation. The half-life of naltrexone's major metabolite, β-naltrexol, is similar, with an initial phase of 12 hours and a terminal phase of 18 hours (Crabtree 1984; Verebely et al. 1976).

■ Adverse Effects

Cardiovascular

No clinically significant cardiovascular toxicity has been reported with naltrexone therapy.

Central Nervous System

Naltrexone is a pure opiate antagonist and does not produce euphoria; however, there have been reports that it produces dysphoria, depression, fatigue, anxiety, irritability, and confusion (Crowley et al. 1985; Hollister et al. 1981; Mendelson et al. 1979).

Endocrinological

Naltrexone elevates plasma levels of luteinizing hormone (LH), follicle-stimulating hormone (FSH), adrenocorticotropic hormone (ACTH), cortisol, and catecholamines acutely, but with chronic dosing, plasma levels return to normal. Naltrexone has no effect, acutely or chronically, on plasma levels of prolactin, growth hormone, thyroid-stimulating hormone (TSH), insulin, glucagon, vasopressin, or gut hormones (Atkinson 1984).

Gastrointestinal

Nausea, abdominal pain and cramps, and vomiting have been reported in more than 10% of patients, and constipation and diarrhea in less than 10% ("Naltrexone—An Investigational Narcotic Antagonist," 1982; ReVia® Product Information 1995). Anorexia and weight loss have also been reported (Kosten and Kleber 1984).

Hepatic damage has been reported in patients receiving doses of naltrexone in the range of 300 mg/day. Serum AST and ALT levels have been reported to be elevated initially with naltrexone doses between 50 and 300 mg, with a return to normal levels with continued use (ReVia® Product Information 1995).

■ Opiate Use

Naltrexone is a competitive inhibitor of opiates at the opiate receptor and thus should be discontinued for at least 48 hours before elective surgery involving opiate analgesia. In patients receiving naltrexone who require emergency analgesia, regional analgesia combined with conscious sedation using a benzodiazepine, nonopiate analgesia, or general anesthesia should be considered (ReVia® Product Information 1995). If opiate analgesia is required, the opiate dose needed will be higher than normal. Because respiratory depression may, therefore, be greater and deeper than usual, a short-acting opiate is preferred and should be used in a setting in which the patient is continuously monitored by personnel trained in cardiopulmonary resuscitation. Non–opiate-receptor effects of the opiate, such as itching, bronchoconstriction, and facial swelling (due to histamine release), may be intense (ReVia® Product Information 1995) and should be anticipated.

Patients chronically using or abusing opiates may have a severe opiate withdrawal reaction beginning 5 minutes after receiving naltrexone and lasting up to 48 hours. Nausea, vomiting, severe diarrhea, confusion, irritability, and hallucinations may occur. Although symptomatic treatment with nonopiate medication usually suffices, carefully titrated doses of short-acting opiates, with monitoring of cardiopulmonary function, may be necessary (ReVia® Product Information 1995).

■ Rational Prescribing

1. Naltrexone may be a useful medication in the alcohol-dependent patient who is likely to be compliant with medication and who is actively involved in a treatment program providing supportive, educational, and/or relapse-prevention components.
2. Naltrexone may be a useful therapy for opiate-dependent patients who are willing or required to take the medication. It may be especially beneficial in patients whose job, social status, or probation from prison is threatened by continued opiate use.
3. Naltrexone is contraindicated in patients who are receiving opiate analgesics or who have significant liver disease.
4. Naltrexone should not be initiated until 7–10 days after the last dose of chronically administered opiates.
5. Patients should carry a card indicating that they are taking naltrexone in case they are involved in an emergency requiring the use of opiates.
6. The longer-term (i.e., beyond 12 weeks) efficacy of naltrexone therapy for alcohol dependence is under active investigation but has not as yet been reported. Continuation beyond this period requires close monitoring of naltrexone and alcohol use.
7. Total abstinence, although desirable, is often not achievable. Slips and relapses should be anticipated and do not necessarily require discontinuation of naltrexone.

Methadone and L-Alpha-Acetyl Methadol

■ Indications

Although opiates were used for the treatment of opiate dependence in the early decades of this century, such use was proscribed by legislation, court decisions, and public attitudes from the mid-1920s until 1972, when the FDA approved methadone for the treatment of opiate dependence (Lowinson et al. 1992). LAAM, an opiate agonist closely related chemically and pharmacologically to methadone, was approved by the FDA for use in the treatment of opiate dependence in 1993 (Bigelow and Preston 1995). Both methadone and LAAM are orally active, need to be taken once per day (methadone) or less often (LAAM), and, in sufficient maintenance doses, block the effects of self-administered opiates without producing euphoria, sedation, or analgesia (Lowinson et al. 1992).

■ Efficacy

Methadone-treated opiate-dependent patients have been demonstrated in a number of studies to be retained in treatment longer, to have lower use of illicit opiates and other drugs, to exhibit a decrease in antisocial behavior, and to display an increase in social stability (employment, school attendance) compared with themselves before treatment, untreated patients, and those treated by other methods (Ball and Ross 1991; Gearing and Schweitzer 1974).

LAAM administered three times per week has been reported to be comparable in efficacy to methadone given once per day when the outcome measures included opiate-positive urines, withdrawal symptoms, and treatment retention (Freedman and Czertko 1981; Jaffe et al. 1970; Senay et al. 1977; Sorenson et al. 1982; Zaks et al. 1972), although in one major study, methadone was somewhat more successful in retaining patients in treatment (Ling et al. 1976).

■ Mechanism of Action

Both methadone and LAAM are opiates that act upon the same μ-opiate receptors as do such illicit and licit opiates as morphine, heroin, fentanyl, and meperidine. When administered in adequate doses, methadone and LAAM occupy these receptors and thus block the reinforcing euphorigenic effects of any other opiate that is administered (Bigelow and Preston 1995).

■ Dosage

Methadone is administered once per day. Initial doses are usually 30–40 mg/day, with gradual increases of 10 mg every 2 or 3 days to a stable maintenance dose (Lowinson et al. 1992). A direct relationship exists between maintenance dose and propensity to relapse to illicit opiate abuse, with doses less than 50 mg/day leading to relapse at a rate five times higher than that for a 70-mg/day dose (Ball and Ross 1991). Although patients vary in their dosage requirements, doses lower than 60 mg/day are usually inadequate for maintenance and prevention of relapse to opiate use, and doses as high as 180 mg/day are sometimes necessary (Hartel et al. 1995; Lowinson et al. 1992; Senay et al. 1977).

LAAM is administered at a starting dose of 20–40 mg three times per week, with gradual increases to 70–90 mg three times per week. Because there is usually a 4- to 6-day delay in the onset of opiate agonist activity, administration of supplemental doses of methadone or another shorter-acting opiate is often required to prevent withdrawal symptoms and relapse to illicit drug use. Every-other-day dosing may be needed in some patients, whereas others may require a higher dose when there will be an interval of 3 rather than 2 days between doses (e.g., a patient receiving LAAM on a Monday/Wednesday/Friday schedule may need doses of 70 mg/ 70 mg/100 mg) (Bigelow and Preston 1995; Tennant et al. 1986).

■ Pharmacokinetics

Methadone is rapidly (although only partially) absorbed after oral administration and reaches peak plasma levels 2–3 hours after ingestion. Its half-life ranges from 13 to 55 hours, with an average of 25 hours (Inturrisi and Verebely 1972a, 1972b; Wolff et al. 1993). Methadone is 70%–85% protein bound (Olsen 1973); its volume of distribution after intravenous administration is 3.6– 6.7 L/kg (Inturrisi et al. 1987; Wolff et al. 1993). Metabolism is four times greater after oral than after intramuscular administration (Inturrisi and Verebely 1972a). Methadone's major metabolite is the N-demethylated derivative, 40% of which is excreted in the urine (Beckett et al. 1968; Verebely and Kutt 1975).

LAAM is well absorbed after oral administration, and peak plasma levels occur 2–4 hours after ingestion. The elimination half-life of LAAM is 35–60 hours (Henderson et al. 1977). LAAM is 80% protein bound (Toro-Goyco et al. 1980). LAAM is extensively metabolized in the liver. Its primary metabolites are nor-levomethadyl acetate (nor-LAAM) and dinor-levomethadyl acetate (dinor-LAAM). Both are pharmacologically active, are more potent than LAAM, and reach higher plasma levels than the parent compound with maintenance therapy. The elimination half-life of nor-LAAM ranges from 30 to 48 hours, whereas that of dinor-LAAM is greater than 100 hours (Henderson et al. 1977). These long elimination half-lives account for the long duration of LAAM's clinical effects, allowing dosing every 48–72 hours.

■ Adverse Effects

Central Nervous System

Methadone and LAAM have been associated with sweating, drowsiness, insomnia, headaches, euphoria, dysphoria, depression, and confusion. Rapid withdrawal is associated with the opiate withdrawal syndrome (Bigelow and Preston 1995; Tennant et al. 1986; see Chapter 10 [page 560] for a discussion of opiate withdrawal syndrome).

Gastrointestinal

Methadone and LAAM are associated with chronic constipation. Little tolerance develops to this side effect (Lowinson et al. 1992; Tennant et al. 1986).

Respiratory

Pulmonary edema and respiratory depression have been reported, although rarely, with therapeutic doses of methadone and LAAM. High doses, as with all opiates, produce respiratory depression to which tolerance develops (Lowinson et al. 1992; Tennant et al. 1986).

Sexual Dysfunction

Impotence and delayed or difficult ejaculation have been reported with methadone and LAAM (Cicero et al. 1975; Ling et al. 1976).

■ Rational Prescribing

1. Methadone and LAAM are useful medications in the opiate-dependent patient who desires maintenance opiate therapy and who persistently relapses with alternative interventions such as behavioral treatment and/or narcotic antagonist therapy.
2. Methadone must be administered daily, and many programs allow patients to take home several days' supply of medication after they are deemed to be stable and reliable. LAAM requires dosing every second or third day; however, it can be dispensed only in a clinic. Thus, LAAM may be more convenient for patients who must attend a clinic to receive opiate-substitution therapy.
3. Sufficient doses of methadone and LAAM are crucial. Doses of less than 60 mg of methadone daily or 80 mg three times per week of LAAM are likely to lead to relapse to illicit opiate use.
4. Patients should carry a card indicating that they are taking methadone or LAAM in case they are involved in an emergency requiring use of opiates.

5. Methadone and LAAM, when used for maintenance therapy, can be dispensed only by specially licensed clinics. Methadone, when used as a pain medication, may be dispensed as would any other Drug Enforcement Administration (DEA) Schedule II opiate. LAAM, however, is available for use only in maintenance programs.
6. Many patients on maintenance therapy require such treatment for long periods, perhaps even for a lifetime. Premature withdrawal—whether voluntary or involuntary—often leads to relapse.

Product List

Disulfiram

*   Oral daily dose range: 125–500 mg; generically available
*   Generic cost index: ≈ 0.09–0.16

Tablets:	**Antabuse**®
250 mg	[$70] Antabuse 250, white, scored
500 mg	[$85] Antabuse 500, white, scored

Levomethadyl Acetate

*   Oral three-times-weekly dosage range: 20–100 mg

Liquid:	**Orlaam**®
10 mg/mL	[$113.30]/474-mL bottle

Methadone

*   Oral daily dose range: 30–180 mg

Liquid:	**Roxane**®
10 mg/mL	[$49.83]/500-mL bottle
5 mg/mL	[$28.77]/500-mL bottle

Naltrexone

*   Oral daily dose: 50 mg

Tablet:	**ReVia**®
50 mg	[$455] ReVia 50, coral, scored

References

Allen JP, Litten RZ: Techniques to enhance compliance with disulfiram. Alcohol Clin Exp Res 16:1035–1041, 1992

Altschuler HL, Phillips PE, Feinhandler DA: Alterations of ethanol self-administration by naltrexone. Life Sci 26:679–688, 1980

Andersen MP: Lack of bioequivalence between disulfiram formulations. Acta Psychiatr Scand 86:31–35, 1992

Ansbacher L, Bosch E, Cancilla P: Disulfiram neuropathy: a neurofilamentous distal axonopathy. Neurology 32:424–428, 1982

446 PDH: Psychotropic Drug Handbook

Atkinson RL: Endocrine and metabolic effects of opiate antagonists. J Clin Psychiatry 45:20–24, 1984

Azrin NH, Sisson RW, Meyers R, et al: Alcoholism treatment by disulfiram and community reinforcement therapy. J Behav Ther Exp Psychiatry 13:105–112, 1982

Ball JC, Ross A: The Effectiveness of Methadone Maintenance Treatment. New York, Springer-Verlag, 1991

Banys P: The clinical use of disulfiram (Antabuse): a review. J Psychoactive Drugs 20:243–261, 1988

Beckett AH, Taylor JF, Casey AF, et al: The biotransformation of methadone in man: synthesis and identification of a major metabolite. J Pharm Pharmacol 20:754–762, 1968

Bennett A, McKeever L, Turk R: Psychotic reactions during tetraethylthiuram disulfide. JAMA 145:483–484, 1951

Bergstrom B, Ohlin H, Lindblom PE, et al: Is disulfiram implantation effective? Lancet 1:49–50, 1982

Bigelow GE, Preston KL: Opioids, in Psychopharmacology: The Fourth Generation of Progress. Edited by Bloom FE, Kupfer DJ. New York, Raven, 1995, pp 1731–1744

Brahen LS, Henderson RK, Capone T, et al: Naltrexone treatment in a jail work-release program. J Clin Psychiatry 45:49–52, 1984

Branchey L, Davis W, Lee KK, et al: Psychiatric complications of disulfiram treatment. Am J Psychiatry 144:1310–1312, 1987

Brewer C: Controlled trials of Antabuse in alcoholism: the importance of supervision and adequate dose. Acta Psychiatr Scand 86:51–58, 1992

Brewer C: Long-term, high dose disulfiram in the treatment of alcohol abuse. Br J Psychiatry 163:687–689, 1993

Brien J, Peachey J, Loomis C: Calcium carbimide–ethanol interaction. Clin Pharmacol Ther 27:426–433, 1980

Bullingham RES, McQuay HJ, Moore RA: Clinical pharmacokinetics of narcotic agonist-antagonist drugs. Clin Pharmacokinet 8:332–343, 1983

Chick J, Erickson CK: Conference summary: consensus conference on alcohol dependence and the role of pharmacotherapy in its treatment. Alcohol Clin Exp Res 20:391–402, 1996

Chick J, Gough K, Falkowski W, et al: Disulfiram treatment of alcoholism. Br J Psychiatry 161:84–89, 1992

Christensen JK, Ronsted P, Vaag UK: Side effects after disulfiram: comparison of disulfiram and placebo in a double-blind multicenter study. Acta Psychiatr Scand 69:165–273, 1984

Cicero TJ, Bell RD, Weist WG, et al: Functions of the male sex organs in heroin and methadone users. N Engl J Med 292:882–887, 1975

Crabtree BL: Review of naltrexone, a long-acting opiate antagonist. Clinical Pharmacy 3:273–280, 1984

Crowley TJ, Wagner JE, Zerbe G, et al: Naltrexone-induced dysphoria in former opioid addicts. Am J Psychiatry 142:1081–1084, 1985

Duckert F, Johnsen J: Behavioral use of disulfiram in the treatment of problem drinking. Int J Addict 22:445–454, 1987

Duckert F, Johnsen J, Peachey J, et al: The disulfiram and calcium carbimide acetaldehyde-mediated reactions. Pharmacol Ther 15:89–97, 1981

Enghusen-Poulsen H, Loft S, Andersen JR, et al: Disulfiram therapy—adverse drug reactions and interactions. Acta Psychiatr Scand 86:59–66, 1992

Faiman M: Biochemical pharmacology of disulfiram, in Biochemistry and Pharmacology of Ethanol, Vol 2. Edited by Majchrowicz E, Noble E. New York, Plenum, 1979, pp 325–348

Fox R: Disulfiram-alcohol side effects. JAMA 204:271–272, 1968

Fram DH, Marmo J, Holden R: Naltrexone treatment—the problem of patient acceptance. J Subst Abuse Treat 6:119–122, 1989

Freedman RR, Czertko G: A comparison of thrice weekly LAAM and daily methadone in employed heroin addicts. Drug Alcohol Depend 8:215–222, 1981

Frisoni GB, DiMonda V: Disulfiram neuropathy: a review (1971–1988) and report of a case. Alcoholism 24:429–437, 1989

Froehlich JC, Harts J, Lumeng L, et al: Naloxone attenuates voluntary ethanol intake in rats selectively bred for high ethanol preference. Pharmacol Biochem Behav 35:385–390, 1990

Fuller RK, Branchey L, Brightwell DR, et al: Disulfiram treatment of alcoholism. JAMA 256:1449–1455, 1986

Gearing FR, Schweitzer MD: An epidemiological evaluation of long term methadone maintenance treatment of heroin addiction. Am J Epidemiol 100:101–112, 1974

Gerrein J, Roseberg CM, Monohan V: Disulfiram maintenance in outpatient treatment of alcoholism. Arch Gen Psychiatry 28:798–802, 1973

Gianoulakis C, Dewaele JP, Thavundayil J: Implications of the endogenous opioid system in excessive ethanol consumption. Alcohol 13:19–23, 1996a

Gianoulakis C, Krishnan B, Thavundayil J: Enhanced sensitivity of pituitary β-endorphins to ethanol in subjects at high risk of alcoholism. Arch Gen Psychiatry 53:250–257, 1996b

Goldfrank LR: Disulfiram and disulfiram-like reactions, in Goldfrank's Toxicologic Emergencies. Edited by Goldfrank LR, Flomenbaum NE, Lewin NA, et al. Norwalk, CT, Appleton & Lange, 1994, pp 899–903

Goldfrank LR, Bresnitz EA, Melinek M, et al: Antabuse. Hospital Physician (December):34–39, 1980

Goldfrank LR, Bresnitz EA, Melinek M, et al: Disulfiram, in Goldfrank's Toxicologic Emergencies. Edited by Goldfrank LR, Flomenbaum NE, Lewin NA, et al. Norwalk, CT, Appleton & Lange, 1990, pp 475–480

Goldstein M, Nakajima K: The effects of disulfiram on catecholamine levels in the brain. J Pharmacol Exp Ther 157:96–102, 1967

Greenstein RA, O'Brien CP, McLellan AT, et al: Naltrexone: a short-term treatment of opiate dependence. Am J Drug Alcohol Abuse 8:291–300, 1981

Haddock NJ, Wilkin JK: Cutaneous reactions to lower aliphatic alcohols before and during disulfiram therapy. Arch Dermatol 118:157–159, 1982

Hald J, Jacobsen E: A drug sensitizing the organism to ethyl alcohol. Lancet 2:1001–1004, 1948

Hart BW, Faiman MD: In vivo pharmacodynamic studies of the disulfiram metabolite S-methyl N,N-diethylthiocarbanate sulfoxide: inhibitors of liver aldehyde dehydrogenase. Alcohol Clin Exp Res 18:340–345, 1994

Hartel DM, Shoenbaum EE, Selwyn PA, et al: Heroin use during methadone maintenance treatment: the importance of methadone dose and cocaine use. Am J Public Health 85:1995

Heath R, Nesselhof W, Bishop M, et al: Behavioral and metabolic changes associated with administration of tetraethylthiuram disulfide (Antabuse). Diseases of the Nervous System 26:99–105, 1965

Henderson GL, Wilson K, Lau DHM: Plasma L-alpha-acetylmethadol (LAAM) after acute and chronic administration. Clin Pharmacol Ther 21:16–25, 1977

Hernberg S, Partanen L, Nordman C, et al: Coronary heart disease among workers exposed to carbon disulphide. British Journal of Industrial Medicine 27:313–325, 1970

Hollister LE, Johnson K, Boukhabza D, et al: Aversive effects of naltrexone in subjects not dependent on opiates. Drug Alcohol Depend 8:37–41, 1981

Iber FL, Lee KK, Lacoursiere R, et al: Liver toxicity encountered in the Veterans Administration trials of disulfiram in alcoholics. Alcohol Clin Exp Res 11:301–304, 1987

Inturrisi CE, Verebely K: Disposition of methadone in man after a single oral dose. Clin Pharmacol Ther 13:923–930, 1972a

Inturrisi CE, Verebely K: The levels of methadone in plasma in methadone maintenance. Clin Pharmacol Ther 13:633–637, 1972b

Inturrisi CE, Colburn WA, Kaiko RF, et al: Pharmacokinetics and pharmacodynamics of methadone in patients with chronic pain. Clin Pharmacol Ther 41:392–401, 1987

Jaffe JH, Shuster CR, Smith MM, et al: Comparison of acetylmethadol and methadone in the treatment of long-term heroin users—a pilot study. JAMA 211:1834–1836, 1970

Jensen SB: Sexual function and dysfunction in young married alcoholics. Acta Psychiatr Scand 69:543–549, 1984

Johnsen J, Morland J: Depot preparations of disulfiram: experimental and clinical results. Acta Psychiatr Scand 86:27–30, 1992

Kosten TR, Kleber HD: Naltrexone induced appetite suppression and weight loss. Int J Psychiatry Med 14:153–155, 1984

Kristensen M: Toxic hepatitis induced by disulfiram in nonalcoholics. Acta Med Scand 209:335–336, 1981

Kristenson H: Long-term Antabuse treatment of alcohol-dependent patients. Acta Psychiatr Scand 86:41–45, 1992

Kwentus J, Major LF: Disulfiram and the treatment of alcoholism: a review. J Stud Alcohol 40:428–446, 1981

Larson EW, Oliney A, Rummans TA, et al: Disulfiram treatment of patients with both alcohol dependence and other psychiatric disorders: a review. Alcohol Clin Exp Res 16:125–130, 1992

Lindros KO, Stowell A, Pikkarainen P, et al: The disulfiram (Antabuse) alcohol reaction in male alcoholics: its efficient management by 4-methylpyrazole. Alcohol Clin Exp Res 5:528–530, 1981

Ling W, Charuvastra VC, Kain SC, et al: Methadyl acetate and methadone as maintenance treatments of heroin addicts: a Veterans Administration cooperative study. Arch Gen Psychiatry 33:709–720, 1976

Liskow B, Nickel E, Tunley N: Alcoholics' attitudes toward and experiences with disulfiram. Am J Drug Alcohol Abuse 16:147–160, 1990

Lowinson JH, Marion IJ, Joseph H, et al: Methadone maintenance, in Substance Abuse: A Comprehensive Textbook. Edited by Lowinson JH, Ruiz P, Millman RB. Baltimore, MD, Williams & Wilkins, 1992, pp 550–561

Lundwall L, Baekland F: Disulfiram treatment of alcoholism—a review. J Nerv Ment Dis 153:381–394, 1971

Major L, Goyer P: Effects of disulfiram and pyridoxine on serum cholesterol. Ann Intern Med 88:53–56, 1978

Mendelson JH, Ellingboe J, Keuhnle JC, et al: Effects of naltrexone on mood and neuroendocrine function in normal adult males. Psychoneuroendocrinology 3:231–236, 1979

Metzger DS, Cornish J, Woody GE, et al: Naltrexone in federal probationers, in Problems of Drug Dependence 1989 (NIDA Research Monograph 95). Edited by Harris LS. Rockville, MD, National Institute on Drug Abuse Committee on Problems of Drug Dependence, 1990, pp 465–466

Mokri B, Ohnishi A, Dyck P: Disulfiram neuropathy. Neurology 31:730–735, 1981

Morland J, Johnson J, Bache-Wiig JL, et al: Lack of pharmacological effects of implanted disulfiram. in Pharmacological Treatments for Alcoholism. Edited by Edwards G, Littleton J. New York, Methuen, 1984, pp 573–578

Myers RD, Borg S, Mossberg R: Antagonism by naltrexone of voluntary alcohol selection in the chronically drinking macaque monkey. Alcohol 3:383–388, 1986

Naltrexone—an investigational narcotic antagonist. Hospital Pharmacy 17:687–688, 1982

National Research Council Committee on Clinical Evaluation of Narcotic Antagonists: Clinical evaluation of naltrexone treatment of opiate-dependent individuals. Arch Gen Psychiatry 35:335–340, 1978

Nora A, Nora J, Blu J: Limb-reduction anomalies in infants born to disulfiram-treated alcoholic mothers (letter). Lancet 2:664, 1977

Norton A, Walsh F: Disulfiram-induced optic neuritis. Transactions—American Academy of Ophthalmology and Otolaryngology 76:1263–1265, 1972

O'Brien CP: Treatment of alcoholism as a chronic disorder. Alcohol 11:433–437, 1994

O'Brien CP, Greenstein R, Ternes J, et al: Clinical pharmacology of narcotic antagonists. Ann N Y Acad Sci 311:232–240, 1978

O'Brien CP, Volpicelli LA, Volpicelli JR: Naltrexone in the treatment of alcoholism. Alcohol 13:35–39, 1996

O'Farrell TJ, Bayog RD: Antabuse contracts for married alcoholics and their spouses: a method to maintain Antabuse ingestion and decrease conflict about drinking. J Subst Abuse Treat 3:1–8, 1986

Olsen G: Methadone binding to human plasma proteins. Clin Pharmacol Ther 14:338–339, 1973

O'Malley SS, Jaffe AJ, Chang G, et al: Naltrexone and coping skills therapy for alcohol dependence. Arch Gen Psychiatry 49:881–887, 1992

O'Malley SS, Jaffe AJ, Chang G: Six-month follow-up of naltrexone and psychotherapy for alcohol dependence. Arch Gen Psychiatry 53:217–224, 1996

Palliyat SK, Schwartz BD: Disulfiram neuropathy: electrophysiological study. Electromyogr Clin Neurophysiol 28:245–247, 1988

Palliyat SK, Schwartz BD, Gant L: Peripheral nerve functions in chronic alcoholic patients on disulfiram: a 6-month follow-up. J Neurol Neurosurg Psychiatry 53:227–230, 1990

Peachey J, Sellers E: The disulfiram and calcium carbimide acetaldehyde-mediated reactions. Pharmacol Ther 15:89–97, 1981

Peachey J, Brien J, Roach C, et al: A comparative review of the pharmacological and toxicological properties of disulfiram and calcium carbimide. J Clin Psychopharmacol 1:21–26, 1981

Petersen EN: The pharmacology and toxicology of disulfiram and its metabolites. Acta Psychiatr Scand 86:7–13, 1992

Phillips M: Disulfiram-induced fulminating hepatitis and monitoring guidelines (letter). J Clin Psychiatry 51:168, 1990

Phillips M, Greenberg J: Dose-ranging study of depot disulfiram in alcohol abusers. Alcohol Clin Exp Res 16:964–967, 1992

Rainey J: Disulfiram toxicity is carbon disulfide poisoning. Am J Psychiatry 134:371–378, 1977

Resnick R, Schuyten-Resnick E, Washton AM: Narcotic antagonists in the treatment of opioid dependence: review and commentary. Compr Psychiatry 20:116–125, 1979

ReVia® [naltrexone] Product Information. Wilmington, DE, DuPont Pharmaceuticals, 1995

Schuckit MA: A one-year follow-up of men alcoholics given disulfiram. J Stud Alcohol 46:191–195, 1985

Sellers E, Naranjo C, Peachey J: Drugs to decrease alcohol consumption. N Engl J Med 305:1255–1262, 1981

Senay EC, Dorus W, Renault PF: Methadyl acetate and methadone. JAMA 237:138–142, 1977

Snyder S, Karacan I, Salis P: Disulfiram and nocturnal penile tumescence in the chronic alcoholic. Biol Psychiatry 16:399–406, 1981

Sorenson JL, Hargreaves WA, Weinberg JA: Withdrawal from heroin in three or six weeks—comparison of methadyl acetate and methadone. Arch Gen Psychiatry 39:167–171, 1982

Tennant FS, Rawson RA, Pumphrey E, et al: Clinical experiences with 959 opioid-dependent patients treated with levo-alpha-acetylmethadol (LAAM). J Subst Abuse Treat 3:195–202, 1986

Toro-Goyco E, Martin BR, Harris LS: Binding of L-alpha-acetyl-methadol and its metabolites to blood constituents. Biochem Pharmacol 29:1897–1902, 1980

Verebely K, Kutt H: Methadone plasma levels in maintenance patients (abstract). Research Communications in Chemical Pathology and Pharmacology 11:373, 1975

Verebely K, Volavka J, Mule SJ, et al: Naltrexone disposition, metabolism, and effects after acute and chronic dosing. Clin Pharmacol Ther 20:315–328, 1976

Vescovi PP, Coiro V, Volpi R, et al: Plasma β-endorphins but not met-enkephalin levels are abnormal in chronic alcoholics. Alcohol Alcohol 27:471–475, 1992

Volpicelli JR, Alterman AI, Hayashida M, et al: Naltrexone in the treatment of alcohol dependence. Arch Gen Psychiatry 49:876–880, 1992

Volpicelli JR, Clay KL, Watson NT, et al: Naltrexone in the treatment of alcoholism: predicting response to naltrexone. J Clin Psychiatry 56 (suppl):39–44, 1995

Wall ME, Brine DR, Perez-Reyes M: Metabolism and disposition of naltrexone in man after oral and intravenous administration. Drug Metab Dispos 9:369–375, 1981a

Wall ME, Brine DR, Perez-Reyes M: The metabolism of naltrexone in man. NIDA Res Monogr 28:105–131, 1981b

Washton AM, Pottash AC, Gold MS, et al: Naltrexone in addicted business executives and physicians. J Clin Psychiatry 45:39–41, 1984

Wilson A, Davidson WJ, Blanchard R: Disulfiram implantation: a trial using placebo implants and two types of controls. J Stud Alcohol 41:429–436, 1980

Wilson A, Blanchard R, Davidson W, et al: Disulfiram implantation: a dose-response trial. J Clin Psychiatry 45:242–247, 1984

Wolff K, Hay AW, Raistrick D, et al: Steady state pharmacokinetics of methadone in opioid addicts. Eur J Clin Pharmacol 44:189–194, 1993

Wright C, Moore RD: Disulfiram treatment of alcoholism. Am J Med 88:647–655, 1990

Wright C, Vafier JA, Lake CR: Disulfiram-induced fulminating hepatitis: guidelines for liver-panel monitoring. J Clin Psychiatry 49:430–434, 1988

Wright C, Moore RD, Grodin DM, et al: Screening for disulfiram-induced liver test dysfunction in an inpatient alcoholism program. Alcohol Clin Exp Res 17:184–186, 1993

Zaks A, Fink M, Freedman AM: Levomethadyl in maintenance treatment of opiate dependence. JAMA 220:811–813, 1972

8

Drug Interactions

The drug interactions described in this chapter have been assigned to one of two severity categories of clinical significance using the criteria described in *Drug Interaction Facts* (Tatro 1996). *Major-severity* drug interactions are defined as either potentially life-threatening or capable of resulting in permanent injury to the patient. *Moderate-severity* drug interactions may cause deterioration in the patient's clinical status, necessitating additional treatment, hospitalization, or prolongation of hospitalization. *Minor* drug interactions are less significant and—because documentation is poor, the potential for harm to the patient is slight, or the incidence of the interaction is quite low—are not delineated in this chapter. The majority of psychotropic drug interactions fall into this latter category. Because of the great number of interactions, only major- and moderate-severity interactions are described in this chapter. A number of moderate interactions occur that are not listed here because poor documentation did not justify their inclusion. For a complete listing of drug interactions, we refer readers to *Drug Interactions and Updates* (Hansten and Horn 1995) and *Drug Interaction Facts* (Tatro 1996).

Cytochrome P450 Hepatic Isoenzymes

The cytochrome P450 oxidative hepatic isoenzymes are the most active family of drug-metabolizing enzymes. Most psychotropic drugs (lithium is an exception) are metabolized to some degree by one or more of the P450 enzymes. There are four cytochrome P450 (CYP) families. CYP1, CYP2, and CYP3 oxidize xenobiotics, while CYP4 hydrolyzes long-chain fatty acids. Each cytochrome family has subfamilies designated by an uppercase letter. The major drug-metabolizing subfamilies are CYP1A, CYP2C, CYP2D, and CYP3A. Individual CYP enzymes are designated by a number (e.g., CYP2D6). Additionally, genetic polymorphs may exist for some of the individual enzymes (e.g., CYP2D6, CYP2C19) such that patients may be classified as superfast, fast, or slow metabolizers (Gonzalez and Idle 1994).

Table 8–1 lists the various drugs metabolized by CYP450 isoenzymes 1A2, 2A6, 2B6, 2C8, 2C9, 2C19, 2D6, 2E1, and 3A4, as well as the drugs that inhibit these enzymes. Many of these potential drug interactions have not been studied; however, they are predictable from a theoretical basis. Thus, although a theoretical drug interaction may be obvious according to Table 8–1, it may not be described in this chapter either because it is of minor significance or because it has not been studied (DeVane 1994; Gelenberg 1995; Gonzalez and Idle 1994; Harvey and Preskorn 1996a, 1996b; Ishaid et al. 1996; Slaughter and Edwards 1995; Wrighton and Stevens 1992). Concurrently administered drugs metabolized by the same P450 enzymes can demonstrate competitive inhibition of one another's metabolism.

Antipsychotics

■ Guanethidine (Major Severity)

Chlorpromazine doses greater than 100 mg/day have been found to reverse the antihypertensive effects of guanethidine (Janowsky et al. 1973). Haloperidol 6–9 mg/day and thiothixene 60 mg/day were found to produce a similar effect (Janowsky et al. 1973). Chlorpromazine blocks the presynaptic neuronal amine uptake pump, thereby denying guanethidine its site of action. Thus, the use of guanethidine is contraindicated in patients receiving antipsychotic medications.

■ Anticholinergics (Moderate Severity)

Controlled studies have indicated that the beneficial effects of both chlorpromazine and haloperidol, especially in regard to cognitive function and social behavior, are reversed by anticholinergic drugs (Singh and Kay 1979). The authors have suggested that the central anticholinergic effects are responsible for this antagonism. However, another study has shown that anticholinergics can reduce plasma levels of oral chlorpromazine by enhancing metabolism in the gut (Rivera-Calimlin et al. 1976). Because of these potential interactions, it is recommended that antiparkinsonian (anticholinergic) drug doses be kept to a minimum when treating extrapyramidal reactions secondary to antipsychotic medications.

Table 8–1. Potential CYP450 drug interactions for U.S.–marketed drugs

P450 isoenzyme	Metabolized by	Inhibited by	Induced by
1A2	acetominophen, amitriptyline, antipyrine, caffeine, clomipramine, clozapine, enoxacin, fluvoxamine, haloperidol, imipramine, olanzapine, ondansetron, phenacetin, propranolol, tacrine, theophylline, R(-)warfarin, verapamil	cimetidine, erythromycin, fluroquinolones, grapefruit juice (naringenin), methoxsalen, paroxetine, sertraline	charbroiled meat, cruciferous vegetables (e.g., broccoli, cabbage, sprouts), omeprazole, tobacco
2A6	coumarin		
2B6	cyclophosphamide		
2C8	arachidonic acid, paclitaxel, retinoic acid, warfarin		
2C9	cyclophosphamide, diclofenac, hexobarbital, ibuprofen, mefanamic acid, naproxen, phenytoin, piroxicam, tenoxicam, thiotepa, tolbutamide, TCAs, torsemide, S(-)warfarin	sertraline	rifampin, barbiturates

(continued)

Table 8–1. Potential CYP450 drug interactions for U.S.–marketed drugs (continued)

P450 isoenzyme	Metabolized by	Inhibited by	Induced by
2C19	clomipramine, diazepam, hexobarbital, imipramine, lansoprazole, mepheny-toin, mephobarbital, moclobemide, omeprazole, proguanil, propranolol	felbamate, fluoxetine, fluvoxamine, fluconazole, sertraline	
2D6	**Antiarrhythmics** encainide, flecainide, mexiletine, propafenone	alfentanil, amiodarone	rifampin
	Antipsychotics clozapine, haloperidol, perphenazine, reduced haloperidol, risperidone, thioridazine	cimetidine, fentanil	
	β-blockers bufuralol, metoprolol, propranolol, timolol	fluvoxamine, norfluoxetine	

Opiates
codeine, dextromethorphan, hydromorphone, methadone, oxycodone, tramadol

propoxyphene, quinidine

TCAs
amitriptyline, clomipramine, desipramine, imipramine, norclomipramine, nortriptyline, trimipramine

SSRIs
fluoxetine, paroxetine

sertraline, yohimbine

Miscellaneous antidepressants
maprotiline, nefazodone, venlafaxine

Miscellaneous
debrisoquin, methylenedioxymethamphetamine (Ecstasy), ondansetron, phenformin, sparteine, tacrine, terfenadine, tropisetron, verapamil

2E1   acetominophen, chlorzoxazone, ethanol, enflurane, halothane

disulfiram

Table 8–1. Potential CYP450 drug interactions for U.S.–marketed drugs (*continued*)

P450 isoenzyme	Metabolized by	Inhibited by	Induced by
3A4	**Antiarrhythmics** amiodarone, lidocaine, propafenone, quinidine **Antidepressants** bupropion, sertraline, TCAs (amitriptyline, clomipramine, desipramine, imipramine, norclomipramine, nortriptyline, trimipramine), venlafaxine **Benzodiazepines** alprazolam, diazepam, midazolam, triazolam **Calcium channel blockers** diltiazem, felodipine, nifedipine, nimodipine, nisoldipine, verapamil	cimetidine, ciprofloxacin, anhydroerythromycin, fluvoxamine, grapefruit juice (naringenin), itraconazole, ketoconazole, nefazodone, norfluoxetine, sertraline, troleandomycin	barbiturates, carbamazepine, glucocorticoids, phenytoin, rifampin, rifabutin

Nonsedating antihistamines

astemizole, terfenadine

Miscellaneous

acetaminophen, alfentanil, amiodarone, codeine, cyclosporin A/G, carbamazepine, cyclophosphamide, cortisol, dapsone, dexamethasone, dextromethorphan, doxorubicin, erythromycin (N-CH$_3$), ethinylestradiol, etoposide, fentanyl, felodipine, ifosfamide, lansoprazole, lidocaine, lomustine, lovastatin, omeprazole, ondansetron, progesterone, tamoxifen, taxol, testosterone, triacetyloleandomycin (TAO), vincristine, vinblastine, vinolrebine, warfarin

Note. SSRIs = selective serotonin reuptake inhibitors; TCAs = tricyclic antidepressants.

■ Barbiturates (Moderate Severity)

Phenobarbital, by virtue of its ability to induce liver microsomal oxidizing enzymes, lowered *chlorpromazine* blood levels and shortened its half-life during a 3-week trial (Loga et al. 1975). Patients receiving chlorpromazine who require a barbiturate for treatment of a seizure disorder may need higher doses of the phenothiazine after starting barbiturate therapy.

In a single case report, *haloperidol* serum levels decreased after phenobarbital administration. A reduction of the phenobarbital dose resulted in an increase in the haloperidol levels (Prakash et al. 1984). A similar effect was reported in a study of 30 patients (Linnoila et al. 1980). However, the results were confounded by the concurrent administration of phenytoin in many of the patients. A higher haloperidol dose may be required in patients also receiving barbiturates.

■ Benzodiazepines (Moderate Severity)

Two cases of cardiorespiratory collapse have been associated with the addition of clozapine to a diazepam regimen (Sassim and Grohmann 1988). Nonetheless, many patients have been treated concomitantly with the two drugs without adverse consequences. Patients already receiving benzodiazepines for whom clozapine is to be initiated should have their vital signs monitored closely for the first few days after clozapine is started.

■ β-Adrenergic–Blocking Agents (Moderate Severity)

In one study, the oral bioavailability of propranolol was increased 25%–32% by *chlorpromazine* due to a decrease in first-pass hepatic metabolism (Vestal et al. 1979). Propranolol plasma concentrations were increased in three of five subjects. Additionally, increased isoproterenol antagonism and lower plasma renin activity were observed. Apparently, a competitive inhibition of hepatic metabolism exists between the two drugs, given that the chlorpromazine plasma concentrations also increased. A randomized, crossover-design study found that the addition of propranolol to a chlorpromazine dosing regimen produced a fivefold increase in the chlorpromazine plasma concentrations (Peet et al. 1981). This drug interaction is of clinical significance, since propranolol in 30- to 80-mg/day doses is now being used to treat antipsychotic-induced akathisia.

A single case report, in a patient receiving haloperidol 10–20 mg/day and propranolol 40–80 mg/day, of three severe hypotensive episodes, two of which required cardiopulmonary resuscitation, has been described (Alexander et al. 1984). This may have been an idiosyncratic reaction. However, because propranolol is the drug of choice for treating akathisia in patients receiving haloperidol, clinicians should warn patients about possible hypotensive effects.

■ Bromocriptine (Moderate Severity)

Antipsychotic drugs and bromocriptine have opposing effects on dopamine. This interaction acquires clinical significance when bromocriptine is used to treat prolactin-secreting pituitary adenomas. Prolactin levels increased 2.5- to 10-fold when the drugs were combined (Robbins et al. 1984). When used concurrently, both drugs should be monitored for reduced pharmacological effect.

■ Carbamazepine (Moderate Severity)

The concomitant administration of *haloperidol* and carbamazepine decreased haloperidol plasma concentrations by as much as 60%, resulting in breakthrough symptoms of psychomotor agitation, obsessive-compulsive rituals, withdrawn behavior, auditory hallucinations, delusions, and inappropriate affect (Arana et al. 1986; Fast et al. 1986). In two cases of rapid-cycling bipolar disorder, concomitant administration of carbamazepine and haloperidol resulted in the development of delirium (Kanter et al. 1984; Yerevanian and Hodgman 1985). Suspected carbamazepine–haloperidol interactions can be managed by increasing the haloperidol dose.

Carbamazepine and *clozapine* should not be administered together because of the increased risk of bone marrow suppression. A survey of patients taking clozapine versus clozapine plus carbamazepine found a prevalence rate of granulocytopenia ($<1,500$ mm^3 neutrophils) of 4% (5 of 133) and 21% (3 of 14), respectively, although agranulocytosis (<500 mm^3 neutrophils) did not occur (Junghan et al. 1993). Additionally, carbamazepine stimulates the hepatic metabolism of clozapine. Discontinuation of carbamazepine therapy in patients taking clozapine resulted in a 71%–100% increase in the clozapine plasma concentrations (Raitasuo et al. 1993).

■ Central Nervous System Stimulants (Moderate Severity)

Amphetamines and, quite probably, all central nervous system (CNS)–active sympathomimetics (e.g., cocaine, methylphenidate, phenylpropanolamine) in large doses precipitate psychotic reactions that are indistinguishable from paranoid schizophrenia (Ellinwood 1967). Schizophrenic patients who received amphetamines for dieting (West 1974) or methylphenidate experimentally (Janowsky et al. 1974) experienced a worsening of their schizophrenic symptomatology. Thus, CNS-active sympathomimetic drugs such as amphetamine, methylphenidate, and the over-the-counter diet pill phenylpropanolamine are contraindicated in schizophrenic patients, regardless of whether they are receiving antipsychotic drugs.

■ Epinephrine (Moderate Severity)

Acute intravenous infusions of epinephrine in patients receiving maintenance oral doses of chlorpromazine have produced hypotension and tachycardia as a result of ephedrine's β-adrenergic agonist activity being unopposed while the α-adrenergic effects were being blocked by the antipsychotic. It is probably wise to avoid the use of chlorpromazine and thioridazine in schizophrenic patients who may require epinephrine in the future (Sletten et al. 1965). The use of the piperazine phenothiazines or the butyrophenone antipsychotic haloperidol is a more rational therapeutic choice.

■ Fluoxetine (Moderate Severity)

The coadministration of **haloperidol** and fluoxetine was associated with severe extrapyramidal side effects (EPS) in a single case. The patient had previously developed mild EPS on haloperidol 2–5 mg/day for 2 years prior to starting fluoxetine. When the two drugs were administered concomitantly, the patient developed severe tongue stiffness, drug-induced parkinsonism, and akathisia. These side effects reversed when both agents were discontinued (Tate 1989). Fluoxetine competitively inhibits hepatic oxidative enzyme CYP2D6 such that haloperidol plasma levels increase by approximately 20% (Goff et al. 1991a). Clinicians should monitor patients for this interaction and switch them to a tricyclic antidepressant if EPS worsen.

Fluoxetine inhibits the metabolism of **clozapine** and is reported to produce a mean 76% increase in clozapine plasma concentrations (Centorrino et al. 1994). This effect, coupled with fluoxetine's ability to downregulate serotonin (5-hydroxytryptamine type 2 [5-HT$_2$]) receptors, may explain why fluoxetine augmentation has produced clinical improvement of negative and depressive symptoms in chronic schizophrenic patients receiving antipsychotics (Spina et al. 1994).

■ Histamine$_2$-Blocking Agents (Moderate Severity)

Cimetidine has been reported to noncompetitively inhibit the metabolism of antipsychotics. In one study, the addition of cimetidine to clozapine therapy caused an increase in the clozapine plasma concentration and the number of clozapine adverse drug reactions (ADRs) (Szymanski et al. 1991). This interaction has been used clinically as a method of reducing the cost of clozapine.

■ Levodopa (Moderate Severity)

Antipsychotic drugs and levodopa have opposing effects on dopamine. When possible, the combined use of these agents should be avoided. If levodopa and an antipsychotic must be administered concurrently, both drugs should be monitored for reduced pharmacological effects (Yaryura-Tobias et al. 1970).

■ Lithium (Moderate Severity)

An intoxication syndrome purportedly caused by *haloperidol* and lithium, characterized by extrapyramidal symptoms, decreased sensorium, hyperthermia, weakness, lethargy, tremor, dystonias, tardive dyskinesia, leukocytosis, elevated serum enzymes (creatine phosphokinase [CPK], lactate dehydrogenase [LDH], alkaline phosphatase [AP]), and elevated blood urea nitrogen (BUN) has been described (W. J. Cohen and Cohen 1974; Loudon and Waring 1976; Sandyk and Hurwitz 1983). However, two retrospective reviews of 425 patients (Baastrup et al. 1976) and 55 patients (Juhl et al. 1977), as well as two controlled, prospective studies with a total of 158 patients (Biederman et al. 1979; Goldney and Spence 1986), found no similar cases.

In a review of 39 case reports of neurotoxicity resulting from a lithium and phenothiazine combination, 82% of the patients developed confusion, disorientation, and unconsciousness; 74%, extrapyramidal effects (rigidity, tremor, akinesia, akathisia, dystonia); 26%, cerebellar signs; 18%, fever; 16%, pyramidal symptoms; and 90%, slow-wave electroencephalogram (EEG) changes (Prakash et al. 1982). In 35 of the patients, the symptoms reversed on discontinuation of one or both drugs.

Although this combination has been used safely and successfully in acutely manic patients, clinicians should be aware of its potential to precipitate a sudden deterioration in a patient's mental and neurological status. Until more definitive data are available, clinicians are advised to recognize the possibility of this interaction, but not to discontinue using the combination in treating an acute manic patient unless that patient becomes intoxicated. If the patient is not psychotic, substitution of a benzodiazepine for the antipsychotic is a potential alternative.

■ Meperidine (Moderate Severity)

A controlled study in healthy subjects demonstrated excessive and/or prolonged respiratory depression as well as hypotension and CNS toxicity in patients receiving chlorpromazine and meperidine concurrently (Stambaugh and Wainer 1981). Thus, despite uncontrolled observations that phenothiazines can potentiate the analgesic effects of the opiates, this combination should be avoided.

■ Phenytoin (Moderate Severity)

As a result of enzyme induction caused by phenytoin, serum clozapine concentrations decreased by an average of 81% after the addition of phenytoin to two patients' medication regimens (D. D. Miller 1991). In both cases, worsening of the psychosis resulted.

Antidepressants

■ Tricyclic Antidepressants

Sympathomimetics (Major Severity)

In patients receiving *tricyclic antidepressants (TCAs),* intravenous infusions of epinephrine, norepinephrine, and phenylephrine have resulted in two- to fourfold, four- to eightfold, and two- to threefold increases, respectively, in the pressor response to these sympathomimetic drugs due to the antidepressant's additive effect in blocking the reuptake of monoamines (i.e., norepinephrine) (Boakes et al. 1973). Sensitivity to partial indirect-acting sympathomimetics (e.g., tyramine, ephedrine, metaraminol) is decreased such that a reduced pressor response is observed (Ghose 1980). Thus, depending on the interacting agent, an increase or decrease in the sympathomimetic dose may be warranted if significant changes in blood pressure are noted in a patient already receiving a tricyclic.

Anticholinergics (Moderate Severity)

Potent anticholinergic TCAs will produce additive peripheral anticholinergic effects of dry mouth, blurred vision, constipation, and urinary retention, especially when administered with other anticholinergic drugs. In addition, patients receiving multiple anticholinergic agents are at increased risk of experiencing CNS anticholinergic delirium, which presents as mental status changes such as hallucinations, delusions, decreased memory, disorientation, and decreased sensorium (Arnold et al. 1981). If a TCA is being used, clinicians are advised to restrict their TCA prescribing to nortriptyline and desipramine, especially in elderly patients.

Barbiturates (Moderate Severity)
Barbiturates appear to stimulate tricyclic metabolism by hepatic microsomal enzyme induction and, thus, can decrease blood levels of the monomethylated tricyclics (e.g., nortriptyline). Whether this is also true of the dimethylated tricyclics (e.g., amitriptyline) is not clear (Ballinger et al. 1974). Additionally, in toxic doses, the respiratory-depressant effects of the tricyclics are additive to those of the barbiturates (Borden and Rostrand 1968).

β-Adrenergic–Blocking Agents (Moderate Severity)
A study using healthy volunteers found that labetalol caused imipramine clearance to decrease by 38% and peak concentrations to increase by 83%. Because the hydroxylated metabolites of imipramine were significantly decreased, it was concluded that labetalol inhibited the microsomal hepatic enzyme CYP2D6 (Hermann et al. 1992). If labetalol is added to a patient's therapy, TCA treatment should be monitored in anticipation of increased ADRs.

Carbamazepine (Moderate Severity)
Carbamazepine induces the metabolism of TCAs, necessitating about a twofold increase in the tricyclic dose requirement (Brosen and Kragh-Sorensen 1993; Brown et al. 1990). Additionally, a single case report documented carbamazepine toxicity resulting from a doubling of the drug's concentration after the addition of desipramine to the patient's therapy (Lesser 1984). Clinicians should expect to increase the TCA dosage if carbamazepine is added to a patient's tricyclic therapy.

Cimetidine (Moderate Severity)
A single case report has described a patient in whom the imipramine half-life increased from 23 to 44 hours with the addition of cimetidine (D. D. Miller and Macklin 1983). A controlled study in six healthy subjects has confirmed this observation (Abernethy et al. 1984). In this investigation, the imipramine half-life increased from 16 to 22 hours, bioavailability increased from 40% to 75%, and clearance decreased from 1,048 to 623 mL/minute. The authors proposed that cimetidine inhibited both demethylation and hydroxylation of imipramine by its interaction with the liver's

cytochrome P450 enzyme system (Abernethy et al. 1984). This interaction is not apparent with ranitidine (Abernethy et al. 1984). Thus, plasma tricyclic levels should be monitored in depressed patients receiving TCAs and cimetidine concomitantly, or ranitidine may be substituted for cimetidine.

Ethanol (Moderate Severity)

Acute ethanol ingestion inhibits the metabolism of TCAs, and prolonged ingestion stimulates the hepatic metabolism of TCAs (Ciraulo et al. 1988). It is thought that the metabolic-induction effect may last a few months. Thus, depressed alcoholic individuals who remain abstinent while taking TCAs may experience an increase in TCA ADRs a few months after initiation of drug therapy once their hepatic enzymes return to normal.

Guanethidine (Moderate Severity)

An interaction study in five hypertensive patients demonstrated that the addition of therapeutic doses of desipramine or protriptyline to the patients' guanethidine therapy resulted in a 27-mm Hg rise in mean blood pressure (J. R. Mitchell et al. 1967). Blood pressure returned to baseline 5 days after discontinuation of the antidepressants. The TCAs inhibit the presynaptic neuronal uptake of guanethidine. In depressed hypertensive patients, the use of an antihypertensive agent other than guanethidine is recommended.

Monoamine Oxidase Inhibitors (Moderate Severity)

If a tricyclic is added to a monoamine oxidase inhibitor (MAOI), or vice versa, there exists the possibility of a toxic reaction manifested by nausea, dizziness, excitability, hyperpyrexia, dyspnea, cardiovascular instability, and seizures. This reaction is more likely to occur if the TCA is added to the MAOI or the TCA is immediately substituted for the MAOI. However, a TCA–MAOI combination can be used safely and effectively if the drugs are begun simultaneously. The patient should be MAOI-free for at least 14 days and tricyclic-free for 7–10 days. It is hypothesized that the toxic reaction stems from a significant increase (caused by both drugs) in the action of the monoamines present in the CNS, resulting in a synergistic augmentation of existing CNS amines (Ponto et al. 1977). Amitriptyline is preferred over imipramine because it produces less sensitization of the norepinephrine receptor (Ponto et al. 1977).

Oral Anticoagulants (Moderate Severity)

Chronic treatment with amitriptyline and nortriptyline did not alter the half-life of warfarin but did produce some inconsistent increases in the half-life of dicumarol (Pond et al. 1975). The bioavailability of dicumarol appeared to be increased. In some subjects, the increased bioavailability was associated with significant increases of the dicumarol half-life as a result of its dose-dependent kinetics. Thus, prothrombin levels should be monitored closely and the anticoagulant dose adjusted accordingly.

Quinidine (Moderate Severity)

Quinidine inhibits the hepatic oxidative enzyme CYP2D6, thus resulting in a significant reduction of TCA clearance (e.g., 35% for imipramine, 85% for desipramine) (E. Steiner et al. 1988). The increase in TCA blood levels combined with the type Ia antiarrhythmic effects of both drugs can result in the development of potentially fatal ventricular arrhythmias. TCAs and quinidine should not be administered together.

Selective Serotonin Reuptake Inhibitors (Moderate Severity)

Fluoxetine may cause inhibition of the hepatic microenzymes responsible for the metabolism of some antidepressants. Three cases have been reported of increased TCA adverse effects and serum levels after the administration of fluoxetine. In one patient, fluoxetine increased nortriptyline concentrations from 88 to 162 ng/mL (Vaughan 1988). In another patient, fluoxetine 20 mg/day raised the plasma desipramine level from 131 to 212 ng/mL, and 40 mg/day raised the level from 131 to 419 ng/mL (I. R. Bell and Cole 1988). A controlled trial compared the effects of fluoxetine and sertraline on desipramine concentrations (Preskorn et al. 1994). After 3 weeks of coadministration, desipramine concentrations had increased by nearly 400% with fluoxetine versus only 34% with sertraline. Although few justifications exist for administering two antidepressants together, a clinical situation could occur in which a fluoxetine-refractory patient needs to be switched to a TCA. In such a circumstance, the relatively long half-life of fluoxetine and its metabolite may produce an exaggerated but transient rise in the plasma TCA concentration.

▪ Monoamine Oxidase Inhibitors

Amine-Containing Foods (Major Severity)

See *Hypertensive crisis* [page 163] under *Cardiovascular* adverse effects of **Monoamine Oxidose Inhibitors** in Chapter 2.

Meperidine (Major Severity)

Fatalities have occurred in patients taking an MAOI and meperidine. The interaction is marked by sweating, rigidity, hypertension or hypotension, and coma and can occur even if the MAOI has been discontinued for several weeks. Caution should be exercised with the other narcotics as well, given that few data are available. Intravenous corticosteroids may be useful in reversing toxicity (Evans-Prosser 1968). Additionally, there is a report that selegiline, the antiparkinsonian MAOI, caused agitation and delirium when coadministered with meperidine (Zornberg et al. 1991).

Selective Serotonin Reuptake Inhibitors and Serotonin Agonists (Major Severity)

Selective serotonin reuptake inhibitors (SSRIs) and serotonin agonists (e.g., clomipramine, fluvoxamine, sertraline, paroxetine, trazodone, fluvoxamine, citalopram, L-tryptophan) taken with MAOIs have resulted in a number of sudden deaths due to the induction of a hyperserotonemic state, a syndrome manifested by signs and symptoms of confusion, restlessness, myoclonus, hyperreflexia, diaphoresis, shivering, and tremor (Graber et al. 1994). If a patient is currently not responding to an MAOI, the drug should be discontinued for at least 2 weeks before reinitiating therapy with any of the potent serotonin-agonist drugs. Likewise, if a patient has not responded to a SSRI, five half-lives (for both the parent drug and its active metabolites) should elapse before beginning MAOI therapy.

Sympathomimetics (Major Severity)

The MAOIs increase the concentration of norepinephrine in presynaptic adrenergic storage vesicles. The subsequent administration of sympathomimetic amines (e.g., amphetamines, ephedrine, metaraminol, methylphenidate, norepinephrine, phenylephrine, phenylpropanolamine, pseudoephedrine) results in the release of greater-than-normal concentrations of norepinephrine to react with the postsynaptic receptor. Fatalities and near-fatalities, manifested by hyperpyrexia, headache, hypertension, cerebral vascular hemorrhage, and/or cardiac arrhythmias, have been reported. Phentolamine, an α-blocker, is recommended for the emergency treatment of this interaction (Boakes et al. 1973). Selegiline, an MAOI-B inhibitor used in parkinsonian patients, may be used safely at dosages less than 20 mg/day in combination with levodopa or levodopa/carbidopa (Heinonen and Lammintausta 1991).

Dextromethorphan (Moderate Severity)
Dextromethorphan appears to block the reuptake of serotonin. Thus, it is not surprising that reactions—including a fatality similar to the MAOI–SSRI interaction (serotonin syndrome)—have been associated with dextromethorphan. Nausea, coma, hypotension, and hyperpyrexia are seen in this interaction (Sovner and Wolfe 1988). Concurrent use of SSRIs and dextromethorphan should be avoided.

Insulin/Oral Sulfonylureas (Moderate Severity)
MAOIs may enhance and/or prolong the hypoglycemic response to insulin and oral sulfonylureas (Adnitt 1968). Patients with diabetes who are being treated for depression with an MAOI may require lower doses of insulin and sulfonylureas. Therefore, such patients should have their fasting blood glucose checked more frequently.

Levodopa (Moderate Severity)
Levodopa is a precursor of dopamine, which, in turn, is a precursor of norepinephrine. The MAOIs reduce the degradation of dopamine and norepinephrine, thereby increasing the risk of a hypertensive episode (Hunter et al. 1970). The concurrent use of carbidopa 300–400 mg/day has been reported to totally or partially block this pressor response (Teychenne et al. 1975). The manufacturer recommends a 14-day washout of the MAOI before starting any levodopa-containing product.

Tricyclic Antidepressants (Moderate Severity)
See subsection on TCA–MAOI interaction (*Monoamine Oxidase Inhibitors* under "Tricyclic Antidepressants," page 466).

■ Selective Serotonin Reuptake Inhibitors

Monoamine Oxidase Inhibitors (Major Severity)
See subsection on MAOI–SSRI interaction (*Selective Serotonin Reuptake Inhibitors and Serotonin Agonists* under "Monoamine Oxidase Inhibitors," page 468).

β-Adrenergic–Blocking Agents (Moderate Severity)
Metoprolol appears to be metabolized by CYP2D6, and case reports of concomitant therapy with fluoxetine have been associated with increased frequencies of bradycardia (Riesenman 1995). Fluvoxamine produces nearly a fivefold increase in the concentration of propranolol because of its noncompetitive inhibition of CYP2C19 (Riesenman 1995).

Cimetidine (Moderate Severity)

When coadministered with paroxetine, cimetidine has been reported to cause substantial increases in serum concentrations of that drug (the systemic bioavailability increased by 50%) through noncompetitive enzyme inhibition (Bannister et al. 1989). No data are available for the other SSRIs.

Cyproheptadine (Moderate Severity)

Anecdotal case reports have documented the loss of SSRI (i.e., fluoxetine, paroxetine) antidepressant activity after the addition of cyproheptadine to therapy for the treatment of SSRI-induced sexual dysfunction (Christensen 1995; Feder 1991). Cyproheptadine, a serotonin antagonist, can reverse the SSRI agonist antidepressant activity. Cyproheptadine should be discontinued if a loss of antidepressant activity is observed in a patient who previously responded to an SSRI.

Diuretics (Moderate Severity)

A number of reports have linked fluoxetine and sertraline with the syndrome of inappropriate secretion of antidiuretic hormone (SIADH) by an unknown mechanism (B. J. Cohen et al. 1990; Crews et al. 1993; Hwang and Magraw 1989). Electrolytes should be monitored closely in patients receiving SSRIs, especially those who are receiving diuretics concomitantly. Electrolyte status should also be monitored more closely in patients taking lithium and a SSRI concomitantly.

Lithium (Moderate Severity)

Lithium neurotoxicity resulting from SSRI augmentation has been reported (Evans and Marwick 1990; Salama and Shafey 1989). However, short-term studies with healthy control subjects have suggested that the SSRIs do not affect lithium clearance (Breuel et al. 1995; Stellamans 1991; Wilner 1991). Thus, these cases of neurotoxicity are hypothesized to result from hyponatremia caused by the SSRI-induced SIADH syndrome, which precipitates lithium neurotoxicity.

Oral Anticoagulants (Moderate Severity)

Sertraline induces a slight increase in the hypoprothrombinemic response to warfarin (Wilner 1991), but fluoxetine and paroxetine have not been demonstrated to produce this effect. The addition of paroxetine to the medication regimens of patients receiving anticoagulants has caused them to develop a predisposition to bleeding episodes without exhibiting elevations in warfarin concentrations or any alterations in the prothrombin time (Bannister et al. 1989). Warfarin's concentration increases by approximately 98%, with an associated increase in prothrombin time, when fluvoxamine is added ("Fluvoxamine," 1996). Anticoagulants may increase the risk of bleeding in some patients receiving SSRIs (Bannister et al. 1989; Claire et al. 1991; Rowe et al. 1978).

Theophylline (Moderate Severity)

Fluvoxamine has been demonstrated in an in vitro study to have a significant inhibitory effect on CYP1A2 (Brosen et al. 1993). Reports show that the combination of fluvoxamine and theophylline can produce a threefold increase in serum theophylline concentration after the sixth day of concomitant administration, resulting in nausea, supraventricular tachycardia, generalized tonic-clonic seizures, and coma (Van den Brekel and Harrington 1994). It is recommended that theophylline dosages be reduced by one-third if that drug is coadministered with fluvoxamine (Ereshefsky et al. 1996).

Tricyclic Antidepressants (Moderate Severity)

See subsection on TCA–SSRI interaction (*Selective Serotonin Reuptake Inhibitors* under "Tricyclic Antidepressants," page 467).

L-Tryptophan (Moderate Severity)

A single uncontrolled trial in five patients suggested that a drug interaction occurs with L-tryptophan augmentation of fluoxetine treatment of obsessive-compulsive disorder. No ADRs were noted on fluoxetine 50–100 mg/day, but symptoms of agitation, aggressiveness, restlessness, worsening of obsessive-compulsive behavior, nausea, and vomiting occurred after the addition of 1–4 g/day of L-tryptophan in all five patients. These symptoms may be construed as a mild serotonin syndrome. The symptoms disappeared on discontinuation of L-tryptophan (W. Steiner and Fontaine 1986). Because of the deaths associated with serotonin syndrome, concomitant L-tryptophan use is not recommended in patients being treated with fluoxetine. L-tryptophan is currently unavailable in the United States but is available in Canada.

Nefazodone

■ Nonsedating Antihistamines (Major Severity)

The nonsedating antihistamines astemizole and terfenadine, in elevated serum concentrations, can potentially cause QT prolongation and torsade de pointes–type ventricular tachycardia that may be fatal. These antihistamines are metabolized by hepatic microsomal isoenzyme CYP3A4. Nefazodone may slow the hepatic metabolism of these drugs through the noncompetitive inhibition of CYP3A4 (Serzone® Product Information 1995).

■ Cytochrome P450 Isoenzyme System (Moderate Severity)

As presented in Table 8–1, nefazodone is a potent inhibitor of cytochrome P450 isoenzyme CYP3A4 and thus can theoretically result in an increase in the plasma concentrations of medications metabolized by this route (e.g., nonsedating antihistamines [terfenadine and astemizole], triazolobenzodiazepines [triazolam, alprazolam, and midazolam]). Coadministration of nefazodone with a CYP3A4-metabolized drug results in increased plasma concentrations of that drug, with no reported increase in nefazodone plasma concentrations.

■ Benzodiazepines (Moderate Severity)

When nefazodone is administered with either triazolam or alprazolam, up to a fourfold increase in plasma concentration may occur, resulting in significant potentiation of the psychomotor effects of the benzodiazepine. Only benzodiazepines metabolized by CYP3A4 have this potential interaction with nefazodone; those metabolized by glucuronidation (e.g., lorazepam, oxazepam) do not (Barbhaiya et al. 1995; Ellingrod and Perry 1995). A single-dose study in which 12 subjects received 0.25 mg of triazolam before and after taking nefazodone 200 mg twice per day reported increases of 1.7-fold, threefold, and fourfold in triazolam's C_{max}, half-life, and area under the curve (AUC), respectively (Riesenman 1995). It is therefore recommended that the triazolam dosage be decreased by 75% when triazolam and nefazodone are coadministered (Riesenman 1995). In a separate study, nefazodone produced a twofold increase in the concentration of alprazolam, suggesting that the alprazolam dosage should be reduced by 50% when that drug is administered with nefazodone (Riesenman 1995).

■ Digoxin (Moderate Severity)

The effects of nefazodone on digoxin pharmacokinetics were assessed in an open-label, randomized, multiple-dose, three-way crossover study in 18 healthy male subjects. Nefazodone 200 mg bid and digoxin 0.2 mg qd were administered both separately and concurrently. When coadministered, nefazodone's kinetic parameters were not affected, but the C_{max}, C_{min}, and AUC for digoxin were increased by 29%, 27%, and 15%, respectively. Although few or no electrocardiogram (ECG) changes were noted, monitoring of digoxin levels (because of its narrow therapeutic range) is recommended (Ellingrod and Perry 1995).

■ Haloperidol (Moderate Severity)

When haloperidol is coadministered with nefazodone, the AUC of haloperidol is 36% higher, whereas the pharmacokinetic parameters of nefazodone and its metabolites are unchanged. The change in haloperidol's AUC is statistically significant; however, because of the variability in patient response, the increase may not always be of sufficient magnitude to warrant decreasing the haloperidol dose when the two drugs are coadministered (Ellingrod and Perry 1995).

Venlafaxine

■ Cytochrome P450 Isoenzyme System (Moderate Severity)

Metabolism of venlafaxine is mediated by the CYP2D6 isoenzyme system. Thus, drugs that inhibit this isoenzyme (e.g., quinidine) (see Table 8–1) may precipitate increases in venlafaxine plasma concentrations and decreases in O-desmethylvenlafaxine (ODV) concentrations. Venlafaxine is also a weak inhibitor of CYP2D6, although the clinical significance of this observation is unknown. Theoretically, given that venlafaxine is metabolized by CYP2D6, it is possible that other drugs that are also metabolized by this enzyme could cause competitive inhibition of metabolism. Some of the medication classes that could cause these potential drug interactions include the β-blockers (e.g., propranolol, metoprolol, timolol), other antidepressants (e.g., amitriptyline, nortriptyline, clomipramine, imipramine, desipramine), antiarrhythmics (e.g., propafenone, encainide), codeine, and dextromethorphan (Ellingrod and Perry 1994). However, no significant drug interactions have yet been reported.

Lithium

■ Thiazide Diuretics (Major Severity)

Thiazides can cause a reduction of lithium clearance, with a consequent increase in the serum lithium level, within several days of diuretic therapy initiation (Jefferson 1979). This interaction is primarily due to the thiazide diuretic–induced increase in sodium and water excretion, which results in an increase in lithium reabsorption. The effect on lithium may be transient, lasting only for a few weeks, at which time the original lithium dose may need to be resumed. Initially, thiazide administration may require a 50% reduction in the lithium dose (Chambers et al. 1977). Lithium levels should be monitored closely in patients beginning thiazide treatment. Furosemide, a loop diuretic, does not affect lithium in this manner (Jefferson 1979).

■ Angiotensin-Converting-Enzyme Inhibitors (Moderate Severity)

Two reports have implicated the angiotensin-converting-enzyme inhibitor (ACEI) lisinopril as the precipitant of lithium-induced neurotoxicity (Douste-Blazy et al. 1986; Navis et al. 1989). ACEIs cause hyponatremia, which, in turn, causes a lithium clearance to decrease. In these two cases, serum lithium concentrations increased approximately fourfold after ACEI therapy was begun. Thus, neurological status and lithium serum concentrations must be monitored closely in patients on lithium who concomitantly receive ACEIs.

■ Carbamazepine (Moderate Severity)

Lithium-induced neurotoxicity reactions (e.g., ataxia, nystagmus, tremors, hyperreflexia, and muscle fasciculations) have been described in patients whose bipolar affective illness was being treated with lithium and carbamazepine (Chaudhry and Waters 1983; Shulka et al. 1984). The mechanism for this reaction stems from carbamazepine's ability to act as a vasopressin (antidiuretic hormone [ADH]) agonist, thereby occasionally causing hyponatremia and water intoxication. The neurotoxicity resulting from accidental lithium intoxication usually originates from hyponatremia precipitated by thiazides, influenza (i.e., vomiting, diarrhea), or concomitant ingestion of a vasopressin-agonist drug such as carbamazepine, thus allowing significantly more lithium to be reabsorbed by the proximal tubules. When combining lithium and carbamazepine to treat refractory manic patients, clinicians should be aware of the increased potential for lithium intoxication.

Lithium reverses carbamazepine-induced neutropenia to such an extent that the neutrophil count exceeds the baseline count observed before the initiation of carbamazepine treatment (Kramlinger and Post 1990). Thus, using lithium to treat carbamazepine-induced neutropenia is significantly more cost effective than resorting to granulocyte colony–stimulating factor (G-CSF).

■ Iodide Salts (Moderate Severity)

Case reports suggest that lithium and iodine possibly have either an additive or a synergistic action in precipitating hypothyroidism (Spaulding et al. 1977). If hypothyroidism occurs in a patient receiving this combination, the clinician should either discontinue the iodide salts or begin thyroid replacement therapy.

■ Methyldopa (Moderate Severity)

Four case reports have described neurotoxic reactions in patients receiving methyldopa and lithium at levels less than 1.5 mEq/L (Osanloo and Deglin 1980). If such reactions occur, consideration should be given to lowering the lithium dose or discontinuing the methyldopa.

■ Osmotic Diuretics (Moderate Severity)

In a single-dose study, the osmotic diuretics urea and mannitol were shown to increase lithium clearance in healthy subjects (Thomsen and Schou 1968). These agents have also been used in treating lithium intoxications (Shneerson 1978).

■ Prostaglandin Inhibitors (Moderate Severity)

Multiple studies have demonstrated that the addition of diclofenac, ibuprofen, indomethacin, naproxen, piroxicam, or ketorolac can decrease lithium clearance significantly within 5 to 10 days, resulting in serum-lithium-concentration increases ranging from 16% to 150% (Tatro 1996). It is thought that renal tubular prostaglandins are involved in the proximal tubular secretion of lithium and that the nonsteroidal antiinflammatory drugs (NSAIDs) inhibit this excretory process. Serum concentrations return to baseline within 7 days of discontinuation of the NSAID. Thus, use of NSAIDs concomitantly with lithium requires more vigorous blood-level monitoring. Aspirin does not affect lithium clearance (Reiman et al. 1983).

■ Theophylline (Moderate Severity)

A controlled study demonstrated a 20% mean decrease in serum lithium levels as a result of theophylline's induction of increases in lithium clearance (Perry et al. 1984). A controlled trial found that an intravenous theophylline infusion producing levels of 14 µg/mL increased lithium clearance by 51% (Holstad et al. 1988). Patients should have their lithium levels monitored closely if theophylline is added to their therapy, especially patients whose levels are in the low-normal range.

■ Urinary Alkalinizers (Moderate Severity)

Lithium clearance increased after the administration of single doses of bicarbonate and acetazolamide (Thomsen and Schou 1968). The authors attributed the interaction to an increase in sodium load to the kidney rather than to the alkalinization of the urine.

■ Verapamil (Moderate Severity)

Despite verapamil's being suggested as a potentially useful agent in the treatment of mania, two cases have been described in which patients' serum lithium concentrations were reduced after the initiation of verapamil therapy. One patient experienced a manic relapse; the second patient's lithium clearance was noted to increase by 35% (Weinrauch et al. 1984). In another case, lithium neurotoxicity developed at therapeutic lithium levels after coadministration of verapamil. This finding was confirmed by rechallenge with verapamil (Price and Shalley 1987). The onset of manic symptoms in a patient receiving these drugs concomitantly should prompt the clinician to investigate and rule out the possibility of a drug interaction.

Carbamazepine

■ Macrolide Antibiotics (Major Severity)

Because erythromycin and troleoandomycin can inhibit carbamazepine metabolism, the anticonvulsant dose may require as much as a 50% reduction in patients treated with these antibiotics (Mesdjian et al. 1980; Y. Y. Wong et al. 1983). Signs and symptoms of carbamazepine neurotoxicity have been reported to occur within 24 to 48 hours of the start of troleoandomycin treatment (Mesdjian et al. 1980). Thus, the carbamazepine dose should be decreased at the beginning of antibiotic therapy and then returned to the original dose at the termination of antimicrobial treatment.

■ Antipsychotics (Moderate Severity)

See subsection on antipsychotic–carbamazepine interaction ("Carbamazepine" under **Antipsychotics** [page 461]).

■ Bupropion (Moderate Severity)

Carbamazepine induces the hepatic microsomal enzyme CYP3A4 to the extent that bupropion is oxidized to hydroxybupropion at a faster rate (Ketter et al. 1995). Bupropion serum concentrations may be decreased sufficiently thereby to result in a loss of antidepressant activity.

■ Calcium Channel–Blocking Agents (Moderate Severity)

At least 15 patients experienced carbamazepine-induced neurotoxicity after the calcium channel blockers diltiazem and verapamil were added to their therapy (Bahls ct al. 1991). However, this effect was not noted with nifedipine (Brodie and MacPhee 1986). Impaired hepatic metabolism is postulated as the mechanism for this interaction. If symptoms of neurotoxicity occur, clinicians should measure the carbamazepine concentration and adjust the dosage accordingly. In another study, the bioavailability of felodipine was reduced by approximately 94% in 10 epileptic patients receiving the anticonvulsants carbamazepine, phenytoin, and/or phenobarbital (Capewell et al. 1988).

■ Cimetidine (Moderate Severity)

Although data in uncontrolled studies are conflicting, a possibility exists that cimetidine, but not ranitidine, could inhibit the hepatic metabolism of carbamazepine (Dalton et al. 1985; Webster et al. 1984). It is also unlikely that the interaction would occur with famotidine or nizatidine. Cimetidine increases serum carbamazepine concentrations for the first few days of treatment, but the carbamazepine levels return to baseline after a week (Dalton et al. 1986). This transient effect of carbamazepine metabolism probably results from the autometabolism property associated with carbamazepine. Thus, if cimetidine is added to the drug regimen of a patient already receiving carbamazepine, the clinician should monitor the patient for potential signs and symptoms of carbamazepine intoxication (e.g., ataxia, nystagmus, sedation, and confusion) during the first week of therapy.

■ Corticosteroids (Moderate Severity)

A controlled trial found that carbamazepine increased prednisolone clearance by 42% (Olivesi 1986). Thus, patients requiring
prophylactic corticosteroid medication will require an upward adjustment of their medication if they begin carbamazepine treatment. Additionally, carbamazepine induces the metabolism of
dexamethasone, thereby increasing the chances of a false-positive
dexamethasone suppression test (Privitera et al. 1982).

■ Cyclosporine (Moderate Severity)

Carbamazepine induces the hepatic metabolism and increases the
clearance of cyclosporine. Cyclosporine blood levels are significantly reduced within several days of starting carbamazepine and
do not return to baseline until carbamazepine has been discontinued for 2–3 weeks (Yee and McGuire 1990). In patients for whom
an anticonvulsant is indicated, valproic acid may be substituted for
carbamazepine.

■ Danazol (Moderate Severity)

Carbamazepine neurotoxicity manifesting as lethargy and ataxia
was reported in five of six women after danazol (for fibrocystic
breast disease) was added to their chronic carbamazepine treatment regimens. Within 30 days of coadministration, carbamazepine levels increased 38%–123%; other antiepileptic drug levels
remained unaffected (Zielinski et al. 1987). This interaction is due
to danazol's inhibition of carbamazepine's conversion to certain
metabolites (Kramer et al. 1986). Management includes monitoring for clinical signs of carbamazepine toxicity and elevated carbamazepine levels.

■ Doxycycline (Moderate Severity)

Two studies have found the elimination half-life of doxycycline to
be reduced in patients receiving chronic carbamazepine therapy
(Neuvonen et al. 1975; Penttila et al. 1974). This interaction is
probably the result of increased hepatic metabolism of doxycycline
but has not been observed with the other tetracyclines. The clinical
significance of this finding has not been established.

■ Isoniazid (Moderate Severity)

Signs and symptoms of carbamazepine-induced neurotoxicity were
noted in 10 of 13 patients after initiation of isoniazid treatment

(Valsalan and Cooper 1982). Carbamazepine serum levels were available for three of the patients and were in the toxic range. It was theorized that carbamazepine hepatic metabolism was inhibited by isoniazid. In another patient, coadministration of the two drugs resulted in elevated liver enzymes, which continued to increase 3 days after isoniazid discontinuation but eventually returned to baseline. This interaction was thought to be a result of a carbamazepine-induced increase in the degradation of isoniazid to hepatotoxic metabolites (Wright et al. 1982). Because isoniazid is also a MAOI, the potential for such an interaction should be considered in treatment-refractory depressed patients receiving the combination of carbamazepine and an MAOI.

■ Lithium (Moderate Severity)

See subsection on lithium–carbamazepine interaction ("Carbamazepine" under **Lithium,** page 474).

■ Mebendazole (Moderate Severity)

In a series of patients, analyzed retrospectively, who received mebendazole alone or in combination with carbamazepine, those who received the combination had lower mebendazole levels. On carbamazepine discontinuation, the mebendazole levels increased in each case (Luder et al. 1986). This type of drug interaction may be explained by carbamazepine's ability to induce hepatic microenzymes.

■ Methadone (Moderate Severity)

Carbamazepine may induce the hepatic metabolism of methadone to concentrations associated with an increased likelihood of withdrawal symptoms (J. Bell et al. 1988). Methadone-maintenance patients receiving enzyme inducing drugs (e.g., carbamazepine, phenytoin, barbiturates) may require larger methadone doses.

■ Neuromuscular Blocking Agents (Moderate Severity)

The neuromuscular blocking action of nondepolarizing muscle relaxants may be reduced following chronic carbamazepine therapy. Compared with control subjects, nine surgical patients who had been receiving carbamazepine for at least 1 month demonstrated significantly shorter recovery times after the administration of pancuronium 0.1 mg/kg iv. The recovery times at the 25%, 50%, 75%, and 90% levels of recovery were approximately 65% shorter in the carbamazepine group. Additionally, the recovery index (i.e., the time between 25% and 75% recovery) was 17 minutes in the carbamazepine group versus 46 minutes in the control group. The recovery time appeared to be inversely correlated with carbamazepine dose (Roth and Ebrahim 1987). Dosage requirements of nondepolarizing muscle relaxants may be increased in patients also receiving carbamazepine, and close monitoring is required. Although this interaction has not been reported in patients receiving succinylcholine, a depolarizing muscle relaxant, caution is warranted in patients on carbamazepine who receive succinylcholine for electroconvulsive therapy (ECT).

■ Oral Anticoagulants (Moderate Severity)

In seven patients, warfarin concentrations were decreased and prothrombin times increased after initiation of carbamazepine therapy (J. M. Hansen et al. 1971; Kendall and Boivin 1981; Massey 1983). This interaction is postulated to result from hepatic microsomal enzyme induction by carbamazepine. Warfarin doses may need to be increased in patients initiating carbamazepine therapy.

■ Oral Contraceptives (Moderate Severity)

A retrospective study reported that 3 of 41 (7%) patients taking oral contraceptives and anticonvulsants became pregnant (Coulam and Annegers 1979). A single-dose pharmacokinetic study found that carbamazepine reduced the bioavailability of ethinyl estradiol by 42% and of levonorgestrel by 40% (Crawford et al. 1990). This metabolic enzyme induction has also been associated with norgestrel subdermal capsules (Norplant®) (Haukkamaa 1986). To reduce the risk of unplanned pregnancy, patients receiving enzyme-inducing anticonvulsants with potential teratogenic effects (e.g., carbamazepine) should use another form of birth control.

■ Propoxyphene (Moderate Severity)

Two uncontrolled trials found that the addition of propoxyphene to patients' carbamazepine regimens resulted in a 66% increase in the anticonvulsant's serum concentrations, probably as a result of propoxyphene's inhibition of carbamazepine's hepatic metabolism (Dam et al. 1977; B. S. Hansen et al. 1980). NSAIDs are probably the analgesics of choice in this situation.

■ Theophylline (Moderate Severity)

Carbamazepine has been reported, in a single case, to decrease plasma theophylline levels and elimination half-life from 5.3 to 2.8 hours (Rosenberry et al. 1983). In another case, theophylline 5 mg/kg every 6 hours decreased carbamazepine concentrations from 30 to 16 mmol/L after seven doses of theophylline and resulted in loss of seizure control (E. A. Mitchell et al. 1986). Dosage adjustments based on plasma levels are indicated for both drugs if carbamazepine and theophylline are used together.

■ Thyroid (Moderate Severity)

Carbamazepine induces the metabolism of thyroxine (T_4) and triiodothyronine (T_3) (Joffe et al. 1984). It also interferes with the increase in circulating thyrotropin (thyroid-stimulating hormone [TSH]) that occurs after the reduction of the thyroid hormones (Aanderud et al. 1981). Thus, patients receiving thyroid replacement therapy may become hypothyroid if carbamazepine is added to their regimens.

■ Tricyclic Antidepressants (Moderate Severity)

See subsection on TCA–carbamazepine interaction (*Carbamazepine* under "Tricyclic Antidepressants," page 465).

■ Valproic Acid (Moderate Severity)

Carbamazepine and valproic acid appear to alter each other's kinetics. In one study, carbamazepine decreased minimum steady-state valproic acid by 21% and increased metabolic clearance by 31% without altering the half-life (Bowdle et al. 1979). In another study, valproic acid increased the carbamazepine half-life by 12%, the unbound carbamazepine half-life by 16%, and the free plasma carbamazepine by 13% (MacPhee et al. 1988). Additionally, increases in the carbamazepine epoxide metabolite, which is associated with toxicity, occur (Rambeck et al. 1990). Because the clinical effects of these changes are difficult to predict, closer plasma monitoring is indicated when using this combination.

Valproic Acid

■ Barbiturates (Moderate Severity)

In one controlled study, to maintain therapeutic phenobarbital concentrations, the barbiturate dose was decreased by 46% after the addition of valproic acid to the therapeutic regimen (Wilder et al. 1978). Because valproic acid can inhibit the hepatic metabolic conversion of phenobarbital to its hydroxylated metabolite (Bruni et al. 1980), patients receiving valproic acid and barbiturates are predisposed to barbiturate intoxication marked by sedation, nystagmus, ataxia, and confusion.

■ Carbamazepine (Moderate Severity)

See subsection on carbamazepine–valproic acid interaction ("Valproic Acid" under **Carbamazepine,** page 481).

■ Phenytoin (Moderate Severity)

Valproic acid and phenytoin have an unpredictable interaction, requiring valproic acid and free phenytoin–level monitoring. Valproic acid has been variously reported to increase, decrease, and have no effect on total phenytoin levels (Henriksen and Johannessen 1982; Tsanaclis et al. 1984). The free fraction of phenytoin is increased due to displacement from serum proteins (Monks and Richens 1980). However, this effect is sometimes offset by decreases in the total phenytoin level. In addition, although enhanced phenytoin toxicity at therapeutic levels has been reported with valproic acid coadministration (Palm et al. 1984), phenytoin appears to decrease valproic acid serum levels (Henriksen and Johannessen 1982). Obviously, close monitoring of the blood levels is indicated because of the idiosyncratic nature of this interaction.

■ Salicylates (Moderate Severity)

Three cases of probable valproic acid toxicity manifesting as tremor, drowsiness, ataxia, nystagmus, and personality changes have been reported after aspirin coadministration (Goulden et al. 1987). In a series of reports of six patients receiving valproic acid, the free levels increased by 49% and free clearance decreased by 28%. A similar effect on total valproic acid concentrations and clearance was observed (Abbott et al. 1986; Farrell et al. 1982; Orr et al. 1982). Aspirin may also alter valproic acid metabolic pathways, thereby producing more potentially hepatotoxic metabolites (Abbott et al. 1986). In patients receiving these drugs together, serum valproic acid levels—including free fraction, clinical signs of valproic acid toxicity, and liver enzymes—should be monitored.

Verapamil

▪ Barbiturates (Moderate Severity)

In a randomized, crossover study of seven volunteers, phenobarbital decreased oral bioavailability and increased systemic clearance of verapamil probably through induction of verapamil metabolism. Administration of phenobarbital 100 mg/day for 3 weeks increased total oral verapamil clearance fourfold and free oral clearance threefold after administration of a single 80-mg oral dose of verapamil or of 80 mg every 6 hours for 5 days (Rutledge et al. 1988). Manic patients receiving chronic barbiturates may require a higher dose of verapamil to control their symptoms.

▪ β-Adrenergic–Blocking Agents (Moderate Severity)

In treating hypertension, verapamil and β-blockers are often used together for their additive or synergistic hypotensive effects. However, the combination may potentiate cardiovascular ADRs (e.g., bradycardia, hypotension) due to the additive effects of the two drugs. These ADRs are more likely to occur in patients with left-ventricular dysfunction or atrioventricular (AV) conduction defects or with intravenous administration of verapamil (Bailey and Carruthers 1991). Verapamil increases the serum concentrations of some β-blockers by as much as 300% (McLean et al. 1985).

▪ Calcium Salts—Vitamin D (Moderate Severity)

Administration of calcium and ergocalciferol to a patient receiving verapamil for atrial fibrillation resulted in recurrence of the arrhythmia (Bar-Or and Gasiel 1981). Administration of iv calcium has been used to treat cases of verapamil overdose and acts by antagonizing verapamil's effects (Perkins 1978). Unless employed as a treatment for verapamil toxicity, calcium salts should be used cautiously in patients receiving verapamil.

▪ Cyclosporine (Moderate Severity)

In a series of five patients, verapamil 120–360 mg/day caused marked increases in cyclosporine levels within 1 week of the start of coadministration. Rechallenge produced the same effect on cyclosporine levels in one patient (Lindholm and Henricsson 1987). In another case report, a verapamil dosage increase from 240 to 360 mg/day resulted in a 360% increase in cyclosporine levels, resulting in shaking and sore gums in the patient (Maggio and

Bartels 1988). If this interaction is suspected, a decrease in cyclo-sporine dose based on blood levels is indicated.

■ Digitalis Glycosides (Moderate Severity)

Over 7–10 days, verapamil decreased digoxin clearance by approximately one-third, resulting in an average 70% increase in blood levels (Klein et al. 1982; Pedersen et al. 1981; Schwartz et al. 1982). A similar effect has been reported with digitoxin (Kuhlmann and Marcin 1985). Not surprisingly, increased digoxin ADRs, including premature ventricular contractions, have been reported (Schwartz et al. 1982). The magnitude of the increase in the drug level is dose dependent (Klein et al. 1982). This interaction may be managed by adjusting the dose of the digitalis glycoside based on blood levels.

■ Neuromuscular Blocking Agents (Moderate Severity)

Verapamil may enhance the neuromuscular blocking effects of nondepolarizing muscle relaxants by blocking the calcium channels at the postsynaptic muscle membrane site of skeletal muscle. In one case, a patient receiving chronic verapamil was given pancuronium for surgery, resulting in prolonged muscle paralysis that failed to respond to neostigmine (Jones et al. 1985). In another case, extended residual neuromuscular blockade was noted upon coadministration of pancuronium, *d*-tubocurarine, and chronic verapamil (Carlos and Erill 1986). If this combination cannot be avoided, the muscle-relaxant dose should be adjusted based on close monitoring of respiratory function.

■ Quinidine (Moderate Severity)

Coadministration of verapamil and quinidine has been associated with severe hypertension, pulmonary edema, ventricular tachycardia, bradycardia, AV block, diaphoresis, and blurred vision (Epstein and Rosing 1981; Trohman et al. 1986). In a study of six volunteers, verapamil increased the quinidine half-life by approximately one-third, possibly explaining some of the reported ADRs (Edwards et al. 1987). These drugs should be used together only if no other alternatives exist, and if toxicity occurs, one or both drugs should be discontinued and symptomatic treatment administered.

■ Rifampin (Moderate Severity)

In a study of six healthy volunteers, 15 days of rifampin administration decreased oral bioavailability of verapamil by 92% and increased iv verapamil clearance (Barbarash et al. 1988). This effect was probably due to induction of verapamil metabolism. If an interaction is suspected in a patient requiring rifampin therapy, the use of a different antimanic agent is indicated.

■ Theophylline (Moderate Severity)

In a study of healthy volunteers, the clearance of a single oral dose of theophylline decreased by 18% after 7 days of verapamil administration (Sirmans et al. 1988). In another study of nine volunteers, theophylline disposition was not altered by verapamil 80 mg every 8 hours for 4 days (Robson et al. 1988). Theophylline levels should be measured if signs of theophylline toxicity occur.

Anxiolytic-Hypnotics

■ Barbiturates

The barbiturates are a class of drugs notorious for interacting with other drugs. In the vast majority of cases, the interaction results from barbiturate induction of hepatic microsomal enzymes, which results in increased clearance of many drugs metabolized by the liver (see Table 8–1). This effect may also substantially increase the first-pass effect for orally administered drugs and thereby decrease their bioavailability. Hepatic enzyme induction is an effect of chronic administration of barbiturates and usually requires at least 2–3 weeks to reach full effect. Because barbiturates currently are only used commonly in psychiatry for the amobarbital interview and for ECT anesthesia, they generally are not involved in many interactions. Barbiturate interactions with the drugs commonly used in psychiatric patients are described in this chapter. However, barbiturate interactions with drugs less frequently used in psychiatric patients are not described. If a drug interaction is suspected in a patient receiving a barbiturate, we recommend consulting a standard drug interaction text such as *Drug Interactions and Updates* (Hansten and Horn 1995).

■ Benzodiazepines

Azole Antifungal Agents (Moderate Severity)
Itraconazole and ketoconazole inhibit the hepatic microsomal oxidative isoenzyme CYP3A4, thereby causing up to 22-fold increases in midazolam and triazolam blood levels (Greenblatt et al. 1995; Olkkola et al. 1994; Varhe et al. 1994). For patients being treated

with an azole antifungal, either oxazepam or lorazepam—benzodiazepines not requiring oxidation—is recommended.

Diltiazem (Moderate Severity)
A controlled study in healthy volunteers found that diltiazem increased the half-life of midazolam by 49%, resulting in prolonged deep sedation of the subjects (Backman et al. 1994). As shown in Table 8–1, a number of benzodiazepines and calcium channel blockers are oxidized by CYP3A4, thus suggesting competitive inhibition as the mechanism of the interaction. Lower doses of benzodiazepines are recommended in patients concomitantly receiving calcium channel blockers.

Disulfiram (Moderate Severity)
The metabolism of benzodiazepines that undergo *N*-demethylation by the microsomal enzyme system in the liver (e.g., chlordiazepoxide, clorazepate, diazepam, flurazepam, halazepam, prazepam) is inhibited by disulfiram (MacLeod et al. 1978). Chlordiazepoxide and diazepam clearance decreased by 54% and 41%, respectively, in the presence of steady-state concentrations of disulfiram. The clearance of oxazepam was not affected (MacLeod et al. 1978). Nonetheless, alcoholic individuals receiving disulfiram probably should not take benzodiazepines because of these agents' addictive potential.

Erythromycin (Moderate Severity)
A controlled trial found that erythromycin treatment inhibited midazolam metabolism such that the serum concentrations increased by 170% and the $t_{1/2}$ increased from 89 to 153 minutes (Olkkola et al. 1993). Thus, erythromycin-medicated patients may not recover from midazolam sedation as quickly as might be expected.

In studies of healthy volunteers, erythromycin and troleandomycin have been reported to increase peak triazolam plasma levels by 50% (Phillips et al. 1986) and 107% (Warot et al. 1987), respectively, and to decrease oral triazolam clearance by 51% (Phillips et al. 1986) and 74% (Warot et al. 1987), respectively. Triazolam doses probably will need to be decreased during a standard course of these antibiotics.

Ethanol (Moderate Severity)
The additive CNS-depressant effects of benzodiazepines and ethanol result in impaired psychomotor functioning and oversedation (Linnoila and Hakkinen 1974; Linnoila et al. 1990). Kinetic studies

suggest that ethanol enhances benzodiazepine's absorption, decreases its volume of distribution, and impairs its elimination. Patients should be instructed to drink only moderately (if at all) when taking a benzodiazepine.

Histamine$_2$-Blocking Agents (Moderate Severity)

A controlled study in six subjects found that ranitidine decreased steady-state diazepam concentrations by 25% without altering the elimination rate. The oral clearance of diazepam was decreased by 30%, whereas the iv clearance was unchanged (Klotz et al. 1983). Thus, it was hypothesized that the gastrointestinal absorption of diazepam is decreased by ranitidine.

The metabolism of benzodiazepines that undergo N-dealkylation (phase I reaction) by the mixed-function oxidative enzyme system in the liver (e.g., chlordiazepoxide, clorazepate, diazepam, flurazepam, halazepam, desmethyldiazepam, alprazolam, triazolam, prazepam) is significantly inhibited by the concurrent administration of cimetidine (Greenblatt et al. 1983; Klotz and Reimann 1981). Addition of cimetidine to the drug regimen of a patient receiving a benzodiazepine could result in a CNS intoxication reaction. Ranitidine can be substituted for cimetidine because it does not impair diazepam metabolism and, in fact, decreases diazepam bioavailability.

Probenecid (Moderate Severity)

Probenecid was reported to decrease lorazepam clearance by 50% and to increase the drug's half-life from 14 to 33 hours following administration of lorazepam 2 mg iv in a randomized, crossover study of nine subjects (Abernethy et al. 1985). In another study, involving 106 patients receiving midazolam 3 mg/kg iv, the mean time to loss of consciousness was 85 seconds in the 54 patients also given probenecid 1 g, as compared with 109 seconds in the 52 patients not receiving probenecid (Dundee et al. 1986). This effect was thought to be due to displacement of the midazolam from protein binding sites.

Protease Inhibitors (Moderate Severity)

Manufacturer in vitro studies indicate that indinavir and ritonavir are oxidized by CYP3A4 (Crixivan® Product Information 1996; Norvir® Product Information 1996). Thus, it is recommended that benzodiazepines metabolized by the CYP3A4 isoenzyme not be administered to patients receiving protease inhibitors, and that oxazepam and lorazepam be used instead.

Rifampin (Moderate Severity)

Triple therapy with isoniazid, ethambutol, and rifampin was found to increase total body clearance of diazepam, thereby offsetting the opposite effect on clearance produced by isoniazid (Ochs et al. 1981). The increased clearance probably resulted from hepatic microsomal induction caused by the rifampin alone. Thus, patients receiving triple therapy may require larger benzodiazepine doses when being treated, for example, for alcohol withdrawal.

■ Buspirone

Haloperidol (Moderate Severity)

Buspirone 180 mg/day has been reported to benefit antipsychotic-induced extrapyramidal ADRs, including tardive dyskinesia (Moss et al. 1993). The effect on tardive dyskinesia—at least on that caused by haloperidol—may be related to buspirone's induction of increased antipsychotic blood levels, resulting in temporary masking of the dyskinetic movements. Buspirone 10–30 mg/day for 6 weeks was found to increase haloperidol concentrations by 26% (Goff et al. 1991b). Although buspirone's beneficial effect on the tardive dyskinesia was not significant at 10–30 mg, higher doses (i.e., 180 mg/day) may produce a large enough increase in the haloperidol concentration to mask the dyskinetic symptoms.

■ Chloral Hydrate

Ethanol (Moderate Severity)

Increased CNS depression and, sometimes, the unexpected ADRs of facial flushing, tachycardia, and headache can occur when ethanol is ingested with chloral hydrate (Sellers et al. 1972). It appears that the alcohol increases trichloroethanol transformation from chloral hydrate, although ethanol metabolism may be inhibited to a minor degree (L. K. Wong 1978). Ethanol should be avoided in patients using chloral hydrate.

Oral Anticoagulants (Moderate Severity)

Approximately 25% of patients receiving warfarin experience a significant but transient potentiation of the hypoprothrombinemic effect of warfarin after chloral hydrate administration (R. R. Miller and Greenblatt 1976). This interaction, a result of the displacement of warfarin from its albumin binding sites by chloral hydrate's inactive metabolite trichloroacetic acid, can occur as early as 12 hours after a 1,000-mg chloral hydrate dose (Udall 1975). Patients receiving oral anticoagulants should use a benzodiazepine rather than chloral hydrate if a hypnotic is required.

Anticholinergic/Antiparkinsonian Agents

■ Amantadine (Moderate Severity)

Amantadine has been reported to potentiate adverse effects of anticholinergic drugs, resulting in nocturnal confusion and hallucinations that resolve on reduction of the anticholinergic dose (Schwab et al. 1969). Thus, patients taking a combination of amantadine and an antiparkinsonian agent for treatment of their EPS should be closely monitored for signs and symptoms of anticholinergic delirium.

■ Antipsychotics (Moderate Severity)

See subsection on antipsychotic–anticholinergic interaction ("Anticholinergics" under **Antipsychotics**, page 454).

■ Tricyclic Antidepressants (Moderate Severity)

See subsection on TCA–anticholinergics interaction (*Anticholinergics* under "Tricyclic Antidepressants," page 464).

Amantadine

■ Anticholinergic/Antiparkinsonian Agents (Moderate Severity)

Amantadine combined with anticholinergic medications increases the risk of anticholinergic delirium (Postma and Van Tilburg 1975). (See subsection on anticholinergic/antiparkinsonian agent–amantadine interaction ["Amantadine" under **Anticholinergic/Antiparkinsonian Agents,** above].)

Disulfiram

■ Ethanol (Major Severity)

Normally, ethanol is metabolized in the liver, first to acetaldehyde by alcohol dehydrogenase and then to acetate by aldehyde dehydrogenase. Disulfiram inhibits aldehyde dehydrogenase and, hence, when used in the presence of alcohol, causes an increase in blood acetaldehyde levels. It is postulated that these increased acetaldehyde levels produce the toxic disulfiram-ethanol reaction, which consists of flushing, diaphoresis, tachycardia, palpitations, increased pulse pressure, shortness of breath, anxiety, nausea and vomiting, and, when more severe, decreased blood pressure, severe hypotension with shock, loss of consciousness, and death. The etiology of the disulfiram-ethanol reaction and acetaldehyde poisoning has been questioned, because acetaldehyde poisoning causes hyper-, not hypotension. It is generally concluded, however, that acetaldehyde is involved in the reaction in some as-yet-unspecified manner (Kitson 1977).

■ Benzodiazepines (Moderate Severity)

See subsection on BZD–disulfiram interaction *(Disulfiram* under "Benzodiazepines," page 486).

■ Chlorzoxazone (Moderate Severity)

In a controlled study in healthy subjects, a single oral dose of disulfiram increased the half-life of chlorzoxazone from 0.9 to 5.1 hours (Kharasch et al. 1993). Disulfiram is a noncompetitive inhibitor of the hepatic isoenzyme CYP2E1, which is at least partially responsible for the oxidative metabolism of chlorzoxazone. If excessive CNS activity is noted during concurrent administration of disulfiram and chlorzoxazone, dosage reduction of the latter drug is probably necessary.

■ Isoniazid (Moderate Severity)

The combination of disulfiram and isoniazid may result in a neurotoxicity manifested by ataxia, dizziness, lethargy, hypomania or dysphoria, and/or delirium. Both drugs inhibit two of three known metabolic pathways for dopamine, thereby increasing norepinephrine levels. Patients receiving these agents concurrently should be monitored for signs of neurotoxicity as well as mental status changes (Whittington and Grey 1969).

■ Metronidazole (Moderate Severity)

Of 29 patients receiving the combination of disulfiram and metronidazole, six developed an intoxication reaction manifesting either as delirium or as an acute psychotic reaction, whereas none of 29 patients receiving disulfiram and placebo became intoxicated (Rothstein and Clancy 1969). Thus, this combination should be avoided.

■ Oral Anticoagulants (Moderate Severity)

Disulfiram enhances the hypoprothrombinemic action of warfarin, thereby necessitating the use of lower warfarin doses. Because warfarin blood levels are not affected by disulfiram, it is hypothesized that disulfiram directly affects the hepatic mechanism responsible for hypoprothrombinemia (O'Reilly 1981).

■ **Phenytoin (Moderate Severity)**

The concurrent administration of phenytoin and disulfiram results in increases in phenytoin blood levels and possible toxicity as a result of the noncompetitive hepatic microsomal enzyme inhibition of phenytoin metabolism by disulfiram (Taylor et al. 1981). Phenytoin doses should be lowered before starting a patient on disulfiram.

■ **Theophylline (Moderate Severity)**

As the result of inhibition of the hepatic microsomal enzyme, the clearance of theophylline was decreased by 21% and 31% in patients taking disulfiram 250 mg/day and 500 mg/day, respectively (Loi et al. 1989). Patients receiving theophylline should expect to decrease their dose if disulfiram is added to their therapy.

References

Aanderud S, Myking OL, Strandjord RE: The influence of carbamazepine on thyroid hormones and thyroxine binding globulin in hyperthyroid patients substituted with thyroxine. Clin Endocrinol 15:247–252, 1981

Abbott FS, Kassam J, Orr JM, et al: The effect of aspirin on valproic acid metabolism. Clin Pharmacol Ther 40:94–100, 1986

Abernethy DR, Greenblatt DJ, Shader RI: Imipramine-cimetidine interaction: impairment of clearance and enhanced absolute bioavailability. J Pharmacol Exp Ther 229:702–705, 1984

Abernethy DR, Greenblatt DJ, Ameer B, et al: Probenecid impairment of acetaminophen and lorazepam clearance: direct inhibition of ether glucuronide formation. J Pharmacol Exp Ther 234:345–349, 1985

Adnitt PI: Hypoglycemic action of monoamine oxidase inhibitors. Diabetes 17:628–633, 1968

Alexander HE, McCarty K, Giffen MB: Hypotension and cardiopulmonary arrest associated with concurrent haloperidol and propranolol therapy. JAMA 252:87–88, 1984

Arana GW, Goff DC, Friedman H, et al: Does carbamazepine-induced reduction of plasma haloperidol levels worsen psychotic symptoms? Am J Psychiatry 143:650–651, 1986

Arnold SE, Kahn RJ, Faldetta LL, et al: Tricyclic antidepressant and peripheral anticholinergic activity. Psychopharmacology (Berl) 74:325–328, 1981

Baastrup PC, Hollnagel P, Sorenson R, et al: Adverse reactions in treatment with lithium carbonate and haloperidol. JAMA 236:2645–2646, 1976

Backman JT, Olkkola KT, Aranko K, et al: Dose of midazolam should be reduced during diltiazem and verapamil treatments. Br J Clin Pharmacol. 37:221–225, 1994

Bahls F, Ozuna J, Ritchie DE: Interactions between calcium channel blockers and the anticonvulsants, carbamazepine and phenytoin. Neurology 41:740–742, 1991

Bailey DG, Carruthers SG: Interaction between oral verapamil and β-blockers during submaximal exercise: relevance of ancillary properties. Clin Pharmacol Ther 49:370–376, 1991

Ballinger BR, Presly A, Reid AH, et al: The effects of hypnotics on imipramine treatment. Psychopharmacologia 39:267–274, 1974

Bannister SJ, Houser VP, Hulse JD, et al: Evaluation of the potential for interactions of paroxetine with diazepam, cimetidine, warfarin, and digoxin. Acta Psychiatr Scand 80 (suppl 350):102–106, 1989

Bar-Or D, Gasiel Y: Calcium and calciferol antagonise effect of verapamil in atrial fibrillation. BMJ 282:1585–1586, 1981

Barbarash RA, Bauman JL, Fischer JH, et al: Near total reduction in verapamil bioavailability by rifampin: electrocardiographic correlates. Chest 94:954–959, 1988

Barbhaiya RH, Shukla UA, Kroboth PD, et al: Coadministration of nefazodone and benzodiazepines, II: a pharmacokinetic interaction study with triazolam. J Clin Psychopharmacol 15:320–326, 1995

Bell IR, Cole JO: Fluoxetine induces elevation of desipramine level and exacerbation of geriatric nonpsychotic depression (letter). J Clin Psychopharmacol 8:447–448, 1988

Bell J, Seres V, Bowron P, et al: The use of serum methadone levels in patients receiving methadone maintenance. Clin Pharmacol Ther 43:623–629, 1988

Biederman J, Lerner Y, Belmaker RH: Combination of lithium carbonate and haloperidol in schizo-affective disorder. Arch Gen Psychiatry 36:327–333, 1979

Boakes AJ, Laurence DR, Teoh PC, et al: Interactions between sympathomimetic amines and antidepressant agents in man. BMJ 1:311–315, 1973

Borden EC, Rostrand SG: Recovery from massive amitriptyline overdosage (letter). Lancet 1:1256, 1968

Bowdle TA, Levy RH, Cutler RE: Effects of carbamazepine on valproic acid kinetics in normal subjects. Clin Pharmacol Ther 26:629–634, 1979

Breuel HP, Muller-Oerlinghausen B, Nickelsen T, et al: Pharmacokinetic interactions between lithium and fluoxetine after single and repeated fluoxetine administration in young healthy volunteers. Int J Clin Pharmacol Therap 33:415–419, 1995

Brodie MJ, MacPhee GJ: Carbamazepine neurotoxicity precipitated by diltiazem. BMJ 292:1170–1171, 1986

Brosen K, Kragh-Sorensen P: Concomitant intake of nortriptyline and carbamazepine. Ther Drug Monit 15:258–260, 1993

Brosen K, Skjelbo E, Rasmussen BB, et al: Fluvoxamine is a potent inhibitor of cytochrome P450 1A2. Biochem Pharmacol 45:1211–1214, 1993

Brown CS, Wells BG, Cold JA, et al: Possible influence of carbamazepine on plasma imipramine concentration in children with attention-deficit hyperactivity disorder. J Clin Psychopharmacol 10:359–362, 1990

Bruni J, Wilder BJ, Perchalski RJ, et al: Valproic acid and plasma levels of phenobarbital. Neurology 30:94–97, 1980

Capewell S, Freestone S, Critchley JA, et al: Reduced felodipine bioavailability in patients taking anticonvulsants. Lancet 2:480–482, 1988

Carlos R, Erill S: Therapeutic rounds: abnormally prolonged responses to neuromuscular blocking agents. Clin Ther 9:22–23, 1986

Centorrino F, Baldessarini RJ, Kando J, et al: Serum concentrations of clozapine and its major metabolites: effects of cotreatment with fluoxetine or valproate. Am J Psychiatry 151:123–125, 1994

Chambers G, Kerry RJ, Owen G: Lithium used with a diuretic. BMJ 3:805–806, 1977

Chaudhry RP, Waters BG: Lithium and carbamazepine interaction: possible neurotoxicity. J Clin Psychiatry 44:30–31, 1983

Christensen RC: Adverse interaction of paroxetine and cyproheptadine (letter). J Clin Psychiatry 56:433–434, 1995

Ciraulo DA, Barnhill JG, Jaffe JH: Clinical pharmacokinetics of imipramine and desipramine in alcoholics and normal volunteers. Clin Pharmacol Ther 43:509–518, 1988

Claire RJ, Servis ME, Cram DL Jr: Potential interaction between warfarin sodium and fluoxetine (letter). Am J Psychiatry 148:1604, 1991

Cohen BJ, Mahelsky M, Adler L: More cases of SIADH with fluoxetine (letter). Am J Psychiatry 147:948–949, 1990

Cohen WJ, Cohen NH: Lithium carbonate, haloperidol and irreversible brain damage. JAMA 230:1283–1287, 1974

Coulam CB, Annegers JF: Do anticonvulsants reduce the efficacy of oral contraceptives? Epilepsia 20:519–525, 1979

Crawford P, Chadwick DJ, Martin C, et al: The interaction of phenytoin and carbamazepine with combined oral contraceptive steroids. Br J Clin Pharmacol 30:892–896, 1990

Crews JR, Potts NL, Schreiber J, et al: Hyponatremia in a patients treated with sertraline (letter). Am J Psychiatry 150:1564, 1993

Crixivan® [indinavir] Product Information. West Point, PA, Merck, 1996

Dalton MJ, Powell JR, Messenheimer JA: The influence of cimetidine on single-dose carbamazepine pharmacokinetics. Epilepsia 26:127–130, 1985

Dalton MJ, Powell JR, Messenheimer JA, et al: Cimetidine and carbamazepine: a complex drug interaction. Epilepsia 27:533–538, 1986

Dam M, Kristensen CB, Hansen BS, et al: Interaction between carbamazepine and propoxyphene in man. Acta Neurol Scand 56:603–607, 1977

DeVane CL: Pharmacokinetics of newer antidepressants. Am J Med 97 (suppl 6A):13S–23S, 1994

Douste-Blazy P, Roustin M, Livarek B, et al: Angiotensin converting enzyme inhibitors and lithium treatment (letter). Lancet 1:1488, 1986

Dundee JW, Halliday NJ, McMurray TJ: Aspirin and probenecid pretreatment influences the potency of thiopentone and the onset of action of midazolam. Eur J Anaesthesiol 3:247–251, 1986

Edwards DJ, Lavoie R, Beckman H, et al: The effect of coadministration of verapamil on the pharmacokinetics and metabolism of quinidine. Clin Pharmacol Ther 41:68–73, 1987

Ellingrod VL, Perry PJ: Venlafaxine: a heterocyclic antidepressant. Am J Hosp Pharm 51:3033–3046, 1994

Ellingrod VL, Perry PJ: Nefazodone: a new antidepressant or another "me too" drug? American Journal of Health-System Pharmacy 52:2799–2812, 1995

Ellinwood EH: Amphetamine psychosis, I: description of the individual and the process. J Nerv Ment Dis 144:273–283, 1967

Epstein SE, Rosing DR: Verapamil: its potential for causing serious complications in patients with hypertrophic cardiomyopathy. Circulation 64:437–441, 1981

Ereshefsky L, Riesenman C, Lam YF: Serotonin selective reuptake inhibitor drug interactions and the cytochrome P450 system. J Clin Psychiatry 57:17–25, 1996

Evans M, Marwick P: Fluvoxamine and lithium: an unusual interaction (letter). Br J Psychiatry 156:286, 1990

Evans-Prosser CDG: The use of pethidine and morphine in the presence of MAO inhibitors. British Journal of Anaesthesia 40:279–282, 1968

Farrell K, Orr JM, Abbott FS, et al: The effect of acetylsalicylic acid on serum free valproate concentrations and valproate clearance in children. J Pediatr 101:142–144, 1982

Fast DK, Jones BD, Kusalic M, et al: Effect of carbamazepine on neuroleptic plasma levels and efficacy (letter). Am J Psychiatry 143:117–118, 1986

Feder R: Reversal of antidepressant activity of fluoxetine by cyproheptadine in three patients. J Clin Psychiatry 52:163–164, 1991

Fluvoxamine, in Physicians' Desk Reference, 50th Edition. Montvale, NJ, Medical Economics Data Production, 1996, pp 2544–2548

Gelenberg A: The P450 family. Biological Therapies in Psychiatry 18:29–31, 1995

Ghose K: Assessment of peripheral adrenergic activity and its interaction with drugs in man. Eur J Clin Pharmacol 17:233–238, 1980

Goff DC, Midha KK, Brotman AW, et al: Elevation of plasma concentrations of haloperidol after the addition of fluoxetine. Am J Psychiatry 148:790–792, 1991a

Goff DC, Midha KK, Brotman AW, et al: An open trial of buspirone added to neuroleptics in schizophrenic patients. J Clin Psychopharmacol 11:193–197, 1991b

Goldney RD, Spence ND: Safety of the combination of lithium and neuroleptic drugs. Am J Psychiatry 143:882–884, 1986

Gonzalez FJ, Idle JR: Pharmacogenetic phenotyping and genotyping: present status and future potential. Clin Pharmacokinet 26:59–70, 1994

Goulden KJ, Dooley JM, Camfield PR, et al: Clinical valproate toxicity induced by acetylsalicylic acid. Neurology 37:1392–1394, 1987

Graber MA, Hoehns TB, Perry PJ: Sertraline-phenelzine drug interaction: a serotonin syndrome reaction. Ann Pharmacother 28:732–735, 1994

Greenblatt DJ, Abernethy DR, Divoll M, et al: Old age, cimetidine, and disposition of alprazolam and triazolam (abstract). Clin Pharmacol Ther 33:253, 1983

Greenblatt DJ, von Moltke LL, Harmatz JS, et al: Interaction of triazolam and ketoconazole (letter). Lancet 345:191, 1995

Hansen BS, Dam M, Brandt J, et al: Influence of dextropropoxyphene on steady state serum levels and protein binding of three antiepileptic drugs in man. Acta Neurol Scand 61:357–367, 1980

Hansen JM, Siersboek-Nielsen K, Skovsted L: Carbamazepine-induced acceleration of diphenylhydantoin and warfarin metabolism in man. Clin Pharmacol Ther 12:539–543, 1971

Hansten PD, Horn JR: Drug Interactions and Updates. Malvern, PA, Lea & Febiger, 1995

Harvey AT, Preskorn SH: Cytochrome P450 enzymes: interpretation of their interactions with selective serotonin reuptake inhibitors, part I. J Clin Psychopharmacol 16:273–285, 1996a

Harvey AT, Preskorn SH: Cytochrome P450 enzymes: interpretation of their interaction with selective serotonin reuptake inhibitors, part II. J Clin Psychopharmacol 16:345–355, 1996b

Haukkamaa M: Contraception by Norplant subdermal capsules is not reliable in epileptic patients on anticonvulsant treatment. Contraception 33:559–565, 1986

Heinonen EH, Lammintausta R: A review of the pharmacology of selegiline. Acta Neurol Scand Suppl 136:44–59, 1991

Henriksen O, Johannessen SI: Clinical and pharmacokinetic observations on sodium valproate: 5-year follow-up study in 100 children with epilepsy. Acta Neurol Scand 65:504–523, 1982

Hermann DJ, Krol TF, Dukes GE, et al: Comparison of verapamil, diltiazem, and labetalol on the bioavailability and metabolism of imipramine. J Clin Pharmacol 32:176–183, 1992

Holstad SG, Perry PJ, Kathol RG, et al: The effect of intravenous theophylline infusion versus intravenous sodium bicarbonate infusion on lithium clearance in normal subjects. Psychiatry Res 25:203–211, 1988

Hunter KR, Boakes AJ, Laurence ER: Monoamine oxidase inhibitors and L-dopa. BMJ 3:388, 1970

Hwang AS, Magraw RM: Syndrome of inappropriate secretion of antidiuretic hormone due to fluoxetine (letter). Am J Psychiatry 146:399, 1989

Ishaid Y, Branch RA, Adedoyin A: Metabolic interactions of putative cytochrome P4503A substrates with alternative pathways of dapsone metabolism in human liver microsomes. Drug Metab Dispos 24:164–171, 1996

Janowsky DS, El-Yousef MK, Davis JM, et al: Antagonism of guanethidine by chlorpromazine. Am J Psychiatry 130:808–812, 1973

Janowsky DS, El-Yousef MK, Davis JM, et al: Provocation of schizophrenic symptoms by intravenous administration of methylphenidate. Arch Gen Psychiatry 28:185–191, 1974

Jefferson JW: Serum lithium levels and long-term diuretic use. JAMA 241:1134–1136, 1979

Joffe RT, Gold PW, Uhde TW, et al: The effects of carbamazepine on the thyrotropin response to thyrotropin-releasing hormone. Psychiatry Res 12:161–166, 1984

Jones RM, Cashman JN, Casson WR, et al: Verapamil potentiation of neuromuscular blockade: failure of reversal with neostigmine but prompt reversal with edrophonium. Anesthesia and Analgesia 64:1021–1025, 1985

Juhl RP, Tsuang MT, Perry PJ: Concomitant administration of haloperidol and lithium in acute mania. Diseases of the Nervous System 38:675–680, 1977

Junghan U, Albers M, Woggon B: Increased risk of hematological side effects in psychiatric patients treated with clozapine and carbamazepine? (letter). Pharmacopsychiatry 26:262, 1993

Kanter GL, Yerevanian BI, Ciccone JR: Case report of a possible interaction between neuroleptics and carbamazepine. Am J Psychiatry 141:1101–1102, 1984

Kendall AG, Boivin M: Warfarin-carbamazepine interaction (letter). Ann Intern Med 94:280, 1981

Ketter TA, Jenkins JB, Schroeder DH, et al: Carbamazepine but not valproate induces bupropion metabolism. J Clin Psychopharmacol 15:327–333, 1995

Kharasch ED, Jenkins JB, Mhyre J, et al: Single-dose disulfiram inhibition of chlorzoxazone metabolism: a clinical probe for P450 2E1. Clin Pharmacol Ther 53:643–650, 1993

Kitson TM: The disulfiram–ethanol reaction: a review. J Stud Alcohol 38:96–113, 1977

Klein HO, Lang R, Weiss E, et al: The influence of verapamil on serum digoxin concentration. Circulation 65:988–1003, 1982

Klotz U, Reimann I: Elevation of steady-state diazepam levels by cimetidine. Clin Pharmacol Ther 30:513–517, 1981

Klotz U, Reimann IW, Ohnhaus EE: Effect of ranitidine on the steady state pharmacokinetics of diazepam. Eur J Clin Pharmacol 24:357–360, 1983

Kramer G, Theisohn M, von Unruh GE, et al: Carbamazepine-danazol drug interaction: its mechanism examined by a stable isotope technique. Ther Drug Monit 8:387–392, 1986

Kramlinger KG, Post RM: Addition of lithium carbonate to carbamazepine: hematological and thyroid effects. Am J Psychiatry 147:615–620, 1990

Kuhlmann J, Marcin S: Effects of verapamil on pharmacokinetics and pharmacodynamics of digitoxin in patients. Am Heart J 110:1245–1250, 1985

Lesser I: Carbamazepine and desipramine: a toxic reaction (letter). J Clin Psychiatry 45:360, 1984

Lindholm A, Henricsson S: Verapamil inhibits cyclosporin metabolism (letter). Lancet 1:1262–1263, 1987

Linnoila M, Hakkinen S: Effects of diazepam and codeine, alone and in combination with alcohol on simulated driving. Clin Pharmacol Ther 15:368–373, 1974

Linnoila M, Viukari M, Vaisanen K, et al: Effect of anticonvulsants on plasma haloperidol and thioridazine levels. Am J Psychiatry 137:819–821, 1980

Linnoila M, Stapleton JM, Lister R, et al: Effects of adinazolam and diazepam, alone and in combination with ethanol on psychomotor and cognitive performance and on the autonomic nervous system reactivity in healthy volunteers. Eur J Clin Pharmacol 38:371–377, 1990

Loga S, Curry S, Lader M: Interactions of orphenadrine and phenobarbitone with chlorpromazine: plasma concentrations and effects in man. Br J Clin Pharmacol 2:197–208, 1975

Loi CM, Day JD, Jue SG, et al: Dose dependent inhibition of theophylline metabolism by disulfiram in recovering alcoholics. Clin Pharmacol Ther 45:476–486, 1989

Loudon JB, Waring H: Toxic reactions to lithium and haloperidol (letter). Lancet 2:1088, 1976

Luder PJ, Siffert B, Witassek F, et al: Treatment of hydatid disease with high oral doses of mebendazole: long-term follow-up of plasma mebendazole levels and drug interactions. Eur J Clin Pharmacol 31:443–448, 1986

MacLeod SM, Sellers EM, Giles HG, et al: Interaction of disulfiram with benzodiazepines. Clin Pharmacol Ther 24:583–589, 1978

MacPhee GJ, Mitchell JR, Wiseman L, et al: Effect of sodium valproate on carbamazepine disposition and psychomotor profile in man. Br J Clin Pharmacol 25:59–66, 1988

Maggio TG, Bartels DW: Increased cyclosporine blood concentrations due to verapamil administration. Drug Intelligence and Clinical Pharmacy 22:705–707, 1988

Massey EW: Effect of carbamazepine on Coumadin metabolism (letter). Ann Neurol 13:691–692, 1983

McLean AJ, Knight R, Harrison PM, et al: Clearance-based oral drug interaction between verapamil and metoprolol and comparison with atenolol. Am J Cardiol 55:1628–1629, 1985

Mesdjian E, Dravet C, Cenraud B, et al: Carbamazepine intoxication due to triacetyloleandomycin administration in epileptic patients. Epilepsia 21:489–496, 1980

Miller DD: Effect of phenytoin on plasma clozapine concentrations in two patients. J Clin Psychiatry 52:23–25, 1991

Miller DD, Macklin M: Cimetidine–imipramine interaction: a case report. Am J Psychiatry 140:351–352, 1983

Miller RR, Greenblatt DJ: Hypnotics, in Drug Effects in Hospitalized Patients. Edited by Miller RR, Greenblatt DJ. New York, Wiley, 1976, pp 171–191

Mitchell EA, Dower JC, Green RJ: Interaction between carbamazepine and theophylline (letter). N Z Med J 1:69–70, 1986

Mitchell JR, Arias L, Oates JA: Antagonism of the antihypertensive action of guanethidine sulfate by desipramine hydrochloride. JAMA 202:973–976, 1967

Monks A, Richens A: Effect of single doses of sodium valproate on serum phenytoin levels and protein binding in epileptic patients. Clin Pharmacol Ther 27:89–95, 1980

Moss LE, Neppe VM, Drevets WC: Buspirone in the treatment of tardive dyskinesia. J Clin Psychopharmacol 13:204–209, 1993

Navis GT, deJong PD, deZeeuw D: Volume homeostasis, angiotensin-converting enzyme inhibition and lithium therapy. Am J Med 86:621, 1989

Neuvonen PJ, Penttila O, Lehtovaara R: Effect of antiepileptic drugs on the elimination of various tetracycline derivatives. Eur J Clin Pharmacol 9:147–154, 1975

Norvir® [ritonavir] Product Information. Chicago, IL, Abbott Laboratories, 1996

Ochs HR, Greenblatt AJ, Roberts GM, et al: Diazepam interaction with antituberculosis drugs. Clin Pharmacol Ther 29:671–678, 1981

Olivesi A: Modified elimination of prednisolone in epileptic patients on carbamazepine monotherapy and in women using low dose contraceptives. Biomed Pharmacother 40:301–308, 1986

Olkkola KT, Aranko K, Luurila H, et al: A potentially hazardous interaction between erythromycin and midazolam. Clin Pharmacol Ther 53:298–305, 1993

Olkkola KT, Backman JT, Neuvonen PJ: Midazolam should be avoided in patients receiving the systemic antimycotics ketoconazole or itraconazole. Clin Pharmacol Therap 55:481–485, 1994

O'Reilly RA: Dynamic interaction between disulfiram and separated enantiomorphs of racemic warfarin. Clin Pharmacol Ther 29:232–236, 1981

Orr JM, Abbott FS, Farrell K, et al: Interaction between valproic acid and aspirin in epileptic children: serum protein binding and metabolic effects. Clin Pharmacol Ther 31:642–649, 1982

Osanloo E, Deglin JH: Interaction of lithium and methyldopa. Ann Intern Med 92:433–434, 1980

Palm R, Silseth C, Alvan G: Phenytoin intoxication as the first symptom of fatal liver damage induced by sodium valproate. Br J Clin Pharmacol 17:597–599, 1984

Pedersen KE, Dorph-Pedersen A, Hvidt S, et al: Digoxin-verapamil interaction. Clin Pharmacol Ther 30:311–316, 1981

Peet M, Middlemiss DN, Yates RA: Propranolol in schizophrenia, II: clinical and biochemical aspects of combining propranolol with chlorpromazine. Br J Psychiatry 139:112–117, 1981

Penttila O, Neuvonen PJ, Aho K, et al: Interaction between doxycycline and some antiepileptic drugs. BMJ 2:470–472, 1974

Perkins CM: Serious verapamil poisoning: treatment with intravenous calcium gluconate. BMJ 2:1127, 1978

Perry PJ, Calloway RA, Cook BL, et al: Theophylline precipitated alterations in lithium clearance. Acta Psychiatr Scand 69:528–537, 1984

Phillips JP, Antal EJ, Smith RB: A pharmacokinetic drug interaction between erythromycin and triazolam. J Clin Psychopharmacol 6:297–299, 1986

Pond SM, Graham GG, Birkett DJ, et al: Effects of tricyclic antidepressants on drug metabolism. Clin Pharmacol Ther 18:191–199, 1975

Ponto LB, Perry PJ, Liskow BI, et al: Tricyclic antidepressant and monoamine oxidase inhibitor combination therapy. Am J Hosp Pharm 34:954–961, 1977

Postma JU, Van Tilburg W: Visual hallucinations and delirium during treatment with amantadine. J Am Geriatr Soc 23:212–215, 1975

Prakash R, Kelwala S, Ban TA: Neurotoxicity with combined administration of lithium and a neuroleptic. Compr Psychiatry 23:567–571, 1982

Prakash R, Reed RM, Bass AD: Combination of phenobarbital and haloperidol in resistant schizophrenia. J Clin Psychopharmacol 4:362–363, 1984

Preskorn SH, Alderman J, Chung M, et al: Pharmacokinetics of desipramine coadministered with sertraline or fluoxetine. J Clin Psychopharmacol 14:90–98, 1994

Price WA, Shalley JE: Lithium-verapamil atoxicity in the elderly (letter). J Am Geriatr Soc 35:177–178, 1987

Privitera M, Greden JF, Gardner RW, et al: Interference by carbamazepine with the dexamethasone suppression test. Biol Psychiatry 17:611–620, 1982

Raitasuo V, Lehtovaara R, Huttunen MO: Carbamazepine and plasma levels of clozapine (letter). Am J Psychiatry 150:169, 1993

Rambeck B, Salke-Treumann A, May T, et al: Valproic acid induced carbamazepine-10-11-epoxide toxicity in children and adolescents. Eur Neurol 30:79–83, 1990

Reiman IW, Diener U, Frolich JC: Indomethacin but not aspirin increases plasma lithium ion levels. Arch Gen Psychiatry 40:283–286, 1983

Riesenman C: Antidepressant drug interactions and the cytochrome P450 system: a critical appraisal. Pharmacotherapy 15:84S–99S, 1995

Rivera-Calimlin L, Nasrallah H, Strauss J, et al: Clinical response plasma levels: effects of dose, dosage schedules, and drug interactions on plasma chlorpromazine levels. Am J Psychiatry 133:646–652, 1976

Robbins RJ, Kern PA, Thompson TL: Interactions between thioridazine and bromocriptine in a patient with a prolactin-secreting pituitary adenoma. Am J Med 76:921–923, 1984

Robson RA, Miners JO, Birkett DJ: Selective inhibitory effects of nifedipine and verapamil on oxidative metabolism: effect on theophylline. Br J Clin Pharmacol 25:397–400, 1988

Rosenberry KR, Defusco CJ, Mansmann HC, et al: Reduced theophylline half-life induced by carbamazepine therapy. J Pediatr 102:472–474, 1983

Roth S, Ebrahim ZY: Resistance to pancuronium in patients receiving carbamazepine. Anesthesiology 66:691–693, 1987

Rothstein E, Clancy DD: Toxicity of disulfiram combined with metronidazole. N Engl J Med 280:1006–1007, 1969

Rowe H, Carmichael R, Lemberger L: The effect of fluoxetine on warfarin metabolism in the rat and man. Life Sci 23:808–811, 1978

Rutledge DR, Pieper JA, Mirvis DM: Effects of chronic phenobarbital on verapamil disposition in humans. J Pharmacol Exp Ther 246:7–13, 1988

Salama AA, Shafey M: A case of severe lithium toxicity induced by combined fluoxetine and lithium carbonate (letter). Am J Psychiatry 146:278, 1989

Sandyk R, Hurwitz MD: Toxic irreversible encephalopathy induced by lithium carbonate and haloperidol: a report of two cases. S Afr Med J 64:875–876, 1983

Sassim N, Grohmann R: Adverse drug reactions with clozapine and simultaneous application of benzodiazepines. Pharmacopsychiatry 21:306–307, 1988

Schwab RS, England AC, Poskanzer DC, et al: Amantadine in the treatment of Parkinson's disease. JAMA 208:1168–1170, 1969

Schwartz JB, Keefe D, Kates RE, et al: Acute and chronic pharmacodynamic interaction of verapamil and digoxin in atrial fibrillation. Circulation 65:1163–1170, 1982

Sellers EM, Carr G, Bernstein JG, et al: Interaction of chloral hydrate and ethanol in man, II: hemodynamics and performance. Clin Pharmacol Ther 13:50–58, 1972

Serzone® [nefazodone] Product Information. Princeton, NJ, Bristol-Meyers Squibb, 1995

Shneerson JM: Acute lithium intoxication. Br J Clin Pract 32:232, 1978

Shulka S, Godwin CD, Long LE, et al: Lithium-carbamazepine neurotoxicity and risk factors. Am J Psychiatry 141:1604–1606, 1984

Singh MM, Kay SR: Therapeutic antagonism between anticholinergic antiparkinsonian agents and neuroleptics in schizophrenia: implications for a neuropharmacological model. Neuropsychobiology 5:74–86, 1979

Sirmans SM, Pieper JA, Lalonde RL, et al: Effect of calcium channel blockers on theophylline disposition. Clin Pharmacol Ther 44:29–34, 1988

Slaughter RL, Edwards DJ: Recent advances: the cytochrome P450 enzymes. Ann Pharmacother 29:619–624, 1995

Sletten IW, Lang WJ, Brown ML, et al: Chronic chlorpromazine administration: some pharmacological and psychological effects in man. Clin Pharmacol Ther 6:575–586, 1965

Sovner R, Wolfe J: Interaction between dextromethorphan and monoamine oxidase inhibitor therapy with isocarboxazid (letter). N Engl J Med 319:1671, 1988

Spaulding SW, Burrow EN, Ramey JN, et al: Effect of increased iodine intake on thyroid function in subjects on chronic lithium therapy. Acta Endocrinol 84:290–296, 1977

Spina E, DeDomenico P, Ruello C, et al: Adjunctive fluoxetine in the treatment of negative symptoms in chronic schizophrenic patients. International Clinical Psychopharmacology 9:281–285, 1994

Stambaugh JE, Wainer IW: Drug interaction: meperidine and chlorpromazine, a toxic combination. J Clin Pharmacol 21:140–146, 1981

Steiner E, Dumont E, Spina E, et al: Inhibition of desipramine 2-hydroxylation by quinidine and quinine. Clin Pharmacol Ther 43:577–581, 1988

Steiner W, Fontaine R: Toxic reaction following the combined administration of fluoxetine and L-tryptophan: five case reports. Biol Psychiatry 21:1067–1071, 1986

Stellamans G: A study to investigate efficacy, adverse events, safety, and pharmacokinetic effects of co-administration of paroxetine and lithium (abstract). Biol Psychiatry 29:628S, 1991

Szymanski S, Lieberman JA, Picou D, et al: A case report of cimetidine-induced clozapine toxicity. J Clin Psychiatry 52:21–22, 1991

Tate JL: Extrapyramidal symptoms in a patient taking haloperidol and fluoxetine (letter). Am J Psychiatry 146:399–400, 1989

Tatro DS: Drug Interaction Facts. St. Louis, MO, Facts & Comparisons, 1996

Taylor JW, Alexander B, Lyon LW: Mathematical analysis of phenytoin-disulfiram interaction. Am J Hosp Pharm 38:93–95, 1981

Teychenne PF, Calne DB, Lewis PJ, et al: Interactions of levodopa with inhibitors of monoamine oxidase and L-aromatic amino acid decarboxylase. Clin Pharmacol Ther 18:273–277, 1975

Thomsen K, Schou M: Renal lithium excretion in man. Am J Physiol 215:823–827, 1968

Trohman RG, Estes DM, Castellanos A, et al: Increased quinidine plasma concentrations during administration of verapamil: a new quinidine-verapamil interaction. Am J Cardiol 57:706–707, 1986

Tsanaclis LM, Allen J, Perucca E, et al: Effect of valproate on free plasma phenytoin concentrations. Br J Clin Pharmacol 18:17–20, 1984

Udall JA: Clinical implications of warfarin interaction with five sedatives. Am J Cardiol 35:67–71, 1975

Valsalan VC, Cooper G: Carbamazepine intoxication caused by interaction with isoniazid. BMJ 285:261–262, 1982

Van den Brekel, Harrington L: Toxic effects of theophylline caused by fluvoxamine. Can Med Assoc J 151:1289–1290, 1994

Varhe A, Olkkola KT, Neuvonen PJ: Oral triazolam is potentially hazardous to patients receiving systemic antimycotics ketoconazole or itraconazole. Clin Pharmacol Therap 56 (6 part 1):601–607, 1994

Vaughan DA: Interaction of fluoxetine with tricyclic antidepressants (letter). Am J Psychiatry 145:1478, 1988

Vestal RE, Kornhauser DM, Hollifield JW, et al: Inhibition of propranolol metabolism by chlorpromazine. Clin Pharmacol Ther 25:19–24, 1979

Warot D, Bergougnan L, Lamiable D, et al: Troleoandomycin-triazolam interaction in healthy volunteers: pharmacokinetic and psychometric evaluation. Eur J Clin Pharmacol 32:389–393, 1987

Webster LK, Mihaly GW, Jones DB, et al: Effect of cimetidine and ranitidine on carbamazepine and sodium valproate pharmacokinetics. Eur J Clin Pharmacol 27:341–343, 1984

Weinrauch LA, Belok S, Delia JA: Decreased serum lithium during verapamil therapy. Am Heart J 108:1378–1380, 1984

West AP: Interaction of low-dose amphetamine use with schizophrenia in outpatients: three case reports. Am J Psychiatry 131:321–322, 1974

Whittington HG, Grey L: Possible interaction between disulfiram and isoniazid. Am J Psychiatry 125:1725–1729, 1969

Wilder BJ, Willmore LJ, Bruni J, et al: Valproic acid: interaction with other anticonvulsant drugs. Neurology 28:892–896, 1978

Wilner KD: The effects of sertraline on the pharmacodynamics of warfarin in healthy volunteers (abstract). Biol Psychiatry 29:345S, 1991

Wong LK: A study of drug interaction by gas chromatography mass spectrometry synergism of chloral hydrate and alcohol. Biochem Pharmacol 27:1019–1022, 1978

Wong YY, Ludden TM, Bell RD: Effect of erythromycin on carbamazepine kinetics. Clin Pharmacol Ther 33:460–464, 1983

Wright JM, Stokes EF, Sweeney VP: Isoniazid-induced carbamazepine toxicity and vice versa: a double drug interaction. N Engl J Med 307:1325–1327, 1982

Wrighton SA, Stevens JC: The human hepatic cytochromes P450 involved in drug metabolism. Crit Rev Toxicol 22:1–21, 1992

Yaryura-Tobias JA, Wolpert A, Dana L, et al: Action of L-dopa in drug-induced extrapyramidalism. Diseases of the Nervous System 31:60–63, 1970

Yee GC, McGuire TR: Pharmacokinetic drug interactions with cyclosporin, part I. Clin Pharmacokinet 19:319–332, 1990

Yerevanian BI, Hodgman CH: A haloperidol-carbamazepine interaction in a patient with rapid-cycling bipolar disorder (letter). Am J Psychiatry 142:785–786, 1985

Zielinski JJ, Lichten EM, Haidukewych D: Clinically significant danazol-carbamazepine interaction. Ther Drug Monit 9:24–27, 1987

Zornberg GL, Bodkin JA, Cohen BM: Severe adverse interaction between pethidine and selegiline (letter). Lancet 337:246, 1991

9

Management and Treatment of Drug Overdose

Many factors affect clinical course after an overdose. In addition to the specific toxicity of a drug, its pharmacokinetic properties may enhance or ameliorate this toxicity. For example, an overdose of a drug may result in delayed absorption of the drug due to formation of an insoluble mass and/or decreased gastric motility. The decrease in motility, despite delaying absorption, may increase the amount of drug absorbed. A drug that normally is rapidly metabolized by the liver may, when taken in overdose amounts, saturate the hepatic enzyme system responsible for its breakdown, causing a higher percentage of the drug to reach the systemic circulation. In a similar fashion, a drug that normally is strongly plasma protein bound may, in overdose, saturate the protein binding sites, thereby increasing the percentage of unbound drug and hence the drug's clinical effects. A drug and/or its active metabolites may be excreted in the bile and be reabsorbed, thus leading to cyclic increases and decreases in blood levels and clinical effects (Jarvis 1991; Rosenberg et al. 1981; Rumack et al. 1996).

In addition, cardiovascular and pulmonary status, acid-base balance, renal and hepatic functions, and temperature regulation may all affect clinical course after an overdose as well as be affected by the specific drugs used in the overdose. Despite these complex reciprocal interactions among drug toxicity, pharmacological activity, and physiological condition, there are several basic procedures common to the management of almost all overdose situations. These are discussed in the following section.

Basic Procedures

1. **Support respiration.** If the patient is not breathing adequately, oxygenate and maintain an adequate tidal volume and, if necessary, intubate or create an artificial airway (Boehnert et al. 1985; Flomenbaum et al. 1994; Nicholson 1983; Rumack et al. 1996).

2. **Establish intravenous access.** Begin an iv line with dextrose 5% in water after drawing blood for complete blood count (CBC), blood urea nitrogen (BUN), electrolytes, and toxicology tests. Obtain arterial blood gases if necessary. If the patient is hypotensive and lungs are clear, place the patient in the Trendelenburg position and give lactated Ringer's solution or normal saline (Flomenbaum et al. 1994).

3. **Administer naloxone.** This will help reverse opiate overdose and will not harm (and may help) patients whose coma is from other causes (Badawy and Evans 1983; Jordan et al. 1980; Kulig and Rumack 1983). An initial dose of 2 mg iv is preferred by some authorities (Flomenbaum et al. 1994) to the usual recommendation of 0.4–0.8 mg because the larger dose causes no harm and will more effectively reverse intoxication with opiates such as codeine and propoxyphene.

4. **Administer glucose and thiamine.** Fifty to 100 mL of 50% glucose will reverse hypoglycemia-induced coma (e.g., due to insulin overdose) and will not harm patients comatose from other causes. Thiamine 100 mg iv should be given in advance of or concurrently with glucose to prevent glucose, which requires thiamine for its metabolism, from inducing Wernicke's syndrome in a predisposed patient. Such patients are usually alcoholic with low thiamine reserves. Wernicke's is caused by thiamine deficiency and can occur acutely when thiamine reserves are depleted by the administration of glucose (Flomenbaum et al. 1994; R. S. Hoffman and Goldfrank 1995; Nicholson 1983; Rumack et al. 1996).

5. **Conduct a brief physical and obtain an electrocardiogram (ECG).** Results from these will establish the need to investigate other medical problems that may require immediate attention in treating a patient who has overdosed (Flomenbaum et al. 1994).

6. **Empty the stomach.** It is best to begin doing this within 4 hours of a significant oral overdose, the sooner the better. Emptying the stomach is accomplished with ipecac syrup in the conscious patient and with gastric lavage in the patient who is not alert. Ipecac induces vomiting by stimulating both peripheral sensory receptors in the gastrointestinal (GI) tract and the chemoreceptor trigger zone in the central nervous system (CNS) (Howland 1994a). Because ipecac has cardiovascular (ECG irregularities), GI (persistent vomiting and diarrhea), and neuromuscular (tremor, seizures) toxicity of its own (Manno and Manno 1977), it is recommended that only 30 mL of

the syrup be given and that this dosage be repeated only once if emesis does not occur within 30 to 60 minutes. The onset of vomiting is not affected by administration of water before or after administration of ipecac and is likewise unaffected by the temperature of the fluid or by movement (e.g., walking) on the part of the patient (Howland 1994a). Milk, on the other hand, does delay the emetic response and should not be given after ipecac (Varipapa and Oderda 1977).

Some authorities advise that activated charcoal should not be given until emesis occurs, as it adsorbs the ipecac and delays the emetic response. However, one study found that no reduction in emetic response occurred when activated charcoal was given 10 minutes after ipecac and before emesis (Freeman et al. 1987). In this study, a second dose of activated charcoal was also administered after emesis. Another study—a prospective, randomized clinical trial in 200 patients with acute toxic ingestions—compared activated charcoal alone with ipecac plus activated charcoal (Albertson et al. 1989). This investigation concluded that in mild to moderate overdoses, activated charcoal alone was preferable to charcoal plus ipecac because the former resulted in a significantly lower complication rate, and because hospitalization rate and amount of time spent in the hospital did not differ for the two treatments. This study and others have led to less routine use of ipecac in the conscious overdose patient in the emergency room (Howland 1994a). However, ipecac is still recommended as a home first-aid treatment for poisoning, with the caveat that it be used only at the advice of a physician or poison control center (Howland 1994a).

Emesis from ipecac usually occurs two to three times over a 30- to 60-minute period. A normal diet, if not contraindicated by the overdose, may be resumed 1 hour after the last emesis (King 1980). Ipecac should not be used in a comatose patient or in one who has lost the gag reflex; its use is also contraindicated after ingestion of acids, alkalies, and petroleum distillates. In an overdose involving a rapidly acting CNS depressant or convulsant, ipecac is relatively contraindicated because of the possibility that a quickly developing coma and/or a seizure will lead to aspiration during subsequent emesis (Boehnert et al. 1985). Ipecac is also contraindicated in patients with esophageal varices and/or decreased platelets and in patients who have ingested sharp objects such as glass or razor blades (Flomenbaum et al. 1994).

Although probably not as effective in emptying the stomach as emesis induced by ipecac (Boehnert et al. 1985), gastric lavage with a large-bore nasogastric tube (French size of 36'40)—with the patient intubated (with endotracheal cuff inflated) and positioned on the left side, in head-down position—should be used in comatose patients. After determining that the tip of the tube is in the stomach, 150–200 mL of water or saline solution is instilled and then drained by gravity or by suction using a large-bore syringe. This process should be repeated until 1–2 liters of fluid have been instilled and drained or until no particulate matter is seen and the drained fluid is clear. Lavage is not recommended in the awake patient, and clinicians should be aware that some researchers feel that lavage has been both overused and inappropriately used as a punitive measure (Blake et al. 1978; Flomenbaum et al. 1994; Matthew 1971; Nicholson 1983). The conclusion that lavage and gastric emptying are overused has been strengthened by a recent randomized study that compared the use of gastric emptying (via ipecac or lavage) plus activated charcoal with activated charcoal alone in 876 overdose patients. No difference in outcome between the two treatments was found, even when patients were stratified by severity of overdose or time of presentation to the emergency room after the overdose (Pond et al. 1995). The authors concluded that gastric emptying could be safely omitted as a treatment in adults after acute overdoses.

7. **Administer activated charcoal.** Fifty to 100 g can be given as a 20%–25% suspension (20–25 g/100 mL of saline or sorbitol cathartics, or water) by mouth or through a nasogastric tube (the tube used for lavage may be used for this purpose). Charcoal is nontoxic, adsorbs a wide range of drugs, and is indicated in all overdoses except alcohol, lithium, and iron (Howland 1994b). Its efficacy in overdoses involving heavy metals or aliphatic hydrocarbons is controversial (Howland 1994b; Smilkstein and Flomenbaum 1994). Efficacy is inversely related to the amount of time elapsed between ingestion of the overdose and charcoal and is directly related to the amount of charcoal given. Hence, the sooner after an overdose charcoal is given the better, although it may be effective up to 24 hours after an overdose of anticholinergics, sustained-release formulations, or enteric-coated products. Activated charcoal may be given after vomiting induced by ipecac, shortly after giving ipecac (it does not appear to prevent vomiting [Badawy and Evans 1983]),

after gastric lavage, or as the only intervention when removal of stomach contents is either of no value or unnecessary (Howland 1994b). Some drugs and/or their metabolites are excreted into the GI tract in gastric fluid (e.g., phencyclidine [PCP]) or bile (e.g., tricyclics), and it has been suggested that activated charcoal be administered q4h in such situations until blood levels of the drug return to normal (Kulig 1986). Activated charcoal also appears to attract certain drugs (e.g., theophylline, phenobarbital) out of the bloodstream and into the gastrointestinal tract (a process termed **GI** *dialysis*) and thus can rapidly lower blood levels of the drug when the charcoal is instilled into the GI tract (Berg et al. 1982; Berlinger et al. 1983; Goldberg and Berlinger 1982; Neuvonen and Elonen 1980; Smilkstein and Flomenbaum 1994). In general, drugs used in overdose that have a small volume of distribution (e.g., are not very fat soluble), low intrinsic clearance, and low plasma protein binding, and that are secreted into the stomach or by the biliary system, should respond to repeated doses of activated charcoal (Chyka 1995). When such drugs have been ingested, activated charcoal should be given every 1–6 hours until blood levels of the drug are within normal limits (Howland 1994b). Some authors have suggested that the total dose of activated charcoal is more important than the frequency of administration and have proposed an activated charcoal–to–drug ratio of 10 to 1 (Howland 1994b; Smilkstein and Flomenbaum 1994; Vale and Proudfoot 1993).

8. **Administer cathartics.** These agents are usually coadministered with activated charcoal and are given to increase the speed of elimination of the toxin. Although cathartics are widely recommended, their benefit has not been clearly established (Chin et al. 1981; Easom et al. 1982; Stewart 1983). Contraindications to their use include adynamic ileus, severe diarrhea, abdominal trauma, intestinal obstruction, and, in the case of saline and magnesium cathartics, renal failure (Flomenbaum et al. 1994; Rumack et al. 1996). The usual dose is 30 g of sodium or magnesium sulfate in 250 mL of water or 75 g of sorbitol as a 35%–70% solution. Some authorities believe that sodium sulfate and sodium phosphate (also used as a cathartic) have limited use, because these agents offer no advantages over magnesium sulfate or sorbitol and are associated with a higher incidence of serious fluid and electrolyte disturbances (Smilkstein and Flomenbaum 1994). Reports that magnesium salts used with multiple doses of activated charcoal have resulted in

magnesium toxicity have led some investigators to suggest that sorbitol be preferred over magnesium cathartics (Garrelts et al. 1989). However, severe fluid and electrolyte problems have been related to multiple doses of sorbitol (Farley 1986). It has therefore been suggested that if multiple doses of activated charcoal are given, the coadministration of cathartics should occur only with the first dose of charcoal or only until the first charcoal stool appears (Flomenbaum et al. 1994; Picchioni et al. 1982; Rumack et al. 1996; Smilkstein and Flomenbaum 1994). However, the need for even this use of cathartics is questionable, given the studies that have demonstrated that activated charcoal produces the same therapeutic outcome regardless of whether it is used alone or in combination with a single dose of sorbitol or magnesium sulfate (Howland 1994c; McNamara et al. 1988). Whole-bowel irrigation with a nonabsorbable solution (Golytely®) composed of polyethylene glycol and electrolytes has been reported to be successful in the management of iron, theophylline, verapamil, zinc, and lead overdoses. The utility of this treatment in the management of psychotropic drug overdoses is largely unexplored, as is the solution's interaction with activated charcoal (Howland 1994d).

9. **Control seizures.** If convulsions occur, give diazepam 10 mg iv, administering slowly over 3–5 minutes while closely monitoring respirations. Rapid iv injection of diazepam can lead to respiratory arrest. Repeat the dose every 10–15 minutes, as needed, to a maximum of 30 mg. If diazepam is ineffective, dilute 50 mg/mL of phenytoin solution in 100 mL of 0.9% saline and administer by slow intravenous push. Administration should be at a rate not exceeding 50 mg/minute and should be performed with ECG monitoring. The initial loading dose is 15–18 mg/kg. Serum levels of phenytoin should be monitored over the next 24 hours to maintain therapeutic blood levels (Nicholson 1983; Rumack et al. 1996). Alternatively, phenobarbital 300–800 mg (10–15 mg/kg) in 100 mL of 0.9% saline can be given intravenously at the rate of 25–50 mg/minute. Additional doses of 120–240 mg may be given every 20 minutes to a maximum of 1–2 g daily. If phenytoin and phenobarbital do not control seizures, pentobarbital 5–8 mg/kg given as a 2.5% solution at the rate of 25 mg/minute may be given, followed by 3 mg/kg per hour titrated to control seizures. If seizures remain refractory, general anesthesia, combined if necessary with neuromuscular blocking agents, should be considered (Nicholson 1983; Rumack et al. 1996).

These basic procedures should be followed in all significant overdoses. In the next section we address management of patients who overdose with specific classes of psychotropic drugs.

Antipsychotics

■ Presentation

The initial effects of intoxication with antipsychotics often include a period of hyperactivity, agitation, delirium, and seizures followed by a period of severe psychomotor retardation, hypotension, hypothermia, respiratory failure, and coma. Anticholinergic symptoms such as tachycardia, urinary retention, and hyperthermia may occur. Quinidine-like effects on the heart may be produced, including prolonged PR, QRS, and QTc intervals; blunt T waves; depressed ST segments; and ventricular tachycardia. These effects are more likely with thioridazine than with other antipsychotics (Buckley et al. 1995). Extrapyramidal effects, especially dystonias, may also be noted (Allen et al. 1980; Lewin and Wang 1994; Rumack et al. 1996).

Patients with cardiovascular symptoms should be admitted and monitored; they should be discharged only after resolution of acute abnormal ECG findings for 24 hours. Patients who are asymptomatic initially can be discharged after a 6-hour uneventful monitored period (Ellenhorn and Barceloux 1988; Rumack et al. 1996).

Neuroleptic malignant syndrome, which may occur hours to months after initiation of antipsychotic therapy, and occasionally after an overdose, appears most commonly following haloperidol and injectable fluphenazine. It is characterized by severe dystonic symptoms, hyperthermia, profuse sweating, and markedly elevated creatine phosphokinase (Levenson 1985).

Insufficient data are available regarding overdose with the new antipsychotic risperidone to assess the drug at this time.

■ Treatment

Basic Procedures
See **Basic Procedures** section at beginning of this chapter.

Cardiovascular System

1. Arrhythmias caused by depressed intraventricular conductivity and associated with a prolonged QT interval may be treated with phenytoin or lidocaine (Ellenhorn and Barceloux 1988).

A loading dose of phenytoin may be given at a rate not exceeding 0.5 mg/kg/minute up to a total dose of 1,000 mg or until the arrhythmia is abolished. Blood levels should then be maintained at 10–20 μg/mL (blood should drawn just before administering the dose of phenytoin). This can usually be accomplished by giving approximately 2 mg/kg of phenytoin iv q12h.

Lidocaine may be administered with a loading dose of 50–100 mg given over 3 minutes, which may be repeated in 5 minutes. Maintenance infusion can then be initiated at a rate of 1–4 mg/minute (Rumack et al. 1996).

If phenytoin and lidocaine are unsuccessful, cardioversion and/or cardiac pacing may be necessary.

Because of the quinidine-like effects of phenothiazines on the heart, quinidine, procainamide, and disopyramide should be avoided (Rumack et al. 1996).

Tachycardia may develop into torsade de pointes, which can be treated with isoproterenol, 2–8 μg/minute, and magnesium (Lewin and Wang 1994).

2. Hypotension often can be managed successfully by placing the patient in the Trendelenburg position and administering isotonic fluids. If a vasopressor is necessary, avoid the use of epinephrine, because it may induce severe hypotension. This occurs because the antipsychotics block peripheral α-receptors and result in unopposed β-agonist activity by epinephrine (Lewin and Wang 1994; Risch et al. 1981a). If a vasopressor is necessary, a pure α-agonist such as levarterenol should be given.

Central Nervous System

1. Dystonic disorders can be treated with diphenhydramine 50 mg iv given over 2 minutes, benztropine 2 mg iv given over 2 minutes, or diazepam 5 mg iv (Gagrat et al. 1978; Lee 1979; Lewin and Wang 1994). If the patient is hyperthermic, diazepam is preferred.
2. Hypothermia may be treated with a warming blanket, and hyperthermia, with a cooling blanket (Rumack et al. 1996).
3. Neuroleptic malignant syndrome may be treated with a cooling blanket and, according to case reports, with dantrolene sodium 1 mg/kg po q12h up to 50 mg/dose or bromocriptine mesylate 5 mg po q8h (May et al. 1983; Mueller et al. 1983).

Renal

1. Hemodialysis or hemoperfusion are ineffective because the phenothiazines, butyrophenones, and thioxanthines are less than 90% protein bound and have a large volume of distribution (Lewin and Wang 1994; Rumack et al. 1996).
2. Monitor input, output, and electrolytes and correct any imbalances.

■ Contraindications

Avoid giving CNS depressants, such as anxiolytic-hypnotics, alcohol, narcotics, and anesthetics, because antipsychotics potentiate the respiratory- and CNS-depressant effects of these agents (Hansten 1979).

■ Toxic Dosages

Antipsychotic overdoses are seldom fatal unless they occur concomitantly with other drugs such as alcohol, sedative-hypnotics, antihistamines, or tricyclic antidepressants (TCAs). In cases reported, the acute lethal dose depends on the specific antipsychotic and has ranged from 15 to 150 mg/kg (Lewin and Wang 1994; Rumack et al. 1996).

Tricyclic and Other Non–Monoamine Oxidase Inhibitor Antidepressants

■ Presentation

The most serious consequences of *tricyclic* overdoses relate to their cardiovascular effects. Supraventricular tachycardia, multifocal premature ventricular contractions (PVCs), ventricular tachycardia, flutter, and/or fibrillation can result in severe hypotension and/or shock. Electrocardiographic abnormalities with overdose include prolonged PR interval, widened QRS complex, QT prolongation, T-wave flattening or inversion, ST-segment depression, right bundle branch block, complete heart block, and cardiac standstill (Langou et al. 1980; Risch et al. 1981b; Weisman et al. 1994).

Anticholinergic effects are also common with overdose and include dry mouth, hyperthermia, mydriasis, urinary retention, tachycardia, decreased GI motility, agitation, disorientation, and hallucinations (Callaham 1979; Weisman et al. 1994).

The mortality associated with overdoses of tricyclics is 7%–10% (Marshall and Forken 1982), and 70% of persons who die from tricyclic overdoses are pronounced dead before receiving medical assistance (Frommer et al. 1987). Because many of the symptoms may be delayed due to enterohepatic circulation of tricyclics and their slowed absorption from the GI tract (i.e., as a result of the anticholinergic activity of TCAs), patients must be observed and monitored for at least 6 hours after an overdose of one of these agents. If a patient remains asymptomatic during this time, significant toxicity is unlikely. However, if the patient displays toxic signs during the observation period, he or she must be observed until asymptomatic for at least 24 hours (Callaham 1979; Rumack et al. 1996; Tokarski and Young 1988). Signs reported to be correlated with severe adverse outcomes are a QRS duration on the ECG equal to or greater than 100 msec (Hansten 1979; Tokarski and Young 1988), an R at lead aVR of the ECG of 3 mm or more, arrhythmias, seizures, respiratory depression, altered mental state, and/or a plasma tricyclic level greater than or equal to 1,000 ng/mL (Foulke 1995; Liebelt et al. 1995; Marshall and Forken 1982). However, other studies have disputed the predictive value of the QRS duration (Foulke et al. 1986) and of tricyclic blood levels (Boehnert and Lovejoy 1985), and have indicated that depth of coma (measured by rating instruments) is a better predictor of outcome than either QRS duration or tricyclic blood levels (Hulten et al. 1992).

The symptoms of *amoxapine* overdose are different from those of overdoses with other tricyclics in that seizures and coma are more prominent features and cardiovascular toxicity is minimal (Kulig et al. 1982). Seizures were observed in 36% of the amoxapine overdoses but in only 4% of overdoses with the other cyclic drugs (Litovitz and Troutman 1983). Acute renal failure, probably secondary to rhabdomyolysis and myoglobinuria, has been reported in 16% of amoxapine overdoses (Gelenberg 1983; Pumariega et al. 1982). A higher mortality rate for overdoses of amoxapine, as compared with those of other tricyclics (except amitriptyline), per million prescriptions issued has been noted (Henry et al. 1995); in another study, the mortality rate for amoxapine overdoses was 15%, as compared with a 0.7% rate for other cylic antidepressant overdoses (Litovitz and Troutman 1983).

A comparison of overdoses with *maprotiline,* a tetracyclic antidepressant, with cases of TCA poisoning found that delirium and seizures were more common with maprotiline, and that the incidence of cardiotoxicity with maprotiline was equal to and perhaps greater than that with tricyclics (Hayes and Kristoff 1986; Park and Proudfoot 1977). Physostigmine reportedly increases the risk of seizures when used for maprotiline overdose (Hayes and Kristoff 1986). Mortality rates associated with maprotiline and TCA overdose have been reported to be equivalent (Knudsen and Heath 1984).

Overdoses with ***trazodone,*** a chemically unique antidepressant that is neither a tricyclic nor a tetracyclic compound, frequently produce hypotension, drowsiness, lethargy, ataxia, nausea, and vomiting, with minimal serious CNS and cardiovascular toxicity (Gamble and Peterson 1986; Hassan and Miller 1985). However, there have been reports of cardiac arrhythmias in patients taking trazodone who had preexisting cardiac disease (Janowsky et al. 1983). Only one death from trazodone overdose has been reported in which trazodone was the only agent taken (Litovitz et al. 1986).

Bupropion, fluoxetine, sertraline, paroxetine, venlafaxine, nefazodone, and ***fluvoxamine*** do not have significant cardiovascular or anticholinergic properties and are thought to be relatively safe in overdose, with few reported deaths from these agents when used by themselves (Borys et al. 1992; Boyer and Feighner 1992; Cooper 1988; Doogan 1991; Fontaine 1993; Granier et al. 1993; Lau and Horowitz 1996; Marcus 1996; Rudolph and Derivan 1996; Somni et al. 1987; Spiller et al. 1994; "Venlafaxine: A New Dimension in Antidepressant Pharmacotherapy" 1993; Wenger and Stern 1983; Wilde et al. 1993). However, many of these medications (fluvoxamine, nefazodone, venlafaxine) have been marketed for too brief a time to permit a definitive understanding of their characteristics in overdose.

■ Treatment

Basic Procedures

(See **Basic Procedures** section at beginning of this chapter.) Up to 15% of tricyclics are excreted in bile and gastric secretions and reabsorbed in the intestines. Therefore, total body clearance may be enhanced with multiple doses of activated charcoal every 2–6 hours (Karkkainen and Neuvonen 1986; Swartz and Sherman 1984).

The use of ipecac is considered to be contraindicated in tricyclic overdose because of the possibility of a precipitous deterioration in mental status and airway protective reflexes (Weisman et al. 1994).

Saline lavage plus activated charcoal (regardless of whether the charcoal was given after lavage or before and after lavage) has been found to be no more effective than activated charcoal alone; hence, the need for lavage in tricyclic overdose is unsubstantiated (Bosse et al. 1995).

Cardiovascular System

1. Because of the possibility of sudden, fatal, late-occurring arrhythmias, all individuals who are symptomatic should be carefully monitored for 48 hours and should not be considered
   for discharge until they have been asymptomatic and arrhythmia free for at least 24 hours (Marshall and Forken 1982;
   Rumack et al. 1996; Weisman et al. 1994). Ventricular arrhythmias (multifocal PVCs, ventricular tachycardia, flutter,
   and fibrillation) may be treated with phenytoin 100 mg iv,
   administered over 3 minutes and repeated q5m until the arrhythmia ceases or a 1,000-mg total dose is reached. It should
   be noted that the usefulness of phenytoin for treatment of
   ventricular dysrhythmia and conduction defects in tricyclic
   overdose has been questioned (Callaham et al. 1988; Mayron
   and Ruiz 1986). Serum should be alkalinized, as this measure improves cardiac conduction, decreases heart rate, and
   lessens ventricular arrhythmias (J. R. Hoffman et al. 1993).
   Alkalinization can be accomplished by giving an initial bolus
   of sodium bicarbonate 1–2 mEq/kg followed by an infusion
   of 100–150 mEq of sodium bicarbonate in 1 L of 5% dextrose titrated over 4–6 hours to maintain a blood pH of 7.5–
   7.55 (Lewin 1994b). Ventricular arrhythmias that do not
   respond to alkalinization and phenytoin may respond to lidocaine 1 mg/kg/dose, repeated q20m if needed. A lidocaine
   maintenance dose of 10–40 µg/kg/minute by continuous iv
   infusion may be started concurrently with the loading dose.
   Quinidine, disopyramide, and procainamide, which have effects on cardiac conduction and are myocardial depressants
   similar to the TCAs, are contraindicated for treating arrhythmias accompanying tricyclic overdose. For patients who are
   still unresponsive, administration of physostigmine 1–2 mg iv
   over 1–3 minutes, repeated q20m if necessary, has been suggested by some. However, other authorities recommend that
   physostigmine not be used for any ventricular arrhythmias
   or ventricular conduction disturbances because these disturbances may be converted to heart block or asystole by physostigmine (Lewin 1994a). Finally, if necessary, propranolol may
   be used at a dose of 1 mg iv q2–5m until a response is seen
   or until a maximum of 20 mg has been given. Careful attention
   to hemodynamic functions is necessary because propranolol
   may depress the myocardium and precipitate congestive heart
   failure and/or hypotension (Weisman et al. 1994).

Patients with supraventricular arrhythmias generally do not need to be treated unless their heart rate exceeds 160 beats/minute, in which case propranolol may be given in the dose indicated above. Physostigmine is not recommended for this purpose.

Bradycardia may occur with trazodone overdose. If it is significant or if heart block occurs, atropine may be indicated, at a dose of 15 µg/kg (up to 0.4–0.6 mg/dose).

2. Serious conduction defects, such as prolonged PR interval, prolonged QTc interval, and widened QRS complex, should be treated with alkalinization of blood as indicated above and possibly with phenytoin at the dosages indicated above (Rumack et al. 1996; Weisman et al. 1994).

3. Hypotension can often be managed successfully by placing the patient in the Trendelenburg position and administering lactated Ringer's or normal saline. If a vasopressor is necessary, a predominantly α-adrenergic agonist such as levarterenol should be administered. Because tricyclic overdose results in α-adrenergic blockade, combination α- and β-adrenergic agonists, such as dopamine, should be avoided, as they may result in predominantly β effects that could exacerbate hypotension. In addition, dopamine is mainly an indirect-acting agent (i.e., it acts by releasing catecholamines from presynaptic storage sites and not by acting directly on postsynaptic receptors) and may be ineffective because the tricyclic overdose may have depleted catecholamines (Weisman et al. 1994).

Central Nervous System

1. Pseudoseizures (myoclonic jerks and choreoathetoid movements without electroencephalographic [EEG] activity) occur in as many as 50% of tricyclic overdoses; these are due to the anticholinergic properties of tricyclics and are responsive to treatment with physostigmine (Risch et al. 1981b; Weisman et al. 1994). They should not be interpreted as true seizures and treated with CNS barbiturates and diazepam, as these agents may further depress the CNS.

2. True seizures refractory to diazepam may respond to physostigmine in doses up to 2 mg iv over 2 minutes (Rumack et al. 1996).

3. Excitation and hallucinations are correlated with TCA blood level (Paderson et al. 1982). Delirium may occur and, if severe, may be treated with physostigmine in doses up to 2 mg iv over 5 minutes (Rumack et al. 1996).

Physostigmine

Specific indications for physostigmine include seizures, severe hallucinations accompanied by disorientation, and possibly severe arrhythmias unresponsive to standard antiarrhythmic agents (Lewin 1994a; Rumack et al. 1996; Weisman et al. 1994). Reversal of these symptoms often occurs within minutes after administration of physostigmine if the diagnosis of tricyclic overdose is correct. The usual dose for a therapeutic trial is 2 mg iv given slowly over 5 minutes, which may be repeated at 20 minutes if no reversal has occurred. This dose may be repeated at 30- to 60-minute intervals if life-threatening symptoms recur. A continuous drip should not be used. Physostigmine is metabolized within 30 to 60 minutes, and, therefore, repeated doses may be necessary. When giving physostigmine, an atropine dose one-half that of physostigmine should be kept ready so as to reverse any toxic cholinergic effects that might result from a physostigmine overdose. Such an overdose may be manifested by salivation, lacrimation, involuntary urination or defecation, bronchoconstriction, sinus bradycardia, heart block, cardiac standstill, and/or seizures. If physostigmine is injected too rapidly, seizures and/or asystole may result. Therefore, physostigmine should be used only in situations involving a life-threatening emergency (Lewin 1994a). Relative contraindications to the use of physostigmine include bronchospastic disease, peripheral vascular disease, gangrene, cardiovascular disease, and mechanical obstruction of the GI or urogenital tract. The presence of ventricular conduction abnormalities or ventricular arrhythmias is also considered a contraindication by some authorities (Lewin 1994a; Rumack et al. 1996).

Renal

1. Neither hemodialysis nor hemoperfusion is effective in tricyclic overdoses, because tricyclics are more than 85%–98% protein bound and have a large volume of distribution (Weisman et al. 1994).
2. Monitor input, output, and electrolytes, and correct any imbalances.

■ Toxic Dosages

The TCAs are the major cause of life-threatening overdoses worldwide (Frommer et al. 1987). Although the risk of suicide attempts does not differ among antidepressants, the tricyclics (including maprotiline and amoxapine) are associated with a higher death rate in overdose than are the nontricyclic antidepressants. For unknown reasons, in the United States, the risk of death after an overdose is greater with desipramine hydrochloride than with other tricyclics (Kapur et al. 1992).

Doses of 10–20 mg/kg of most TCAs are frequently accompanied by coma and cardiovascular symptoms. Doses of 35–50 mg/kg are usually fatal. A QRS complex of more than 100 msec in the first 24 hours after an overdose is usually indicative of a serious overdose (Marshall and Forken 1982; Spiker and Biggs 1976), although, as noted above, the predictive value of this ECG abnormality has been disputed (Foulke et al. 1986).

Children appear to be more sensitive to the toxic effects of antidepressants, and a fatal outcome has occurred in a child after the ingestion of imipramine 250 mg (Biederman 1991; Rumack et al. 1996).

Monoamine Oxidase Inhibitors

■ Presentation

Symptoms following an overdose of a monoamine oxidase inhibitor (MAOI) may not be evident for 6–12 hours after ingestion. Symptoms include tremors, rigidity, neuromuscular weakness and incoordination, flushing, diaphoresis, agitation, mental confusion, tachypnea, hypertension, tachycardia, hyperthermia, miosis, increased deep-tendon reflexes, involuntary movements, seizures, headache, dizziness, and precordial pain. Severe toxicity leads to coma, profound hypotension, bradycardia, and asystolic arrest. The clinical course may be due to a phase of catecholamine excess followed by a phase of catecholamine depletion. If the MAOI has been combined with tyramine-containing foods (e.g., aged cheese and meats, red wine, Italian broad beans) or a sympathomimetic (e.g., phenylephrine, phenylpropanolamine, amphetamine, cocaine, ephedrine, dopamine, tryptophan), severe hypertension may occur (Ciocatto et al. 1972; Rumack et al. 1996; Sauter 1994; Tollefson 1983). Serious and fatal interactions have also been reported between MAOIs and meperidine, dextromethorphan (used in cold medications), and selective serotonin reuptake inhibitors (SSRIs) such as fluoxetine. Symptoms of such combinations include disorientation, severe hyperthermia, muscular rigidity, hypertension or hypotension, coma, and seizures. The syndrome is thought to result from excess levels of serotonin (caused by the blockade of serotonin metabolism by MAOIs) combined with blockade of the reuptake of serotonin from the synaptic cleft (Nierenberg and Semprebon 1993; Sauter 1994).

■ Treatment

Basic Procedures
See **Basic Procedures** section at beginning of this chapter.

Cardiovascular System

1. Hypotension is treated by placing the patient in the Trendelenburg position and administering intravenous fluids. Pressor agents should be used with extreme caution because of the potential for precipitating a hypertensive crisis. If a pressor agent must be used, a direct-acting adrenergic agonist, such as epinephrine, norepinephrine, or isoproterenol, is preferable because they act without releasing intracellular amines (Rumack et al. 1996; Sauter 1994).

2. Hypotensive crises are best treated with a rapidly reversible vasodilator, such as nitroprusside. Although longer-acting agents such as the α-adrenergic-blocker phentolamine, the β-blocker labetalol, and the calcium channel blocker nifedipine have been used successfully (Abrams et al. 1985; Clary and Schweizer 1987; Sauter 1994), some authorities recommend that these agents be used with extreme caution, if at all, because MAOI-associated hypertensive crisis often leads to severe hypotension, which can be exacerbated and difficult to reverse if a long-acting hypotensive agent has been given (Sauter 1994). However, patients who present with hypertension soon after the onset of an MAOI-drug or dietary interaction may be treated initially with a rapid-acting oral or parental calcium channel or α-blocking agent such as nifedipine or labetalol. Methyldopa and guanethidine are contraindicated, as they may potentiate hypertension (Rumack et al. 1996).

3. If ventricular arrhythmias—which constitute an ominous sign—occur, they should be treated with lidocaine or procainamide. Bretylium should be avoided, as it may lead to increased release of norepinephrine, followed by catecholamine depletion and orthostatic hypotension (Sauter 1994).

Central Nervous System

1. Excitation, if severe, can be treated with 2–10 mg of diazepam iv. Phenothiazines should be avoided because they may aggravate hypotension (Rumack et al. 1996; Sauter 1994).

2. Hyperthermia should be managed with a cooling blanket or other means of external cooling. Phenothiazines should not be used, because they can precipitate irreversible shock (Rumack et al. 1996; Sauter 1994).

Renal

The excretion of tranylcypromine is increased sevenfold by decreasing urinary pH from 8 to 5 (Turner et al. 1967). However, some authorities believe that the benefits of acidifying patients' urine to increase the excretion of toxic substances seldom justify the risks (Rumack et al. 1996; Sauter 1994). Hemodialysis has been associated with rapid recovery from tranylcypromine (Matter et al. 1965) and phenelzine (Versaci et al. 1964) intoxications.

■ **Toxic Dosages**

Data on lethal doses in humans are difficult to evaluate because of the possibility that drug interactions could have produced the same symptoms seen in overdose. Nonetheless, six deaths have been reported from phenelzine at doses of 385–750 mg, and four deaths have been reported from tranylcypromine at doses of 170–7,850 mg (Rumack et al. 1996; Tollefson 1983).

Lithium

■ **Presentation**

Symptoms of lithium intoxication generally occur at serum lithium levels greater than 2 mEq/L. Lithium poisoning may be caused by 1) the intake of a single, large overdose with suicidal intent or 2) a reduction of renal lithium clearance without a corresponding reduction of dosage. Renal lithium clearance may be reduced as a result of 1) kidney disease or 2) sodium deficiency. The sodium deficiency may be caused by 1) a low-salt diet, 2) a weight-reduction diet without salt supplementation, 3) treatment with diuretic drugs, 4) extrarenal sodium loss (e.g., sweating from a fever), or 5) a rise of the serum lithium concentration above a certain patient-specific, critical level (Schou 1978).

Mild lithium intoxication is characterized by increasing lethargy, drowsiness, fine tremors of the hands, anorexia, nausea, vomiting, and diarrhea. As the intoxication becomes more severe, increasing CNS involvement occurs, including marked impairment of consciousness; restlessness; hyperreflexia; coarse, generalized tremors; muscle fasciculations; myoclonic and choreoathetoid movements; ataxia; dysarthria; seizures; and coma (Hansen and Amdisen 1978).

Various ECG abnormalities have been occasionally reported, including first-degree heart block, prolonged QT interval, nonspecific ST–T-wave changes, and intraventricular conduction delay. These cardiac changes are rare, however, and are seldom specifically treated, although one case of ventricular arrhythmia was treated successfully with iv magnesium sulfate (Mateer and Clark 1982).

■ Treatment

Basic Procedures

(See **Basic Procedures** section at beginning of this chapter.) No clinical data exist to indicate that activated charcoal is of value in treating lithium overdose, whereas in vitro data have indicated that it is of no benefit (Favin et al. 1988). However, because mixed overdoses frequently occur and because activated charcoal does no harm in pure lithium overdose, some authorities recommend its routine use in lithium overdose (Henry et al. 1994).

Sodium polystyrene given orally and repeatedly over 24 hours has been reported useful in case reports and small studies in lowering serum lithium levels in overdose (Belanger et al. 1992; Roberge et al. 1993; Tomaszewski et al. 1992). It is not considered a substitute for hemodialysis in severe cases.

Sustained-release forms of lithium have been found to exhibit delayed toxicity after overdose (Bosse and Arnold 1992; Dupuis et al. 1996). Whole-bowel irrigation beginning 1 hour after lithium ingestion has been reported to be useful in rapidly lowering lithium serum concentrations (Smith et al. 1991).

Renal

1. Sodium that has been lost by dehydration, diuretics, or disease states should be replaced, because low total-body sodium levels decrease lithium clearance (Henry et al. 1994; Rumack et al. 1996).
2. Saline diuresis, achieved by administering 150–300 cc/hour of 0.9% sodium chloride intravenously, may be useful in enhancing lithium elimination only in the sodium-depleted patient (Henry et al. 1994; Rumack et al. 1996).
3. Osmotic diuretics (e.g., mannitol, urea) and phosphodiesterase inhibitors (e.g., aminophylline) have produced increases in lithium clearance of 30%–60%. However, limited data are available regarding the use of these agents in treating lithium

overdose (Perry et al. 1984; Schou 1980; Thomsen and Schou 1975), and they are not recommended by some authorities because of their propensity to cause dehydration and subsequent retention of sodium and lithium (Henry et al. 1994).

4. Dialysis should be considered in patients who are comatose and/or have a serum lithium level greater than 4 mEq/L 6 hours or longer after ingestion. For patients who have chronically overdosed and who exhibit neurological toxicity, hemodialysis has been suggested for lithium levels greater than 1.5 mEq/L. With chronic overdose, much of the lithium is intracellular and not immediately available for removal by hemodialysis. Hemodialysis is more effective than peritoneal dialysis; the latter, which is no more beneficial than normal urinary elimination, should be considered—if at all—only when hemodialysis is not available. Hemodialysis should be continued until the lithium concentration is less than 1 mEq/L 8 hours after dialysis. It should be kept in mind that, although serum concentrations of lithium may fall rapidly during dialysis, these concentrations often rebound, peaking 6–8 hours after dialysis has been stopped. Hemodialysis with a bicarbonate rather than a conventional acetate dialysate may prevent such a rebound and may be more effective in removing intracellular lithium rapidly, although data are limited (Henry et al. 1994; Rumack et al. 1996).

■ Toxic Dosages

Mild to moderate lithium intoxications occur at serum levels between 1.5 and 2.5 mEq/L; severe intoxications, at between 2.5 and 3.5 mEq/L; and fatalities, at greater than 3.5 mEq/L. However, there is often little correlation between serum lithium levels and severity of intoxication. In patients not chronically taking lithium, levels as high as 3–6 mEq/L have been noted without intoxication symptoms. On the other hand, intoxications during chronic therapy have been described with serum levels in the normal therapeutic range of 0.6–1.5 mEq/L (Hansen and Amdisen 1978; Henry et al. 1994).

Carbamazepine and Valproic Acid

■ Presentation

Carbamazepine is an anticonvulsant also used in the treatment of bipolar disorder. It is chemically related both to the TCA imipramine and to phenytoin, and its symptoms of toxicity are similar in some respects to those observed with these compounds. Toxic cardiovascular effects occur with carbamazepine but are less frequent than with tricyclics (Schmidt and Schmitz-Buhl 1995; Spiller et al. 1990). When more-serious cardiovascular effects do occur, they are more likely to be in elderly women who develop bradyarrhythmias and conduction delays with only moderately elevated carbamazepine levels (Kasarskis et al. 1992). Sinus tachycardia occurs frequently in overdose. Prolonged PR, QRS, and QT intervals; conduction defects; bradycardia; and hypotension may also occur (Spiller et al. 1990). Neurological toxic effects include nausea, vomiting, dizziness, lethargy, dysarthria, nystagmus, ophthalmoplegia, ataxia, dyskinesia, dystonia, choreoathetoid movements, disorientation, convulsions, and coma. Hyponatremia occurs in 10%–15% of patients. Rare toxic manifestations include oliguria, subepidermal bullae formation, hypothermia, and respiratory depression (Drenck and Risbo 1980; Lehrman and Bauman 1981; Leslie et al. 1983; Osborn 1994; Rumack et al. 1996; Seymour 1993; Sullivan et al. 1981).

Valproic acid is a branched-chain carboxylic acid used both as an anticonvulsant and as an antimanic agent. In overdoses, symptoms have included nausea, vomiting, disorientation, extrapyramidal movements, and cardiac disturbances. Although liver-function tests may be abnormal, hepatotoxicity has not been associated with acute overdose (Osborn 1994).

■ Treatment

Basic Procedures
(See **Basic Procedures** section at beginning of this chapter.) Repeated doses of activated charcoal may be particularly beneficial in carbamazepine overdoses because of carbamazepine's enterohepatic recirculation (Osborn 1994). However, although the value of repeated dosing with activated charcoal in decreasing the half-life of carbamazepine has been demonstrated, the utility of this method in improving time to clinical recovery has not been established (Wason et al. 1992). Repeated dosing with activated charcoal has also been recommended for valproic acid overdose, but with few data to provide guidance (Osborn 1994).

Cardiovascular System
1. Monitor ECG and vital signs carefully for 24 hours. Treat symptomatically. Specific therapy for cardiac events are not

well reported, but, at least for carbamazepine, are probably similar to treatment reported for tricyclics (Osborn 1994).

2. Hypotension can often be managed by placing the patient in the Trendelenburg position and giving isotonic intravenous fluids. If the patient is unresponsive and a vasopressor is necessary, a direct-acting α-agonist such as levarterenol can be administered (Osborn 1994).

Central Nervous System

Despite carbamazepine's anticholinergic properties and other similarities to tricyclics, no reports exist of physostigmine treatment of seizures and coma caused by carbamazepine overdose.

Renal

1. Hemodialysis for the treatment of acute overdose with carbamazepine has not been reported; however, given carbamazepine's high protein binding in the serum, hemodialysis would not be expected to be effective (Osborn 1994; Rumack et al. 1996).

2. Charcoal hemoperfusion has been used successfully in treating carbamazepine overdose. Indications are a deteriorating clinical state and failure to respond to supportive medical care (Osborn 1994; Rumack et al. 1996).

3. In one case report involving an overdose of valproic acid, both hemodialysis and hemoperfusion were reported to be beneficial in rapidly lowering serum levels of the drug and improving the patient's clinical condition (Tank and Palmer 1993).

■ Toxic Dosages

Signs of carbamazepine intoxication, including ataxia and nystagmus, occur at blood levels greater than 12 μg/mL (therapeutic levels 8–12 μg/mL). At least one study found a correlation between carbamazepine serum levels and toxicity, with levels greater than 40 μg/mL associated with coma, seizures, respiratory failure, cardiac conduction defects, and/or death, and levels less than 40 μg/mL associated with uneventful recovery (Hojer et al. 1993). However, another study did not find such correlations (Spiller et al. 1990). Patients have been reported to have survived doses as high as 34 g.

Valproic acid appears relatively safe in other-than-massive overdose, with few fatalities reported (Andersen and Ritland 1995; Dupuis et al. 1990).

Central Nervous System Depressants (Other Than Benzodiazepines)

■ Presentation

Barbiturates, ethanol, and nonbarbiturate hypnotics (ethchlorvynol, glutethimide, methyprylon, methaqualone, paraldehyde, chloral hydrate, meprobamate), act as depressants to the CNS. At therapeutic doses, patients may be drowsy or asleep but can easily be aroused. With increasing doses, individuals become comatose and cannot be aroused, although they will withdraw from painful stimuli. Reflexes can be hyperactive, depressed, or absent and are of no diagnostic value. As coma deepens, individuals will not respond to painful stimuli. As coma deepens further with increasing dosage, hypothermia, respiratory depression, and hypotension occur, and finally, circulatory failure and cardiac arrest ensue (McCarron et al. 1982; Osborn and Goldfrank 1994).

Hemorrhagic bullae, most often on hands, buttocks, and knees, may occur in patients who have overdosed with barbiturates.

Patients who have been chronically intoxicated with depressants for 1–2 months or more may experience withdrawal symptoms if the drugs are suddenly stopped (see section on anxiolytic-hypnotic withdrawal [page 569] in Chapter 10).

■ Treatment

Basic Procedures

(See **Basic Procedures** section at beginning of this chapter.) Multiple oral doses of activated charcoal administered every 2–4 hours have been demonstrated to significantly decrease the half-life while increasing the total body clearance of phenobarbital (Pond et al. 1984), a process referred to as *GI dialysis.* Activated charcoal has also been reported to adsorb meprobamate and glutethimide. Whether this favorable effect on the elimination of phenobarbital from the body is paralleled by a more favorable clinical course has not yet been determined (Osborn and Goldfrank 1994).

Cardiovascular System

Hypotension can often be managed successfully by placing the patient in the Trendelenburg position and administering isotonic fluids. If a vasopressor is necessary, either dopamine or levarterenol may be administered. Dopamine is considered by some to be the drug of choice, as it increases cardiac output while preserving renal blood flow (Rumack et al. 1996).

Renal

1. Short-acting barbiturates (e.g., pentobarbital, secobarbital):
   a. Forced diuresis is of no value, because it increases excretion by only 2%–5% and can result in congestive heart failure and fluid overload (Osborn and Goldfrank 1994).
   b. Alkalinization of the urine does not affect renal excretion of these drugs (Harvey 1985; Osborn and Goldfrank 1994; Rumack et al. 1996).
   c. Hemodialysis (with a lipid dialysate) and hemoperfusion have been reported to hasten the removal of some short-acting barbiturates from the blood, although the literature in this area is sparse (DeBroc 1986; Osborn and Goldfrank 1994; Rumack et al. 1996).
2. Long-acting barbiturates (e.g., phenobarbital):
   a. Alkalinizing the urine will increase the excretion of pheno-barbital. Sufficient sodium bicarbonate should be given intravenously to produce a urine flow of 3–6 mL/kg/hour and to maintain urine pH at about 8. This may be achieved with 2–3 ampules (88–132 mEq/L) of sodium bicarbonate in dextrose 5% in water, with 20–40 mEq/L of potassium chloride added when necessary. Additional sodium bicar-bonate and potassium chloride (20–40 mEq/L) may be needed to achieve an alkaline urine. Renal function and fluid electrolyte balance must be carefully assessed before and during alkalinization, and caution against giving potas-sium to an oliguric or anuric patient must be maintained (Osborn and Goldfrank 1994; Rumack et al. 1996).
   b. Hemodialysis or hemoperfusion may be of value in patients in deep coma who fail to respond to general supportive measures and alkaline diuresis (Rumack et al. 1996).
3. The literature on the treatment of nonbarbiturate hypnotic overdose is sparse. Several of these drugs are very lipid soluble (e.g., ethchlorvynol, glutethimide) and are redistributed from serum to tissue and then slowly released back to serum, leading to prolonged and cyclic coma (Osborn and Goldfrank 1994). Use of hemodialysis and/or hemoperfusion has been suggested for overdoses with these agents; however, few data exist to support the utility of this intervention. Most nonbarbiturate hypnotics respond to some extent to hemodialysis and/or hemoperfusion. Peritoneal dialysis may also be used if hemodia-lysis or hemoperfusion is not available, but it is only 10%–25% as effective (Pond 1994).

4. Ethanol is rapidly metabolized by the liver at a constant rate. For severe overdoses, hemodialysis will rapidly decrease the blood levels of ethanol.

■ Toxic Dosages

1. In adults, short-acting barbiturates can produce fatal intoxications at a dose of 3 g when taken alone. Serum levels above 14 µg/mL result in stupor and coma in the nondependent patient. The highest barbiturate level for which recovery has been reported is 580 µg/mL. Toxicity is increased greatly when a barbiturate is taken with other anxiolytic-hypnotics, including alcohol, or with antihistamines. The degree of CNS depression is often not a good guide to the amount of ingested barbiturate (and other depressants), inasmuch as the patient may be tolerant to some of the depressant effects. Very little tolerance develops to the lethal dose of anxiolytic-hypnotics, however, and hence, patients who are chronic users may be close to a lethal dose without clinically manifesting severe intoxication (Harvey 1985; Osborn and Goldfrank 1994; Rumack et al. 1996).

2. Long-acting barbiturates generally are associated with some degree of toxic symptomatology if the dose exceeds 8 mg/kg, although dependent patients have been known to use dosages greater than 1,000 mg/day without experiencing severe toxicity (Rumack et al. 1996).

3. Nonbarbiturate hypnotics have been reported to be fatal in overdoses of 10–15 times the therapeutic dose (Rumack et al. 1996).

4. Alcohol blood levels in excess of 400 mg% have been reported to be fatal (Rumack et al. 1996).

Benzodiazepines, Zolpidem, and Buspirone

■ Presentation

Benzodiazepines are unique anxiolytic-hypnotics in that they are not very toxic; however, two recent studies have called attention to the possibility that although benzodiazepines are not very toxic as a group, differences in toxicity may exist among individual drugs in the group. In the first study, in England, temazepam and flurazepam were associated with more overdose deaths per million prescriptions than any other benzodiazepines (Serfaty and Masterson 1993). In the second study, in Australia, temazepam was associated with more sedation after overdose than were other benzodiazepines (Buckley 1995). However, in general, even large doses (e.g., diazepam 1,500 mg) cause only minor toxic symptoms (e.g., ataxia, lethargy, slurred speech). Deep coma, characterized by unresponsiveness to painful stimulation or by respiratory depression, is uncommon in benzodiazepine overdose and, if present, should suggest the possibility that other drugs have been taken in addition to the benzodiazepines (Divoll et al. 1981; Greenblatt et al. 1977; Osborn and Goldfrank 1994; Rumack et al. 1996).

Although respiratory depression is uncommon with overdose of benzodiazepines, it should be noted that respiratory arrest has occurred after rapid intravenous injection of these drugs.

Abrupt withdrawal of benzodiazepines taken in therapeutic doses for several months can result in a withdrawal syndrome (see section on anxiolytic-hypnotic withdrawal [page 569] in Chapter 10).

Zolpidem is chemically distinct from the benzodiazepines but pharmacologically acts at the benzodiazepine receptor. Symptoms of overdose appear similar in quality and severity to those of the benzodiazepines and are more serious when zolpidem is combined in overdose with alcohol and other drugs (Wyss et al. 1996).

Buspirone, used as an antianxiety agent but chemically distinct from the benzodiazepines, appears to have mild toxicity in overdose, as judged from the limited number of cases reported. Drowsiness appears to be the main symptom. Buspirone is less sedating than other benzodiazepines and interacts less with alcohol (Rumack et al. 1996).

■ **Treatment**

Basic Procedures
(See **Basic Procedures** section at beginning of this chapter.) Repeated oral charcoal every 2–6 hours may enhance total body clearance and elimination of benzodiazepines (Traeger and Haug 1984).

Cardiovascular System
Hypotension can often be managed successfully by placing the patient in the Trendelenburg position and administering isotonic fluids. If a vasopressor is necessary, either dopamine or levarterenol can be administered (Divoll et al. 1981; Rumack et al. 1996).

Central Nervous System
Even large doses result in agitation, ataxia, drowsiness, dysarthria, and lethargy, but rarely significant coma. Deep coma, marked hypotension, or respiratory depression should prompt the suspicion

that drugs in addition to benzodiazepines have been ingested and/ or that additional CNS pathology exists (Divoll et al. 1981; Osborn and Goldfrank 1994; Rumack et al. 1996).

Renal
Neither hemodialysis nor forced diuresis is an effective means of removing benzodiazepines (Osborn and Goldfrank 1994). The value of hemodialysis in zolpidem or buspirone overdoses has not been evaluated.

Antidote
Flumazenil, a specific benzodiazepine antagonist, rapidly reverses benzodiazepine-induced coma after intravenous injection, with effects lasting from 1 to 4 hours. The initial dose is 1 mg given over 1 minute, with additional doses of 1 mg given every minute until the desired response occurs or a maximum of 8 mg is given. If no response occurs after 5 mg, further doses are unlikely to be successful. If partial response occurs, up to 8 mg may be given (Spivey et al. 1993). If re-sedation occurs, the dose may be repeated at 20-minute intervals, with a maximum of 3 mg/hour (Gelman and Rumack 1994).

Flumazenil should be used with caution in persons with a history of benzodiazepine abuse, as it may precipitate benzodiazepine withdrawal, including seizures. It is considered by some authorities to be contraindicated in mixed overdoses involving cyclic antidepressants, because of an increased incidence of cardiac arrhythmias and seizures (Spivey 1992).

In patients with suspected multiple-drug overdose, flumazenil probably reverses sedation only to the degree that benzodiazepines are involved in the overdose and may exacerbate the clinical condition if cyclic antidepressants are involved. Hence, some authorities do not recommend its use routinely as a therapeutic or diagnostic tool in a comatose patient presenting to the emergency room. Specifically, these authors suggest that flumazenil's use should be avoided in patients with an obstructed airway, cardiac arrhythmias, seizure disorder, signs of cyclic antidepressant overdose, or severe hypotension (Geller et al. 1991; Howland 1994e). However, in one double-blind placebo study of 105 patients presenting unconscious to an emergency room with suspected multiple-drug ingestion, patients given flumazenil substantially improved on a coma rating scale within 5 minutes of injection, compared with placebo patients. No patient, even among those who were later shown to have overdosed with cyclic antidepressants, experienced seizures or arrhythmias (Hojer et al. 1990). Two later studies of unconscious patients presenting to an emergency room, both double-blind and controlled, one with 326 patients and one with 170, confirmed the value and relative safety of flumazenil in doses up to 10 mg (given at the rate of 1 mg/minute). However, 4 and 3 patients, respectively, experienced seizures and/or arrhythmias. Of these 7 patients, 4 had ingested significant amounts of tricyclics in addition to benzodiazepines (Flumazenil in Benzodiazepine Intoxication Multicenter Study Group 1992; Spivey et al. 1993).

Two more recent clinical studies—involving a series of mixed-overdose patients seen in the emergency room and given flumazenil—that attempted to resolve the controversy of flumazenil's utility in treating such patients reached opposite conclusions. The first study found that flumazenil was safe and effective, even in patients overdosing with tricyclics (Weinbroum et al. 1996), whereas the second concluded that patients with serious mixed overdoses had a higher incidence of seizures after receiving flumazenil (Gueye et al. 1996).

In summary, the value of flumazenil as a routine diagnostic and therapeutic tool in a comatose patient requires further study, but this agent may have a place in pure benzodiazepine overdose. Major side effects, besides seizures and arrhythmias, include injection-site pain, agitation, vomiting, dizziness, and headache (Spivey et al. 1993).

■ Toxic Dosages

Diazepam doses as high as 1,355 mg have been taken without significant toxicity. There are no well-documented fatalities of oral overdoses of benzodiazepines alone (Thompson et al. 1975). However, unlike oral ingestion, intravenous administration of diazepam is associated with a 1.7% incidence of life-threatening reactions, including hypotension and respiratory or cardiac arrest (Litovitz 1983). Benzodiazepines can be very toxic when combined with other CNS depressants such as alcohol and may result in severe coma, respiratory depression, and death (Osborn and Goldfrank 1994; Rumack et al. 1996).

No fatalities involving zolpidem used alone in overdose have been reported, and only mild symptoms have been observed in overdoses as high as 600 mg (Wyss et al. 1996). One case report indicated flumazenil to be of value in treating zolpidem overdose (Lheureux et al. 1990).

No fatalities with buspirone used alone have been reported. With overdoses up to 375 mg, the most common side effect was drowsiness (Goetz et al. 1989). The lethal dose for 50% of animals tested (LD_{50}) is 586 mg/kg in dogs and 356 mg/kg in monkeys (Rumack et al. 1996).

Opiates

■ Presentation

Acute overdose with any of the opiates can lead to coma, pulmonary edema, and respiratory arrest. Overdose with an opiate with a long half-life, such as methadone, can lead to 24–48 hours of severe respiratory depression. Because the opiates cause delayed gastric emptying, coma and respiratory depression may improve initially only to worsen later (Goldfrank and Weisman 1994; Khantzian and McKenna 1979; Rumack et al. 1996).

Classically, pinpoint pupils are observed, although severe acidosis and hypoxia due to respiratory depression may cause pupils to dilate. Pinpoint pupils do not always occur with meperidine overdose (Goldfrank and Weisman 1994).

Seizures may occur with meperidine, fentanyl, and proxyphene overdoses. Intraventicular conduction delays, heart block, bigeminy, ventricular tachycardia, and ventricular fibrillation can occur with propoxyphene overdose. These cardiotoxic effects of propoxyphene are not reversible by naloxone (Goldfrank and Weisman 1994).

Common signs and symptoms of opiate overdose include urinary retention, muscle spasm, itching, hyperpyrexia, leukocytosis, and hyperamylasemia. Chronic abusers may present with abscesses, arrhythmias, cellulitis, osteomyelitis, endocarditis, postanoxic encephalopathy, rhabdomyolysis, acute tubular necrosis, glomerulonephritis, and thrombophlebitis (Goldfrank and Weisman 1994; Khantzian and McKenna 1979). Individuals who have been using opiates chronically may experience withdrawal if these agents are suddenly discontinued (see section on opiate withdrawal [page 560] in Chapter 10).

■ Treatment

Basic Procedures
See **Basic Procedures** section at beginning of this chapter.

Central Nervous System

Meperidine, fentanyl, and propoxyphene overdoses have been associated with seizures. These seizures may be prevented by treatment with naloxone (Goldfrank and Weisman 1994). Illicit meperidine use has been associated with a syndrome resembling idiopathic Parkinson's disease (Rumack et al. 1996).

Respiratory System

Pulmonary edema may occur with overdose or with small amounts of narcotics injected intravenously. Management of such edema is the same as that of narcotic overdose. If PO_2 drops below 50 mm Hg when 60% oxygen by face mask is used, continuous positive airway pressure (CPAP) or intubation and positive end expiratory pressure (PEEP) may be needed (Goldfrank and Weisman 1994; Rumack et al. 1996).

Antidote

Naloxone (Narcan®), a pure narcotic antagonist with no agonist (and hence no respiratory-depressant) effects, is capable of reversing opiate overdoses. It is the drug of choice in mixed unknown overdoses because it will reverse coma and respiratory depression caused by opiates without harming the patient if other agents are also involved ("Diagnosis and Management of Acute Drug Abuse Reactions" 1983; Evans et al. 1973; Rumack et al. 1996; Weisman 1994). There is evidence that naloxone may actually aid in the reversal of coma induced by ethanol, diazepam, or clonidine (Badawy and Evans 1983; Jordan et al. 1980; Kulig and Rumack 1983). If the coma and respiratory depression are from other causes, naloxone will do no harm.

Naloxone may induce vomiting; hence, comatose patients should be intubated before receiving the drug. Opiate withdrawal may be precipitated in patients dependent on opiates and consists of irritability, vomiting, agitation, abdominal pain, diaphoresis, and piloerection. Because of the short half-life of naloxone, this reaction is transient and never life-threatening.

The initial dose in a patient with respiratory depression is 2.0 mg; in a patient with CNS depression without respiratory depression, it is 0.4–0.8 mg, which should be given intravenously if a vein is available, or, if not, given intramuscularly or subcutaneously. The dose may be repeated q5m; the drug is relatively safe, and intravenous doses of 24 mg have been given without any apparent ill effects. If 10 mg have been given without effect, opiate overdose becomes questionable. However, it has been reported that higher-than-usual doses of naloxone are necessary to reverse propoxyphene, pentazocine, methadone, fentanyl, diphenoxylate, nalbuphine, and butorphanol overdoses. Buprenorphine may exhibit a delayed or partial response to naloxone (Flomenbaum et al. 1994; Goldfrank and Weisman 1994).

Continuous intravenous naloxone may be given to treat an overdose of a long-acting narcotic such as methadone or propoxyphene. Naloxone 4–6 mg can be added to each liter of dextrose 5% in water and given at the rate of 100 mL/hour, thus delivering 0.4–0.6 mg/hour. Such mixtures should be used within 24 hours of being prepared. The infusion rate may be increased or decreased as needed to maintain the patient in an arousable state with a respiratory rate of 10–20 respirations per minute. If continuous infusion is not initiated, repeat boluses every 20–60 minutes may be necessary (Goldfrank and Weisman 1994; Rumack et al. 1996). More-complex continuous-dosing regimens have been proposed but not as yet tested in clinical situations (Goldfrank et al. 1986). Even if patients improve rapidly, they must be carefully observed and supported for 24–48 hours.

■ Toxic Dosages

Unlike the anxiolytic-hypnotics, significant tolerance develops to the lethal dose of opiates. Relatively small doses, sometimes in the therapeutic range, have proved fatal for children, whereas very large doses of opiates have been well tolerated without fatal outcome in tolerant opiate-dependent individuals (Rumack et al. 1996).

Central Nervous System Stimulants

■ Presentation

These drugs include amphetamine, methamphetamine, phenmetrazine, methylphenidate, most diet pills, and cocaine. Early CNS toxic effects include restlessness, irritability, and insomnia. As toxicity develops, the patient, although fully oriented, experiences a cluster of schizophrenia-like symptoms that include paranoid delusions, ideas of reference, and/or auditory, visual, tactile, or olfactory hallucinations. Compulsive behavior and dyskinesias (bruxism, tics) and seizures may occur. Peripheral toxic effects include mydriasis, diaphoresis, hyperpyrexia, nausea, vomiting, and diarrhea. Cardiovascular effects include tachycardia, palpitations, arrhythmias, hypertension, and, possibly, circulatory collapse (Chiang and Goldfrank 1994; Lewin et al. 1994; Rumack et al. 1996; D. E.

Smith 1969). Acute myocardial infarction and ventricular and atrial tachyarrhythmias have been reported in cocaine abuse and overdoses in patients without underlying heart disease or myocarditis (Isner et al. 1986; H. W. B. Smith et al. 1987; Virmani et al. 1988). Cerebral hemorrhage and infarction associated with cocaine and with methamphetamine use have been described (Levine et al. 1987; Rockrock et al. 1988; Tuchman et al. 1987).

Chronic intoxication often leads to marked weight loss and malnutrition due to anorexia. Withdrawal from chronic use of stimulants usually leads to profound depression, often accompanied by suicidal ideation and behavior. This depression may last for several weeks to months but may be responsive to tricyclic antidepressant medication. There is no clear-cut physiological withdrawal from stimulants, although the acute depression and concomitant suicidal ideation make withdrawal potentially fatal (Gold et al. 1985; D. E. Smith 1969).

■ Treatment

Basic Procedures
See **Basic Procedures** section at beginning of this chapter.

Central Nervous System

1. Acute psychosis manifested by delusions and auditory hallucinations is effectively treated with antipsychotics. If the patient is hypertensive in addition to being psychotic, chlorpromazine is an effective medication for both problems (Espelin and Done 1968). If hypertension is not a problem and there is concern regarding the cardiovascular effects of chlorpromazine, haloperidol, which has minimal cardiovascular effects, may be used (Angrist et al. 1974). Haloperidol 5 mg im or po q2–4h is a safe and effective treatment for reversing stimulant psychosis (Gagrat et al. 1978). Chlorpromazine may be used in a dose of 25–50 mg im or of 100 mg po q2–4h until the psychosis is controlled (Gagrat et al. 1978). However, chlorpromazine, especially when administered intramuscularly, may cause significant hypotension and possibly cardiac arrhythmias. If a patient is psychotic due to ingestion of an unknown drug, it is preferable to use an anxiolytic-hypnotic such as diazepam 10–20 mg po rather than an antipsychotic, because some illicit drugs have significant anticholinergic effects that are often made worse by the addition of an antipsychotic. If it is certain, however, that a pure stimulant is the drug being abused, many

authorities consider antipsychotics the drugs of choice (Rosenberg et al. 1981; Rumack et al. 1996). Other authorities, however, prefer to use benzodiazepines and to avoid all antipsychotics, even in pure-stimulant overdoses, because they feel that the antipsychotics may further adversely affect thermoregulation and lower the seizure threshold (Chiang and Goldfrank 1994; Lewin et al. 1994).

2. Seizures refractory to diazepam may occur and may be treated with phenytoin and phenobarbital. If seizures remain refractory, general anesthesia with thiopental or halothane should be considered (Rumack et al. 1996).

3. Hyperthermia may occur during overdose, perhaps as a result of increased muscular activity, vasoconstriction, and/or a direct effect of the stimulant on the hypothalamus. A syndrome in seven cocaine-related deaths consisting of hyperthermia, delirium, agitation, and muscular rigidity has been reported (Welti and Fishbain 1985) and is suggestive of neuroleptic malignant syndrome.

Treatment of hyperthermia, depending on severity, involves placing the patient in a cool room, minimizing physical activity, sponging the patient with tepid water, and/or placing the patient on a hypothermic blanket or, in severe cases (i.e., temperatures greater than 40°C), in an ice bath (Schwartz and Oderda 1980). Temperatures higher than 40°C are associated with a poor prognosis. In cases suggestive of neuroleptic malignant syndrome, the use of bromocriptine, a dopamine agonist, has been advocated (Kosten and Kleber 1987). In a retrospective study of 634 patients with neuroleptic malignant syndrome, patients given bromocriptine, dantrolene, or amantadine had lower fatality rates than those not receiving these medications (Sakkas et al. 1991).

Cardiovascular System
Hypertension is often short lived, especially with cocaine, and, even when untreated, may be followed by significant hypotension (Schwartz and Oderda 1980). If treatment is needed, hypertension usually responds to the doses of chlorpromazine indicated earlier (see #1 under *Central Nervous System* in "Treatment," above). If the hypertension does not respond, phentolamine (Regitine®), phenoxybenzamine (Dibenzyline®), sodium nitroprusside (Nipride®), or iv chlorpromazine may be used. If iv chlorpromazine is used, a slow infusion of approximately 0.1 mg/kg should be given over 15 minutes. More-rapid administration may result in a sudden and dangerous drop in blood pressure. Propranolol, used to treat stimu-

lant hypertension, has been associated with "paradoxical hypertension," perhaps due to unopposed α-adrenoreceptor stimulation (Ramoska and Sacchetti 1985). Hence, labetalol, which has α- and β-adrenoreceptor–blocking properties, may be preferable (Gay and Loper 1988). Hypotension, which may result either from treatment or as a late consequence of stimulant toxicity, should be treated with intravenous fluids and the Trendelenburg position, with pressor amines being used only in very refractory cases (Chiang and Goldfrank 1994; Lewin et al. 1994; Rumack et al. 1996).

Renal

Rhabdomyolysis can occur with overdose of stimulants (Menashe and Gottlieb 1988), and hence, the patient's urinary myoglobin and serum creatinine phosphokinase (CPK) should be monitored.

Acidification of the patient's urine will result in more rapid excretion of stimulants such as amphetamines, which have a high acid dissociation constant (pKa) (Anggard et al. 1973), although some authorities feel that it is never appropriate because it does not improve mortality and morbidity significantly and it frequently leads to medically serious metabolic acidosis (Pond 1994). Acidification should not be attempted in the presence of rhabdomyolysis, because renal failure may result. Urine may be acidified by giving ammonium chloride 8–12 g/day po in divided doses or 1–2 g q6h iv. Urine pH should be monitored and kept between 4.5 and 5.5 (Rumack et al. 1996).

■ Toxic Dosages

The lethal dose of methamphetamine and amphetamine is considered to be approximately 20–25 mg/kg; however, the lethal and toxic doses are highly variable because of the development of tolerance in chronic abusers, who have been known to use amphetamine 5,000 mg/day or cocaine 10,000 mg/day without significant toxic effects. On the other hand, fatalities have been reported after ingestions as low as 1.3 mg/kg of amphetamine or 25 mg of cocaine. Hyperpyrexia greater than 40°C after overdose has been reported to indicate a poor prognosis (Chiang and Goldfrank 1994; Lewin et al. 1994; Rumack et al. 1996).

Lysergic Acid Diethylamide and Marijuana

■ Presentation

Lysergic acid diethylamide (LSD) in a dose as low as 30 μg reliably alters perception and can induce kaleidoscopic visual and auditory hallucinations, illusions, delusions, hyperacusis, synesthesia, paresthesias, derealization, depersonalization, mood disturbances, marked fluctuations in time sense and mood, deranged kinesthetic sense, and disordered thought processes. These mental changes may be accompanied by peripheral changes that include nausea, salivation, lacrimation, tremors, muscle weakness, mydriasis, hypertension, tachycardia, hyperreflexia, slight ataxia, and facial flushing. Hyperthermia, convulsions, coma, and respiratory arrest have been reported with massive overdoses of LSD (Pradhan and Hollister 1977; Rumack et al. 1996).

The psychoactive ingredient of marijuana is tetrahydrocannabinol (THC). Marijuana is a mixture of the flowers, stems, and seeds of the plant *Cannabis sativa* and is generally smoked, but may be ingested, usually mixed with food. Hashish, which contains a higher concentration of THC, is the resin secreted by the plant. Effects occur within minutes of smoking and within 30 to 60 minutes of ingestion and last 3–4 hours after smoking and 8–12 hours after ingestion. Low doses lead to relaxation, a sense of heightened sensory awareness, tachycardia, and injected conjunctivae (red sclera). In higher doses, short-term memory disturbances, tremor, diaphoresis, muscular weakness, orthostatic hypotension, and ataxia may occur. In yet-higher doses, a toxic confusional state with hallucinations and delusions may occur that resembles hallucinogenic intoxication (Nahas and Goldfrank 1994).

■ Treatment

Prevention of Absorption
LSD is rapidly and completely absorbed from the GI tract, and hence, the usual procedures of inducing emesis and using activated charcoal and cathartics to prevent further absorption of the drug are of questionable value (Aaron and Ferm 1994; Rumack et al. 1996).

Marijuana is generally smoked, in which case GI procedures are of no benefit. There is no information on the value of GI procedures when marijuana is ingested; however, given marijuana's relatively benign and short-lived toxic-symptom profile, such procedures are probably of limited value (Nahas and Goldfrank 1994).

Central Nervous System
Patients who are experiencing a frightening psychotic or acute anxiety reaction to LSD or marijuana may respond to simple verbal reassurance. If such reassurance is not effective or cannot be provided, diazepam 5–10 mg po is useful in decreasing panic reactions.

It is best to avoid the use of antipsychotics, because they tend to worsen the effects of other drugs, which may have been taken instead of or along with the LSD or marijuana (Aaron and Ferm 1994; Nahas and Goldfrank 1994; Pradhan and Hollister 1977; Rumack et al. 1996).

Antidote
L-5-hydroxytryptophan (5-HTP) 400 mg/day and carbidopa 100 mg/day have been reported to reverse psychotic symptoms of LSD in a single case report (Abraham 1983).

■ Toxic Dosages

Only one LSD-overdose death has been reported (Griggs and Ward 1977). Doses as high as 1–2 g have been survived, although suicides and accidents under the influence of the drug have been reported (Smart and Bateman 1967).

There have been no documented deaths attributable to marijuana overdose per se, although injuries and/or fatalities resulting from accidents while under the influence of marijuana have been reported (Nahas and Goldfrank 1994).

Phencyclidine

■ Presentation

Acute organic brain syndromes resulting from smoking, snorting, or ingesting "low" (<5 mg) doses of PCP may appear within minutes and may continue for 1–72 hours (more typically, 4–6 hours). Symptoms often begin as a cataleptic state with catatonic rigidity. Mild agitation and excitement may ensue as subjects experience depersonalization, paranoid ideation, changes in body image, diplopia, paresthesias, tremulousness, analgesia, and other generalized sensory disturbances. Often the individual will appear to be inebriated, demonstrating euphoria, decreased concentration, drowsiness, confusion, ataxia, and slurred speech. Seizures may occur (Aronow et al. 1980; Goldfrank et al. 1994; Rumack et al. 1996; D. E. Smith et al. 1978).

Physical examination may reveal a diminished or absent response to pinprick as well as other sensory impairment (taste, vision, and audition). Systolic and diastolic blood pressures fluctuate from normal to moderately elevated levels. This is often accompanied by other sympathomimetic effects such as flushing, diaphoresis, and tachycardia. Ophthalmological effects include rotatory horizontal and vertical nystagmus and pupils of variable size but usually

miotic. Other signs that might be present include tremor, myoclonus, opisthotonos, torticollis, grimacing, hyperthermia, ptosis,
excessive salivation, and variable but usually hyperactive deep-
tendon reflexes. The presence of abdominal cramps, hematemesis,
and diarrhea may be a result of by-products that were not completely separated during the illicit synthesis of PCP. Rhabdomyolysis with myoglobinuria and acute renal failure have been reported after PCP overdoses (Aronow et al. 1980; Goldfrank et
al. 1994; McCarron 1986; Patal et al. 1980; Rumack et al. 1996).

■ Treatment

Basic Procedures
(See **Basic Procedures** section at beginning of this chapter.) Although not verified clinically, the value of multiple doses of activated charcoal every 2–6 hours in enhancing the elimination
of PCP is probable, given that PCP is secreted into the stomach
from all routes of administration (Goldfrank et al. 1994; Rumack
et al. 1996). Continuous gastric suction may also be of value for
this reason but should be reserved for those comatose patients in
whom electrolytes can be carefully monitored and replaced (Goldfrank et al. 1994).

Central Nervous System
1. Psychotic symptoms should initially be treated by minimizing
    all sensory stimuli; the patient should be placed in a quiet,
    dimly lighted, nonthreatening setting. Such reduction in sen-
    sory stimuli can markedly reduce the psychotomimetic effects
    of the drug. If such setting is not possible or is not effective,
    patients may be given diazepam 10 mg po or slowly iv. Diaze-
    pam may be repeated iv q10m until agitation is controlled.
    If agitation and psychotic symptoms are severe and/or diaze-
    pam is ineffective, patients may be given haloperidol 5–10 mg
    im or po q2–4h (Clinton et al. 1987). PCP's psychotomimetic
    effects are partially due to its anticholinergic properties, and
    hence, antipsychotics, such as chlorpromazine, which have
    a great deal of intrinsic anticholinergic activity, are contraindi-
    cated in treating PCP psychosis. Restraints should be avoided
    if possible, as they may contribute to rhabdomyolysis (Aronow
    et al. 1980; Rumack et al. 1996; D. E. Smith et al. 1978).
2. Hyperthermia, which may be observed in severe overdoses,
    may be managed with a cooling blanket or by sponging.

Cardiovascular System

Hypertensive crisis may be treated with intravenous infusions of nitroprusside as needed, or with phentolamine until the hypertension is controlled, and then q2–4h as needed (Goldfrank et al. 1994; Rumack et al. 1996).

Renal

1. Urinary acidification, maintaining a pH between 4.5 and 5.5, increases the renal clearance of PCP. Urine may be acidified by administering ammonium chloride 8–12 g/day po in divided doses or 1–2 g iv q6h. Acidification should be avoided in patients with rhabdomyolysis, as myoglobin may precipitate in the kidneys and cause acute renal failure (Aronow and Done 1978; Barton et al. 1980; Perez-Reyes 1982). Although acidification of the urine is widely used, its value has been questioned (Fauman 1981; McCarron 1986; Rumack 1980; Rumack et al. 1996), and it is considered by some authorities to be contraindicated in all overdoses, given its unfavorable risk-benefit ratio (Pond 1994). In addition, considering that PCP is only 10% excreted by the kidneys and 90% metabolized by the liver, little is to be gained by acidifying the urine, especially in view of the risk of inducing systemic acidoses and/or myoglobin precipitation (Goldfrank et al. 1994).

2. Hemoperfusion and hemodialysis are of little value in treating PCP overdoses, as would be expected given the drug's large volume of distribution, substantial protein binding, high lipid solubility, and limited renal excretion (Goldfrank et al. 1994).

■ Toxic Dosages

The lethal dose of PCP in humans is not clearly established, but doses greater than 20 mg may be fatal (Young et al. 1987). Blood levels of PCP between 30 and 100 ng/mL have been associated with coma, myoclonus, and seizures (Rumack et al. 1996).

Anticholinergics

■ Presentation

Anticholinergic intoxications are characterized by various neuropsychiatric signs, including disorientation, confusion, recent memory loss, agitation, dysarthria, incoherent speech, push of speech (pressure to keep talking), hallucinations, delusions, ataxia, periods of hyperactivity alternating with periods of somnolence, paranoia, anxiety, seizures, and coma. Hallucinations associated with anticholinergic overdose are usually visual but may also be auditory or tactile or all three. The visual hallucinations are characterized by the patient's picking, plucking, grasping, or gathering imaginary objects seen on clothing or suspended in space. Tactile hallucinations of crawling insects are occasionally noted (Perry et al. 1978; Rumack et al. 1996).

Physical signs resulting from postganglionic, parasympathetic blockade (antimuscarinic action) include widely dilated, poorly reactive pupils; warm, dry skin; facial flushing; decreased secretions of the mouth, pharynx, nose, and bronchi; foul-smelling breath; fever; tachycardia; hypertension; decreased bowel activity; hyperreflexia; and urinary retention (Perry et al. 1978; Rumack et al. 1996).

Such symptoms may be seen in overdose from a variety of anticholinergic medications, including antihistamines, antiparkinsonian agents, antipsychotics, antispasmodics, tricyclic antidepressants, mydriatic ophthalmological products, mushrooms, and skeletal muscle relaxants (Weisman and Goldfrank 1994).

■ Treatment

Basic Procedures
See **Basic Procedures** section at beginning of this chapter.

Central Nervous System
In the presence of seizures, delirium, and/or severe hallucinations and in the absence of ventricular conduction abnormalities or ventricular arrhythmias, a trial of physostigmine may be initiated. The CNS toxic effects should be reversed in minutes if the diagnosis is correct and the patient has not ingested other substances and has not sustained anoxic damage.

In a therapeutic trial, physostigmine 2 mg is given iv over several minutes. If physostigmine is given too rapidly, seizures and/or asystole may result. If reversal has not occurred within 20 minutes, another 1–2 mg may be tried. The dose may be repeated by slow intravenous administration if life-threatening symptoms recur. Physostigmine may be used every several hours by iv injection, because it is metabolized within 30 to 60 minutes. It should not be administered as an iv drip. Physostigmine should be used to correct or prevent life-threatening complications and not simply to keep a patient awake (Lewin 1994a; Rumack 1973; Rumack et al. 1996; Weisman and Goldfrank 1994; Weisman et al. 1994).

In addition to ventricular cardiac abnormalities, bronchospastic disease, peripheral vascular disease, gangrene, cardiovascular disease, and mechanical obstruction of the GI or genitourinary tract are relative contraindications to the use of physostigmine. Whenever physostigmine is used, atropine 1 mg for possible iv injection should be available to reverse a cholinergic crisis, which may be induced by physostigmine (Lewin 1994a; Rumack et al. 1996).

If physostigmine is not successful in controlling seizures, the methods outlined for seizure control in the **Basic Procedures** section at the beginning of this chapter should be used.

Cardiovascular System

Sinus tachyarrhythmias do not require treatment unless there are signs of cardiac failure or instability. Some authorities suggest that life-threatening arrhythmias and/or hypertension be treated with physostigmine according to the guidelines listed above, whereas others counsel against the drug's use in these circumstances because of its propensity to cause heart block and asystole (Lewin 1994a; Rumack et al. 1996). If physostigmine is considered to be contraindicated or is ineffective, propranolol 1 mg iv q2–5m or labetalol 20 mg iv q10m may be administered until a response occurs or until a maximum of 20 mg of propranolol or 300 mg of labetolol has been given. However, because β-blockers may depress myocardial function and precipitate congestive heart failure or severe hypotension, hemodynamic function must be monitored carefully in patients receiving these agents (Lewin 1994a; Rumack et al. 1996; Weisman et al. 1994).

Renal

1. Because most anticholinergics have a large volume of distribution, little free drug is present in the plasma, and hence, peritoneal dialysis and hemodialysis and hemoperfusion are of no value.

2. Monitor input, output, and electrolytes and correct any imbalance.

■ Toxic Dosages

Although rare, deaths have resulted directly or indirectly from anticholinergic intoxications (Johnson 1967; Slovis et al. 1971). Fever and delirium in serious anticholinergic overdosage may progress to coma and, ultimately, to cardiac and respiratory depression (Granacher and Baldessarini 1976). Death may occur, especially in children, possibly as a result of hyperpyrexia or brain stem depression (Heiser and Gillin 1971). Five deaths resulted indirectly from stramonium intoxication in which the delirious individuals died from exposure or drowning (Gowdy 1972). Thus, intoxicated patients often must be hospitalized for their own safety until their sensoriums have cleared.

References

Aaron CK, Ferm RP: Lysergic acid diethylamide and other psychedelics, in Goldfrank's Toxicologic Emergencies. Edited by Goldfrank LR, Flomenbaum NE, Lewin NA. Norwalk, CT, Appleton & Lange, 1994, pp 881–887

Abraham HD: L-5 hydroxytryptophan for LSD-induced psychosis. Am J Psychiatry 140:456–458, 1983

Abrams JM, Schulman P, White WB: Successful treatment of monoamine oxidase inhibitor-tyramine hypertensive emergency with labetalol (letter). N Engl J Med 313:52, 1985

Albertson TE, Derlet RW, Foulke GE, et al: Superiority of activated charcoal alone compared with ipecac and activated charcoal in the treatment of acute toxic ingestions. Ann Emerg Med 18:56–59, 1989

Allen MD, Greenblatt DJ, Noel BJ: Overdose with antipsychotic drugs. Am J Psychiatry 137:234–236, 1980

Andersen GO, Ritland S: Life threatening intoxication with sodium valproate. J Toxicol Clin Toxicol 33:279–284, 1995

Anggard E, Jonsson L, Hogmark A, et al: Amphetamine metabolism in amphetamine psychosis. Clin Pharmacol Ther 14:870–880, 1973

Angrist B, Lee HK, Gershon S: The antagonism of amphetamine-induced symptomatology by a neuroleptic. Am J Psychiatry 131:817–821, 1974

Aronow R, Done A: Phencyclidine overdose. JACEP 7:56–59, 1978

Aronow R, Micali JN, Done AK: A therapeutic approach to the acutely overdosed PCP patient. Journal of Psychedelic Drugs 12:259–267, 1980

Badawy AA, Evans M: Naloxone in ethanol intoxication (letter). Ann Intern Med 98:672, 1983

Barton CH, Sterling ML, Vaziri ND: Rhabdomyolysis and acute renal failure associated with phencyclidine intoxication. Arch Intern Med 40:568–569, 1980

Belanger DR, Tierney MG, Dickinson G: Effect of sodium polystyrene sulfonate on lithium bioavailability. Ann Emerg Med 21:1312–1315, 1992

Berg MJ, Berlinger WJ, Goldberg MJ, et al: Acceleration of the body clearance of phenobarbital by oral activated charcoal. N Engl J Med 307:642–644, 1982

Berlinger WJ, Spector R, Goldberg MJ, et al: Enhancement of theophylline clearance by oral activated charcoal. Clin Pharmacol Ther 33:351–354, 1983

Biederman J: Sudden death in children treated with a tricyclic antidepressant. J Am Acad Child Adolesc Psychiatry 30:495–498, 1991

Blake DR, Bramble MG, Evans JG: Is there excessive use of gastric lavage in the treatment of self-poisoning? Lancet 2:1362–1364, 1978

Boehnert MT, Lovejoy FN: Value of the QRS duration versus the serum drug level in predicting seizures and ventricular arrhythmias after acute overdose of tricyclic antidepressants. N Engl J Med 313:474–479, 1985

Boehnert MT, Lewander WJ, Gaudreault P, et al: Advances in clinical toxicology. Pediatr Clin North Am 32:193–211, 1985

Borys DJ, Setzer SC, Ling LJ, et al: Acute fluoxetine overdose: a report of 234 cases. Am J Emerg Med 10:115–120, 1992

Bosse GM, Arnold TC: Overdose with sustained-release lithium preparations. J Emerg Med 10:719–721, 1992

Bosse GM, Barefoot JA, Pfeifer MP, et al: Comparison of three methods of gut decontamination in tricyclic antidepressant overdose. J Emerg Med 13:203–209, 1995

Boyer WF, Feighner JP: An overview of paroxetine. J Clin Psychiatry 53 (2, suppl):21–26, 1992

Buckley NA: Relative toxicity of benzodiazepines in overdose. BMJ 310:219–221, 1995

Buckley NA, Whyte IM, Dawson AH: Cardiotoxicity more common in thioridazine overdose than with other neuroleptics. J Toxicol Clin Toxicol 33:199–204, 1995

Callaham M: Tricyclic antidepressant overdose. JACEP 8:413–425, 1979

Callaham M, Schumaker H, Pentel P: Phenytoin prophylaxis of cardiotoxicity in experimental amitriptyline poisoning. J Pharmacol Exp Ther 245:216–220, 1988

Chiang WK, Goldfrank LR: Amphetamines, in Goldfrank's Toxicologic Emergencies. Edited by Goldfrank LR, Flomenbaum NE, Lewin NA, et al. Norwalk, CT, Appleton & Lange, 1994, pp 509–515

Chin L, Picchioni AL, Gillespie T: Saline cathartics and saline cathartics plus activated charcoal as antidotal treatments. Clinical Toxicology 18:865–871, 1981

Chyka PA: Multiple-dose activated charcoal and enhancement of systemic drug clearance: summary of studies in animals and human volunteers. J Toxicol Clin Toxicol 33:399–405, 1995

Ciocatto E, Fagiano G, Bava GL: Clinical features and treatment of overdosage of monoamine oxidase inhibitors and their interaction with other psychotropic drugs. Resuscitation 1:69–72, 1972

Clary C, Schweizer E: Treatment of MAOI hypertensive crisis with sublingual nifedipine. J Clin Psychiatry 48:249–250, 1987

Clinton JE, Sterner S, Steimachers Z, et al: Haloperidol for sedation of disruptive emergency patients. Ann Emerg Med 16:319–322, 1987

Cooper GL: The safety of fluoxetine: an update. Br J Psychiatry 153 (suppl 3):77–86, 1988

DeBroc ME: Hemoperfusion: a useful therapy for the severely poisoned patient? Human Toxicology 5:11–14, 1986

Diagnosis and management of acute drug abuse reactions. Medical Letter 25:85–88, 1983

Divoll M, Greenblatt DJ, Lacasse Y, et al: Benzodiazepine overdosage: plasma concentrations and clinical outcome. Psychopharmacology 73:381–383, 1981

Doogan DP: Toleration and safety of sertraline: experience worldwide. International Clinical Psychopharmacology 6 (suppl 2):47–56, 1991

Drenck NE, Risbo A: Carbamazepine poisoning, a surprisingly severe case. Anaesth Intensive Care 8:203–205, 1980

Dupuis RE, Lichtman SN, Pollack GM: Acute valproic acid overdose. Clinical course and pharmacokinetic disposition of valproic acid and metabolites. Drug Saf 5:65–71, 1990

Dupuis RE, Cooper AA, Rosamond LJ, et al: Multiple delayed peak lithium concentrations following acute intoxication with an extended release product. Ann Pharmacother 30:356–359, 1996

Easom JM, Caraccio TR, Lovejoy FM: Evaluation of activated charcoal and magnesium citrate in the prevention of aspirin absorption in humans. Clin Pharmacol 1:154–156, 1982

Ellenhorn MJ, Barceloux DG: Neuroleptic drugs, in Medical Toxicology Diagnosis and Treatment of Human Poisoning. New York, Elsevier, 1988, pp 478–490

Espelin DE, Done AK: Amphetamine poisoning, effectiveness of chlorpromazine. N Engl J Med 278:1361–1365, 1968

Evans LEJ, Roscoe P, Swainson CP, et al: Treatment of drug overdosage with naloxone, a specific narcotic antagonist. Lancet 1:452–455, 1973

Farley T: Severe hypernatremic dehydration after use of an activated charcoal-sorbitol suspension. J Pediatr 109:719–722, 1986

Fauman BJ: Treatment of phencyclidine overdose (letter). Ann Emerg Med 10:165, 1981

Favin FD, Klein-Schwartz W, Oderda GM: In vitro study of lithium carbonate adsorption by activated charcoal. J Toxicol Clin Toxicol 256:443–450, 1988

Flomenbaum NE, Goldfrank LR, Weisman RS, et al: General management of the poisoned or overdosed patient, in Goldfrank's Toxicologic Emergencies. Edited by Goldfrank LR, Flomenbaum NE, Lewin NA, et al. Norwalk, CT, Appleton & Lange, 1994, pp 25–41

Flumazenil in Benzodiazepine Intoxication Multicenter Study Group: Treatment of benzodiazepine overdose with flumazenil. Clin Ther 14:978–995, 1992

Fontaine R: Novel serotonergic mechanisms and clinical experience with nefazodone. Clin Neuropharmacol 16 (suppl 3):S45–S50, 1993

Foulke GE: Identifying toxicity risk early after antidepressant overdose. Am J Emerg Med 13:123–126, 1995

Foulke GE, Albertson TE, Walby WF: Tricyclics antidepressant overdose: emergency department findings as predictions of clinical course. Am J Emerg Med 4:496–500, 1986

Freeman GE, Pasternak S, Krenzelok EP: A clinical trial using syrup of ipecac and activated charcoal concurrently. Ann Emerg Med 16:164–166, 1987

Frommer DA, Kulig KW, Marx JA, et al: Tricyclic antidepressant overdose: a review. JAMA 257:521–526, 1987

Gagrat D, Hamilton J, Belmaker RH: Intravenous diazepam in the treatment of neuroleptic-induced acute dystonia and akathisia. Am J Psychiatry 135:1232–1233, 1978

Gamble DK, Peterson LG: Trazodone overdose: four years of experience from voluntary reports. J Clin Psychiatry 47:544–546, 1986

Garrelts JC, Watson WA, Holloway KD, et al: Magnesium toxicity secondary to catharsis during management of theophylline poisoning. Am J Emerg Med 7:34–37, 1989

Gay GR, Loper KA: The use of labetalol in the management of cocaine crisis. Ann Emerg Med 17:282–283, 1988

Gelenberg AJ: And still more about overdoses with amoxapine (Asendin). Biological Therapies in Psychiatry 6:10–11, 1983

Geller E, Crome P, Schaller MD, et al: Risks and benefits of therapy with flumazenil in mixed drug intoxications. Eur Neurol 31:241–250, 1991

Gelman CR, Rumack BH (eds): Flumazenil. Denver, CO, DRUGDEX® Information System, MICROMEDEX, Inc., 1994

Goetz CM, Krenzelok EP, Lopez G, et al: Buspirone toxicity: a prospective study (Abstract 167). Vet Hum Toxicology 31:371, 1989

Gold MS, Washton AM, Dackis CA: Cocaine abuse: neurochemistry, phenomenology, and treatment, in Cocaine Use in America (National Institute on Drug Abuse [NIDA] Research Monograph 61; DHMS Publ No [ADM] 85-1414). Edited by Kozel NJ, Adams EH. Washington, DC, Superintendent of Documents, U.S. Government Printing Office, 1985

Goldberg MJ, Berlinger WG: Treatment of phenobarbital overdoses with activated charcoal. JAMA 247:2400–2401, 1982

Goldfrank LR, Weisman RS: Opioids, in Goldfrank's Toxicologic Emergencies. Edited by Goldfrank LR, Flomenbaum NE, Lewin NA, et al. Norwalk, CT, Appleton & Lange, 1994, pp 769–783

Goldfrank LR, Weisman RS, Errick JK, et al: A dosing nomogram for continuous infusion intravenous naloxone. Ann Emerg Med 15:566–570, 1986

Goldfrank LR, Lewin NA, Osborn H: Phencyclidine, in Goldfrank's Toxicologic Emergencies. Edited by Goldfrank LR, Flomenbaum NE, Lewin NA, et al. Norwalk, CT, Appleton & Lange, 1994, pp 875–880

Gowdy JM: Stramonium intoxication: review of symptomatology in 212 cases. JAMA 221:585–587, 1972

Granacher RP, Baldessarini RJ: Physostigmine treatment of delirium induced by anticholinergics. Am Fam Physician 13:99–103, 1976

Granier R, Azoyan P, Chataigner D, et al: Acute fluvoxamine poisoning. J Int Med Res 21:197–208, 1993

Greenblatt DJ, Allen MD, Noel BJ, et al: Acute overdosage with benzodiazepine derivatives. Clin Pharmacol Ther 21:497–514, 1977

Griggs E, Ward M: LSD toxicity: a suspected cause of death. J Ky Med Assoc 75:172–173, 1977

Gueye PN, Hoffman JR, Taboulet P, et al: Empiric use of flumazenil in comatose patients: limited applicability of criteria to define low risk. Ann Emerg Med 27:730–735, 1996

Hansen HE, Amdisen A: Lithium intoxication (report of 23 cases and review of 100 cases from the literature). Quarterly Journal of Medicine 47:123–144, 1978

Hansten PD: Drug Interactions: Clinical Significance of Drug–Drug Interactions and Drug Effects on Clinical Laboratory Results. Philadelphia, PA, Lea & Febiger, 1979

Harvey SC: Hypnotics and sedatives, in The Pharmacological Basis of Therapeutics, 7th Edition. Edited by Gilman AG, Goodman LS, Rall TW, et al. New York, Macmillan, 1985, pp 339–371

Hassan L, Miller DO: Toxicity and elimination of trazodone after overdose. Clinical Pharmacy 4:97–100, 1985

Hayes PE, Kristoff CA: Adverse reactions to five new antidepressants. Clinical Pharmacy 5:471–480, 1986

Heiser JF, Gillin JC: The reversal of anticholinergic drug-induced delirium and coma with physostigmine. Am J Psychiatry 127:1050–1054, 1971

Henry GC, Osborn H, Weisman RS: Lithium, in Goldfrank's Toxicologic Emergencies. Edited by Goldfrank LR, Flomenbaum NE, Lewin NA, et al. Norwalk, CT, Appleton & Lange, 1994, pp 761–768

Henry JA, Alexander CA, Sener EK: Relative mortality from overdose of antidepressants. BMJ 310:221–224, 1995

Hoffman JR, Votey SR, Bayer M, et al: Effect of hypertonic sodium bicarbonate in the treatment of moderate-to-severe cyclic antidepressant overdose. Am J Emerg Med 4:336–341, 1993

Hoffman RS, Goldfrank LR: The poisoned patient with altered consciousness: controversies in the use of a "coma control." JAMA 274:562–569, 1995

Hojer J, Baehrendtz S, Matell G, et al: Diagnostic utility of flumazenil in coma with suspected poisoning: a double-blind, randomized controlled study. BMJ 301:1308–1311, 1990

Hojer J, Malmlund HO, Berg A: Clinical features in 28 consecutive cases of laboratory confirmed massive poisoning with carbamazepine alone. J Toxicol Clin Toxicol 31:449–458, 1993

Howland MA: Syrup of ipecac, in Goldfrank's Toxicologic Emergencies. Edited by Goldfrank LR, Flomenbaum NE, Lewin NA, et al. Norwalk, CT, Appleton & Lange, 1994a, pp 63–65

Howland MA: Activated charcoal, in Goldfrank's Toxicologic Emergencies. Edited by Goldfrank LR, Flomenbaum NE, Lewin NA, et al. Norwalk, CT, Appleton & Lange, 1994b, pp 63–73

Howland MA: Cathartics, in Goldfrank's Toxicologic Emergencies. Edited by Goldfrank LR, Flomenbaum NE, Lewin NA, et al. Norwalk, CT, Appleton & Lange, 1994c, pp 72–73

Howland MA: Whole-bowel irrigation, in Goldfrank's Toxicologic Emergencies. Edited by Goldfrank LR, Flomenbaum NE, Lewin NA, et al. Norwalk, CT, Appleton & Lange, 1994d, pp 74–75

Howland MA: Flumazenil, in Goldfrank's Toxicologic Emergencies. Edited by Goldfrank LR, Flomenbaum NE, Lewin NA. Norwalk, CT, Appleton & Lange, 1994e, pp 805–810

Hulten BA, Adams R, Askenasi R, et al: Predicting severity of tricyclic overdose. J Toxicol Clin Toxicol 30:161–170, 1992

Isner JM, Estes M, Thompson PD, et al: Acute cardiac events temporally related to cocaine abuse. N Engl J Med 315:1438–1443, 1986

Janowsky D, Curtis G, Zosook S, et al: Trazodone-aggravated ventricular arrhythmia. J Clin Psychopharmacol 3:372–376, 1983

Jarvis MR: Clinical pharmacokinetics of tricyclic antidepressant overdose. Psychopharmacol Bull 27:541–550, 1991

Johnson CE: Mystical force of the nightshade. International Journal of Neuropsychiatry 3:268–275, 1967

Jordan C, Lehane JR, Jones JG: Respiratory depression following diazepam: reversal with high-dose naloxone. Anesthesiology 53:293–298, 1980

Kapur S, Mieczkowski T, Mann JJ: Antidepressant medications and the relative risk of suicide attempt and suicide. JAMA 268:3441–3445, 1992

Karkkainen S, Neuvonen PJ: Pharmacokinetics of amitriptyline influenced by oral charcoal and urine pH. International Journal of Clinical Pharmacology, Therapy, and Toxicology 24:326–332, 1986

Kasarskis EJ, Kuo CS, Berger R, et al: Carbamazepine-induced cardiac dysfunction: characterization of two distinct clinical syndromes. Arch Intern Med 152:186–191, 1992

Khantzian EJ, McKenna GJ: Acute toxic and withdrawal reactions associated with drug use and abuse. Ann Intern Med 90:361–372, 1979

King WD: Syrup of ipecac: a drug review. Clinical Toxicology 17:353–358, 1980

Knudsen K, Heath A: Effects of self-poisoning with maprotiline. BMJ 288:601–603, 1984

Kosten TR, Kleber HD: Sudden death in cocaine abusers: relation to neuroleptic malignant syndrome. Lancet 1:1198–1199, 1987

Kulig K: Management of poisoning associated with "newer" antidepressant agents. Ann Emerg Med 15:1039–1045, 1986

Kulig K, Rumack BH: Efficacy of naloxone in clonidine poisoning (letter). American Journal of Diseases of Children 137:807, 1983

Kulig K, Rumack B, Sullivan J, et al: Amoxapine overdose: coma, seizures without cardiotoxic effects. JAMA 248:1092–1094, 1982

Langou RA, Van Dyke C, Tahan SR, et al: Cardiovascular manifestations of tricyclic antidepressant overdose. Am Heart J 100:458–464, 1980

Lau GT, Horowitz BZ: Sertraline overdose. Acad Emerg Med 3:132–136, 1996

Lee A: Treatment of drug-induced dystonic reactions. JACEP 8:453–457, 1979

Lehrman SN, Bauman ML: Carbamazepine overdose. American Journal of Diseases of Children 135:768–769, 1981

Leslie PJ, Heyworth R, Prescott LF: Cardiac complication of carbamazepine intoxication: treatment by hemoperfusion (letter). BMJ 286:1018, 1983

Levenson JL: Neuroleptic malignant syndrome. Am J Psychiatry 142:1137–1145, 1985

Levine SR, Washington JM, Jefferson MF, et al: "Crack" cocaine–associated stroke. Neurology 37:1849–1853, 1987

Lewin NA: Physostigmine salicylate, in Goldfrank's Toxicologic Emergencies. Edited by Goldfrank LR, Flomenbaum NE, Lewin NA, et al. Norwalk, CT, Appleton & Lange, 1994a, pp 607–608

Lewin NA: Sodium bicarbonate, in Goldfrank's Toxicologic Emergencies. Edited by Goldfrank LR, Flomenbaum NE, Lewin NA. Norwalk, CT, Appleton & Lange, 1994b, pp 735–737

Lewin NA, Wang RY: Neuroleptic agents, in Goldfrank's Toxicologic Emergencies. Edited by Goldrank LR, Flomenbaum NE, Lewin NA, et al. Norwalk, CT, Appleton & Lange, 1994, pp 739–747

Lewin NA, Goldfrank LR, Hoffman RS: Cocaine, in Goldfrank's Toxicologic Emergencies. Edited by Goldfrank LR, Flomenbaum NE, Lewin NA, et al. Norwalk, CT, Appleton & Lange, 1994, pp 847–862

Lheureux P, Debailleul G, DeWitt O, et al: Zolpidem intoxication mimicking narcotic overdose: response to flumazenil. Human Exp Toxicol 9:105–107, 1990

Liebelt EL, Francis PD, Woolf AD: ECG lead aVR versus QRS interval in predicting seizures and arrhythmias in acute tricyclic antidepressant toxicity. Ann Emerg Med 26:195–201, 1995

Litovitz T: Benzodiazepines, in Clinical Management of Poisoning and Drug Overdose. Edited by Haddad LM, Winchester JF. Philadelphia, PA, WB Saunders, 1983, pp 475–487

Litovitz TL, Troutman WG: Amoxapine overdose: seizures and fatalities. JAMA 250:1069–1071, 1983

Litovitz TL, Norman SA, Veltri JC: 1985 Annual Report of the American Association of Poison Control Centers National Data Collection System. Am J Emerg Med 4:427–458, 1986

Manno BR, Manno JE: Toxicology of ipecac: a review. Clinical Toxicology 10:221–222, 1977

Marcus RN: Safety and tolerability of nefazodone. J Psychopharmacology 10 (suppl 1):11–17, 1996

Marshall JB, Forken AD: Cardiovascular effects of tricyclic antidepressant drugs: therapeutic usage, overdose, and management of complications. Am Heart J 103:402–414, 1982

Mateer JR, Clark MR: Lithium toxicity with rarely reported ECG manifestations. Ann Emerg Med 11:208–211, 1982

Matter BJ, Donat PE, Bril ML, et al: Tranylcypromine sulfate poisoning: successful treatment of hemodialysis. Arch Intern Med 116:18–20, 1965

Matthew H: Acute poisoning: some myths and misconceptions. BMJ 1:519–522, 1971

May DC, Morris SW, Stewart RM, et al: Neuroleptic malignant syndrome: response to dantrolene sodium. Ann Intern Med 98:183–184, 1983

Mayron R, Ruiz E: Phenytoin: does it reverse tricyclic antidepressant–induced cardiac conduction abnormalities? Ann Emerg Med 15:876–880, 1986

McCarron MM: Phencyclidine overdose, in Phencyclidine: An Update. Edited by Clonet DH. NIDA Research Monograph 64. DMHS Publ No (ADM) 86-1443. Washington, DC, Superintendent of Documents, U.S. Government Printing Office, 1986

McCarron MM, Schulze BW, Walberg CB, et al: Short-acting barbiturate overdosage. JAMA 248:55–61, 1982

McNamara R, Aaron C, Gembory SM, et al: Sorbitol catharsis does not enhance efficacy of charcoal on a simulated acetaminophen overdose. Ann Emerg Med 17:243–246, 1988

Menashe PI, Gottlieb JE: Hyperthermia, rhabdomyolysis, and renal failure after recreational use of cocaine. South Med J 81:379–380, 1988

Mueller PS, Vester JW, Fermaglich J: Neuroleptic malignant syndrome: successful treatment with bromocriptine. JAMA 249:386–388, 1983

Nahas GG, Goldfrank LR: Marijuana, in Goldfrank's Toxicologic Emergencies. Edited by Goldfrank LR, Flomenbaum NE, Lewin NA, et al. Norwalk, CT, Appleton & Lange, 1994, pp 889–898

Neuvonen PJ, Elonen E: Effect of activated charcoal on absorption and elimination of phenobarbital, carbamazepine and phenylbutazone in man. Eur J Clin Pharmacol 17:51–57, 1980

Nicholson DP: The immediate management of overdose. Med Clin North Am 67:1279–1293, 1983

Nierenberg DW, Semprebon M: The central nervous system serotonergic syndrome. Clin Pharmacol Ther 53:84–88, 1993

Osborn H: Phenytoin and other anticonvulsants, in Goldfrank's Toxicologic Emergencies. Edited by Goldfrank LR, Flomenbaum NE, Lewin NA, et al. Norwalk, CT, Appleton & Lange, 1994, pp 589–600

Osborn H, Goldfrank LR: Sedative-hypnotic agents, in Goldfrank's Toxicologic Emergencies. Edited by Goldfrank LR, Flomenbaum NE, Lewin NA, et al. Norwalk, CT, Appleton & Lange, 1994, pp 787–804

Paderson OL, Gram LF, Kaistensen CB, et al: Overdosage of antidepressants: clinical and pharmacokinetic aspects. Eur J Clin Pharmacol 23:513–521, 1982

Park J, Proudfoot AT: Acute poisoning with maprotiline hydrochloride (letter). BMJ 1:573, 1977

Patal R, Das M, Palazzolo M, et al: Myoglobinuric acute renal failure in phencyclidine overdose: report of observation in eight cases. Ann Emerg Med 9:549–553, 1980

Perez-Reyes M: Urine pH and phencyclidine excretion. Clin Pharmacol Ther 32:535–541, 1982

Perry PJ, Wilding DC, Juhl RP: Anticholinergic psychosis. Am J Hosp Pharm 35:725–727, 1978

Perry PJ, Calloway RA, Cook BL, et al: Theophylline precipitated alterations of lithium clearance. Acta Psychiatr Scand 69:528–537, 1984

Picchioni A, Chin L, Gillespie T: Evaluation of activated charcoal-sorbitol suspension as an antidote. Clinical Toxicology 29:433–444, 1982

Pond SM: Techniques to enhance elimination of toxic compounds, in Goldfrank's Toxicologic Emergencies. Edited by Goldfrank LR, Flomenbaum NE, Lewin NA, et al. Norwalk, CT, Appleton & Lange, 1994, pp 73–83

Pond SM, Olson KR, Osterloh JH, et al: Randomized study of the treatment of phenobarbital overdose with repeated doses of activated charcoal. JAMA 251:3104–3108, 1984

Pond SM, Lewis-Driver DJ, Williams GM, et al: Gastric emptying in acute overdose: a prospective randomized controlled trial. Med J Aust 163:345–349, 1995

Pradhan SN, Hollister LE: Abuse of LSD and other hallucinogenic drugs, in Drug Abuse: Clinical and Basic Aspects. Edited by Pradhan SN, Dultra SN. St. Louis, MO, CV Mosby, 1977, pp 274–289

Pumariega AJ, Muller B, Rivers-Bulkeley N: Acute renal failure secondary to amoxapine overdose. JAMA 248:3141–3142, 1982

Ramoska E, Sacchetti AD: Propanolol-induced hypertension in treatment of cocaine intoxication. Ann Emerg Med 14:1112–1113, 1985

Risch SC, Groom GP, Janowsky DS: Interfaces of psychopharmacology and cardiology, part II. J Clin Psychiatry 42:47–59, 1981a

Risch SC, Groom GP, Janowsky DS: Interfaces of psychopharmacology and cardiology, part I. J Clin Psychiatry 42:22–34, 1981b

Roberge RJ, Martin TG, Schneider SM: Use of sodium polystyrene in a lithium overdose. Ann Emerg Med 22:1911–1915, 1993

Rockrock JF, Rubenstein R, Lyden PD: Ischemic stroke associated with methamphetamine inhalation. Neurology 38:589–592, 1988

Rosenberg J, Benowitz NL, Pond S: Pharmacokinetics of drug overdose. Clin Pharmacokinet 6:161–192, 1981

Rudolph RL, Derivan RT: The safety and tolerability of venlafaxine hydrochloride: analysis of the clinical trials database. J Clin Psychopharmacol 16 (suppl 2):54S–61S, 1996

Rumack BH: Anticholinergic poisoning: treatment with physostigmine. Pediatrics 52:449–451, 1973

Rumack BH: Phencyclidine overdose: an overview (editorial). Ann Emerg Med 9:595, 1980

Rumack BH, Hess AJ, Gelman CR (eds): POISINDEX® System. Englewood, CO, Micromedex, Inc., 1996

Sakkas P, Davis JM, Janicak PG, et al: Drug treatment of the neuroleptic malignant syndrome. Psychopharmacol Bull 27:381–384, 1991

Sauter D: Monoamine oxidase inhibitors, in Goldfrank's Toxicologic Emergencies. Edited by Goldfrank LR, Flomenbaum NE, Lewin NA, et al. Norwalk, CT, Appleton & Lange, 1994, pp 749–759

Schmidt S, Schmitz-Buhl M: Signs and symptoms of carbamazepine overdose. J Neurol 242:169–173, 1995

Schou M: Preclinical and clinical pharmacology of lithium, in Principles of Psychopharmacology. Edited by Clark WG, del Giudice J. New York, Academic Press, 1978, pp 343–356

Schou M: The recognition and management of lithium intoxication, in Handbook of Lithium Therapy. Edited by Johnson FN. Lancaster, England, MTP Press, 1980, pp 394–402

Schwartz WK, Oderda GM: Management of cocaine intoxication. Clinical Toxicology Consultant 2:45–58, 1980

Serfaty M, Masterson G: Fatal poisonings attributed to benzodiazepines in Britain during the 1980s. Br J Psychiatry 163:386–393, 1993

Seymour JF: Carbamazepine overdose: features of 33 cases (review). Drug Saf 8:81–88, 1993

Slovis TL, Ott JE, Teitelbaum DT, et al: Physostigmine therapy in acute tricyclic antidepressant poisoning. Clinical Toxicology 4:451–459, 1971

Smart RF, Bateman R: Unfavorable reactions to LSD: a review and analyses of the available case reports. Canadian Medical Association Journal 97:1214–1221, 1967

Smilkstein MJ, Flomenbaum NE: Techniques used to prevent absorption of toxic compounds, in Goldfrank's Toxicologic Emergencies. Edited by Goldfrank LR, Flomenbaum NE, Lewin NA, et al. Norwalk, CT, Appleton & Lange, 1994, pp 47–59

Smith DE: The characteristics of dependence in high dose methamphetamine abuse. Int J Addict 4:453–459, 1969

Smith DE, Wesson DR, Buxton ME, et al: The diagnosis and treatment of the PCP abuse syndrome, in Phencyclidine (PCP) Abuse: An Appraisal. Edited by Petersen RC, Stillman RC. Rockville, MD, NIDA Research Monograph 21, DHEW Publ No (ADM) 78-728, 1978, pp 224–240

Smith HWB III, Liberman HA, Brod SL, et al: Acute myocardial infarction temporally related to cocaine use. Ann Intern Med 107:13–18, 1987

Smith SW, Ling LJ, Halstenson CE: Whole-bowel irrigation as a treatment for lithium overdose. Ann Emerg Med 20:536–539, 1991

Somni RW, Crimson ML, Bowden CL: Fluoxetine: a serotonin-specific second-generation antidepressant. Pharmacotherapy 7:1–15, 1987

Spiker D, Biggs J: Tricyclic antidepressants—prolonged plasma levels after overdose. JAMA 236:1711–1712, 1976

Spiller HA, Krenzelok EP, Cookson E: Carbamazepine overdose: a prospective study of serum levels and toxicity. J Toxicol Clin Toxicol 28:445–458, 1990

Spiller HA, Ramoska EA, Krenzelok EP, et al: Bupropion overdose: a 3-year multicenter retrospective analysis. Am J Emerg Med 12:43–45, 1994

Spivey WH: Flumazenil and seizures: an analysis of 43 cases. Clin Ther 24:292–305, 1992

Spivey WH, Roberts JR, Derlet RW: A clinical trial of escalating doses of flumazenil for reversal of suspected benzodiazepine overdose in the emergency department. Ann Emerg Med 22:1813–1821, 1993

Stewart JJ: Effects of emetic and cathartic agents on the gastrointestinal tract and the treatment of toxic ingestion. J Toxicol Clin Toxicol 20:199–253, 1983

Sullivan JB, Rumack BH, Peterson RG: Acute carbamazepine toxicity resulting from overdose. Neurology 31:621–624, 1981

Swartz CM, Sherman A: The treatment of tricyclic antidepressant overdose with repeated charcoal. J Clin Psychopharmacol 4:336–340, 1984

Tank JE, Palmer BF: Simultaneous "in series" hemodialysis and hemoperfusion in the management of valproic acid overdose. Am J Kidney Dis 22:341–344, 1993

Thompson WL, Johnson AD, Maddrey WL: Diazepam and paraldehyde for treatment of severe delirium tremens: a controlled trial. Ann Intern Med 82:175–180, 1975

Thomsen K, Schou M: The treatment of lithium poisoning, in Lithium Research and Therapy. Edited by Johnson FN. London, Academic Press, 1975, pp 227–236

Tokarski GF, Young MJ: Criteria for admitting patients with tricyclic antidepressant overdose. J Emerg Med 6:121–124, 1988

Tollefson GD: Monoamine oxidase inhibitors: a review. J Clin Psychiatry 44:280–288, 1983

Tomaszewski C, Musso C, Pearson JR, et al: Lithium absorption prevented by sodium polystyrene sulfonate in volunteers. Ann Emerg Med 21:1308–1311, 1992

Traeger SM, Haug MT: Reduction of diazepam serum half-life and reversal of coma by activated charcoal in a patient with severe liver disease. Clinical Toxicology 24:329–337, 1984

Tuchman AJ, Daras M, Zalzal P, et al: Intracranial hemorrhage after cocaine abuse (letter). JAMA 257:1175, 1987

Turner P, Young JH, Paterson J: Influence of urinary pH on the excretion of tranylcypromine sulfate. Nature 215:881–882, 1967

Vale JA, Proudfoot AT: How useful is activated charcoal? BMJ 306:78–79, 1993

Varipapa RJ, Oderda G: Effect of milk on ipecac-induced emesis. N Engl J Med 296:112–113, 1977

Venlafaxine: a new dimension in antidepressant pharmacotherapy. J Clin Psychiatry 54:119–126, 1993

Versaci AA, Nakamoto S, Koloff WJ: Phenelzine intoxication: report of a case treated by hemodialysis. Ohio State Medical Journal 60:770–771, 1964

Virmani R, Robinowitz M, Smialek JE, et al: Cardiovascular effects of cocaine: an autopsy study of 40 patients. Am Heart J 115:1068–1076, 1988

Wason S, Baker RC, Carolan P, et al: Carbamazepine overdose—the effects of multiple dose activated charcoal. J Toxicol Clin Toxicol 30:39–48, 1992

Weinbroum A, Rudick V, Sorkine P, et al: Use of flumazenil in the treatment of drug overdose: a double blind and open clinical study in 110 patients. Crit Care Med 24:199–206, 1996

Weisman RS: Naloxone, in Goldfrank's Toxicologic Emergencies. Edited by Goldfrank LR, Flomenbaum NE, Lewin NA, et al. Norwalk, CT, Appleton & Lange, 1994, pp 784–786

Weisman RS, Goldfrank LR: Antihistamines, in Goldfrank's Toxicologic Emergencies. Edited by Goldfrank LR, Flomenbaum NE, Lewin NA. Norwalk, CT, Appleton & Lange, 1994, pp 601–606

Weisman RS, Howland MA, Hoffman RS, et al: Cyclic antidepressants, in Goldfrank's Toxicologic Emergencies. Edited by Goldfrank LR, Flomenbaum NE, Lewin NA, et al. Norwalk, CT, Appleton & Lange, 1994, pp 725–734

Welti CV, Fishbain DA: Cocaine-induced psychosis and sudden death in recreational cocaine users. J Forensic Sci 30:873–880, 1985

Wenger TL, Stern WC: The cardiovascular profile of bupropion. J Clin Psychiatry 44:176–182, 1983

Wilde MI, Plosker GL, Benfield P: Fluvoxamine: an updated review of its pharmacology and therapeutic use in depressive illness. Drugs 46:895–924, 1993

Wyss PA, Radovanovic D, Meierabt PJ: Acute overdose of zolpidem. Schweitzerische Medizinische Wochenschrift 126:750–756, 1996

Young T, Lawson GS, Gacono CB: Clinical aspects of phencyclidine (PCP). Int J Addict 22:1–15, 1987

10

Management of Withdrawal

The following schedules are presented individually as reviews of alcohol, opiate, anxiolytic-hypnotic, nicotine, and central nervous system (CNS) stimulant withdrawal. This chapter addresses the medical management of acute withdrawal syndromes and not maintenance treatment. The long-term management of alcohol and drug dependence is discussed in Chapter 7.

It is important to note that polysubstance abuse is common (Harrison et al. 1984). For example, 50% of heroin users may abuse cocaine, whereas 25%–50% may use alcohol to excess (Kreek 1987). As many as 30% of alcoholic patients admitted for management of withdrawal are concurrently abusing alcohol and benzodiazepines (Benzer and Cushman 1980). Because the morbidity and mortality risk is greater with anxiolytic-hypnotics than with opiates or CNS stimulants, the primary treatment of the patient with mixed substance abuse should be directed toward anxiolytic-hypnotic withdrawal.

Alcohol Withdrawal and Withdrawal Schedule

■ Presentation

Tolerance to and *physical dependence* on ethanol are probably manifestations of compensatory neurophysiological changes that offset the depressant effect of alcohol on neuronal excitability, impulse conduction, and transmitter release. When alcohol ingestion is abruptly discontinued or rapidly decreased, the compensatory changes are maladaptive and give rise to the signs and symptoms of the withdrawal reaction (Sellers and Kalant 1976).

The severity of the reaction varies with the intensity and duration of the preceding alcohol exposure. It is generally accepted that if 16 oz of whiskey (40%–55% ethanol) is ingested daily for 2–3 weeks, physical dependence will occur (Liskow and Goodwin 1987). As the amount of ethanol ingested daily and the duration of exposure increases, so does the likelihood of severe withdrawal. In one study, individuals ingesting a fifth (26 oz) of whiskey per day or its equivalent for 7 weeks or longer were at an increased risk of developing severe withdrawal (Isbell et al. 1955). This finding was confirmed in a later study in which up to 40 oz of whiskey ingested for 24 days resulted in severe withdrawal (Mendelson and LaDou 1964).

Withdrawal symptoms occur on a continuum. The withdrawal syndrome is classified as minor or major and may present with any or all of the signs and symptoms noted (Sellers and Kalant 1976).

Minor Withdrawal

This phase is characterized by the onset of signs and symptoms 8–12 hours after reduction or discontinuation of alcohol intake. Individuals may experience tremor, irritability, anorexia, nausea, vomiting, epigastric distress, diaphoresis, mild to moderate elevation of vital signs, and insomnia. Symptoms reach a peak within 24 hours and may begin to subside within 48–72 hours. Visual hallucinations in a clear sensorium may be observed during this phase (Sellers and Kalant 1976).

Seizures during withdrawal are typically generalized, nonfocal, and two to six in number; 90% occur within 7 to 48 hours of cessation of drinking (Guthrie 1989; Reed and Liskow 1987; Sellers and Kalant 1976). Seizures have been reported to occur in 7%–15% of individuals; they require treatment if they are repeated, continuous, or life-threatening. Seizures occurring after 48 hours and status epilepticus seizures are unusual, as are seizures occurring after the onset of delirium tremens. Seizures occurring after 48 hours may suggest withdrawal from a drug other than or in addition to alcohol (e.g., long-acting benzodiazepines). (See **Anxiolytic-Hypnotic Withdrawal and Withdrawal Schedule** [page 569].)

Major Withdrawal

The minor phase of withdrawal may progress to major withdrawal (delirium tremens), which is manifested by worsening of tremors *(tremens)* and marked elevation of vital signs, incontinence, insomnia, increased psychomotor activity, visual and (infrequently) auditory hallucinations, and profound disorientation *(delirium).* Signs of major withdrawal are most evident between 48 and 60 hours after alcohol discontinuation and generally last about 60 hours. Delirium tremens occurs in less than 5% of hospitalized patients. Estimates of the mortality rate of delirium tremens have ranged from 45% in 1910 to 2% in 1986 (Guthrie 1989; Sellers and Kalant 1976).

Death may result from hyperthermia, peripheral vascular collapse, and/or infection. In many cases, the cause of death is not apparent (Isbell et al. 1955).

The alcohol withdrawal syndrome is self-limited. If the patient does not die, *recovery* occurs within 5 to 7 days without treatment (Reed and Liskow 1987; Sellers and Kalant 1976).

■ Treatment

Although many older treatments have been used for management of alcohol withdrawal, benzodiazepines remain the treatment of choice (Bird and Makela 1994; Erstad and Cotugno 1995; Sellers and Kalant 1976). Newer treatments investigated in alcohol withdrawal include α-blockers (e.g., clonidine), β-blockers (e.g., propranolol, atenolol), and *valproate* (Erstad and Cotugno 1995; Keck et al. 1992). Although blood pressure and pulse may be controlled with α- and β-blockers, the ability of the newer treatments to prevent seizures and delirium tremens has not been adequately studied. Typically, studies of newer treatments have not included enough patients to detect differences in these adverse effects (Guthrie 1989; Reed and Liskow 1987). Also, the benefit of combining one of these newer treatments with a benzodiazepine has not been investigated. *Carbamazepine* has shown promise in the treatment of alcohol withdrawal but requires further study (Erstad and Cotugno 1995; Guthrie 1989; Keck et al. 1992; Stuppaeck et al. 1992).

Although *oral* and *intravenous ethanol* have been advocated for treatment of ethanol withdrawal, the efficacy and safety of these agents have been compared with those of benzodiazepines in only a few studies involving limited numbers of patients (Craft et al. 1994). Further investigation is required to determine the utility of intravenous ethanol in the prevention of withdrawal in trauma and medically ill patients.

Antipsychotics do not prevent alcohol withdrawal signs and symptoms, but may be useful in the management of major withdrawal (see Delirium Tremens [page 558] under *Complicated Withdrawal,* below) (Liskow and Goodwin 1987).

General Management

Multivitamin preparations are commonly given, although their value is unproven. Typically, *thiamine* 50–100 mg is given parenterally in the management of Wernicke's encephalopathy. There is no evidence to justify the routine daily oral administration of thiamine, but it is advisable to give at least a single parenteral dose to all hospitalized patients who have a history of significant ethanol intake (Erstad and Cotugno 1995). *Hydration* may be required, although often, in withdrawal, overhydration may be present. *Elec-

trolyte disturbances should be managed, as should their resultant medical problems (Erstad and Cotugno 1995; Guthrie 1989; Reed and Liskow 1987; Sellers and Kalant 1976). There is no evidence that magnesium alone will prevent seizures or delirium tremens (Erstad and Cotugno 1995; Reed and Liskow 1987).

Uncomplicated Withdrawal

Only 15%–30% of hospitalized patients will require pharmacological management for withdrawal (Naranjo et al. 1983; Shaw et al. 1981; Wartenberg et al. 1990; Whitfield et al. 1978). One strategy for separating patients who require pharmacological management from those who do not is to monitor for minor signs of withdrawal. Changes in several of the following parameters would indicate a patient potentially at risk for severe withdrawal: elevated systolic (i.e., >160 mm Hg) and diastolic (i.e., >90 mm Hg) blood pressure, pulse (i.e., >90), and temperature (i.e., >38°C) as well as nausea, vomiting, diaphoresis, or tremor present 8–15 hours after the cessation or reduction of alcohol intake. Several scales have been developed and modified for assessing a patient's need for pharmacological management, but none have been universally accepted (Wartenberg et al. 1990).

Unfortunately, it is not possible to separate patients who will experience only minor withdrawal symptoms from those likely to develop delirium tremens.

▶ Benzodiazepines

Benzodiazepines (BZDs) are superior to placebo for prevention of alcohol withdrawal and are the treatment of choice (Guthrie 1989; Liskow and Goodwin 1987; Reed and Liskow 1987).

Provided that appropriate doses and schedules are maintained, any BZD should be equally successful in withdrawing a patient from alcohol. Chlordiazepoxide (Librium®, generic), diazepam (Valium®, generic), lorazepam (Ativan®, generic), oxazepam (Serax®, generic), alprazolam (Xanax®, generic), and clorazepate (Tranxene®, generic) have been studied in alcohol withdrawal (Guthrie 1989; Reed and Liskow 1987). However, most literature involves chlordiazepoxide and diazepam. (For approximate equivalent oral doses of benzodiazepines, see the Product List in Chapter 4.)

Short-acting BZDs (e.g., oxazepam, lorazepam) are proposed to be of benefit in patients with liver disease because the metabolism of these agents is less impaired. However, it has been suggested that these drugs might increase the risk of withdrawal if a proper dose and schedule are not maintained (Bird and Makela 1994). If a short-acting BZD is used, close attention to dose and interval is necessary. Generally, in uncomplicated patients, a long-acting BZD (i.e., chlordiazepoxide, diazepam, clorazepate) is preferred in alcohol withdrawal (Bird and Makela 1994; Guthrie 1989; Reed and Liskow 1987). (For information on the pharmacokinetics of benzodiazepines, see Chapter 4.)

Chlordiazepoxide is routinely used for withdrawal; a suggested withdrawal protocol for individuals able to take oral medications is presented in Table 10–1. "Symptom-triggered" treatment, in which a BZD is administered on an "as-needed" basis, has been reported to be as efficacious as routinely administered drug, although it requires less drug and is associated with a shorter withdrawal time (Saitz et al. 1994). However, this approach has been studied only on an acute alcohol detoxification unit with experienced staff and a high staff–patient ratio. The utility of this schedule, which requires close monitoring of patients, may be reduced in a busy general medical or surgical ward.

Orders should also indicate that doses are to be held if a patient is asleep or is showing signs of BZD excess (e.g., nystagmus, slurred speech, ataxia, hypersomnia). As-needed (prn) orders are not recommended, as they may leave the patient undertreated. Likewise, the physician should evaluate each dosage period and write new orders, if necessary. Generally, the suggested regimen is adequate for most individuals undergoing withdrawal. Most patients do not need 300 mg on day 1, but usually require 100–200 mg. Occasionally, the dose will need to be adjusted upward (if withdrawal symptoms occur) or decreased (if intoxication symptoms develop).

If the patient displays breakthrough signs or symptoms between oral doses, especially during the first 24 hours, a supplemental parenteral dose of lorazepam 2–4 mg im or iv or of diazepam 10–15 mg iv should be given q30m–2h rather than altering the oral administration schedule.

Table 10–1. Ethanol withdrawal with chlordiazepoxide

Treatment day	Dose (mg)	Schedule
1	50	q4h
2	50	q6h
3	25	q4h
4	25	q6h
5	—	—

Source. Guthrie 1989; Sellers and Kalant 1976.

An alternative protocol to the tapering schedule presented in Table 10–1 uses loading doses of diazepam or chlordiazepoxide (Guthrie 1989; Wartenberg et al. 1990). Diazepam 20 mg po q1–2h or chlordiazepoxide 100 mg initially, followed by 50 mg q1h po, is administered until the patient demonstrates signs of intoxication (e.g., ataxia, dysarthria, sustained nystagmus, sedation). Generally, the patient receives no further medication. This protocol warrants further research.

▶ Barbiturates

Barbiturates have been replaced by the BZDs in the treatment of alcohol withdrawal. Although the barbiturates are cross-tolerant with ethanol, the BZDs offer a wider therapeutic index (i.e., a higher threshold for toxicity). Initial doses of **secobarbital** and **pentobarbital** in the management of withdrawal range from 600 to 1,200 mg in the first 24 hours; these doses are tapered over the next 5 days. These drugs should be administered on a q6h schedule. **Phenobarbital,** which is longer acting (half-life 4–5 days) than secobarbital and pentobarbital, has been administered in doses ranging from 180 to 360 mg in the first 24 hours of withdrawal. Although its half-life suggests that tapering would not be necessary, phenobarbital is usually tapered over 4–5 days (Jaffe 1980).

Barbiturates, as well as other anxiolytic and hypnotic drugs, should not be administered to an intoxicated patient because of potentiation of CNS-depressant effects.

Complicated Withdrawal

▶ Patient NPO/Vomiting

If the patient is unable to follow the oral withdrawal protocol outlined in Table 10–1, diazepam 10–15 mg iv or lorazepam 2–4 mg im or iv may be substituted for chlordiazepoxide 50 mg as equivalent doses. If the patient is vomiting, often only one or two doses are needed, after which the oral schedule can be instituted.

▶ Delirium Tremens

Patients should be examined for injuries and major medical illnesses, such as pneumonia and meningitis. If any such conditions are found, the patient should be medically managed as discussed previously (see *General Management* [page 555]). In addition, to reduce agitation and autonomic hyperactivity and to prevent exhaustion, the patient should receive pharmacological treatment.

Traditionally, in those patients in whom **induction of a calm state** is required for medical and nursing care, diazepam 10 mg iv is given initially, followed by 5 mg iv q5m until the patient is **quiet but** *awake* (Reed and Liskow 1987; Thompson et al. 1975). In one study, the *diazepam* dose required to produce this state was 15–215 mg (mean 46 mg). The time to induction of a calm state varied from 0.5 to 3 hours (mean 1.5 hour) (Thompson et al. 1975). However, diazepam doses as high as 2,000 mg have been required in a 24-hour period (Reed and Liskow 1987). *Lorazepam* 2–4 mg iv may be substituted for diazepam. Once the patient is stabilized, the BZD dose should be tapered over 3–4 days.

Sodium amobarbital may be given to calm an agitated patient if diazepam or lorazepam cannot be used (Jaffe 1980). The drug may be given iv or im. Each im injection should contain less than 5 mL, and a dose of amobarbital less than 500 mg is recommended. A single iv dose should not exceed 1,000 mg. The rate of iv injection of amobarbital should not exceed 1 mL/minute. Too-rapid injection may lead to respiratory depression and hypotension. After a calm state is achieved, the patient's barbiturate should be tapered over 3–4 days. In patients with compromised pulmonary function, barbiturates should be administered with extreme caution.

Although anxiolytics will decrease autonomic symptoms of alcohol withdrawal, decrease agitation, and increase sleep, the symptoms of disorientation and visual hallucinations usually remain for an average of 29 and 45 hours, respectively, regardless of the treatment (Thompson et al. 1975). Therefore, once a patient is in delirium tremens, dosing of the anxiolytic is based on vital signs and total hours of rest or sleep, not on the presence of hallucinations or the patient's orientation status.

Minimal experience exists with the combination of *antipsychotics* and *benzodiazepines* in the management of delirium tremens. The authors have had positive outcomes in several patients with the combination of haloperidol 5 mg and lorazepam 2–4 mg im administered every 2 hours (B. I. Liskow and B. Alexander, "The Combined Use of a Benzodiazepine and Antipsychotic in the Management of Delirium Tremens" [unpublished data], August 1996). The time to resolution of agitation, disorientation, and psychotic symptoms appeared to be reduced with this regimen, as several patients' signs and symptoms resolved within 24 hours. However, this clinical experience needs to be supported by others' experience and with controlled trials.

▶ **Seizures**

Prophylactic anticonvulsant therapy is unnecessary in the alcoholic patient with *no* prior seizure history (Guthrie 1989; Reed and Liskow 1987).

Patients with a *history of withdrawal seizures* are at an increased risk for recurrent seizures during alcohol withdrawal, although this risk is not great (Guthrie 1989; Reed and Liskow 1987). Study results are conflicting regarding the necessity of adding an anticonvulsant to the withdrawal regimen (Rothstein 1973; Sampliner and Iber 1974; Wilber and Kulik 1981). If an anticonvulsant is used, the recommended regimen is phenytoin 300 mg/day for 5 days in addition to the BZD. Chronic therapy with phenytoin is unnecessary in this group of patients.

If a history of *seizures unrelated to alcohol withdrawal* is obtained and the patient has inadequate anticonvulsant blood levels, a loading dose of phenytoin 15 mg/kg should be given (Reed and Liskow 1987). The total loading dose should be divided into three doses and administered orally over 12 hours. Maintenance treatment of 300 mg/day with blood-level adjustment of the dose is recommended.

Seizures appearing in the course of alcohol withdrawal that are multiple (i.e., *status epilepticus*) should be treated initially by diazepam, followed by an iv loading dose of phenytoin 15 mg/kg. Because of the potential adverse effects of parenteral phenytoin, this procedure requires specialized nursing and medical care.

Opiate Withdrawal and Withdrawal Schedule

■ Presentation

Opiate withdrawal is typically a nonfatal syndrome that occurs after daily use of an opiate (Farrell 1994; Kosten 1990a). However, morbidity may be significant and, if withdrawal is present, may warrant pharmacological management.

Morphine and Heroin
Generally, a severe abstinence syndrome occurs if an individual has received morphine 250 mg/day or heroin 80–120 mg/day for 18–20 days. A milder morphine abstinence syndrome may occur with lower doses (e.g., 30 mg) and/or shorter durations of use (e.g., 10 days).

The *abstinence syndrome* is characterized by restlessness, lacrimation, rhinorrhea, yawning, perspiration, gooseflesh ("cold turkey"), restless sleep, and mydriasis during the first 24 hours (onset usually 8–12 hours after a reduction in dose or cessation of use). As the syndrome progresses, these symptoms become more severe and may be accompanied by muscle twitching and spasms; kicking movements, severe aches in the back, abdomen, and legs; abdominal and muscle cramps; hot and cold flashes; insomnia; nausea, vomiting, and diarrhea; coryza and severe sneezing; and increases in body temperature, blood pressure, respiratory rate, and heart rate. These symptoms reach peak intensity in 36–72 hours following withdrawal of the drug or injection of a narcotic antagonist. Without treatment, the syndrome runs its course in 5–7 days, even though craving for the drug may continue for months (Fraser et al. 1961; Guthrie 1990).

Buprenorphine

Buprenorphine is a partial agonist/antagonist that is available only for parenteral administration. It is 25–50 times more potent than morphine and has a much longer duration of action, as it will block morphine's effect for 30 hours after a single dose (Jasinski et al. 1978).

Although animal studies suggest that buprenorphine has less potential for abuse than does morphine, the drug has been abused by former opiate abusers. Physical dependence occurred with abrupt discontinuation of buprenorphine 8 mg/day (equivalent to 240 mg morphine) administered iv for 1–2 months (Jasinski et al. 1978). Withdrawal signs and symptoms were similar to those of morphine but were less severe. They appeared over 3–10 days, peaked at 14 days, and declined over the next 1–2 weeks.

Butorphanol

Butorphanol, like pentazocine, buprenorphine, and nalbuphine, has both agonist and antagonist properties. Its analgesic effect is about 3–7 times as potent as that of morphine and 40 times as potent as that of meperidine.

When butorphanol 48 mg/day (equivalent to morphine 240 mg) was given to former opiate abusers for 35 days, the subjects experienced the usual effects associated with opiates. Abrupt withdrawal of butorphanol resulted in symptoms that began within 4 to 24 hours and progressed in severity to a peak at 48 hours. Withdrawal symptoms were similar to but more intense than those produced by pentazocine. Naloxone, a narcotic antagonist, also produced typical opiate withdrawal symptoms when administered to these subjects (Vandam 1980).

Codeine

Codeine, as an analgesic, is one-tenth to one-twelfth as potent as morphine. In one study, codeine 240–600 mg qid given parenterally was needed to substitute for parenteral morphine 50–150 mg/day (Himmelsbach 1934). When codeine was discontinued abruptly in the patients in this study, mild morphine-like abstinence symptoms occurred over the first 30 hours, followed by suddenly severe symptoms that lasted until the fourth or fifth day, at which point recovery began. The average daily dose of codeine attained by eight former opiate abusers within 18 days was about 1,500 mg (range 1,200–1,800 mg) (Fraser et al. 1960). Nalorphine, a narcotic antagonist, given after 30–45 days of drug administration, precipitated mild to moderate abstinence, as did abrupt withdrawal at 60 days. However, with general use, the risk of primary codeine abuse and dependence is low (Rowden and Lopez 1989).

Hydrocodone

Hydrocodone's dosage range is 20–60 mg/day, and its duration of action ranges from 4 to 8 hours. It is commercially available in the United States only in combination(s) with acetaminophen, aspirin, and/or caffeine. It is important to consider that acetaminophen-induced liver damage may be present in patients taking these over-the-counter preparations. Hydrocodone's withdrawal signs and symptoms fall between those of codeine and morphine in severity (Jaffe and Martin 1985).

Hydromorphone

This compound, a semisynthetic derivative of morphine, is eight times as potent as morphine; however, its duration of action is somewhat shorter. Withdrawal symptoms from hydromorphone, although qualitatively similar to those from morphine, are not usually as severe (Pradhan and Dutta 1977).

Levomethadyl Acetate

Levomethadyl acetate[1] (Orlaam®), or L-alpha acetyl methadol[2] (LAAM), is an oral long-acting opiate agonist (Guthrie 1990; Kosten 1990b). Doses of 60–100 mg three times weekly are approximately equivalent in efficacy and adverse effects to methadone 50–100 mg daily.

Levomethadyl acetate is extensively metabolized by the liver to two active metabolites, norlevomethadyl acetate and dinorlevomethadyl acetate (Henderson et al. 1977). The half-lives of the parent drug and the nor- and dinor- metabolites are 35–60 hours, 30–48 hours, and more than 100 hours, respectively. Abrupt with-

---

[1] Generic name used by manufacturer.
[2] Generic name used in older drug literature.

drawal of levomethadyl produces a syndrome qualitatively similar to methadone withdrawal except that it develops more slowly and is more prolonged (however, it is usually less intense if equivalent doses are compared) (Judson et al. 1983). Gradual reduction by 4%–8% per week (a 23-week taper schedule), as compared with abrupt discontinuation, of levomethadyl acetate resulted in successful transition to naltrexone treatment in 28% and 46% of patients, respectively. Therefore, abrupt discontinuation was more successful than a tapering schedule in discontinuing levomethadyl.

Levorphanol
Levorphanol is chemically related to hydromorphone. Its duration of action is 6–8 hours, and the usual dose is 2–3 mg. Levorphanol's withdrawal symptoms are similar to those of morphine (Jaffe and Martin 1985).

Meperidine
Meperidine is one-eighth to one-tenth as potent an analgesic as morphine, and its duration of action extends from 2 to 4 hours (Pradhan and Dutta 1977). The abstinence syndrome usually develops within 3 hours after the last dose, reaches its peak within 8 to 12 hours, and then declines. Withdrawal symptoms worse than those from morphine include muscle twitching, restlessness, and nervousness, whereas nausea, vomiting, and diarrhea tend to be less severe than those from morphine (Isbell and White 1953).

Methadone
Methadone is qualitatively and quantitatively similar to morphine except that its duration of action is longer on repeated administration (Kosten 1990a; Martin et al. 1973).

Abrupt withdrawal of methadone produces a syndrome that is qualitatively similar to morphine withdrawal, but it develops more slowly and is more prolonged, although usually less intense. Symptoms do not start until 24–48 hours after the last dose and peak in intensity at about the third day. The symptoms may not subside until the third week. This early abstinence syndrome is followed by a secondary, or protracted, abstinence syndrome of physiological and psychological disturbances that may last for months (Kosten 1990a).

Nalbuphine
Nalbuphine, like pentazocine, buprenorphine, and butorphanol, has both agonist and antagonistic properties. It is equipotent to morphine in analgesic effect and is available only in injectable form.

The potential for abuse of nalbuphine is equal to that of pentazocine and possibly less than that of propoxyphene or codeine. Nalbuphine 147–240 mg/day administered for up to 51 days produced withdrawal symptoms that were similar to but more intense than those produced by pentazocine abstinence (Jaffe and Martin 1985).

Oxycodone
Oxycodone is a modified codeine compound whose analgesic potency and duration of action are similar to those of morphine (Pradhan and Dutta 1977). Oxycodone is available in the United States as 5-mg tablets and in combination with either aspirin or acetaminophen. It is important to consider that acetaminophen-induced liver damage may exist in these patients.

Oxycodone's addiction liability and withdrawal syndrome are similar to those of morphine (Pradhan and Dutta 1977).

Oxymorphone
Oxymorphone is an opiate similar to hydromorphone. It is eight times more potent in its analgesic effects than morphine, and its duration of action is 4–5 hours. Withdrawal signs and symptoms are similar to those of morphine (Jaffe and Martin 1985).

Pentazocine
Pentazocine is one of many compounds that was synthesized as part of an attempt to develop an effective analgesic that had little or no abuse potential. It has both agonistic actions and weak opiate antagonistic activity. In terms of analgesic effect, a 30- to 50-mg dose given parenterally is approximately equal to morphine 10 mg. As regards peak effect, pentazocine is approximately one-fourth as potent orally as parenterally.

Former opiate abusers given high doses of pentazocine spaced closely enough to produce continuous action (e.g., 60–90 mg q4h) consistently develop physical dependence that can be demonstrated by abrupt withdrawal or precipitated by naloxone (Jasinski et al. 1970). The withdrawal syndrome after chronic doses of more than 500 mg/day is similar to opiate withdrawal, although milder. Withdrawal symptoms include abdominal cramps, chills, elevated temperature, vomiting, sweating, lacrimation, anxiety, and drug-seeking behavior.

In contrast to morphine and other opiates, pentazocine does not prevent or ameliorate the morphine withdrawal syndrome. Instead, when high doses of pentazocine are given to subjects who are physically dependent on morphine, pentazocine's antagonistic actions, although weak, will precipitate withdrawal symptoms.

Pentazocine is also available as a tablet that contains pentazocine 50 mg and naloxone hydrochloride 0.5 mg (Talwin® Nx). Naloxone, a narcotic antagonist with no agonistic properties, has no pharmacological effect when administered orally at this dose, and thus does not alter the analgesic properties of pentazocine when taken as recommended. If intravenous administration of the pentazocine–naloxone formulation used in the tablets is attempted, the narcotic effects of pentazocine will be blocked and withdrawal symptoms may occur in those persons who are dependent on opiates. However, case reports suggest that this formulation may be abused (Lahmeyer and Craig 1987). The original pentazocine tablet formulation is no longer being manufactured.

Propoxyphene

It is estimated that 90–120 mg of orally administered propoxyphene is required to produce analgesia equal to that of codeine 60 mg or aspirin 600 mg.

Abrupt discontinuation of chronically administered propoxyphene (up to 800 mg/day given for almost 2 months) resulted in mild abstinence symptoms. Higher doses of propoxyphene produced confusion, delusions, and hallucinations. Propoxyphene 800 mg/day reduces the intensity of morphine withdrawal somewhat less effectively than does codeine 1,500 mg/day (Fraser and Isbell 1960).

■ Treatment

Pharmacological treatments for opiate addiction include opiate substitution (e.g., methadone, buprenorphine), adrenergic agents (e.g., clonidine), and combination treatments (e.g., naltrexone/clonidine) (Guthrie 1990; Kosten 1990a, 1990b).

Because opiate abusers often give inconsistent and unreliable drug histories, treatment is warranted only after the initial appearance of the signs and symptoms of physical withdrawal. The appearance of the withdrawal syndrome confirms that the individual is indeed dependent and requires treatment. The use of nasally applied naloxone 1 mg accurately differentiated persons dependent on opiates from control subjects (Loimer et al. 1992). All dependent individuals demonstrated withdrawal symptoms within 10 to 15 minutes. The study authors recommended this procedure in emergency medicine and withdrawal treatment (see *Clonidine/Naltrexone Combination* [page 569]).

The following regimens are designed to manage the acute medical withdrawal symptoms of opiates. If possible, continued treatment in a substance abuse center is highly recommended.

Methadone

The initial methadone dose is determined by the presenting signs and symptoms (Table 10–2). The initial dose is repeated after 12 hours. Supplementary doses of methadone 5–10 mg are provided if withdrawal signs either are not suppressed or reappear during the first 24 hours. Once the initial 24-hour dose is established, it is tapered at a rate of 20% per day (for a short-acting opiate) or every other day (for a long-acting opiate) (Gossop et al. 1989; Kosten 1990a). The methadone is given on a q12h or q8h dosage schedule, with vital signs recorded before each dose. It is unusual for a patient to require more than 40 mg during the initial 24 hours of withdrawal (Fultz and Senay 1975; Khantzian and McKenna 1979).

If the patient is initially unable to tolerate oral medications, methadone 10 mg im should be given and followed as soon as possible with the initial oral dose of methadone, as calculated from the presenting withdrawal grade (i.e., complicated versus uncomplicated).

It is important to note that *federal regulations* require that hospitals or treatment centers that are not specifically licensed to provide methadone detoxification of opiate dependence limit the

Table 10–2.   Methadone dosing schedule for opiate-dependent patients

Grade	Signs and symptoms	Initial methadone dose (mg)
1	Lacrimation, rhinorrhea, diaphoresis, yawning, restlessness, insomnia	5
2	Dilated pupils, piloerection, muscle twitching, myalgia, arthralgia, abdominal pain	10
3	Tachycardia, hypertension, tachypnea, fever, anorexia, nausea, extreme restlessness	15
4	Diarrhea, vomiting, dehydration, hyperglycemia, hypotension	20

Source.   Fultz and Senay 1975; Khantzian and McKenna 1979.

use of methadone for this purpose to 72 hours (Code of Federal Regulations 1983). This period allows the treatment facility to find a center specifically licensed to withdraw the patient if more than 72 hours will be required.

Levomethadyl Acetate

Levomethadyl acetate (Orlaam®) was marketed as an orphan drug for the maintenance treatment of opiate dependence (e.g., heroin) (Guthrie 1990; Kosten 1990b) (see *Levomethadyl Acetate* [page 562] under "Presentation," above). It is a Drug Enforcement Administration (DEA) Schedule II controlled substance and must be dispensed by a clinic approved by the local state agency, the DEA, and the U.S. Food and Drug Administration (FDA). It is recommended that levomethadyl be used for maintenance therapy and not for management of acute withdrawal (see Chapter 7 for a complete discussion of the maintenance treatment of opiate dependence).

Clonidine

In 1978 it was reported that the antihypertensive drug clonidine suppressed symptoms of opiate withdrawal in 10 methadone-dependent patients whose medication was abruptly discontinued (Gold et al. 1978a; Guthrie 1990; Kosten 1990a, 1990b). Subsequent successes have been reported in both controlled and uncontrolled trials (Gold et al. 1978b, 1979, 1980). The studies report that although clonidine eliminates objective signs of withdrawal, at the doses used it does not completely suppress subjective withdrawal complaints such as anxiety, restlessness, insomnia, and muscle aches (Charney and Kleber 1980; Charney et al. 1981; Gold et al. 1980; Riordan and Kleber 1990; Washton and Resnick 1979; Washton et al. 1980). Current reviews of the literature on clonidine treatment of opiate withdrawal are available (Fishbain et al. 1993; Guthrie 1990; Redmond 1981).

Additional reports have supported clonidine's use in the management of withdrawal from meperidine, propoxyphene, levorphanol, oxycodone, and heroin (Bond 1986; Guthrie 1990). In one case report, clonidine was effective in suppressing symptoms of withdrawal from the combined use of codeine and glutethimide (Bond 1986).

It has been shown that clonidine lacks significant affinity for opiate receptors. The data suggest that the opiate withdrawal syndrome is caused by a rebound increase in norepinephrine activity in areas such as the locus coeruleus, which is regulated by α_2-adrenergic and opiate receptors. It is hypothesized that clonidine is an effective pharmacological substitute for opiate-induced inhibition of noradrenergic activity (Gold et al. 1980; Guthrie 1990; Kosten 1990a, 1990b; Redmond 1981). Although clonidine patches have been used in place of oral clonidine, there are no direct-comparison studies demonstrating this formulation's relative efficacy and safety (Fishbain et al. 1993; Milhorn 1992). Clonidine patches are placed for up to 1 week.

▶ **Long-Acting Opiates**

A recommended dosing regimen for withdrawal from a long-acting opiate (e.g., methadone) uses an average clonidine dose of 0.017 mg/kg/day in divided doses (Gold et al. 1979). However, it is important to note that the clonidine doses required and/or tolerated may vary widely. In one study, clonidine doses ranged from 0.009 to 0.025 mg/kg/day (Charney et al. 1981). A typical clonidine protocol is as follows: on the first day of administration, the patient is given a 0.006-mg/kg dose, which is repeated at bedtime (Gold et al. 1980). For the next **10 days,** the patient is given clonidine 0.017 mg/kg/day in divided doses of 0.007 mg/kg at 0800 hours, 0.003 mg/kg at 1600 hours, and 0.007 mg/kg at 2300 hours. Clonidine doses should be held and the daily dose reduced if the diastolic blood pressure falls below 60 mm Hg or marked sedation occurs. Sedation is noted to improve over 2–3 days. On days 11 through 14, the clonidine dose should be decreased by 50%, and on day 15, the drug is discontinued. Clonidine is available as 0.1-, 0.2-, and 0.3-mg tablets.

▶ **Short-Acting Opiates**

A suggested withdrawal protocol for a short-acting opiate (e.g., heroin, morphine, meperidine) could start with an average clonidine dose of 0.017 mg/kg/day. On the first day of administration, the patient is given a 0.006-mg/kg dose, which is repeated at bedtime. For the next 4 days, the patient receives the clonidine dose on the administration schedule described above for long-acting opiates. The dose is titrated against objective withdrawal signs and adverse effects. On days 6 through 8, the clonidine dose can be decreased by 50% and on day 9, the drug can be discontinued. This schedule is based on the observation that short-acting opiates often produce a quicker onset, earlier peak, and shorter duration of withdrawal signs and symptoms than do long-acting opiates (e.g., methadone) (Fishbain et al. 1993; Jaffe and Martin 1985; Kosten 1990a) (see individual agents under "Presentation" at the beginning of this section).

Clonidine/Naltrexone Combination

A combination of clonidine and the orally active long-acting opiate antagonist naltrexone have been used to shorten the duration of the methadone and heroin withdrawal protocol. The rationale for using this combination is that clonidine may prevent the withdrawal symptoms that would be precipitated by naltrexone, while naltrexone "resets" or desensitizes opiate receptors. With this approach, a typical 14-day methadone withdrawal protocol can be shortened to 3–4 days (Fishbain et al. 1993; Kosten 1990a).

One protocol includes a starting dose of naltrexone 12.5 mg/day that is increased to 50 mg/day on day 3. With this naltrexone dosing regimen, clonidine was needed for only 4 days with a total dose of 1.7 mg after a peak dose of 0.6 mg on day 1 of the protocol (Vining et al. 1988). This approach requires further study (Kosten 1990b).

Buprenorphine

Buprenorphine is a mixed opiate agonist/antagonist that is being investigated as an opiate withdrawal and maintenance treatment (Fishbain et al. 1993; Guthrie 1990; Kosten 1990a, 1990b). Although initial studies are promising, more research is required to determine buprenorphine's utility in the management of opiate abuse.

Anxiolytic-Hypnotic Withdrawal and Withdrawal Schedule

Withdrawal and management of withdrawal from anxiolytic-hypnotics (e.g., barbiturates, BZDs, miscellaneous agents) are addressed in this section (Isbell 1950; Wikler 1968) (Table 10–3). The discussion will focus primarily on BZDs because of their widespread use. Withdrawal syndromes that occur with discontinuation of a BZD require pharmacological management for patient comfort and sometimes for prevention of potentially serious medical consequences (Woods and Winger 1995).

Discontinuation of BZDs can lead to relapse, rebound, and/or withdrawal symptoms (Noyes et al. 1988). *Relapse* is defined as the gradual return of the original symptoms of the illness and is estimated to occur in 63%–81% of patients. *Rebound* refers to the reoccurrence of the original symptoms at a level more severe than baseline. *Withdrawal* involves the presentation of new symptoms related solely to discontinuation of the drug. Rebound symptoms, like withdrawal symptoms, will gradually return to a baseline level following BZD discontinuation.

**Table 10–3.   Dose equivalents and half-life classifications
                  for anxiolytic-hypnotic drugs**

Generic name	Half-life (hours)[a]	Dose (mg)[b]
Benzodiazepines		
alprazolam	short	1
chlordiazepoxide	long	25
clonazepam	short	1[c]
clorazepate	long	15
diazepam	long	10
flurazepam	long	15[c]
halazepam	long	40[c]
lorazepam	short	1
oxazepam	short	10
prazepam	long	10
temazepam	short	15
triazolam	short	0.50
Barbiturates		
amobarbital	short	100
aprobarbital	short	25[c]
butabarbital	long	100[c]
butalbital (in Fiorinal)	short	50
mephobarbital	long	50[c]
pentobarbital	short	100
phenobarbital	long	30
secobarbital	short	100
Miscellaneous		
chloral hydrate	short	200[c]
ethchlorvynol	short	200[c]
ethinamate	short	200[c]
glutethimide	short	250
meprobamate	short	400

Note.   This table contains guidelines for initial doses; dosage
adjustments must be made based on clinical observation of the
patient for adequate coverage of withdrawal and excessive
anxiolytic-hypnotic effects.
[a] Short = average half-life <30 hours; long = average half-life
≥30 hours (designation includes half-life of active metabolite[s]).
[b] Equivalent dose; for patients receiving multiple drugs (e.g.,
flurazepam, alprazolam), each drug should be converted to a
diazepam or secobarbital equivalent and totaled.
[c] Estimated.
Source.   Busto et al. 1986; Harrison et al. 1984; Harvey 1985;
Rickels et al. 1990; Smith and Landry 1990; Smith and Wesson 1983;
Sullivan and Sellers 1992.

BZD withdrawal can be classified in several ways: minor versus major withdrawal and low- versus high-dose withdrawal (Albeck 1987; Smith and Landry 1990). The minor/major convention follows the historical classification of ethanol withdrawal and emphasizes the severity of withdrawal signs and symptoms. The low-/high-dose classification will be used here, as daily dose is usually a significant factor in assessing the medical risk of BZD withdrawal. For this discussion, *low dose* will refer to the manufacturer's recommended daily doses (Smith and Landry 1990). Discontinuation of therapeutic doses (e.g., low-dose withdrawal) typically, but not always, results in minor withdrawal symptoms. Likewise, major withdrawal symptoms are primarily associated with high-dose use. (For recommended daily doses for benzodiazepines, see the Product List in Chapter 4.)

Several clinical situations exist that may require management of BZD withdrawal. These include the substance abuse patient without a primary psychiatric illness who is using high doses of a single BZD or multiple anxiolytic-hypnotics and the generalized anxiety or panic disorder patient who is receiving therapeutic or high doses of a BZD (DuPont 1990). Different strategies are necessary to manage these cases.

■ Presentation

Rebound Symptoms

Seven of nine *controlled, short-term* (mean 10 weeks, range 3–34 weeks) studies of *therapeutic* doses reported the occurrence of rebound symptoms. BZDs were abruptly discontinued in all seven of the studies. However, only three of the nine studies reported the actual incidence of rebound symptoms, which ranged from 3% to 44% (Noyes et al. 1988). These three studies are briefly summarized here. In one report, when diazepam was discontinued after being administered for 6 weeks and 14–22 weeks in two groups of patients, rebound symptoms occurred in 3% and 18% of subjects, respectively. In two other studies, diazepam was administered for 4 weeks and alprazolam, for 8 weeks. Discontinuation led to rebound symptoms in 44% and 33% of subjects, respectively. The wide range of reported rebound incidence in these three studies was due to differences in length of treatment, drugs studied, and definition of rebound symptoms. In all seven trials that reported rebound symptoms, *withdrawal* symptoms with BZD discontinuation were noted.

Withdrawal Symptoms

Because reports of BZD discontinuation may or may not include baseline measurements, the frequency of true withdrawal symptoms is difficult to determine. This uncertainty contributes to a significant variability in the reported incidence of withdrawal.

Many reports suggest that BZDs differ with respect to frequency, severity, and time course (e.g., onset, peak, and duration of symptoms) of withdrawal based on the half-life of the drug (Busto et al. 1986; Fontaine et al. 1984; Marriott and Tyrer 1993; Morgan and Oswald 1982; Rickels et al. 1986, 1990; Sellers 1978; R. Tyrer et al. 1981; Woods and Winger 1995) (Table 10–3). (For information on the pharmacokinetics of benzodiazepines, see Chapter 4.)

▶ Low Dose

Signs and symptoms.   Reported signs and symptoms attributed to low-dose withdrawal include nausea, vomiting, irritability, tremor, incoordination, insomnia, restlessness, blurred vision, sweating, anorexia, and/or weakness as well as anxiety (Noyes et al. 1988; Marriott and Tyrer 1993). Depersonalization, heightened perception (especially to light and sound), and illusions are also commonly reported. However, many of these symptoms have also been reported in unmedicated anxiety patients (Rodrigo and Williams 1986).

Incidence and duration of use.   *Uncontrolled* investigations report that almost all patients experience withdrawal syndromes upon discontinuation of therapeutic doses of BZDs after long-term use (Noyes et al. 1988).

Nine *controlled, long-term* (mean 3 years, range 1–16 years) studies examined the effect of BZD discontinuation (Noyes et al. 1988). Six of the nine investigations had abruptly discontinued the BZD, whereas the other three had tapered the drug. Two of the studies reported no withdrawal symptoms upon abrupt discontinuation. Only five of the nine studies reported the actual incidence of withdrawal. Although definitions of withdrawal varied, the mean incidence was 45% (range 0%–100%). The two studies that reported the highest frequency of withdrawal reactions (82% and 100%) included patients who had previously experienced difficulty on discontinuing the BZD (Petursson and Lader 1981; Rickels et al. 1986).

In one group (Rickels et al. 1983) the incidence of withdrawal for **8 months or more** (average 3 years) and for less than 8 months of daily BZD use was 43% and 5%, respectively.

These results are in contrast to the relatively low risk of severe withdrawal reactions occurring after discontinuation of therapeutic doses of a BZD in controlled trials. None of the 494 patients included in discontinuation studies after *short-term administration* (average 10 weeks, range 3–34 weeks) of therapeutic doses of a BZD experienced severe withdrawal symptoms (Fruensgaard 1976; Kahn et al. 1980; Noyes et al. 1985, 1988; Olajide and Lader 1984).

Of 271 patients receiving therapeutic doses for an average of 3 years, 14 (5%) developed severe reactions. One report contributed 10 of these 14 cases (Petursson and Lader 1981). These 10 patients had previously experienced difficulty discontinuing the BZD. Excluding this report, 4 of 255 patients (1.5%) experienced severe reactions.

Time course.   That BZD half-life influences the time course of low-dose drug discontinuation was demonstrated in a double-blind protocol (Busto et al. 1986). Forty patients who had received an average diazepam equivalent dose of 15 ± 10 mg/day for at least 3 months were recruited. The drugs were discontinued by abrupt placebo substitution or by tapering diazepam doses of 1–5 mg/week over 5–6 weeks. Patients in the placebo group experienced more withdrawal symptoms ($P < .0001$), more severe symptoms ($P < .0001$), and an earlier onset of symptoms ($P < .01$) than did subjects in the diazepam-taper group.

In the placebo group, the *onset* of symptoms occurred within 1 day after discontinuation of the short-acting BZD. However, onset of symptoms occurred 5 days after discontinuation of the long-acting BZD. *Peak* withdrawal symptoms with short- and long-acting BZD occurred at 1.0 ± 0.5 days and at 9.6 ± 5.1 days, respectively. Withdrawal symptoms usually *disappeared* within 2 to 4 weeks.

The patients who used short-acting BZDs before the study reported more-intense withdrawal symptoms than did the patients using long-acting drugs. Although this finding was not statistically significant, it is noteworthy that all seven patients who refused to continue taking the "study drug" (e.g., placebo) had been receiving a short-acting BZD prior to the study.

Summary.   Withdrawal symptoms occurred in approximately 50% of patients receiving therapeutic doses of BZDs for an average of 3 years (Noyes et al. 1988). Most symptoms were of mild to moderate intensity. Although discontinuation of a BZD that has been taken daily for less than 8 months produces a small risk of withdrawal symptoms, *rebound* symptoms are common.

▶ **High Dose**

Signs and symptoms.   Qualitatively, BZD withdrawal is similar to withdrawal from the older anxiolytic-hypnotics (i.e., barbiturates) (Albeck 1987; Hollister et al. 1961). Abrupt discontinuation of the drug(s) in a dependent individual can lead to a medically significant withdrawal or abstinence syndrome (Jaffe 1985). Minor withdrawal symptoms (in the approximate order of their appearance) include anxiety, involuntary muscle twitches, coarse intention tremor of the hands and fingers, dilated pupils, progressive weakness, dizziness, visual illusions, nausea, vomiting, insomnia, weight loss, and orthostatic hypotension with an increase in pulse rate of 20 beats/minute on standing. The major withdrawal symptoms consist of tonic-clonic seizures and an acute organic brain syndrome or delirium that resembles alcohol withdrawal delirium tremens (Albeck 1987; Isbell 1950; Wikler 1968). This syndrome may include confusion, disorientation, agitation, markedly elevated vital signs, and visual hallucinations. Hyperpyrexia, which has been primarily described with barbiturate withdrawal, may occur with minor or major withdrawal symptoms and is considered a poor prognostic sign. The probability of a withdrawal reaction is a function of both the daily dose and the duration of drug use.

Incidence and duration of use—barbiturates.   Minor withdrawal symptoms occurred upon abrupt discontinuation in only 6% of subjects receiving *secobarbital* or *pentobarbital* 400 mg/day for 90 consecutive days. However, after abrupt discontinuation, a 50% minor withdrawal rate and an 11% seizure rate was observed in 18 subjects receiving secobarbital 600 mg/day for 7 weeks. In subjects taking either pentobarbital or secobarbital 900–2,200 mg/day for 1–6 months, 100% experienced minor withdrawal symptoms, 78% experienced seizures, and 67% experienced delirium with abrupt discontinuation (Fraser et al. 1958).

Incidence and duration of use—benzodiazepines.   Several early *studies* examined the effect of abrupt discontinuation of high-dose, short-term BZD administration. Minor withdrawal symptoms occurred in 50% (6 of 13) and seizures in 8% of subjects receiving diazepam 120 mg/day for 21 consecutive days (Hollister et al. 1963). In another study, 11 patients were switched to placebo after receiving chlordiazepoxide 300–600 mg/day for 2–6 months (Hollister et al. 1961). Six patients had received 600 mg/day, and 10 of 11 patients had been treated for 5 months or longer. Ten patients experienced withdrawal symptoms, including agitation, insomnia, anorexia, nausea, and depression. Two patients (18%) developed major motor seizures 7 and 8 days, respectively, after chlordiaze-poxide discontinuation. In contrast, however, another study re-ported that the severity of withdrawal reactions after discontin-uation did not differ between diazepam 135 mg/day and 20 mg/day (Hallstrom and Lader 1981). The correlation of BZD dose and duration of use to incidence and severity of BZD withdrawal re-mains difficult to quantify. However, these two factors appear to be primary considerations in predicting the likelihood of a withdrawal reaction.

Today, because of ethical considerations prohibiting prospective studies of abrupt discontinuation of high-dose BZDs, *case reports* are the major source of information regarding severe BZD with-drawal reactions. A similar number of BZD-induced withdrawal *seizures* were reported for the short-acting BZDs lorazepam, oxaz-epam, and alprazolam as were reported for the far more commonly prescribed long-acting BZDs diazepam, chlordiazepoxide, and clor-azepate (Perry and Alexander 1986). (See Table 10–3 [page 570] for BZD half-life classifications.) Twenty-three cases of withdrawal seizures have been reported for the short-acting group and 17 cases for the long-acting group. A total of 14 cases in each group in-volved diazepam and lorazepam. Seizures after discontinuation of *lorazepam* occurred in patients who had been receiving 2–12 mg/day (median 7.5 mg/day) for 3 weeks to 4 months (median 3 months). Only 3 of the 14 patients were receiving doses outside the recommended therapeutic range of 1–10 mg/day. The 14 cases of seizures following abrupt discontinuation of *diazepam* were in patients who had received a dose range of 20–170 mg/day (median 77.5 mg/day) for 3 weeks to 12 years (median 7.5 months). Nine of the 14 patients were receiving dosages outside the recommended therapeutic range of 4–40 mg/day. Assuming that lorazepam 2 mg is approx- imately equivalent to diazepam 10 mg, the following observation can be made (Busto et al. 1986; Smith and Wesson 1983): Lorazepam, a short-acting BZD, appears to provoke with-drawal syndromes after less than half the duration of daily use and at half the equivalent dose of diazepam.

Time course—barbiturates.   The time course of withdrawal for short- and long-acting barbiturates approximates that for short- and long-acting BZDs (Fraser et al. 1958; Jaffe 1985) (see Ta-ble 10–3 [page 570] and *Time course—benzodiazepines,* below).

Time course—benzodiazepines.   Seizures following lorazepam withdrawal occurred within 1–4 days (median 64 hours) after drug discontinuation, whereas those following diazepam withdrawal occurred between 2 and 27 days (median 5 days) (Perry and Alexander 1986). The mean half-life values for lorazepam, diazepam, and diazepam's major metabolite desmethyldiazepam are 14, 31, and 51 hours, respectively (Sellers 1978). The onset of withdrawal symptoms is expected when the drug has been nearly eliminated. Therefore, seizures from withdrawal of a short-acting BZD with a half-life that is 25%–50% of a long-acting BZD occur within half the time of those from the long-acting drug.

If *delirium* developed, it occurred within 2 to 8 days after discontinuing lorazepam, and within 3 to 10 days after abrupt discontinuation of diazepam.

Therefore, knowledge of a drug's elimination half-life may be used to estimate severity and time course of withdrawal even if experience with that drug's withdrawal has not been specifically reported in the literature (Hollister 1980; Jaffe 1985; Perry and Alexander 1986). (See Table 10–3 [page 570] for half-life comparisons of anxiolytic-hypnotics.) As a general rule, drugs with a plasma half-life of 8–20 hours produce the most severe reactions because of a rapid decline in levels. Drugs with a half-life of more than 20 hours (including active metabolites) often produce milder withdrawal reactions as compared with short-acting drugs (if equivalent doses are compared). Severe withdrawal symptoms from drugs with short half-lives may last 5–7 days, while withdrawal symptoms from drugs with long half-lives may last 10–14 days. Therefore, the tapering dose and schedule will be determined by the half-life of the drug. If a patient was taking a combination of short- and long-acting anxiolytic-hypnotics, then, conservatively, the extended withdrawal protocol should be used (see "Treatment," below).

Alprazolam deserves special mention, because the FDA has instructed the manufacturer to include a patient package insert warning patients of possible withdrawal symptoms with discontinuation of this drug. Interestingly, at this time, no other BZD has been singled out for this requirement. Alprazolam withdrawal case reports in the literature through 1985 have been reviewed (Browne and Hauge 1986). The eight patients had received alprazolam 1.5–10 mg/day for durations of 2 to 18 months. Six of the eight patients were receiving alprazolam doses above the manufacturer's recommended therapeutic dose of 4 mg/day. However, doses of 6–10 mg/day have been recommended for treatment of panic disorders. (See *Panic Disorder* [page 310] under "Dosage" of **Benzodiazepines** in Chapter 4.) Withdrawal seizures occurred in four of eight cases at a median dose of 6 mg/day. Delirium/psychosis occurred in the remaining four cases. In all cases, withdrawal signs and symptoms were evident within 72 hours of abstinence.

Summary.   On the average, discontinuation of a short-acting BZD will lead to more significant withdrawal symptoms that occur earlier after drug discontinuation and, overall, last a shorter period of time as compared with a long-acting BZD (Jaffe 1985).

■ Treatment

Protocol design considerations include BZD metabolism (e.g., short- versus long-acting), dose and duration of use, patient diagnostic status (e.g., concurrent psychiatric illness versus no active diagnosis), time course of withdrawal (e.g., onset, peak, and duration of withdrawal symptoms), and concurrent cross-tolerant drug use (e.g., ethanol) (Albeck 1987). Age did not affect the success of a BZD withdrawal protocol in a recent study (Schweizer et al. 1989).

Management of BZD withdrawal is divided into low- and high-dose categories (Marriott and Tyrer 1993; Smith and Landry 1990). A patient with a preexisting (and possibly concurrent) anxiety state adds the confounding variable of relapse to the possibility of rebound and withdrawal (see "Presentation" [page 571], above).

Low-Dose Withdrawal

▶ Benzodiazepine Taper

Conservatively, drugs should not be abruptly discontinued in patients who have received manufacturer-recommended doses of BZDs on a daily basis for more than 1 month (Fontaine et al. 1984; Harrison et al. 1984; Laughren et al. 1982; Petursson and Lader 1981; Smith and Landry 1990; P. Tyrer et al. 1983). Because severe withdrawal symptoms are not expected, gradual tapering of the BZD over a 2- to 4-week period on an outpatient basis should be attempted. Withdrawal symptoms appear to be most intense with the last few doses of drug (Fruensgaard 1976). To help distinguish relapse of symptoms from withdrawal, the patient should remain off BZDs for at least 3 weeks, if possible (Rickels et al. 1990).

Long-acting benzodiazepine.   If the patient is receiving a long-acting BZD (Table 10–3), he or she may remain on the originally prescribed drug. The weekly tapering rate is determined by dividing the total daily dose of BZD by five and rounding the number to a dose attainable with available dosage forms (see the Product List in Chapter 4). Each week, the dose would be reduced by this tapering rate. For example, a patient receiving diazepam 20 mg/day would be tapered at a rate of 4 mg/week (e.g., week 1: 16 mg/day; week 2: 12 mg/day; week 3: 8 mg/day; and week 4: 4 mg/day). This withdrawal protocol covers the time period over which withdrawal symptoms typically occur (Busto et al. 1986; Rickels et al. 1990). If necessary, the tapering schedule can be slowed toward the end of the protocol (i.e., dose reduction by one-eighth of the total weekly dose for the last 2 weeks) (Rickels et al. 1990).

Short-acting benzodiazepine—same-drug method. If the patient is receiving a short-acting BZD (Table 10–3), consideration is given to slowly tapering the dose of the prescribed BZD according to a schedule similar to that described above for a long-acting BZD (Rickels et al. 1990). The manufacturer of alprazolam recommends a tapering schedule not to exceed 0.5 mg every 3 days. (See also *Short-acting benzodiazepine—same-drug method* [page 581] under *High-Dose Withdrawal*, below.)

Short-acting benzodiazepine—substitution method. A cross-tolerant, long-acting BZD may be substituted for a short-acting BZD (Smith and Landry 1990). The rationale for this method is the observation that less-severe withdrawal symptoms are associated with long-acting compounds (Rickels et al. 1990). Although several reports have suggested that such substitution constitutes an acceptable strategy for patients receiving a short-acting drug, this method has not been extensively studied (Albeck 1987; Busto et al. 1986; Harrison et al. 1984; Perry et al. 1981). To accomplish the switch from a short-acting to a long-acting BZD, approximate equivalent doses for BZD have been suggested (Busto et al. 1986; Harrison et al. 1984; Smith and Landry 1990; Smith and Wesson 1983) (Table 10–3). However, inaccuracy in suggested BZD dose equivalents may affect the success of this recommendation. One author suggests (without documentation) that a ratio of two to three times the usual recommended diazepam equivalency (e.g., Table 10–3 equivalents) should be used (Rickels et al. 1990). Although, theoretically, any long-acting BZD could be used, diazepam has been the most widely studied (Busto et al. 1986; Harrison et al. 1984; Perry et al. 1981). Clonazepam has also been reported to be useful (Albeck 1987; Patterson 1990). Presumably, duration of the withdrawal protocol could be shortened by using a long-acting compared with a short-acting BZD (Perry et al. 1981; P. Tyrer et al. 1983).

▶ Nonbenzodiazepine Management
Non-BZDs have been suggested for management of BZD withdrawal. The rationale for this recommendation stems from the desire to remove the patient from the BZDs' reinforcing pharma-

cological effect. However, this approach has not been extensively investigated (Rickels et al. 1990), and more research is required to determine the role of non-BZD drugs in the management of BZD withdrawal.

Antidepressants. Several patients were successfully withdrawn from a BZD while receiving only a tricyclic or monoamine oxidase inhibitor (MAOI) antidepressant (Rickels et al. 1990; P. Tyrer 1985). Both tricyclic antidepressants (TCAs) and MAOIs are effective antipanic drugs. Preliminary results suggest that TCAs and MAOIs might be useful in treating generalized anxiety disorder (see "Efficacy" [page 321] under **Antidepressants** in Chapter 4). If this supposition is confirmed, these agents might be especially beneficial for the patient with a preexisting (and possibly concurrent) anxiety disorder.

One recommendation is to place patients whose original symptoms are likely to reemerge on imipramine 150 mg/day or greater (range 100–300 mg/day) for 4 weeks before BZD withdrawal is initiated (Rickels et al. 1990; P. Tyrer 1985). Although the sedating TCAs (e.g., doxepin, imipramine, amitriptyline) have been recommended for this purpose, research demonstrating differences in efficacy based on relative sedation has not been performed. (For more information on tricyclic antidepressant dosing, pharmacokinetics, and adverse effects, see Chapter 2.)

The second-generation antidepressants amoxapine, bupropion, fluoxetine, sertraline, paroxetine, fluvoxamine, maprotiline, and trazodone have not been extensively investigated in panic disorder or generalized anxiety disorder. Their utility in managing BZD withdrawal is unknown.

Buspirone. Pharmacological studies demonstrate no cross-tolerance between buspirone and the BZDs; therefore, the drug has no value in the treatment of BZD withdrawal (Lader and Olajide 1987; Schweizer and Rickels 1986). However, a preliminary study reported that buspirone 25–45 mg/day started 4 weeks before a 2-week BZD taper was successful in preventing symptom relapse in 85% of patients (Rickels et al. 1990).

Carbamazepine. A double-blind study reported that carbamazepine 200–600 mg/day, when initiated 4 weeks before a 2-week BZD taper, was successful managing withdrawal symptoms in 92% of patients (Rickels et al. 1990).

Clonidine. Clonidine, an α_2-adrenergic agonist, at 0.3–0.6 mg/day po for up to 3 months has been used to treat several cases of low-dose BZD withdrawal, with primarily negative results (Goodman 1986; Kesharan and Crammer 1985; Rickels et al. 1990; Vinogradov et al. 1986).

Propranolol. In one report, 2 weeks of propranolol, a β-adrenergic blocker, at doses of 60–120 mg/day reduced the severity, but not the incidence, of withdrawal symptoms (R. Tyrer et al. 1981).

Trazodone. Ten patients treated concurrently with trazodone 300 mg/day were successfully tapered from their BZD regimens over a 2- to 4-week period (Ansseau and De Roeck 1993). These patients had been receiving diazepam equivalents ranging from 54 to 150 mg/day (average 83 mg/day) for 3–15 years (average 6.4 years). The role of trazodone in management of BZD withdrawal syndromes requires further study.

▶ Nonpharmacological Management
Fifty percent (5 of 10) of panic disorder patients with mild to severe agoraphobia who received an alprazolam taper relapsed and resumed alprazolam treatment within 6 months of drug discontinuation (Spiegel et al. 1994). However, none of the 11 patients who received 12 sessions of cognitive treatment in addition to an alprazolam taper restarted the drug within the 6-month time period. Nonetheless, two other studies have reported that cognitive treatment did not prevent return to medication in a similar situation (Spiegel et al. 1994). The success in the positive study may have been due to a lower alprazolam dose and a slower taper than used in the other studies.

High-Dose Withdrawal
Panic disorder as well as substance abuse patients may be receiving high-dose BZDs. Typically, substance abuse patients present a complicated picture because of questionable dosage/duration information and a mixed anxiolytic-hypnotic or polysubstance abuse history. The following sections discuss several options for management of high-dose BZD discontinuation.

▶ Withdrawal Procedure Without Tolerance Testing
This method assumes that a reasonably accurate history can be obtained. The use of a BZD rather than a barbiturate derivative for withdrawal decreases the likelihood that a patient will experience significant untoward effects if the dose administered is too high compared with the actual amount of drug ingested. Administering too high a dose of a BZD will usually lead to slight intoxication within the first one to three doses of the withdrawal protocol. This oversedation can be quickly reversed by holding and/or decreasing

successive doses. Using too low a dose will often lead to minor withdrawal signs and symptoms that indicate the need for a higher dose.

Short-acting benzodiazepine—same-drug method.   A patient receiving high doses of a short-acting BZD might be withdrawn using the same drug (Albeck 1987). Most experience with short-acting BZD withdrawal procedures involves alprazolam. The manufacturer originally recommended that patients be tapered from the drug at the rate of 1 mg every 3 days. It has updated the package insert, which now recommends that the drug not be tapered faster than 0.5 mg every 3 days. However, a study reported that 14 of 18 patients with panic disorder who were treated for longer than 12 weeks at an average dose of 5.25 mg/day (range 2.5–8.0 mg/day) could not complete this 4- to 5-week withdrawal protocol, primarily because of symptom relapse (Fyer et al. 1987). Nine patients experienced withdrawal symptoms. A similar experience was noted in three case reports of alprazolam withdrawal (Browne and Hauge 1986). The utility of this recommendation, especially with much higher doses in patients without a psychiatric diagnosis, has not been reported. This method is usually not practical for most non-designated substance abuse treatment centers because inpatients taking high doses of alprazolam would require extensive tapering time to achieve abstinence.

Short-acting benzodiazepine—substitution method.   It would be useful to know whether substitution of a long-acting BZD for a short-acting one could shorten the time needed to withdraw a patient. In one study using *diazepam,* 16 of 23 inpatients successfully underwent withdrawal from high-dose BZDs (e.g., alprazolam, bromazepam, diazepam [primary drug], lorazepam, oxazepam, triazolam) ranging from 40 to 500 mg/day (median 150 mg/day) diazepam equivalents without any complications (Harrison et al. 1984). Diazepam was substituted at a dose of 40% of the reported daily consumption and was tapered at a rate of 10% per day. Of the remaining 7 patients, 6 had minor withdrawal symptoms and 1 patient, who was inadequately dosed, experienced major withdrawal symptoms of paranoia and confusion.

It has been suggested that the *triazolobenzodiazepines* alprazolam and triazolam may not be cross-tolerant with other BZDs. In two cases, diazepam substitution did not alleviate *alprazolam's* withdrawal syndrome once it occurred (Browne and Hauge 1986). However, the diazepam doses used in these cases may have been too low.

One patient with *triazolam* withdrawal psychosis responded to lorazepam (Heritch et al. 1987), whereas another patient on triazolam 10 mg/day had a seizure 13 hours after discontinuing the drug despite receiving chlordiazepoxide 600 mg po and diazepam 75 mg iv before the seizure occurred (L. S. Schneider et al. 1987). However, four patients who had ingested triazolam 5–15 mg/day for between 3 months and 5 years were successfully withdrawn using diazepam (Sullivan and Sellers 1992). More information is needed to determine the best approach for treating triazolobenzodiazepine withdrawal. However, initial cases suggest that withdrawal of alprazolam and triazolam may be safety accomplished if adequate doses of cross-tolerant BZDs are used (Rickels et al. 1990). Long-acting BZDs are recommended over short-acting ones (see Table 10–3 [page 570]).

In one study, 41 of 48 patients treated with alprazolam for panic disorder were successfully converted (i.e., no withdrawal, rebound, or relapse symptoms occurred) from alprazolam to *clonazepam* using a 2:1 ratio, respectively (Herman et al. 1987). Clonazepam is a high-potency, long-acting BZD (Table 10–3).

Short-acting benzodiazepine—carbamazepine.   Three patients with panic disorder treated with alprazolam 5–9 mg/day successfully completed a 2-week alprazolam taper after carbamazepine 600–800 mg/ day was instituted 4 weeks before the taper (Klein et al. 1986). One patient was successfully withdrawn from triazolam 15 mg/day ingested for 1 year with carbamazepine (doses not stated) (Sullivan and Sellers 1992).

Long-acting benzodiazepine—same-drug method.   Patients receiving long-acting BZDs prior to admission might be withdrawn with the same drug using the procedure outlined above for short-acting BZDs (e.g., start with 40% of total daily dose on day 1 and taper at 10% per day using diazepam) (Harrison et al. 1984).

Long-acting benzodiazepine—carbamazepine.   A recent open study reported success with carbamazepine 400–800 mg/day in the management of long-acting (e.g., chlordiazepoxide, diazepam, clonazepam) and short-acting (e.g., alprazolam) BZD withdrawal (Ries et al. 1989). Five of 9 patients had used high doses of the BZD, and most patients had been on the BZD for 0.5–5 years. All patients were switched from the BZD to carbamazepine within 1 to 6 days (median 3 days) without significant withdrawal symptoms. Carbamazepine was discontinued 3–14 days after the last BZD dose. Although patients could receive a supplemental BZD 1) if diaphoresis or tremulousness occurred or 2) if their pulse or blood pressure increased by more than 40% of baseline values, no additional BZD doses were required.

❱ Withdrawal Procedure With Tolerance Testing

Although identification and treatment of the drug-dependent person are necessary in order to avoid symptomatic withdrawal, the patient may be unable or unwilling to provide an accurate account of his or her drug intake. Also, the presence of mixed anxiolytic-hypnotic abuse would indicate tolerance testing to determine a total tolerant BZD dose.

Historically, the pentobarbital tolerance test has been used to establish dependence, primarily in patients abusing barbiturates (Albeck 1987; Ewing and Bakewell 1967; Fraser et al. 1958). An increase in BZD prescribing in the 1970s and 1980s led to the need for a BZD tolerance test (Perry et al. 1981). Although barbiturates and BZDs may be cross-tolerant, diazepam is preferred over pentobarbital in tolerance testing. Diazepam can be dosed until the end point of intoxication is reached, whereas pentobarbital must be limited to a maximum dose of 1,000 mg because of the risk of respiratory depression, even in patients tolerant to the drug's hypnotic effects at this large dose. The diazepam tolerance test has been successfully used, albeit in a small number patients (Perry et al. 1981).

The experience of tolerance-testing *alprazolam* patients is limited. One case report described a male patient treated with alprazolam 4 mg/day for 18 months who increased his dosage to 10 mg/day for 2 weeks before being tolerance-tested with diazepam (Votolato et al. 1987). This patient tolerated a diazepam dose more than 2½ times the predicted dose, based on a reported equivalent dose (Table 10–3). Only at 260 mg/day did the patient demonstrate slight ataxia. He was successfully withdrawn with diazepam over an unspecified period of time, and experienced significant insomnia only for the first 5 days of the withdrawal protocol. In an unpublished case, we tolerance-tested a patient who had ingested alprazolam 16 mg/day after he had been tapered to alprazolam 12 mg/day (B. Alexander and B. L. Cook, "Tolerance Testing and Withdrawal of a Patient Receiving Alprazolam 16 mg/day" [unpublished data], August 1996). The patient tolerated more than 2½ times the equivalent diazepam dose. In the future, to avoid the problem of extending the tolerance test into the time of natural sleep, which complicates interpretation of the results, the use of diazepam 40 mg q2h might be considered.

Stabilization procedure.   Patients cannot be tolerance-tested until they cease to show signs of either drug withdrawal or drug intoxication. Because patients are often admitted to the hospital in the middle of the day or at night, tolerance testing usually cannot be conveniently commenced until the following day. Thus, if a patient is lucid and displays no signs of withdrawal or intoxication when initially seen, an order for diazepam 20 mg or pentobarbital 200 mg orally at bedtime may be given and the test begun at 0800 hours the following morning. If the patient exhibits signs of withdrawal when initially seen, he or she should be given diazepam 20 mg or pento-barbital 200 mg every 2 hours (to a maximum of 1,000 mg) until asleep and then receive no medication until the test commences at 0800 hours the following morning. *(Note:* This technique may be used in preparation for a withdrawal protocol in a patient experiencing acute withdrawal symptoms for whom tolerance testing is not planned.) If the patient shows signs of intoxication (e.g., lateral gaze nystagmus, minimal ataxia, slurred speech, positive Romberg sign) when initially seen, no medication need be given until the test dose begins at 0800 hours the following morning. While the patient is being tested, he or she should be npo except for fruit juices.

Tolerance testing.   The procedure for conducting the tolerance test involves repeated doses of diazepam 20 mg or pentobarbital 200 mg administered orally to clinically unintoxicated patients who have been npo except for fruit juices for 2 hours.

Normally, the initial dose of diazepam or pentobarbital is administered at 0800 hours. If a patient exhibits any signs of intoxication (e.g., ataxia, dysarthria, coarse nystagmus, rombergism, excessive sleep) between 0800 and 1000 hours, he or she is considered to be nontolerant, and no further medication is necessary. If alert, the patient is given additional diazepam 20-mg or pentobarbital 200-mg doses every 2 hours (the maximum pentobarbital dose is 1,000 mg) until signs of intoxication are exhibited at any time during the 2 hours after the dose. Patients who become intoxicated with one or two doses (e.g., up to diazepam 40 mg or pentobarbital 400 mg) are considered not at great risk of experiencing severe withdrawal symptoms and, based on the judgment of the clinician, may not require further hospitalization (see Table 10–4). Conservatively, such patients might be placed on a low-dose withdrawal protocol (see *Low-Dose Withdrawal* [page 577] under "Treatment," above).

Withdrawal protocol.   If the tolerance test is positive, the patient is withdrawn with phenobarbital or diazepam. The initial daily requirement of phenobarbital is determined by substituting pheno-barbital 30 mg for every pentobarbital 100 mg administered during the tolerance test. The starting diazepam dose is calculated to be

Table 10–4.   Tolerance test outcomes

Intoxicating or hypnotic dose		
Pentobarbital (mg)	**Diazepam (mg)**	**Tolerance rating**
200	20	none
400	40	minimal
600	60	definite
800	80	marked
1,000	> 100	extreme

Table 10–5.   Sample diazepam withdrawal schedule

Day	Tolerance level
Test dose	160
1	65[*]
2	60
3	55
4	50
5	45
6	40
7	35
8	30
9	25
10	20
11	15
12	10
13	5
14	0

[*]mg/day diazepam calculated as 40% of reported benzodiazepine ingestion; total daily dose divided every 6 hours (depending on available dosage forms).

40% of the test dose (Harrison et al. 1984). During withdrawal, the daily requirement of phenobarbital or diazepam is decreased by 10% from an initial level equal to the intoxicating dose. The tapering schedule (e.g., day 1) begins at midnight on the day after tolerance testing. Sample schedules for diazepam and pentobarbital are provided in Tables 10–5 and 10–6, respectively.

A divided-dosage schedule of q6h is recommended rather than four-times-a-day dosing. Dosing q6h would place one or two doses at a time when a patient would be expected to be sleeping. Typically, a patient experiencing withdrawal has significantly reduced total sleep time. Therefore, if the person is sleeping, those doses

Table 10–6.   Sample pentobarbital-phenobarbital withdrawal schedule

Day	Tolerance level
Test dose	1,000[a]
1	300[b]
2	270
3	240
4	210
5	180
6	150
7	120
8	90
9	60
10	30
11	0

[a] mg pentobarbital. [b] mg phenobarbital; total daily dose divided every 6 hours (depending on available dosage forms).

should be held and not "made up." This dosing schedule allows "self-titration" of the dose.

Monitoring procedures.   Staff should observe the patient for nausea, diaphoresis, and tremor and should take the patient's blood pressure, temperature, and pulse before each dose. The number of hours of sleep per night and any symptoms displayed are recorded. These observations are used to adjust the withdrawal schedule in the event that the patient develop the signs and symptoms of abstinence or intoxication.

An increase in vital signs and/or a decrease in sleep are used as indices of an abstinence syndrome. Additionally, the withdrawal schedule is slowed if symptoms of withdrawal (e.g., tremor, nausea, diaphoresis) occur or if the patient is observed to sleep less than 4 hours per night. Under the diazepam protocol, if *significant* withdrawal symptoms occur between scheduled po doses, diazepam 10 mg iv or lorazepam 2 mg iv can be administered every 20 minutes as necessary to eliminate objective signs of withdrawal. This amount should be added to the scheduled BZD dose and the tapering dose readjusted. If withdrawal symptoms are not serious and the patient is able to take oral medications, diazepam 20 mg every 2 hours should be administered until the withdrawal symptoms cease. Again, the doses should be added to the calculated daily dose and the tapering schedule readjusted.

If the barbiturate protocol is used, pentobarbital 200 mg po q2h (for a total of 1,000 mg/day) or 100 mg iv/im every 10–20 minutes (up to a maximum of 500 mg/day) may be used.

Patients are also monitored throughout the tapering schedule for signs of drug intoxication that might be indicative of tolerance test inaccuracy (e.g., false-positive tests, overestimation of drug tolerance). If, before a scheduled dose, the patient presents with ataxia, dysarthria, coarse nystagmus, rombergism, or persistent drowsiness, doses should be held until these symptoms clear, and the daily dose should be reduced by 1 day's requirement.

Nicotine Withdrawal and Withdrawal Schedule

The cost of nicotine product use, in health-care utilization and lost productivity, is approximately $96 billion per year (Fiore et al. 1994).

■ Presentation

The nicotine withdrawal syndrome includes anger, anxiety, craving, decreased concentration, decreased heart rate, frustration, gastrointestinal (GI) disturbances, headache, increased coughing, insomnia, irritability, restlessness, tremor, and weight gain (Fiore et al. 1992). Although the mechanism of the withdrawal syndrome is unknown, it is suggested to involve CNS adrenergic overactivity (Foote et al. 1983).

After cessation of nicotine use or a reduction in the amount ingested, the onset of withdrawal symptoms may vary from 2 to 24 hours. The intensity of the symptoms will typically decline over the subsequent several days to weeks. However, the craving for nicotine reaches a peak within 24 hours and may continue for several weeks or months (Fiore et al. 1992).

■ Treatment

Although many nonpharmacological treatments have been used to eliminate the use of nicotine, these have not been generally successful in producing long-term abstinence (Fiore et al. 1990). Direct recommendations from a physician produce quit rates of 7%–10% (Fiore et al. 1992). However, in several surveys, only about 50% of physicians asked their patients about tobacco use (Fiore et al. 1992).

Recently, the use of pharmacological treatment to supplement the psychological/educational approaches has been investigated. Withdrawal treatment strategies include nicotine replacement, nicotine antagonists, symptomatic management, and aversive agents (Fiore et al. 1992; Jarvik and Henningfield 1988).

Nicotine Replacement

A meta-analysis of 53 studies lasting more than 6 months and involving 17,703 subjects reported that nicotine replacement with chewing gum (42 studies), patches (9 studies), intranasal spray (1 study), and inhaler (1 study) increased the odds ratio of abstinence:nonabstinence to 1.71 in treated versus control subjects (Silagy et al. 1994). The odds ratios for the different delivery systems were 1.61, 2.07, 2.92, and 3.05, respectively. Interestingly, the addition of behavioral treatment in some of the studies did not increase the rate of smoking cessation.

▶ Nicotine Polacrilex Gum

Pharmacokinetics. Nicotine polacrilex gum (Nicorette®) contains 2 or 4 mg of nicotine per piece and releases approximately 90% of the active ingredient after 30 minutes of chewing (Nemeth-Coslett et al. 1988). When the 2-mg gum is used according to the manufacturer's recommendation, it supplies 30%–64% of precessation nicotine levels (Fiore et al. 1992). Hourly use may be required to maintain adequate serum concentrations (Russell 1988).

Withdrawal effects. The effect of nicotine polacrilex has not been demonstrated to have a significant effect on *withdrawal symptoms* such as alertness, craving, disorientation, and dizziness (Fagerstrom 1988). However, nicotine may have a beneficial effect on anger, anxiety, frustration, irritability, increased appetite or weight gain, reduced concentration, and restlessness.

Efficacy in smoking cessation. A meta-analysis of 14 controlled studies of smokers presenting to a clinic for smoking cessation reported 6-month success rates of 27% for the gum and 18% for placebo treatment (Fiore et al. 1992). However, a review of the use of the gum in general medical practices reported no differences in the success rates of nicotine polacrilex and placebo gum during a 6- to 12-month follow-up (both approximately 11%). Notwithstanding, studies that combine nicotine polacrilex and intensive counseling report success rates of 27%–50%.

Adverse effects. Adverse effects reported in approximately 40% of patients include GI effects (e.g., mouth ulcers, oral burning, nausea, anorexia, jaw soreness, excessive salivation), hiccups, and headache (Benowitz 1988). Use of the gum for longer than 6 months is not recommended, as dependence may occur in 10% of regular users (Nunn-Thompson and Simon 1989).

▶ Nicotine Patches

Nicotine patches were marketed to reduce the compliance problems associated with the gum. The first patch was marketed in 1992 in the United States.

Pharmacokinetics.   The absolute bioavailability of nicotine is approximately 82% (Palmer et al. 1992). Initial plasma concentrations occur within 1 to 4 hours, and peak levels occur between 3 and 12 hours. Steady-state concentrations are reached within 2 to 4 days. Patch discontinuation results in unmeasurable serum nicotine concentrations within 24 hours.

Patches produce a steady release of nicotine and have the advantage over the gum of avoiding peak/trough nicotine concentrations (Fiore et al. 1992). Theoretically, the craving and withdrawal effects are minimized and the habit-reinforcing effects of peak/trough nicotine concentrations, which are produced by smoking and the gum, are avoided.

Withdrawal effects.   Overall, the literature reports conflicting results regarding the efficacy of nicotine patches in preventing the signs and symptoms of nicotine withdrawal (Fiore et al. 1992, 1994). Those studies that report positive effects indicate only a moderate reduction in symptomatology.

Efficacy in smoking cessation.   Overall, in 11 double-blind, placebo-controlled trials, 8-week cessation rates for nicotine patches and placebo were 18%–77% and 7%–53%, respectively (Fiore et al. 1992, 1994). The 6-month rates were 22%–42% and 5%–28%, respectively. Adjunctive treatment programs will approximately double the cessation rate (Fiore et al. 1992).

Adverse effects.   The most common adverse effects seen with patches are time-limited erythema, pruritis, or burning at the site of application in 35%–54% of patients (Fiore et al. 1992). In addition, mild insomnia may occur in up to 23% of patch users.

Although patients with cardiovascular disease may safely receive nicotine patches, they should be warned against smoking while using the patch because of a potentially increased risk of myocardial infarctions (Fiore et al. 1992). Likewise, individuals weighing less than 45 kg and/or smoking fewer than 10 cigarettes per day should receive the second-step nicotine patch dose (i.e., dosage reduction schedule) (Palmer et al. 1992).

Products.   Two products, Habitrol® and Nicoderm®, are available in patch strengths of 21 mg, 14 mg, and 7 mg and have a 24-hour release time (Fiore et al. 1992). These are administered

daily for 2–4 weeks, 2 weeks, and 2 weeks, respectively. Nicotrol®
is available in 15-mg, 10-mg, and 5-mg patches that are designed to
release nicotine over 16 hours. The rationale for the 16-hour patch
is that it more closely mimics the way cigarettes are consumed. The
dosage reduction schedule for Nicotrol® is the same as those for
Habitrol® and Nicoderm®. Pro*Step*® is available in 22-mg and
11-mg 24-hour-release patches. Its administration schedule consists of 3–5 weeks followed by dosage reduction for an additional
3 weeks.

Administering patches for longer than 8 weeks is generally not
recommended (Fiore et al. 1992).

▶ Nicotine Spray

Nicotine spray was marketed because for many, nicotine gum was
hard to use and release of nicotine from transdermal patches was
unacceptability slow.

Pharmacokinetics.   Absorption of nicotine is rapid, especially
during the first 2.5 minutes, with the peak level occurring 5 minutes after administration (Sutherland et al. 1992a). Average nicotine levels of 10.5 ng/mL were achieved with a 2-mg dose of
nicotine base. With prn nicotine spray, nicotine levels averaged
44% of patients' prior smoking levels.

Withdrawal effects.   Nicotine withdrawal symptoms were mod-
estly reduced with the use of nicotine spray compared with placebo
in a double-blind study (Sutherland et al. 1992b).

Efficacy in smoking cessation.   Three recent double-blind, placebo-controlled 6- to 12-month trials examined the effect of nicotine nasal spray on smoking cessation rate (Hjalmarson et al. 1994;
Schneider et al. 1995; Sutherland et al. 1992b). The abstinence
rates for nicotine spray and placebo ranged from 18% to 27% and
8% to 15%, respectively. Thus, active treatment approximately
doubled the success rate.

Adverse effects.   Generally, nicotine spray is well tolerated. Minor nasal mucosa irritant effects are generally reported, but only at
a slightly greater rate with the nicotine spray than with placebo
(Hjalmarson et al. 1994; Schneider et al. 1995; Sutherland et al.
1992b).

Products.   The typical dose is 0.5 mg/spray. The number of doses
per day will depend on the number of cigarettes ingested daily and
the patient's nicotine tolerance. Nicotine spray is sold as Nicotrol®
NS, a 10-mg/mL solution in a 10-mL spray bottle.

▶ **Nicotine Polacrilex Gum Combined With Nicotine Patches**

In a double-blind, placebo-controlled study, subjects receiving the combination of a nicotine patch (15 mg for 12 weeks, tapered to 10 mg and 5 mg for 6 weeks each) plus more than four pieces of gum per day were compared with subjects in two comparison groups (Kornitzer et al. 1995). The first comparison group received a placebo patch plus active gum, and the second received the reverse (i.e., an active patch plus placebo gum). Gum use was restricted to 6 months in all 3 groups. One-year abstinence rates, as verified by carbon monoxide monitoring, were 18.1% for the patch/gum combined-treatment group and 13% for both comparison groups ($P =$ not significant). Only at the 3-month and 6-month assessment periods was the success rate for the combined-treatment group significantly better than that for the comparison groups. No significant differences were observed among the three groups in systemic or local adverse effects. The efficacy of combined nicotine patch/gum treatment requires further study.

Nicotine Antagonist

Mecamylamine is a centrally active nicotine antagonist that was marketed in the 1950s as an antihypertensive agent. The drug has been studied only in two 3-week nonblind, uncontrolled trials in small numbers of patients (Nunn-Thompson and Simon 1989). Adverse reactions observed with 5–50 mg/day included anticholinergic effects. One-third and one-half of patients, respectively, were abstinent at the end of the studies. However, only 14% were still abstinent at 1-month follow-up. Additional controlled studies of mecamylamine need to be performed.

Symptomatic Management

Buspirone, clonidine, lobeline, and tricyclic antidepressants have been investigated for use in management of nicotine withdrawal (Nunn-Thompson and Simon 1989).

Buspirone 15–60 mg/day in a 6-week trial produced a 70% reduction in craving and a 75% reduction in cigarette consumption in seven patients (Gawin et al. 1989). Dizziness occurred with higher doses. Weight gain was not reported.

Clonidine has been studied in double-blind, placebo-controlled trials using oral (10 studies) and transdermal (5 studies) dosage forms (Gourlay and Benowitz 1995; Nunn-Thompson and Simon 1989). Oral doses ranged from 0.10 to 0.700 mg/day. Common adverse effects included sedation, dizziness/hypotension, and dry mouth. Transdermal clonidine was administered as a 0.1-mg patch at a dose of 0.1–0.2 mg/day.

Five of six studies involving durations of 21 days or less reported that clonidine was more effective than placebo (Gourlay and Benowitz 1995). A total of 448 patients were enrolled in the studies; two of the studies involved patches, and four used po administration. However, in nine studies (three patch and six oral) involving 6–12 months of clonidine treatment versus 2–12 weeks of placebo administration, the average success rates were 27% and 17%, respectively (Gourlay and Benowitz 1995). Only one of the nine studies reported a significant difference between clonidine and placebo. It is recommended that clonidine be started 48–72 hours prior to smoking cessation.

The *tricyclic antidepressants* imipramine and doxepin have been investigated as an adjunct to smoking cessation. Imipramine 75 mg/day plus group therapy was ineffective in reducing smoking compared with a control condition of group therapy alone (Jacobs et al. 1971). However, this dose may have been too low to be effective. Doxepin 150 mg/day, in a 7-week, double-blind, placebo-controlled trial and a 5-week open study, had a reported success rate of 50% and 78%, respectively (Whelan and Davis 1990). The drug produced an average weight gain of 11.7 pounds in study patients, as compared with an average 2.5-pound gain in subjects receiving placebo. Other adverse effects included dry mouth and sedation. The study's authors concluded that doxepin may be useful in managing nicotine withdrawal symptoms. Long-term effects of tricyclic antidepressants need to be investigated.

Lobeline is a derivative of *Lobelia inflata*, a plant similar to tobacco that produces primarily GI side effects. A review of placebo-controlled studies concluded that the drug is not effective in the treatment of nicotine withdrawal (Davison and Rosen 1972).

Aversive Treatments
Silver acetate produces an unpleasant metallic taste when combined with nicotine. Available over the counter as a gum containing 6 mg per piece, the usual dose is 6 pieces/day. One blinded, controlled trial reported that after 3 weeks of use, 11% of active-treatment patients and 4% of placebo-treated patients were abstinent (Malcolm et al. 1986). At 4-month follow-up, 7% and 3% of patients, respectively, were not smoking.

In one study, oral (e.g., dry mouth, loss of taste, tongue discoloration) and abdominal (e.g., nausea, heartburn, cramps) adverse effects were reported by 22% and 13.2% of patients, respectively. This compared with rates of 5.7% and 0%, respectively, in placebo-treated subjects. Silver poisoning has also been reported with this agent (Nunn-Thompson and Simon 1989).

Recommendations

Pharmacological treatments should be considered for patients with significant nicotine dependence that have failed to respond to nonpharmacological approaches. At best, the response in short-term studies may approach 70%. The greatest chance for successful cessation of tobacco use is provided by the combination of pharmacological and behavioral therapies. Management of **withdrawal** includes nicotine polacrilex gum, nicotine spray, nicotine patches, clonidine, and doxepin. **Maintenance** treatment with nicotine patches, mecamylamine, or silver acetate gum might be considered (Nunn-Thompson and Simon 1989).

Central Nervous System Stimulant Withdrawal and Withdrawal Schedule

Cocaine, amphetamine, and amphetamine derivatives remain the primary CNS stimulants of abuse. Although this section deals primarily with cocaine abuse, withdrawal presentation and management techniques for amphetamines are similar to those for cocaine (Kosten 1990a; Lago and Kosten 1994).

Cocaine and amphetamines share many pharmacological effects. Cocaine blocks the reuptake of dopamine, serotonin, and norepinephrine (Sitland-Marken et al. 1990). In addition, it may increase the synthesis of dopamine and norepinephrine while blocking the production of serotonin.

■ Presentation

The abstinence syndrome described for *cocaine* has been divided into three phases (Gawin 1989; Gawin and Kleber 1986; Hall et al. 1990). *Phase I,* the crash, is characterized by agitation, significant dysphoria, fatigue, hypersomnolence, hyperphagia, and anorexia that occur within 9 hours of cocaine discontinuation but may last up to 4 days. This period is marked by a loss of cocaine craving. *Phase II,* the withdrawal period, may last from 1 to 10 weeks. The first week of this phase is characterized by normal sleep, euthymia, little anxiety, and minimal cocaine craving. However, this state is replaced with loss of pleasure, diminished energy, and increasing anxiety that lead to significant cocaine craving. Relapse is likely to occur at this point. *Phase III,* the extinction period, begins after

1–10 weeks of abstinence. During this period, cravings may occur when reminders of objects or events associated with past cocaine use are encountered. If the person does not relapse, the desire for cocaine will eventually abate, although the process may require months to years.

A similar pattern has been described for *amphetamines* (Kosten 1990a; Watson et al. 1972).

This "triphasic" withdrawal presentation has been questioned (Lago and Kosten 1994). Two inpatient studies did not report a crash phase, and mood gradually improved for 3–4 weeks of treatment. The difference in these findings may be due to these studies' use of outpatient versus inpatient treatment settings.

■ Treatment

Approaches to the management of cocaine abuse involve psychological and pharmacological strategies (Hall et al. 1990). Only pharmacological strategies are discussed here. Pharmacological management is directed toward reestablishing normal concentrations of neurotransmitters (e.g., dopamine, norepinephrine, serotonin) that were depleted or suppressed with continuous cocaine use (Kosten 1990a; Lago and Kosten 1994). Normalization of neurotransmitters would theoretically reduce or eliminate cocaine craving. Agents that have been investigated for this use include direct- and indirect-acting dopamine agonists and first- and second-generation antidepressants.

Dopamine Agonists
The use of methylphenidate, levodopa/carbidopa, and pemoline in cocaine withdrawal has been investigated in a limited number of open trials. Amantadine and bromocriptine have been studied in one and four controlled trials, respectively (Kosten 1990a). It is important to note that only 53 patients were investigated in these trials. In 0.635- to 1.25-mg single doses, bromocriptine produced a greater reduction in cocaine craving than did placebo (Dackis and Gold 1985; Dackis et al. 1987). In a 10-day study, bromocriptine 7.5 mg/day and amantadine 200 mg/day were equally effective in suppressing cravings for cocaine (Tennant and Sagherian 1987). Bromocriptine 0.625 mg qid for 6 weeks produced significantly greater reduction of craving compared with placebo (Giannini et al. 1987). To minimize side effects, bromocriptine doses lower than 2.5 mg/day might be attempted.

Antidepressants

Antidepressants may decrease presynaptic receptor sensitivity and reduce autoinhibition (Kosten 1990a). Imipramine, desipramine, maprotiline, and trazodone have been studied in open trials (Hall et al. 1990). Only desipramine has been investigated in six placebo-controlled trials (Levin and Lehman 1991). The number of patients treated was 200. Overall, desipramine was more effective than placebo in achieving abstinence; however, there were no differences between the groups in retaining patients in treatment. (See "Dosage" and "Adverse Effects" subsections [pages 141 and 149, respectively] under **Tricyclic Antidepressants** in Chapter 2.)

Lithium

In one controlled trial, the response rates for lithium and placebo were 25% and 17%, respectively, for reductions in cocaine use, craving, and assessment scores (Gawin et al. 1989). More studies need to be performed to assess the efficacy of lithium in CNS stimulant abuse.

Bromocriptine

Five studies involving 41 patients reported some benefit in short-term (e.g., 2–42 days) and long-term (e.g., 9 months) treatment with bromocriptine (Sitland-Marken et al. 1990). However, these studies used different assessment techniques, and most were uncontrolled. Doses ranged from 0.625 to 12.5 mg/day. Almost 90% of patients dropped out of the studies as a result of adverse effects (e.g., headache, sedation, tremor). Double-blind, controlled studies with larger samples sizes and standardized assessments are needed to determine bromocriptine's precise role in the management of withdrawal and abstinence from cocaine use.

■ Summary

Additional pharmacological studies are required to assess the efficacy of various agents in the treatment of cocaine withdrawal. It is important to note that if pharmacological treatment is considered, it should be in conjunction with nonpharmacological approaches performed by trained personnel.

References

Albeck JH: Withdrawal and detoxification from benzodiazepine dependence: a potential role for clonazepam. J Clin Psychiatry 48 (suppl 10):48–49, 1987

Ansseau M, De Roeck J: Trazodone in benzodiazepine dependence. J Clin Psychiatry 54:189–191, 1993

Benowitz NL: Toxicity of nicotine: implications with regard to nicotine replacement therapy, in Nicotine Replacement: A Critical Evaluation. Edited by Pomerleau OF, Pomerleau CS, Fagerstrom K-O, et al. New York, Alan R. Liss, 1988, pp 187–217

Benzer D, Cushman P: Alcohol and benzodiazepines: withdrawal syndromes. Alcohol Clin Exp Res 4:243–247, 1980

Bird RD, Makela EH: Alcohol withdrawal: what is the benzodiazepine of choice? Ann Pharmacother 28:67–71, 1994

Bond WS: Psychiatric indications for clonidine: the neuropharmacologic and clinical basis. J Clin Psychopharmacol 6:81–87, 1986

Browne JL, Hauge KJ: A review of alprazolam withdrawal. Drug Intelligence and Clinical Pharmacy 20:837–841, 1986

Busto U, Sellers EM, Naranjo CA, et al: Withdrawal reaction after long-term therapeutic use of benzodiazepines. N Engl J Med 315:854–859, 1986

Charney DS, Kleber HD: Iatrogenic opiate addiction: successful detoxification with clonidine. Am J Psychiatry 127:989–990, 1980

Charney DS, Sternberg DE, Kleber HD, et al: The clinical use of clonidine in abrupt withdrawal from methadone. Arch Gen Psychiatry 38:1273–1277, 1981

Code of Federal Regulations, Chapter II, Title 21, Section 1306.07, April 1, 1983

Craft PP, Foil MB, Cunningham PR, et al: Intravenous ethanol for alcohol detoxification in trauma patients. South Med J 87:47–54, 1994

Dackis CA, Gold MS: Pharmacological approaches to cocaine addiction. J Subst Abuse Treat 2:139–145, 1985

Dackis CA, Gold MS, Sweeney DR, et al: Single-dose bromocriptine reverses cocaine craving. Psychiatry Res 20:261–264, 1987

Davison GC, Rosen RC: Lobeline and reduction of cigarette smoking. Psychol Rep 31:443–456, 1972

DuPont FL: A practical approach to benzodiazepine discontinuation. J Psychiatr Res 24 (suppl 2):81–90, 1990

Erstad BL, Cotugno C: Management of alcohol withdrawal. American Journal of Health-Systems Pharmacy 52:697–709, 1995

Ewing JA, Bakewell WE: Diagnosis and management of depressant drug dependence. Am J Psychiatry 123:909–917, 1967

Fagerstrom K-O: Efficacy of nicotine chewing gum: a review, in Nicotine Replacement: A Critical Evaluation. Edited by Pomerleau OF, Pomerleau CS, Fagerstrom K-O, et al. New York, Alan R. Liss, 1988, pp 109–128

Farrell M: Opiate withdrawal. Addiction 89:1471–1475, 1994

Fiore MC, Novotny TE, Pierce JP, et al: Methods used to quit smoking in the United States. JAMA 263:2760–2765, 1990

Fiore MC, Jorenby DE, Baker TB, et al: Tobacco dependence and the nicotine patch. JAMA 268:2687–2694, 1992

Fiore MC, Kenford SL, Jorenby DE, et al: Two studies of clinical effectiveness of the nicotine patch with different counseling treatments. Chest 105:524–533, 1994

Fishbain DA, Rosomoff HL, Cutler R, et al: Opiate detoxification protocols: a clinical manual. Ann Clin Psychiatry 5:53–65, 1993

Fontaine R, Chouinard G, Annable L: Rebound anxiety in anxious patients after abrupt withdrawal of benzodiazepine treatment. Am J Psychiatry 141:848–852, 1984

Foote SL, Bloom FE, Aston-Jones G: Nucleus locus coeruleus: new evidence of anatomical and physiological specificity. Physiol Rev 63:844–914, 1983

Fraser HF, Isbell H: Human pharmacology and addiction liability of dl- and d-propoxyphene. Bull Narc 12:9–14, 1960

Fraser HF, Wiler A, Essig CF, et al: Degree of physical dependence induced by secobarbital or pentobarbital. JAMA 166:126–129, 1958

Fraser HF, Isbell H, Van Horn GD: Human pharmacology and addiction liability of norcodeine. J Pharmacol Exp Ther 129:172–177, 1960

Fraser HF, Van Horn GD, Martin WR, et al: Methods for evaluating addiction liability, A: "attitude" of opiate addicts toward opiate-like drugs; B: a short-term "direct" addiction test. J Pharmacol Exp Ther 133:371–387, 1961

Fruensgaard K: Withdrawal psychosis: a study of 30 consecutive cases. Acta Psychiatr Scand 53:105–118, 1976

Fultz JM, Senay EC: Guidelines for the management of hospitalized narcotic addicts. Ann Intern Med 82:815–818, 1975

Fyer AJ, Liebowitz MR, Gorman JM: Discontinuation of alprazolam treatment in panic patients. Am J Psychiatry 144:303–308, 1987

Gawin FH, Kleber HD: Abstinence symptomatology and psychiatric diagnosis in cocaine abusers. Arch Gen Psychiatry 43:107–113, 1986

Gawin F, Compton M, Byck R: Buspirone reduces smoking. Arch Gen Psychiatry 46:288–289, 1989

Gawin FH: Cocaine abuse and addiction. J Fam Pract 29:193–197, 1989

Giannini AJ, Baumgartel P, DiMarzio LR: Bromocriptine therapy in cocaine withdrawal. J Clin Pharmacol 27:267–270, 1987

Gold MS, Redmond DE, Kleber HD: Clonidine in opiate withdrawal (letter). Lancet 1:929–930, 1978a

Gold MS, Redmond DE, Kleber HD: Clonidine blocks acute opiate-withdrawal symptoms (letter). Lancet 2:599–602, 1978b

Gold MS, Pottash AC, Sweeney DR, et al: Opiate withdrawal using clonidine: a safe, effective, and rapid nonopiate treatment. JAMA 243:343–346, 1979

Gold MS, Redmond E, Kleber HD: Noradrenergic hyperactivity in opiate withdrawal supported by clonidine reversal of opiate withdrawal. Am J Psychiatry 137:1121–1122, 1980

Goodman WK: Ineffectiveness of clonidine in the treatment of the benzodiazepine withdrawal syndrome: report of three cases. Am J Psychiatry 143:900–903, 1986

Gossop M, Griffiths P, Bradley B, et al: Opiate withdrawal symptoms in response to 10-day and 21-day methadone withdrawal programmes. Br J Psychiatry 154:360–363, 1989

Gourlay SG, Benowitz NL: Is clonidine an effective smoking cessation therapy? Drugs 50:197–207, 1995

Guthrie SK: The treatment of alcohol withdrawal. Pharmacotherapy 9:131–143, 1989

Guthrie SK: Pharmacologic interventions for the treatment of opioid dependence and withdrawal. DICP Ann Pharmacother 24:721–734, 1990

Hall WC, Talbert RL, Ereshefsky L: Cocaine abuse and its treatment. Pharmacotherapy 10:47–65, 1990

Hallstrom C, Lader M: Benzodiazepine withdrawal phenomena. International Pharmacopsychiatry 16:235–244, 1981

Harrison M, Busto U, Naranjo CA, et al: Diazepam tapering in detoxification for high-dose benzodiazepine abuse. Clin Pharmacol Ther 36:527–533, 1984

Harvey SC: Hypnotics and sedatives, in The Pharmacological Basis of Therapeutics, 7th Edition. Edited by Gilman AG, Goodman LS, Rall TW, et al. New York, Macmillan, 1985, pp 349–354

Henderson GL, Wilson K, Lau DHM: Plasma L-alpha-acetylmethadol (LAAM) after acute and chronic administration. Clin Pharmacol Ther 21:16–25, 1977

Heritch AJ, Capwell R, Roy-Byrne PP: A case of psychosis and delirium following withdrawal from triazolam. J Clin Psychiatry 48:168–169, 1987

Herman JB, Rosenbaum JR, Brotman AW: The alprazolam to clonazepam switch for the treatment of panic disorder. J Clin Psychopharmacol 7:175–178, 1987

Himmelsbach CK: Addiction liability of codeine. JAMA 103:1420–1421, 1934

Hjalmarson A, Franzon M, Westin A, et al: Effect of nicotine nasal spray on smoking cessation: a randomized, placebo-controlled, double-blind study. Arch Intern Med 154:2567–2572, 1994

Hollister LE, Motzenbecker FP, Degan RO: Withdrawal reactions from chlordiazepoxide ("Librium"). Psychopharmacologia 2:63–68, 1961

Hollister LE, Bennett JL, Kimbell I, et al: Diazepam in newly admitted schizophrenics. Diseases of the Nervous System 24:746–748, 1963

Hollister LE: Benzodiazepines 1980—current update: a look at the issues. Psychosomatics 10 (suppl):4–8, 1980

Isbell H: Manifestations and treatment of addiction to narcotic drugs and barbiturates. Med Clin North Am 34:425–438, 1950

Isbell H, White WM: Clinical characteristics of addictions. JAMA 14:558–565, 1953

Isbell H, Fraser HF, Wikler A, et al: An experimental study of the etiology of "rum fits" and delirium tremens. Quarterly Journal of Studies on Alcohol 16:1–33, 1955

Jacobs MA, Spilken AZ, Norman MM, et al: Interaction of personality and treatment conditions associated with success in a smoking control program. Psychosom Med 33:545–556, 1971

Jaffe JH: Drug addiction and drug abuse, in The Pharmacological Basis of Therapeutics, 6th Edition. Edited by Gilman AG, Goodman LS, Gilman A. New York, Macmillan, 1980, pp 535–584

Jaffe JH: Drug addiction and drug abuse, in The Pharmacological Basis of Therapeutics, 7th Edition. Edited by Gilman AG, Goodman LS, Rall TW, et al. New York, Macmillan, 1985, p 571

Jaffe JH, Martin WR: Opioid analgesics and antagonists, in The Pharmacological Basis of Therapeutics, 7th Edition. Edited by Gilman AG, Goodman LS, Rall TW, et al. New York, Macmillan, 1985, pp 504–531, 541–545

Jarvik ME, Henningfield JE: Pharmacologic treatment of tobacco dependence. Pharmacol Biochem Behav 30:279–294, 1988

Jasinski DR, Martin WR, Hoeldtke RD: Effects of short- and long-term administration of pentazocine in man. Clin Pharmacol Ther 11:385–403, 1970

Jasinski DR, Pevnick JS, Griffith JD: Human pharmacology and abuse potential of the analgesic buprenorphine. Arch Gen Psychiatry 35:501–516, 1978

Judson BA, Goldstein A, Inturrisi CE: Methadyl acetate (LAAM) in the treatment of heroin addicts, II: double-blind comparison of gradual and abrupt detoxification. Arch Gen Psychiatry 40:834–840, 1983

Kahn A, Joyce P, Jones AV: Benzodiazepine withdrawal syndromes. N Z Med J 92:94–96, 1980

Keck PE, McElroy SL, Friedman LM: Valproate and carbamazepine in the treatment of panic and posttraumatic stress disorders, withdrawal states, and behavioral dyscontrol syndromes. J Clin Psychopharmacol 12:36S–41S, 1992

Kesharan MS, Crammer JL: Clonidine in benzodiazepine withdrawal. Lancet 1:1325–1326, 1985

Khantzian EJ, McKenna GJ: Acute toxic and withdrawal reactions associated with drug use and abuse. Ann Intern Med 90:361–372, 1979

Klein E, Uhde TW, Post RM: Preliminary evidence for the utility of carbamazepine in alprazolam withdrawal. Am J Psychiatry 143:235–236, 1986

Kornitzer M, Boutsen M, Dramaix M, et al: Combined use of nicotine patch and gum in smoking cessation: a placebo-controlled clinical trial. Prev Med 24:41–47, 1995

Kosten TR: Neurobiology of abuse drugs: opioids and stimulants. J Nerv Ment Dis 178:217–227, 1990a

Kosten TR: Current pharmacotherapies for opioid dependence. Psychopharmacol Bull 26:69–74, 1990b

Kreek MJ: Multiple drug abuse patterns and medical consequences, in Psychopharmacology: The Third Generation of Progress. Edited by Meltzer HY. New York, Raven, 1987, pp 1597–1604

Lader M, Olajide KD: A comparison of buspirone and placebo in relieving benzodiazepine withdrawal symptoms. J Clin Psychopharmacol 7:11–15, 1987

Lago JA, Kosten TR: Stimulant withdrawal. Addiction 89:1477–1481, 1994

Lahmeyer HW, Craig RJ: Pentazocine-naloxone: another "addiction-proof" drug of abuse. Int J Addict 22:1163–1166, 1987

Laughren TP, Battey Y, Greenblatt DJ, et al: A controlled trial of diazepam withdrawal in chronically anxious outpatients. Acta Psychiatr Scand 65:171–179, 1982

Levin FR, Lehman AF: Meta-analysis of desipramine as an adjunct in the treatment of cocaine addiction. J Clin Psychopharmacol 11:374–378, 1991

Liskow BI, Goodwin DW: Pharmacological treatment of alcohol, intoxication withdrawal, and dependence: a critical review. J Stud Alcohol 48:356–370, 1987

Loimer N, Hofmann P, Chaudhry HR: Nasal administration of naloxone for detection of opiate dependence. J Psychiatr Res 26:39–43, 1992

Malcolm R, Currey HS, Mitchell MA, et al: Silver acetate gum as a deterrent to smoking. Chest 90:107–111, 1986

Marriott S, Tyrer P: Benzodiazepine dependence: avoidance and withdrawal. Drug Saf 9:93–103, 1993

Martin WR, Jasinski DR, Haertzen CA, et al: Methadone—a reevaluation. Arch Gen Psychiatry 28:286–295, 1973

Mendelson JH, LaDou J: Experimentally induced chronic intoxication and withdrawal in alcoholics, II: psychophysiological findings. Quarterly Journal of Studies on Alcohol 25 (suppl 2):14–39, 1964

Milhorn HT: Pharmacologic management of acute abstinence syndromes. Am Fam Physician 45:231–239, 1992

Morgan K, Oswald I: Anxiety caused by a short-life hypnotic (letter). Br J Psychiatry 284:942, 1982

Naranjo CA, Sellers EM, Chater K, et al: Nonpharmacologic intervention in acute alcohol withdrawal. Clin Pharmacol Ther 34:214–219, 1983

Nemeth-Coslett R, Benowitz NL, Robenson N: Nicotine gum: chew-rate, subjective effects, and plasma nicotine. Pharmacol Biochem Behav 29:47–51, 1988

Noyes R, Clancy J, Coryell WH, et al: A withdrawal syndrome after abrupt discontinuation of alprazolam. Am J Psychiatry 142:114–116, 1985

Noyes R, Garvey MJ, Cook BL, et al: Benzodiazepine withdrawal: a review of the evidence. J Clin Psychiatry 49:382–389, 1988

Nunn-Thompson CL, Simon PA: Pharmacotherapy for smoking cessation. Clinical Pharmacy 8:710–720, 1989

Olajide D, Lader M: Depression following withdrawal from long-term benzodiazepine use: a report of four cases. Psychol Med 14:937–940, 1984

Palmer KJ, Buckley MM, Faulds D: Transdermal nicotine: a review of its pharmacodynamic and pharmacokinetic properties, and therapeutic efficacy as an aid to smoking cessation. Drugs 44:498–529, 1992

Patterson JF: Withdrawal from alprazolam dependency using clonazepam: clinical observations. J Clin Psychiatry 5 (suppl):47–49, 1990

Perry PJ, Stambaugh RL, Tsuang MT, et al: Sedative-hypnotic tolerance testing and withdrawal comparing diazepam to barbiturates. J Clin Psychopharmacol 1:289–296, 1981

Perry PJ, Alexander B: Sedative/hypnotic dependence: patient stabilization, tolerance testing, and withdrawal. Drug Intelligence and Clinical Pharmacy 20:532–537, 1986

Petursson H, Lader MH: Withdrawal from long-term benzodiazepine treatment. BMJ 283:643–645, 1981

Pradhan SN, Dutta SN: Narcotic analgesics, in Drug Abuse: Clinical and Basic Aspects. Edited by Pradhan SN, Dutta SN. St. Louis, MO, CV Mosby, 1977, pp 59–65

Redmond DE: Central alpha-adrenergic mechanism in opiate withdrawal and other psychiatric syndromes: studies with clonidine. J Clin Psychiatry 43:1–48, 1981

Reed JS, Liskow BI: Current medical treatment of alcohol withdrawal. Rational Drug Therapy 21:1–7, 1987

Rickels K, Case G, Downing RW, et al: Long-term diazepam therapy and clinical outcome. JAMA 250:767–771, 1983

Rickels K, Case WG, Schweizer EE, et al: Low-dose dependence in chronic benzodiazepine users: a preliminary report on 119 patients. Psychopharmacol Bull 22:407–415, 1986

Rickels K, Case WG, Schweizer E, et al: Benzodiazepine dependence: management of discontinuation. Psychopharmacol Bull 26:63–68, 1990

Ries RK, Roy-Byrne PP, Ward NG, et al: Carbamazepine treatment for benzodiazepine withdrawal. Am J Psychiatry 146:536–537, 1989

Riordan CE, Kleber HD: Rapid opiate detoxification with clonidine and naloxone. Lancet 1:2079–2080, 1990

Rodrigo EK, Williams P: Frequency of self-reported "anxiolytic withdrawal" symptoms in a group of female students experiencing anxiety. Psychol Med 16:467–472, 1986

Rothstein E: Prevention of alcohol withdrawal seizures: the roles of diphenylhydantoin and chlordiazepoxide. Am J Psychiatry 130:1381–1382, 1973

Rowden AM, Lopez JR: Codeine addiction. DICP Ann Pharmacother 23:475–477, 1989

Russell MAH: Nicotine replacement: the role of blood nicotine levels, their rate of change, and nicotine tolerance, in Nicotine Replacement: A Critical Evaluation. Edited by Pomerleau OF, Pomerleau CS, Fagerstrom K-O, et al. New York, Alan R. Liss, 1988, pp 63–94

Saitz R, Mayo-Smith MF, Roberts MS, et al: Individualized treatment for alcohol withdrawal: a randomized double-blind controlled trial. JAMA 272:519–523, 1994

Sampliner R, Iber FL: Diphenylhydantoin control of alcohol withdrawal seizures. JAMA 230:1430–1432, 1974

Schneider LS, Syapin PJ, Pawluczyk S: Seizure following triazolam withdrawal despite benzodiazepine treatment. J Clin Psychiatry 48:418–419, 1987

Schneider NG, Olmstead R, Mody FV, et al: Efficacy of a nicotine nasal spray in smoking cessation: a placebo-controlled, double-blind trial. Addiction 90:1671–1682, 1995

Schweizer E, Rickels K: Failure of buspirone to manage benzodiazepine withdrawal. Am J Psychiatry 143:1590–1592, 1986

Schweizer E, Case G, Rickels K: Benzodiazepine dependence and withdrawal in elderly patients. Am J Psychiatry 146:529–531, 1989

Sellers EM: Clinical pharmacology and therapeutics of benzodiazepines. Canadian Medical Association Journal 118:1533–1538, 1978

Sellers EM, Kalant H: Alcohol intoxication and withdrawal. N Engl J Med 294:757–762, 1976

Shaw JM, Kolesar GS, Sellers EM, et al: Development of optimal treatment tactics for alcohol withdrawal, I: assessment and effectiveness of supportive care. J Clin Psychopharmacol 1:382–388, 1981

Silagy C, Mant D, Fowler G, et al: Meta-analysis on efficacy of nicotine replacement therapies in smoking cessation. Lancet 343:139–142, 1994

Sitland-Marken PA, Wells BG, Froemming JH, et al: Psychiatric applications of bromocriptine therapy. J Clin Psychiatry 51:68–82, 1990

Smith DE, Landry MJ: Benzodiazepine dependency discontinuation: focus on the chemical dependency detoxification setting and benzodiazepine-polydrug abuse. J Psychiatr Res 24 (suppl 2):145–156, 1990

Smith DE, Wesson DR: Benzodiazepine dependency syndromes. J Psychoactive Drugs 15:85–95, 1983

Spiegel DA, Bruce TJ, Gregg SF, et al: Does cognitive behavior therapy assist slow-taper alprazolam discontinuation in panic disorder? Am J Psychiatry 151:876–881, 1994

Stuppaeck CH, Pycha R, Miller C, et al: Carbamazepine versus oxazepam in the treatment of alcohol withdrawal: a double-blind study. Alcohol Alcohol 27:153–158, 1992

Sullivan JT, Sellers EM: Detoxification for triazolam physical dependence. J Clin Psychopharmacol 12:124–127, 1992

Sutherland G, Russell MA, Stapleton JA, et al: Nasal nicotine spray: a rapid nicotine delivery system. Psychopharmacology 108:512–518, 1992a

Sutherland G, Stapleton JA, Russell MA, et al: Randomized controlled trial of nasal nicotine spray in smoking cessation. Lancet 340:324–329, 1992b

Tennant FS Jr, Sagherian AA: Double-blind comparison of amantadine and bromocriptine for ambulatory withdrawal from cocaine dependence. Arch Intern Med 147:109–112, 1987

Thompson WL, Johnson AD, Maddrey WL: Diazepam and paraldehyde for treatment of severe delirium tremens: a controlled trial. Ann Intern Med 82:175–180, 1975

Tyrer P: Clinical management of benzodiazepine dependence (letter). BMJ 291:1507, 1985

Tyrer P, Owen R, Dawling S: Gradual withdrawal of diazepam after long-term therapy. Lancet 1:1402–1406, 1983

Tyrer R, Rutherford D, Huggett T: Benzodiazepine withdrawal symptoms and propranolol. Lancet 1:520–522, 1981

Vandam LD: Drug therapy: butorphanol. N Engl J Med 302:381–384, 1980

Vining E, Kosten TR, Kleber HD: Clinical utility of rapid clonidine naltrexone detoxification for opioid abusers. British Journal of Addiction 83:567–575, 1988

Vinogradov S, Reiss AL, Csernansky JG, et al: Clonidine therapy in withdrawal from high dose alprazolam treatment. Am J Psychiatry 143:1188–1191, 1986

Votolato NA, Botcha KJ, Olson SC: Comment: alprazolam withdrawal. Drug Intelligence and Clinical Pharmacy 21:753–754, 1987

Wartenberg AA, Nirenberg TD, Liepman MR, et al: Detoxification of alcoholics: improving care by symptom-triggered sedation. Alcohol Clin Exp Res 14:71–75, 1990

Washton AM, Resnick RB: Clonidine for opiate detoxification: outpatient clinical trials. Am J Psychiatry 136:100–102, 1979

Washton AM, Resnick RB, LaPlaca RW: Clonidine hydrochloride: a non-opiate treatment for opiate withdrawal. Psychopharmacol Bull 16:50–52, 1980

Watson R, Hartmann E, Schildkraut JJ: Amphetamine withdrawal: affective state, sleep patterns, and MHPG excretion. Am J Psychiatry 129:263–269, 1972

Whelan AM, Davis SK: Doxepin in smoking cessation. DICP Ann Pharmacother 24:598–599, 1990

Whitfield CL, Thompson G, Lamb A, et al: Detoxification of 1,024 alcoholic patients without psychoactive drugs. JAMA 239:1409–1410, 1978

Wikler A: Diagnosis and treatment of drug dependence of the barbiturate type. Am J Psychiatry 125:758–765, 1968

Wilber R, Kulik FA: Anticonvulsant drugs in alcohol withdrawal: use of phenytoin, primidone, carbamazepine, valproic acid, and the sedative anticonvulsants. Am J Hosp Pharm 1138–1143, 1981

Woods JH, Winger G: Current benzodiazepines issues. Psychopharmacology 118:107–115, 1995

11

Narcotherapy

Indications and Efficacy

Sodium amobarbital (Amytal™) was first used in psychiatry in 1930 by Bleckwenn to induce sleep in agitated and mute psychotic patients. He found that when previously mute and/or excited patients emerged from sleep induced by intravenous amobarbital, they often spoke and functioned normally for several hours (Bleckwenn 1930). In 1932, Lindemann described similar effects with amobarbital doses less than those necessary to induce sleep. In the late 1930s, uncontrolled studies found the drug to be useful in eliciting information from patients and in obtaining "truth" from criminals (Dysken et al. 1979a). However, in the late 1940s, amobarbital was judged of little use in criminal proceedings when it was demonstrated that normal individuals were able to maintain a false story under the influence of amobarbital (Dysken et al. 1979a; Gerson and Victoroff 1948).

During World War II, amobarbital and pentobarbital were used to treat posttraumatic stress disorder. Soldiers who were able to relive battlefield experiences under the influence of the barbiturates were reported able to return rapidly to combat duty (Grinker and Spiegel 1948).

In the early 1950s, amobarbital was found to be useful in uncovering organic mental symptoms in patients with various forms of underlying organic brain disease. In addition, it was found possible to make a prognosis for these patients by conducting serial amobarbital interviews. If symptoms worsened with succeeding interviews, the prognosis was generally poor (Weinstein et al. 1953, 1954).

In the mid-1960s, Woodruff studied the effect of amobarbital in patients with affective disorder, schizophrenia, and schizoaffective illness (Woodruff 1966). He found that, under the influence of amobarbital, affective-disorder patients were either unchanged or less concerned with their depression; schizophrenic patients displayed additional psychotic symptoms; and schizoaffective patients responded in a varied and inconsistent manner to the drug. Woodruff concluded that patients' diagnoses did not change under

amobarbital and that symptoms improved only in mute and uncommunicative patients.

More recently, in a double-blind, randomized, placebo-controlled
study, Dysken also investigated whether barbiturates helped clarify
patients' diagnoses and whether new and important information
could be gained under the drug's influence (Dysken et al. 1979b).
He reported that diagnostic interviews produced the same results
under barbiturate and saline and that as much new information was
gained with saline as with barbiturate. The only exception was one
catatonic patient who responded to barbiturates but not to saline.

The consensus of these investigations and of several other authors and reviewers is that although much research remains to be
done, the amobarbital interview is probably of value in the following (Kwentus 1981; Lampke 1982; Naples and Hackett 1978; Perry
and Jacob 1982):

1. Differential diagnosis of the mute, uncommunicative, and/or
    catatonic patient. Those patients whose underlying illness is
    depression will often "normalize" and begin to speak and act
    normally and be fully oriented. Patients with underlying schizo-
    phrenia will frequently produce additional psychotic symptoms
    and will be oriented. Patients with organicity may begin talk-
    ing, but will become more confused and disoriented with amo-
    barbital.
2. Diagnosis of patients with suspected organicity. Patients who
    are intact but have underlying central nervous system (CNS)
    pathology may become disoriented under amobarbital. On se-
    rial testing, worsening of the disorientation indicates progres-
    sion of the underlying CNS pathology.

In addition, amobarbital has also been found, in uncontrolled
studies, to be of use in the treatment of posttraumatic stress disorder, in recovery of memory in patients with psychogenic amnesia
and fugue, in establishing a more accurate history in Munchausen's
syndrome, and in recovery of function in patients with conversion
disorder (Grinker and Spiegel 1948; Herman 1938; Lambert and
Reese 1944; McDonald et al. 1979; Ruedrich et al. 1985).

False positives, in which an amobarbital interview produces
mental clearing despite an organic etiology, can occur with alcohol
withdrawal syndrome, seizure disorder, and antipsychotic-induced
muteness. False negatives, in which functional confusion does not
clear with amobarbital, can occur with faulty technique (e.g., injecting too rapidly or too slowly), malingering, and, possibly, hysteria (Lampke 1982; Ward et al. 1978).

Amobarbital has not been used in the treatment of catatonia because its effects are short lived; patients rapidly relapse after initial relief of their catatonic symptoms. Continuous or repetitive treatment of catatonic symptoms with amobarbital has not been reported. However, beginning in the late 1980s, lorazepam 2–4 mg im or po was found to be effective in normalizing patients with acute and chronic catatonia. In some cases, patients were maintained in a catatonia-free state for up to 2 years with continued oral doses of lorazepam 2–4 mg po (Gaind et al. 1994; Greenfield et al. 1987; Ripley and Millson 1988; Salam and Kilzieh 1988; Salam et al. 1987; Yassa et al. 1990). Higher dosages of lorazepam, up to 20 mg/day, have been reported to be necessary for the successful treatment of catatonia in certain patients (Smith and Lebegue 1991). Most case reports indicate success with several doses over several days or weeks of lorazepam (Salam and Kilzieh 1988), but others indicate that for some patients a sustained or increasing dose is necessary over a prolonged period of months for improvement to occur (Gaind et al. 1994).

In one of the two largest series of cases reported (Rosebush et al. 1990), 12 of 15 episodes (80%) of catatonia occurring in patients with a variety of psychiatric and organic illnesses responded completely and dramatically to lorazepam 1–2 mg po or im within 3 hours. The majority of patients relapsed within 24 hours but responded to lorazepam when it was readministered and maintained their improvement while the drug was continued for several weeks. The second large series of cases consisted of 18 patients with catatonia from nonorganic causes. Patients received either intramuscular diazepam or small doses of oral lorazepam . Two patients responded immediately and completely, and 14 showed significant clinical improvement within 48 hours with continued treatment. However, 9 of the latter patients required electroconvulsive therapy (ECT) for further improvement (Ungvari et al. 1994). Although diazepam's beneficial effects on catatonia have also been reported by others (McEvoy and Lohr 1984; Ripley and Millson 1988), oral and intravenous forms of diazepam have been noted to be less effective than lorazepam (Wetzel and Benkert 1988). Clonazepam has been reported to be ineffective in one patient who subsequently responded to lorazepam (Smith and Lebegue 1991).

Mechanism of Action

It has been postulated that amobarbital's and lorazepam's ability to modify catatonic symptoms is related to their propensity to reduce cholinergic and dopaminergic activity and increase γ-aminobutyric acid (GABA) activity in the basal ganglia (Menza 1991; Menza and Harris 1989; Rosebush and Mazurek 1991). Speculation has also involved consideration of catatonia as a type of complex partial seizure that is reversed by known anticonvulsants such as benzodiazepines or barbiturates (Menza 1991; Menza and Harris 1989; Salam and Kilzieh 1988), although existing data do not demonstrate electroencephalographic (EEG) or clinical indications of seizures in catatonic patients (Rosebush and Mazurek 1991). The clinical observation that patients who were catatonic later revealed that they experienced intense anxiety and fear during the catatonic episode has led to the speculation that amobarbital's and lorazepam's efficacy in relieving catatonia is attributable to their anxiolytic properties (Rosebush et al. 1990).

Dosage and Method of Administration of Amobarbital and Lorazepam

1. A solution of sodium amobarbital is prepared by mixing 10 mL of sterile water with sodium amobarbital 500 mg, yielding a solution of sodium amobarbital 50 mg/mL. The solution is then drawn up into a 10-mL syringe. Amobarbital hydrolyses in solution or on exposure to air. Therefore, not more than 30 minutes should elapse from the time the container is opened until its contents are used.

2. A 19-gauge Butterfly needle is inserted into a suitable vein.

3. Amobarbital 1 mL (50 mg) is injected immediately, and the interviewer begins to ask nonthreatening questions, such as the patient's name and where he or she is. The infusion is continued at the rate of 1 mL/minute until sustained lateral-gaze nystagmus, mild slurring of speech, and/or mild drowsiness are noted. This generally occurs when between 150 and 350 mg of amobarbital has been administered, but can occur with much lower doses in the elderly and in patients with organic disease. The narcosis can be maintained with 0.5–1.0 mL (25–50 mg) of amobarbital every 5–10 minutes.

4. If the patient is given slightly too much drug and falls asleep, he or she should begin to awaken in 5–10 minutes, at which time questions can be resumed without additional amobarbital administration. Normally, an interview can be conducted with a maximum of amobarbital 250 mg. Under no circumstances should more than 1,000 mg (20 mL) of amobarbital be used.

5. Amobarbital interviews are no longer commonly performed, and little research has examined their clinical indications in recent years. Benzodiazepines, and especially lorazepam, have gained favor as a first-line treatment for catatonia, whether functional or organic in etiology (Fricchione 1989; Rosebush et al. 1990). Lorazepam is given po, im, or iv at a dose of 1–2 mg. If catatonia is relieved but then recurs, lorazepam is readministered and, if necessary, continued at a dosage of 2–4 mg/day for several weeks or longer. The relative value of these two treatments (amobarbital and benzodiazepines) in other clinical conditions for which amobarbital has proved possibly useful remains unexplored. The sequential use of these agents (using benzodiazepines if amobarbital fails or vice versa) also has not been investigated except for one case in which a patient who dramatically responded to lorazepam but relapsed then dramatically responded to amobarbital (Rosebush et al. 1990).

Pharmacokinetics

See "Pharmacokinetics" (page 373) under **Benzodiazepines and Nonbenzodiazepines** in Chapter 5.

Adverse Effects

Amobarbital must be used with caution in patients with liver and kidney disease and in those with congestive heart failure. It is contraindicated in patients with porphyria and in those allergic to barbituric acid derivatives (Naples and Hackett 1978; Perry and Jacob 1982). Laryngospasm may occur with administration of amobarbital. For this reason, an individual familiar with the treatment of this event should be present when amobarbital is given. Vigorous mechanical respiration will often terminate the laryngospasm. If that fails, succinylcholine 10 mg iv should be given along with continuous mechanical respiration with 100% oxygen until spontaneous respiration returns. (For additional information on the adverse effects of barbiturates and benzodiazepines, see Chapter 5.)

Product List

Amobarbital
*   Parenteral dose range: 100–1,000 mg

Injection:	**Amytal**™
500 mg	[$9/500-mg ampule]

References

Bleckwenn W: Narcosis as therapy in neuropsychiatric conditions. JAMA 95:1168–1171, 1930

Dysken M, Chang S, Casper R, et al: Barbiturate-facilitated interviewing. Biol Psychiatry 14:421–432, 1979a

Dysken M, Kooser J, Haraszti J, et al: Clinical usefulness of sodium amobarbital interviewing. Arch Gen Psychiatry 36:789–794, 1979b

Fricchione G: Catatonia: a new indication for benzodiazepines? Biol Psychiatry 26:761–765, 1989

Gaind GS, Rosebush PI, Mazurek MF: Lorazepam treatment of acute and chronic catatonia in two mentally retarded brothers. J Clin Psychiatry 55:20–23, 1994

Gerson M, Victoroff V: Experimental investigation into the validity of confessions obtained under sodium Amytal narcosis. Clinical Psychopathology 9:359–368, 1948

Greenfield D, Conrad C, Kincare P, et al: Treatment of catatonia with low-dose lorazepam. Am J Psychiatry 144:1224–1225, 1987

Grinker R, Spiegel J: Men Under Stress. Philadelphia, PA, Blakiston, 1948

Herman M: The use of intravenous sodium Amytal in psychogenic amnesic states. Psychiatr Q 12:738–742, 1938

Kwentus J: Interviewing with intravenous drugs. J Clin Psychiatry 42:432–436, 1981

Lambert C, Reese W: Intravenous barbiturates in the treatment of hysteria. BMJ 2:70–73, 1944

Lampke R: Interviewing with intravenous drugs (letter). J Clin Psychiatry 43:344, 1982

Lindemann E: Psychological changes in normal and abnormal individuals under the influence of sodium Amytal. Am J Psychiatry 88:1083–1091, 1932

McDonald A, Kline SA, Billings RF: The limits of Munchausen's syndrome. Can J Psychiatry 24:323–328, 1979

McEvoy JP, Lohr JB: Diazepam for catatonia. Am J Psychiatry 141:284–285, 1984

Menza MA: Lorazepam and catatonia. J Clin Psychiatry 52:186–187, 1991

Menza MA, Harris D: Benzodiazepines and catatonia: an overview. Biol Psychiatry 26:842–846, 1989

Naples M, Hackett T: The Amytal interview: history and current uses. Psychosomatics 19:98–105, 1978

Perry J, Jacob D: Overview: clinical applications of the Amytal interview in psychiatric emergency settings. Am J Psychiatry 139:552–559, 1982

Ripley TL, Millson RC: Psychogenic catatonia treated with lorazepam. Am J Psychiatry 145:764–765, 1988

Rosebush PI, Mazurek MF: A consideration of the mechanism by which lorazepam might treat catatonia. J Clin Psychiatry 52:187–188, 1991

Rosebush PI, Hildebrand AM, Furlong BG, et al: Catatonic syndrome in a general psychiatric inpatient population: frequency, clinical presentation, and response to lorazepam. J Clin Psychiatry 51:357–362, 1990

Ruedrich SL, Chung-Chou C, Wadle CV: The Amytal interview in the treatment of psychogenic amnesia. Hospital and Community Psychiatry 36:1045–1046, 1985

Salam SA, Pillai AK, Beresford TP: Lorazepam for psychogenic catatonia. Am J Psychiatry 144:1082–1083, 1987

Salam SA, Kilzieh N: Lorazepam treatment of psychogenic catatonia: an update. J Clin Psychiatry 49 (12, suppl):16–21, 1988

Smith M, Lebegue B: Lorazepam in the treatment of catatonia (letter). Am J Psychiatry 9:1265, 1991

Ungvari GS, Leung CM, Wong MK, et al: Benzodiazepines in the treatment of catatonic syndrome. Acta Psychiatr Scand 89:285–288, 1994

Ward N, Rowlatt D, Burke P: Sodium amobarbital in the differential diagnosis of confusion. Am J Psychiatry 135:75–78, 1978

Weinstein E, Kahn R, Sugarman L: The diagnostic use of amobarbital sodium in brain disease. Am J Psychiatry 109:889–894, 1953

Weinstein E, Kahn R, Sugarman L, et al: Serial administration of the "Amytal test" for brain disease. Archives of Neurology and Psychiatry 71:217–226, 1954

Wetzel H, Benkert O: Lorazepam for treatment of catatonic symptoms and severe psychomotor retardation. Am J Psychiatry 145:1175–1176, 1988

Woodruff R: The diagnostic use of amylobarbitone interview among patients with psychotic illness. Br J Psychiatry 112:727–732, 1966

Yassa R, Iskandar H, Lalinec M, et al: Lorazepam as an adjunct in the treatment of catatonic states: an open trial. J Clin Psychopharmacol 10:66–68, 1990

12

Electroconvulsive Therapy

Indications

Convulsive therapy was introduced as a treatment for psychoses, especially schizophrenia, by Meduna in 1934. He initiated the treatment in the belief, based on clinical observations of his time, that patients with schizophrenia seldom experienced idiopathic epilepsy and that patients with epilepsy did not develop schizophrenia. He reasoned, therefore, that inducing seizures in patients with schizophrenia might cure their disease. Such an inverse relationship between the presence of schizophrenia and seizures is now known to be erroneous, but Meduna did achieve moderate success in ameliorating symptoms of psychoses by inducing seizures with intravenous camphor (Meduna and Friedman 1939). In 1938, Cerletti and Bini successfully induced seizures in humans with an electrical current passed through the head. The efficacy of electroconvulsive therapy (ECT) for psychotic depression, involutional depression, mania, and, to a lesser extent, schizophrenia was noted in the 1940s. In the late 1940s, modification of the seizure with succinylcholine and short-acting barbiturates markedly decreased serious side effects of ECT and increased its usefulness (Fink 1979). With the introduction of drug therapy for psychoses and depression in the mid-1950s, the use of ECT declined. However, with the growing recognition in the 1970s that drug therapy was not universally effective came a resurgence of interest in ECT among clinicians and researchers that has continued despite significant opposition from the antipsychiatry movement (Fink 1991).

Four major reviews of ECT, three in the United States and one in Great Britain, reaffirmed ECT's value in the treatment of major depression, catatonia, mania, and acute psychotic exacerbation in schizophrenia. These reviews also acknowledged that in the severely psychomotor-retarded patient who has stopped eating and taking fluids and in the actively suicidal patient, ECT is often the only reliable treatment available and, in such cases, may be lifesaving (American Psychiatric Association 1978, 1990; Consensus Conference 1985; Peppard and Ellam 1980).

Efficacy

Two controlled but nonblind studies (comparing ECT with antidepressant medication and placebo) in the mid-1960s established the efficacy of ECT in the treatment of major depressive disorder (Greenblatt et al. 1964; Medical Research Council et al. 1965). Since that time, multiple studies comparing ECT with placebo, antidepressant medication, and simulated ECT have consistently shown ECT to be superior or equivalent to these treatments. No study has shown these treatments to be more effective than ECT. Approximately 70%–80% of patients respond to ECT, 30%–52% to antidepressants, and 25%–45% to placebo (American Psychiatric Association 1990; Crowe 1984). However, a recent review of all studies comparing tricyclic antidepressants with ECT concluded that the data support the equivalence but not the superiority of ECT to tricyclics in the treatment of nonpsychotic depression (Piper 1993).

Much attention has focused on five double-blind, controlled studies conducted since 1978 that compared simulated ECT (in which control patients go through the entire ECT procedure except that they do not receive a dose of electricity) with real ECT in the treatment of depression (Brandon et al. 1984; Clinical Research Centre Division of Psychiatry 1984; Freeman et al. 1978; Johnstone et al. 1980; Lambourn and Gill 1978; West 1981). Although the methodologies of these studies differed significantly, and each has been criticized for diverse reasons, taken together they indicate that depressed patients show a greater improvement with real than with simulated ECT over a 3- to 4-week course of treatment. Three of the five studies (Brandon et al. 1984; Johnstone et al. 1980; Lambourn and Gill 1978) included follow-up assessments ranging from 4 to 28 weeks and were in agreement that the superiority of real over simulated ECT was not sustained. These studies indicate, therefore, that ECT's greatest value is in producing rapid relief of depressive symptoms. Rapidity of effect was also demonstrated to favor ECT compared with antidepressant medication in one double-blind, controlled study (Gangadhar et al. 1982). Although, in that study, response rates for ECT and imipramine were equivalent at 4 weeks, they favored ECT during the first 3 weeks. Subsequent studies have supported the shorter onset of action of ECT in comparison with antidepressants (Segman et al. 1995).

It has long been maintained, based on clinical observation, that ECT is most effective in alleviating depressive illness accompanied by "endogenous" symptoms such as marked depression, psychomotor retardation and/or agitation, terminal insomnia, guilt, diurnal variation of symptoms (worse in the morning), and loss of appetite and weight (Fink 1979; Hamilton 1986). It has also been maintained that ECT is of value in delusional depression (Crow and Johnstone 1986; Kantor and Glassman 1977; Minter and Mandel 1979), which is usually poorly responsive to standard antidepressant and antipsychotic medications alone. Evidence of the benefit of ECT for patients with delusional depression was provided by Kroessler (1985), who reviewed 17 prospective and retrospective studies comparing tricyclic antidepressants (TCAs), antipsychotics, TCA/antipsychotic combinations, and/or ECT in the treatment of delusional depression. He found overall positive response rates of 34% in the TCA group, 51% in the antipsychotic group, 77% in the TCA/antipsychotic group, and 82% in the ECT group. The value of ECT was further enhanced by the finding that many of the patients benefiting from it had been unresponsive to previous medication trials.

Two simulated- versus real-ECT studies have addressed the issue of clinical predictors of response to ECT (Brandon et al. 1984; Clinical Research Centre Division of Psychiatry 1984). Although both confirmed the value of delusions as a predictor of positive response to ECT, one found that endogenous subtype did not predict a positive response (Clinical Research Centre Division of Psychiatry 1984), and the other did not examine endogenous symptoms separately from delusions (Brandon et al. 1984). A later study combined the data in these two studies and concluded that ECT 1) has short-term benefit for depressed patients with psychomotor retardation or delusions, 2) may have a synergistic effect on patients with both delusions and retardation, and 3) does not appear to be of benefit (compared with simulated ECT) in patients with neither of these symptoms (Buchan et al. 1992). However, a subsequent study analyzing data from one of the earlier simulated-ECT studies concluded that the presence of delusions, retardation, or agitation did not predict treatment response, and that patients with and without these symptoms responded equally and positively to real versus simulated ECT (O'Leary et al. 1995). This finding was bolstered in a recent review (Sackeim and Rush 1995) of studies examining the response of melancholic or endogenous depression to ECT. The authors concluded that patients with endogenous or melancholic subtypes of depression are no more or less likely to respond to ECT than are patients who have major depressive disorder without these subtype features. A later study, however, which examined the value of rating scales in predicting response to

ECT, found that psychomotor retardation, agitation, and psychotic features were robust independent predictors of response to ECT, and that the combination of these features predicted the best therapeutic response to ECT (Hickie et al. 1996). In sum, these studies suggest that the presence of delusional depression, and perhaps of endogenous depression, is the best predictor of response to ECT, although the absence of such features does not preclude a positive response to ECT.

Catatonia, often classified as a subtype of schizophrenia but frequently associated with manic-depressive illness, is consistently reported to be very responsive to ECT (Abrams and Taylor 1977; M. A. Taylor 1990), even in its more malignant forms (Geretsegger and Rochawanski 1987; S. C. Mann et al. 1986), although no controlled studies have been done to verify these clinical observations. Retrospective studies, clinical observations, and a recent review of the available literature have indicated that ECT is effective in treating acute mania, including mania that has responded poorly to pharmacotherapy (Fink 1979; McCabe 1976; McCabe and Norris 1977; Mukherjee et al. 1994). ECT in conjunction with antipsychotics may be more beneficial in manic patients than medication alone, as demonstrated in a recent randomized, double-blind study in which 15 manic patients receiving ECT with chlorpromazine 600 mg/day were compared with manic patients receiving simulated ECT and the same dose of chlorpromazine (Sikdar et al. 1994). Patients receiving real ECT and the antipsychotic showed significantly greater and faster improvement than did those receiving simulated ECT and the antipsychotic.

In a randomized, controlled, nonblinded study comparing lithium and ECT in the treatment of mania, weekly ratings revealed that ECT was more effective than lithium during weeks 2 through 8, with this finding reaching statistical significance in weeks 6, 7, and 8. ECT's superiority to lithium was especially apparent in patients with mixed symptoms of mania and depression or with extreme manic excitement. Follow-up assessments after 8 weeks revealed no differences between lithium and ECT (Small et al. 1988, 1991).

ECT has not proven to be of benefit in the treatment of chronic schizophrenia (Fink 1979; Hamilton 1986; Small 1986), especially in those patients with mainly negative symptoms of schizophrenia, such as social withdrawal, affective flattening, and paucity of thought and expression. Schizophrenic patients taking maintenance antipsychotics who exhibit intensified positive psychotic symptoms, such as hallucinations, delusions, and bizarre behavior, have been shown, in a controlled study, to be more responsive to real than to simulated ECT. However, these advantages had dissipated by 8–12 weeks post-ECT (Abraham and Kulhara 1987; P. J. Taylor and Fleminger 1980). Multiple studies have compared neuroleptics plus ECT with neuroleptics alone in the treatment of schizophrenia, and the majority have demonstrated the combination superior both in short-term efficacy and in speed of response (Fink and Sackeim 1996). ECT, therefore, might be of benefit in schizophrenic patients experiencing acute exacerbations of psychotic or depressive symptoms who are unresponsive, or only partly responsive, to medication (Small et al. 1993).

Patients with first-onset psychosis diagnosed as schizophreniform disorder (without good prognostic features), all of whom were given haloperidol, were randomized to a course of six real or sham ECT sessions. Patients showed equal improvement in their psychotic symptoms when rated weekly for 6 weeks and when rated at 6 months' posttreatment, regardless of which ECT treatment (real versus sham) they received (Sarkar et al. 1994). Notwithstanding these findings, it has been proposed that initial treatment of first-episode psychotic patients with ECT instead of neuroleptics might reduce this population's exposure to the adverse effects of antipsychotics. In addition, the possibility that effective treatment of first-episode psychosis can positively alter the course of schizophrenia has led to the suggestion that first-episode patients who do not respond to neuroleptics should receive a course of ECT (Fink and Sackeim 1996).

Medical conditions for which ECT has been reported to be of value include delirium, neuroleptic malignant syndrome, iatrogenic hypopituitarism, intractable epilepsy, and Parkinson's disease (American Psychiatric Association 1990; Kellner et al. 1994; Rasmussen and Abrams 1991).

Psychiatric conditions for which ECT is generally believed to be an ineffective treatment, based on case reports, include personality disorders, substance abuse and dependence, gender identity disorders, somatoform disorders, and anxiety disorders (Fink 1993). Although obsessive-compulsive disorder is usually considered to be nonresponsive to ECT, case reports and series have reported benefits (Maletzky et al. 1994).

Mechanism of Action

The mechanism of action of ECT is unknown. In the past, studies had demonstrated that the means of inducing the seizure was not related to therapeutic efficacy. Furthermore, it had been maintained that a seizure lasting 15–25 seconds or longer was necessary and sufficient for therapeutic efficacy (Brandon et al. 1984; Clinical Research Centre Division of Psychiatry 1984; Freeman et al. 1978; Johnstone et al. 1980; Lambourn and Gill 1978; Ottosson 1962a, 1962b; West 1981). However, a recent investigation has demonstrated that production of a seizure of adequate duration is not necessarily sufficient to achieve therapeutic efficacy (Sackeim et al. 1993). The necessity of producing a seizure to achieve therapeutic efficacy, although still accepted by most researchers, has also been questioned (Sackeim 1994a). Sackeim has postulated that stimulation of deep brain structures may be the necessary and sufficient cause of the antidepressant effects of ECT and that such stimulation may be accomplished without provocation of a seizure, although not with current technology. He hypothesizes that development of high-power, focal magnetic-induction techniques may lead to suitable methods for inducing such deep-brain-structure stimulation.

In searching for a mechanism of action for ECT, much attention has been devoted to biochemical alterations in the central nervous system (CNS). As a consequence of the seizure, major changes occur in the synthesis and turnover of such centrally acting neurotransmitters as serotonin, norepinephrine, γ-aminobutyric acid (GABA), and acetylcholine, and in the up- and downregulation of the receptors for these and other neurotransmitters, although many of the studies done in this area are not in agreement with one another (Kapur and Mann 1993; J. J. Mann and Kapur 1994). Some of the changes in neurotransmitter levels and receptors parallel those seen with administration of antidepressant medication, but there are many differences, especially in relation to serotonin (5-hydroxytryptamine [5-HT]), norepinephrine, and dopamine (D) turnover in human studies and serotonin and dopamine receptor changes in animal studies (Fochtmann 1994; J. J. Mann and Kapur 1994; Rudorfer et al. 1988). For example, whereas changes in human dopamine levels and receptors are not seen with most antidepressants, animal studies have indicated that dopamine levels in various brain regions increase, that these increases persist after repeated electrically induced convulsions, and that D_1 receptors appear to be more involved than D_2 receptors (Nutt and Glue 1993). $5\text{-}HT_2$ receptors, which are downregulated (i.e., decreased in number and function) with most antidepressant medications, are upregulated after electrically induced seizures (Kapur and Mann 1993; J. J. Mann and Kapur 1994; Nutt and Glue 1993; Rudorfer et al. 1988).

ECT also causes markedly increased cerebral vascular permeability, increased plasma β-endorphin levels, probable decreased plasma GABA, and release of anterior pituitary hormones, such as adrenocorticotropic hormone (ACTH), prolactin, and luteinizing hormone (LH). However, release of anterior pituitary hormones have not clearly correlated with therapeutic efficacy of ECT, and, therefore, such release is not at present useful in predicting clinical outcome (Clark et al. 1995; Devanand et al. 1995b; Gleiter and Nutt 1989; Kamil and Joffe 1991; Kety 1974; Lerer and Shapiro 1986; Ottosson 1974; Scott 1989).

Plasma concentrations of peptides (neurophysins) released in association with the release of the posterior pituitary hormones vasopressin and oxytocin are increased by ECT. Of note, several studies have demonstrated that an increase in the peptide associated with oxytocin after a first ECT is correlated with therapeutic outcome at 2 months (Scott 1989; Scott et al. 1991). Increase in this peptide after the first ECT may, therefore, have prognostic significance. Unfortunately, the assay for this peptide is difficult and not likely to be widely available.

It should be noted that two widely studied endocrine challenge tests, the dexamethasone suppression test (DST) and the thyroid-stimulating hormone (TSH) response to thyrotropin-releasing hormone (TRH), have not been demonstrated to correlate with therapeutic outcome (Decina et al. 1987; Joffe and Sokolov 1994; Scott 1989).

To explain the mechanism of action of ECT, Joffe and Sokolov cite a neuroendocrine hypothesis in which ECT directly causes the release of a specific as-yet-unidentified peptide from the hypothalamus, thus leading to behavioral and hormonal changes. This hypothetical peptide has been named "antidepressin," and TRH has been postulated as a possible candidate for the peptide. However, no conclusions regarding the peptide's existence or identity are possible with current evidence (Joffe and Sokolov 1994).

Neurophysiologically, ECT has been noted to have anticonvulsive properties, leading some investigators to hypothesize that ECT potentiates active inhibitory processes that terminate seizure activity. The underlying theory is that psychiatric illnesses responding to ECT are seizure equivalents or share with seizures a common etiological mechanism (Post et al. 1986; Sackeim 1994a; Sackeim et al. 1986, 1987b).

Other theories have been proposed, one of which relates the mechanism of action of ECT to its differential effects on the left and right cerebral hemispheres and another of which postulates that the major therapeutic effects of ECT are attributable to its actions on the diencephalon, leading to a stabilization of hypothalamic function (Sackeim 1994a). Explorations of the mechanism of action of ECT are in their infancy and should be significantly aided by new research approaches resulting from recent findings regarding ECT (Potter 1994; Sackeim 1994a) and from new technologies such as positron-emission tomography (PET), magnetic resonance imaging (MRI), single photon emission computed tomography (SPECT), and computerized electroencephalograms (EEGs) (Coffey 1994; Potter 1994). (For a thorough review of current knowledge and theories regarding the mechanism of action of ECT, see Sackeim 1994a.)

Dosage and Variation in Treatment

Until recently, it was thought that an electrical stimulus with sufficient energy to produce a generalized seizure lasting 20–30 seconds was necessary and sufficient for therapeutic efficacy. However, recent studies indicate that although the production of a generalized seizure is necessary for therapeutic response, it may not be sufficient. Specifically, it has been shown that in order to achieve maximal therapeutic benefit, right unilateral ECT requires electrical energy up to 2.5 times in excess of that needed to produce a generalized seizure. This excess energy is not necessary for bilateral ECT (Sackeim et al. 1987a, 1993).

The minimum dosage of electricity needed to induce a seizure (i.e., the seizure threshold) is higher in older than in younger patients, higher when using bilateral compared with unilateral electrode placement, higher with each succeeding treatment in a series of ECT treatments, higher with increasing head size, higher in African Americans, and higher in men than in women (Coffey et al. 1995a; Colenda and McCall 1996; McCall et al. 1993; Sackeim et al. 1987b). The seizure threshold of males correlates more strongly with age than does that of females. In addition, whereas this correlation holds in males for both right unilateral and bilateral ECT, females show an age effect only for right unilateral ECT (Sackeim et al. 1991). It should be noted that not all investigators have reported a difference in the seizure thresholds of men and women (Beale et al. 1994). The rise in seizure threshold with succeeding treatments is positively correlated with age but not with gender, electrode placement, initial seizure threshold, therapeutic response, or speed of therapeutic response (Coffey et al. 1995b).

Seizure threshold is inversely related to seizure duration (Coffey et al. 1995b; Shapira et al. 1996). Seizures of more than 25 seconds' duration do not enhance the therapeutic efficacy of ECT, and those of less than 25 seconds may be of sufficient duration for therapeutic efficacy in some patients (Sackeim et al. 1991). Although definitive data do not yet exist, it is generally agreed that seizures of less than 15 seconds are unlikely to be effective (Sackeim et al. 1991), and most clinicians continue to accept 25 seconds as a necessary duration for an effective seizure (American Psychiatric Association 1990). However, other ictal variables, such as seizure intensity as measured by EEG, are being actively investigated as potentially better markers of treatment adequacy (Krystal et al. 1993; Shapira et al. 1996).

If maximum doses of electricity do not induce seizures or if seizures are too short in duration, intravenous caffeine sodium benzoate (500–2,000 mg) may be given 5–10 minutes before ECT to reduce the seizure threshold and thus prolong seizures (Coffey et al. 1990; Hinckle et al. 1987; Kelsey and Grossberg 1995; Shapira et al. 1987). However, some have advised caution in administering caffeine because of its tendency to cause hypertension and tachycardia (Acevedo and Smith 1988), and others have indicated that its use does not improve therapeutic outcome (Hicks et al. 1994). Theophylline has also been used as a proconvulsant agent in ECT (Swartz and Lewis 1991), but its potential for causing prolonged seizures and status epilepticus when given in conjunction with ECT has provoked concern (Sackeim et al. 1991).

The number of ECT treatments required for full therapeutic benefit in depression is generally considered to be 6–12 (American Psychiatric Association 1990; Kornhuber and Weller 1995). However, some patients require fewer and some more treatments for maximal clinical improvement. Additional treatments given beyond remission or maximal improvement do not affect relapse rates. Lack of remission or lack of continued improvement may be attributable to the achievement of maximal effect from ECT, in which case treatments should terminate after two sessions from which no benefit is apparent. However, lack of improvement may also be due to the use of suboptimal stimulus intensity, especially in a patient receiving unilateral ECT. In such cases, increasing stimulus intensity or switching to bilateral ECT should be considered (American Psychiatric Association 1990). As noted earlier, for patients receiving unilateral ECT, a stimulus level 2.5 times that needed to induce a seizure results in increased therapeutic efficacy. In addition, for both unilateral and bilateral treatments, suprathreshold (i.e., 2.5 times threshold) stimuli result in a more rapid therapeutic improvement, although such improvement may be at the expense of increased adverse cognitive effects (Sackeim et al. 1993).

In the United States, ECT treatments are generally given three times per week. More-frequent administration causes increased post-ECT confusion and memory loss without improving therapeutic efficacy. Three studies comparing bilateral and right unilateral ECT administered twice versus three times weekly found that when patients were evaluated at comparable times after treatment onset, twice-weekly sessions produced as much therapeutic improvement as did thrice-weekly sessions while causing less cognitive impairment (Gangadhar et al. 1993; Lerer et al. 1995; McAllister et al. 1987). The one study that addressed the issue of speed of improvement demonstrated that patients receiving ECT three times per week responded more rapidly than those receiving it two times per week; however, when patients were assessed 1 week after treatment termination, the two groups showed equal therapeutic improvement and the two-times-per-week group had less cognitive impairment than did the three-times-per-week group (Lerer et al. 1995).

The practice of inducing more than one seizure per ECT session is not widely used, as it appears to enhance the speed of therapeutic response to some degree but with a marked increase in short-term confusion and adverse cognitive effects (Maletzky 1981; Roemer et al. 1990). This practice, however, was stimulated by work suggesting that total seizure time might be the critical variable in determining the adequacy of treatment, with seizure time for an entire course of ECT less than 500 seconds (as measured by EEG evidence of seizures) leading to little improvement and seizure time greater than 1,500 seconds leading to little additional improvement (Maletzky 1981). The issue is of importance because if total seizure time is the critical variable in therapeutic response, patients could be given multiple seizures each ECT session, thereby hastening their recovery—even if at the expense of additional cognitive impairment. Although some clinicians currently use total seizure time as a gauge of therapeutic efficacy, the utility of this measure for that purpose has yet to be demonstrated in randomized, controlled studies (Sackeim et al. 1991). In addition, as demonstrated by the lack of efficacy of low-threshold unilateral therapy, seizure duration is not in itself an adequate index of the adequacy of therapeutic efficacy.

Few data exist regarding the number of ECT sessions required for illnesses other than major depressive disorder. The number often cited as necessary for treatment of mania and schizoaffective disorders is 12–20, and for schizophrenia, 12–40 (Fink 1979; Kalinowsky and Hippius 1969; Maletzky 1981; Roemer et al. 1990). The clinical impression that mania requires a greater number of ECT treatments than that required for depressive illness has not been supported by available retrospective and prospective studies (Mukherjee et al. 1994; Small et al. 1986).

The two electrodes used to induce ECT seizures may be placed on both sides of the head (bilateral), or both electrodes may be placed on one side of the head (unilateral). Bilateral placement is usually bitemporal. However, a recent study reported that bifrontal placement was more effective and caused fewer adverse cognitive effects than did bitemporal or right unilateral placement (Letemendia et al. 1993). Asymmetric bilateral electrode placement (right frontotemporal and left temporal) has also been reported in a small case series to be therapeutically effective and to produce minimal cognitive effects (Manly and Swartz 1994). Unilateral placement is variable (e.g., frontoparietal, temporoparietal, temporo-occipital), but electrodes are most often placed on the side of the nondominant cerebral hemisphere, usually the right side. The majority of studies to date have indicated 1) no difference in therapeutic efficacy between using nondominant unilateral or bilateral electrode placement, 2) less memory loss and less post-ECT confusion with nondominant unilateral ECT, and 3) the probable advantage of temporal-vertex (d'Elia)–type nondominant unilateral electrode placement (d'Elia 1970; d'Elia and Raotoma 1975; Heshe et al. 1978; Maletzky 1981; Pettinati et al. 1986; Reichert et al. 1976; Sand-Stromegren 1973; Squire and Slater 1978; Welch 1982).

Despite these apparent advantages of unilateral ECT, many clinicians still use and prefer to administer bilateral ECT (Farah and McCall 1993), and some investigators support the continued use of bilateral ECT in special situations (Abrams 1986, 1992c; Small et al. 1986). It has been suggested that the controversy may be perpetuated by both the increased incidence of missed seizures with unilateral compared with bilateral ECT (Pettinati and Nilsen 1985) and the fact that threshold-dose unilateral ECT (i.e., inducing a seizure with the minimum current necessary) is markedly less effective than threshold-dose bilateral ECT (Abrams et al. 1991; Sackeim et al. 1986, 1993). The problem of missed seizures may be rectified with the increasing tendency to monitor EEGs. However, presence and adequacy of seizure duration may be difficult to assess with currently used EEG recording methods and devices (Small 1994), as indicated by studies showing poor interrater reliability in determining seizure duration (Guze et al. 1989; Ries 1985). It should be noted that not all studies have indicated such poor interrater reliability (Krystal and Weiner 1995; Warmflash et al. 1987), and that computer-generated determinations of seizure end points have been developed that are reported to have good reliability and validity (Swartz et al. 1994). In summary, although all reports agree that fewer short-term cognitive deficits occur with nondominant unilateral than with bilateral ECT, many researchers and clinicians believe that, in patients who have mania or who require a sure response (because of active suicidal ideation, poor nutrition, or associated serious medical problems), bilateral ECT is preferable to unilateral ECT. In such populations, bilateral ECT can be used either as an initial therapy or as a second-line treatment if four to five unilateral treatments given with suprathreshold stimuli result in an inadequate response.

An increasing percentage of patients given ECT are those who have proven unresponsive to a trial of adequate dosage and duration of one or more antidepressant medications (Sackeim 1994b). Such medication-resistant patients are more likely to be unresponsive to ECT than are patients who have not been shown to be medication resistant (Prudic et al. 1990). It has been suggested that medication-resistant patients may require a more intensive course of ECT (e.g., higher current, more treatments) than do non–medication-resistant patients (Sackeim 1994b).

The relapse rate for depressive disorders after ECT is as high as 50% 6 months after and 59% 1 year after ECT (Barton et al. 1973; Sackeim 1994b). There is evidence that this relapse rate can be markedly reduced by maintaining patients on therapeutic doses of antidepressant medication or lithium for at least 1 year post-ECT (Coppen et al. 1981; Imlah et al. 1965; Kay et al. 1970; Perry and Tsuang 1979; Riddle and Scott 1995; Seager and Bird 1962). However, this evidence is based on a population of patients who were less likely to have demonstrated medication resistance than are today's population of patients receiving ECT (Sackeim 1994b). Sackeim (1994b) has reported that patients who were medication resistant before receiving ECT had a much higher relapse rate post-ECT than did patients who were not medication resistant (64% versus 32%) and that this result was independent of the adequacy of posttreatment pharmacotherapy. Because most of the patients in studies of the value of post-ECT pharmacotherapy were given tricyclics both before and after ECT, it has been suggested that patients who are medication resistant before receiving ECT be placed after ECT on an antidepressant class other than the one to which they have proven resistant (Sackeim et al. 1989, 1990).

Recent concerns regarding the high rate of relapse of patients after ECT has led to the suggestion that abrupt termination of ECT may contribute to this high rate and that perhaps ECT should be tapered over several weeks or months with a gradually increasing time interval between treatments. One retrospective study has shown this strategy beneficial in reducing relapses over the course of 1 year (Petrides et al. 1994).

Strategies for beginning antidepressant medication during a course of ECT rather than waiting until the end of treatment have also been suggested, thus giving the antidepressant time to be effective and possibly preventing early relapse post-ECT (Sackeim 1994b).

For medication-resistant patients especially, the value of maintenance ECT in which one treatment is given at weekly or less-frequent intervals and continued for years has received increased attention. Although not extensively used or studied, maintenance ECT has been noted in case reports and series to prevent relapses for periods as long as 5 years in patients with major depressive and bipolar disorders (Karliner and Wehrheim 1965; Schwarz et al. 1995; Steibel 1995; Stephens et al. 1993; Stevenson and Georghegan 1951; Vanelle et al. 1994).

Adverse Effects

Adverse effects of ECT can be divided into those occurring during or shortly after an ECT session and those persisting after a complete course of ECT. Before the introduction of succinylcholine to modify seizures, fractured long bones and vertebrae were common side effects of ECT. Fear and panic in patients just before receiving ECT were also commonly encountered, but have been largely eliminated by the use of barbiturate anesthesia (Fink 1979).

During and immediately after ECT, blood pressure changes and various cardiac arrhythmias are common although seldom serious; even patients with significant cardiovascular disease can be successfully and safely treated with ECT (Elliott et al. 1982; Rice et al. 1994; Zielinski et al. 1993). Rare, serious complications in this time period include laryngospasm, prolonged apnea, and death. Prolonged apnea occurs in persons with an inherited deficiency of pseudocholinesterase, which is necessary to metabolize succinylcholine. It is estimated to occur in 1 of 3,000 individuals and will, of course, be noted during the first ECT treatment (Fink 1979). The reported fatality rate for ECT has declined steadily from 1 patient per 950 patients treated, reported in 1961, to 1 per 3,000, in 1976 (Asnis et al. 1978; Heshe and Roeder 1976; Perrin 1961).

Most of the deaths occurred in the several hours immediately after ECT and were attributable to cardiovascular or pulmonary complications, most often ventricular arrhythmias or arrest with or without accompanying myocardial infarctions (Crowe 1984; Fink 1979). Actual mortality rates are likely much lower, as judged by the marked improvement in anesthesia mortality rates in the last 20 years as a result of improved anesthesia techniques (Voelker 1995). In a recent study of ambulatory surgery outpatients undergoing a range of anesthesia procedures, many of whom were elderly with multiple medical illnesses, the mortality rate was less than 1 death per 10,000 patients (Warner et al. 1993).

Immediately after treatment, patients experience postictal confusion, which is usually cumulative over a course of therapy, is less severe with nondominant unilateral than with bitemporal therapy, is less severe with low-energy-wave forms of ECT, and clears within 7 to 10 days at most (Price 1982a, 1982b).

Approximately 10% of patients may exhibit an agitated delirium when emerging from anesthesia, and a small percentage may undergo prolonged seizure activity. These symptoms may be rapidly terminated by administering 5–20 mg of intravenous diazepam or 2–8 mg of midazolam. Because the delirium is likely to occur after each subsequent treatment in a patient initially experiencing delirium, some clinicians recommend administering the diazepam or midazolam intravenously to such patients immediately after their seizure ends and spontaneous respirations return (Abrams 1992b; Grogan et al. 1995; Hansen-Grant et al. 1995; Welch 1993).

A post-ECT headache occurs in 25%–50% of patients. It is usually bitemporal or bifrontal, nonthrobbing, and remits in 2–8 hours, often without analgesics. More severe and persistent headaches have also been reported (DeBattista and Mueller 1995; Maletzky 1981).

Miscellaneous posttreatment side effects, including muscle soreness, occur in approximately 30% of patients. The soreness (which may be due to the amount of succinylcholine given and not to the amount of muscle movement during ECT) remits within 24 hours, usually without specific therapy. Nausea occurs in approximately 20% of patients but usually clears in 12–24 hours without specific therapy; this symptom is perhaps caused by air being pushed into the stomach during forced ventilation, or by the drugs used during ECT (Maletzky 1981).

The most notable long-term effect of ECT is memory disturbance. This memory impairment is both retrograde and anterograde, is greater with bitemporal and unilateral dominant than with unilateral nondominant therapy, is cumulative over the course of therapy, and correlates with both pre-ECT cognitive impairment and prolonged postictal disorientation after ECT treatments. Unilateral nondominant ECT impairs mainly nonverbal memory, whereas unilateral dominant impairs verbal memory and bilateral impairs both. Thus, there is often relatively little apparent memory deficit, which is judged mainly by verbal memory, after unilateral nondominant ECT. Patients frequently complain of subjective memory disturbances for months or years post-ECT (most frequently after bilateral ECT). Objectively, however, recovery from anterograde and retrograde amnesia is complete within 6 to 9 months after ECT, although memory for some events surrounding the course of ECT may be permanently lost (Price 1982a, 1982b; Sobin et al. 1995; Squire 1986). A follow-up study found that 55% of patients who received bilateral ECT still complained of memory difficulties 3 years later (Squire and Slater 1983). However, memory as well as somatic complaints are common in depression, and many patients who complain of such problems following ECT are clinically depressed (Cronholm and Ottosson 1963; Devanand et al. 1995a; Frith et al. 1983; Weeks et al. 1980).

Concerns about possible ECT-induced structural brain damage have been allayed by a recent review of the literature on this subject (Devanand et al. 1994), which concluded that such damage does not occur. This conclusion has been further strengthened by a recent prospective MRI study (Coffey et al. 1991) that evaluated patients before ECT and at 2 days and 6 months after ECT and found no relationship between ECT and MRI findings of structural brain abnormalities.

Certain conditions place patients at substantially increased risk of adverse consequences from ECT. These conditions include recent myocardial infarction (within the past 3 months and especially if associated with unstable cardiac function), increased cerebrospinal fluid (CSF) pressure (ECT causes a further rise in CSF pressure, which can lead to herniation if the CSF pressure is already high due to the presence of a space-occupying lesion), severe chronic obstructive pulmonary disease, uncorrected metabolic derangements, infectious disease, recent fractures (within the past 3 months), retinal detachment, severe closed-angle glaucoma, pheochromocytoma, frequent premature ventricular contractions, fulminant congestive heart failure, malignant uncontrolled hypertension, meningitis, acute cerebrovascular accident, acute renal failure, acute hepatic failure, uncontrolled gastrointestinal hemorrhage, and anesthetic risk rated at American Society of Anesthesiologists

(ASA) level IV or V (Abrams 1992a; American Psychiatric Association 1990; Crowe 1984; Maletzky 1981). Patients with porphyria must have a nonbarbiturate anesthetic agent, and patients with pseudocholinesterase deficiency must not be given succinylcholine as a muscle-paralyzing agent (Gleiter and Nutt 1989).

Absolute contraindications to ECT include only nonconsent in a competent patient.

Most authorities advise discontinuing all psychotropics before initiating ECT (Abrams 1992b), although there is evidence that continuing antipsychotics and/or antidepressants may be beneficial in certain patients (Kellner et al. 1991; Sikdar et al. 1994). Reserpine and lithium should be discontinued before ECT because of reports of an increased risk of confusion, memory impairment, and delirium in patients taking these drugs (Abrams 1992b; Kellner et al. 1991), although not all studies concur that continuing lithium during ECT leads to such problems (Jha et al. 1996; Mukherjee 1993). An appreciable drug-free interval before starting ECT is not necessary for any psychotropic agent, monoamine inhibitors included (American Psychiatric Association 1990).

Although medications received for a medical condition are usually continued throughout ECT, special attention should be given to certain medications (American Psychiatric Association 1990; Nobler and Sackeim 1993). Lidocaine and some of its analogs raise the seizure threshold and may lead to abortive seizures; hence, if a patient can be safely switched to a therapeutically comparable antiarrhythmic, this should be done, especially if abortive seizures are noted. Benzodiazepines and various anticonvulsants also raise the seizure threshold and/or shorten seizure duration and may lead to abortive treatments. Such a problem can sometimes be overcome by raising electrical stimulus levels. In general, benzodiazepines are decreased or discontinued before initiating ECT and/or, if possible, patients receiving long-acting agents such as diazepam or clonazepam are switched to shorter-acting agents such as lorazepam or alprazolam. Anticonvulsants used for control of a patient's seizure disorder are generally maintained, whereas anticonvulsants used to control psychiatric disorders such as mania or schizoaffective disorder are discontinued (Sackeim et al. 1991).

Theophylline and caffeine increase seizure duration and may cause prolonged seizures. Consideration should be given to discontinuing theophylline before initiating ECT. Consideration might also be given, if seizures are excessively prolonged, to inquiring about the patient's caffeine intake (Sackeim et al. 1991). Patients receiving ECT and the selective serotonin reuptake inhibitor paroxetine were reported in one case series to have seizure durations double those of patients receiving ECT and tricyclic antidepressants (Curran 1995).

Devices Used in ECT

The three U.S. manufacturers of ECT equipment are MECTA, Somatics, and Medcraft, each of which produces two or more ECT models (Stephens et al. 1991). (A fourth manufacturer, ElCoT, has withdrawn from the market, although several of its devices may still be in use.) All models deliver a constant current (amperage) as a train of brief bidirectional square-wave electrical pulses, which is the preferred method of administering ECT. This method superseded the previous method of constant voltage delivered as a continuous sinusoidal wave. The older method was shown to require more energy for seizure induction and to cause more adverse short-term cognitive effects without producing an improvement in therapeutic efficacy (Stephens et al. 1991; Weiner 1980, 1986).

The extent to which these devices allow the operator to control stimulus energy varies, with the number of adjustable variables ranging from one (stimulus duration) to as many as four variables (pulse frequency, pulse width, stimulus duration, and current). Although little work has been done to assess the value of varying these separate components of stimulus energy, one study (Swartz and Larson 1989) has demonstrated that varying the stimulus duration while holding the total charge constant affects the device's ability to induce a full seizure, and another (Rasmussen et al. 1994) indicated that briefer pulse widths and longer stimulus durations induce seizures at lower energy thresholds than do more standard settings. At present, however, other than for research purposes, the value of being able to change more than one stimulus variable is unproven and adds to the complexity of administration. All manufacturers have at least one model that produces a paper recording of the EEG and electrocardiogram (ECG), which allows verification and recording of seizures and their duration. All ECT devices contain a fail-safe mechanism that prevents current from being delivered if voltage exceeds a preset amount (Stephens et al. 1991).

Devices and models differ in a number of ways, and manufacturers provide manuals and/or videotapes that must be reviewed and understood before operating the individual devices.

Method of Administration

There are a number of methods for administering ECT in a rational and safe manner. The procedures described in this section are those used at Department of Veterans Affairs and university psychiatric services in Kansas and Iowa, where they have proven to be safe and effective. These procedures generally follow the guidelines given in the American Psychiatric Association's task force report on the practice of ECT (American Psychiatric Association 1990).

ECT is administered by a team, each member of which is experienced in the administration of ECT. The team consists of a staff psychiatrist who is credentialed and privileged in the administration of ECT, a psychiatric resident, a nurse, and an anesthesiologist or anesthetist.

■ Pretreatment Procedures

1. All patients receive a complete physical and psychiatric evaluation to determine their appropriateness for ECT. Psychiatric symptoms and cognitive status are clearly recorded, because they will be followed during the course of ECT to monitor therapeutic efficacy and adverse cognitive effects. Pretreatment laboratory tests include complete blood count (CBC), electrolytes, blood urea nitrogen (BUN), creatinine, fasting blood sugar (FBS), chest X ray, and ECG. Abnormalities are evaluated before ECT and specialty consultation obtained as indicated. Spine X rays are optional and are done to detect pre-ECT abnormalities (Milstein et al. 1995).

2. An anesthesia evaluation is performed that addresses the nature and extent of anesthetic risk and any anesthesia modifications thus required.

3. The patient's staff psychiatrist enters a note into the record summarizing indications and risks for ECT; listing additional evaluation procedures undertaken, and their results; describing discussion with and consent of the patient for ECT; and noting any modification in medication and/or ECT technique indicated.

4. The day before the first treatment, the physician completes a checklist that indicates that the patient's physical and mental status is appropriate for ECT, that appropriate lab work has been completed and results are within appropriate ranges, and that the patient and/or the patient's guardian has given informed consent for the administration of ECT.

5. Pretreatment orders:
   a. Either **atropine** 1 mg or **glycopyrrolate** (Robinul®) 0.4 mg is administered subcutaneously or intramuscularly ½ hour before treatment. Alternatively, the atropine or glycopyrrolate may be given intravenously 2 minutes before anesthesia induction (Kramer et al. 1992).
   b. Shampoo and wash hair the evening before treatment.
   c. The patient should have nothing to eat or drink after midnight. ECT is generally administered early in the morning.
   d. A temperature of 99.8°F or higher on the morning of treatment should be investigated by the physician, and ECT should be canceled or continued at the discretion of the physician after appropriate investigation.

■ Treatment Procedures

1. Equipment:
   a. ECT devices should initially be set at the manufacturer's recommendation, also taking into consideration factors affecting seizure threshold, such as patient's age and sex, electrode placement, anesthesia dosage, and concomitant medications.
   b. The following should be present in the ECT room: rubber mouthpieces, airways, oxygen delivery system able to deliver positive-pressure oxygen by face mask or endotracheal tube, ECG, blood-pressure recording device, suction apparatus, intubation equipment, emergency cart, and cardioversion equipment. Peripheral nerve stimulator and pulse oximeter are optional but encouraged.

2. Patient procedures:
   a. Inquiry should be made as to whether the patient has been npo since midnight and whether the patient has voided before treatment. If the patient has not been npo (a sip of water to swallow the medication is allowable), treatment should be canceled; if the patient has not voided, he or she should then be requested to do so.
   b. The patient is placed on the treatment table face up.
   c. Dentures, chewing gum, glass eyes, eyeglasses, contact lenses, bobby pins, and combs should be removed before treatment.
   d. The portion of the patient's head where the recording and treatment electrodes will be placed should be cleansed with

alcohol or acetone. After application of electrode paste if necessary, the two ECG electrodes are placed in the standard ECG positions: bifrontally for bilateral treatment (an alternative placement is mid-forehead and either the right or the left mastoid prominence behind the ear) or both frontally on the side opposite the active ECT electrodes for unilateral treatment. (An alternative placement is frontally and over the mastoid on the side opposite the active ECT electrode.) The EEG electrodes should be far enough apart that the electrode paste from each of the electrodes does not touch. In bilateral and unilateral treatment, it is best to hold the treating electrodes in place manually at the time of treatment. However, a rubber headband may be used, and is applied before the treatment. In either case, electrode jelly or paste is applied to the electrodes.

   e. An iv drip is started with 500 mL of dextrose 5% in water.
   f. If the device being used allows a test of patient impedance, the test should be done at this point. Some clinicians prefer to perform this step immediately after anesthesia induction.
   g. The patient is given 100% pure oxygen to breathe through a face mask.
   h. If the motor seizure is to be monitored, a blood pressure cuff on the arm opposite the one with the iv is inflated to a pressure just above the systolic pressure and held there. If unilateral treatment is to be given, the blood pressure cuff should be on the arm (or leg) on the same side as the side receiving the ECT in order to ensure that a generalized bilateral seizure has occurred.

3. Medication:
   a. If curare is used, it should be given iv at this time.
   b. Atropine 1 mg or glycopyrrolate 0.4 mg, if not given intramuscularly or subcutaneously ½ hour before treatment, is given iv push.
   c. Methohexital is injected iv push.
   d. Once it is ascertained the patient is asleep (by asking the patient questions, observing if the eyes focus when they are opened, or other means), succinylcholine is given iv push and the iv is opened to flush the tubing.

4. Administration of ECT:
   a. After the injection of succinylcholine, a rubber mouthpiece is inserted (Minneman 1995) and the electrodes are placed on the right temple (approximately 3 cm above the mid-

point of a line joining the external auditory meatus and the outer canthus of the eye) and 3 cm to the right of the vertex (for right unilateral ECT), unless the physician specifically wishes to do bilateral ECT, in which case the electrodes are placed bitemporally as described above for the right temple. If bifrontal placement is used, the electrodes should be placed 5 cm above the lateral angle of each orbit on a line parallel to the sagittal plane (Letemendia et al. 1993).

Note: If, after the first unilateral ECT, the patient seems more confused than expected, the next treatment should be given as a left unilateral ECT. This method of assessing cerebral hemispheric dominance was found in one review to lessen post-ECT confusion in a substantial majority of patients (Kopelman 1982) and obviates the need to determine cerebral dominance before initiating ECT.

b. Ventilation with 100% oxygen is begun.

c. After fasciculations cease (or plantar reflexes are no longer obtainable), the stimulus is administered according to the device's instructions. If no seizure occurs (as determined by lack of tonic-clonic movements in the arm or leg that has the blood pressure cuff above systolic pressure or by lack of seizure activity on the EEG), the stimulus is increased 25%–100% and reapplied after a wait of 20–40 seconds to allow for the possibility of a delayed seizure occurring. If a seizure occurs but lasts less than 25 seconds (as determined by tonic-clonic movements or the EEG), 1) the patient is ventilated with oxygen, and 2) the settings on the device are increased by 25%–100% as recommended by the manufacturer. Three minutes are then allowed to elapse from the end of the aborted (<25 seconds) seizure to the readministration of the stimulus. The 3-minute wait is necessary because, for approximately 120 seconds after the end of a seizure, the brain cannot be induced to have another seizure and, for an additional 60 seconds, the brain generally will respond with only an abortive seizure. These time periods are referred to as the ***absolute*** and the ***relative*** refractory periods, respectively (Maletzky 1981). For abortive seizures (i.e., those that occur but last less than 25 seconds), these time periods may be excessive. However, by adhering to the recommended time frame, the possibility that one is in the absolute or relative refractory period is lessened, and the chance for a successful second seizure is increased. In general, no more than four attempts to induce a seizure are made. Additional succinylcholine may be necessary if the patient is beginning to breathe and/or shows spontaneous movements, in which case 50% of the initial succinyl-choline dose is given. Seldom are additional doses of metho-hexital needed.

Note: Because of evidence that 25 seconds of seizure time may be necessary but not sufficient when unilateral treat-ment is administered (for discussion, see "Dosage and Vari-ation in Treatment" [page 618]), an alternative procedure for unilateral ECT is recommended by several ECT authori-ties. The threshold dose of electricity necessary to yield a seizure of 25 seconds or more is established by adjusting the device setting(s) to the lowest level, administering the treatment, and, if an adequate seizure (25 seconds or longer) is not obtained, gradually increasing the setting until an adequate seizure is obtained. The setting for sub-sequent treatments is then positioned at 150%–250% over this threshold level. Some researchers recommend that a similar procedure be used for bilateral therapy and that sub-sequent treatments be set at 50%–100% over the threshold position (Weiner 1994).

d. Immediately after the end of the clonic phase of the seizure, the rubber mouthpiece is replaced by an airway, the patient is ventilated with 100% oxygen, and the blood pressure cuff, which has been kept above systolic pressure, is deflated.

5. Post-ECT procedures:
   a. Immediately after placement of the airway, ventilation with oxygen is continued until spontaneous respiration is re-sumed. It is important during this phase that the patient's neck be hyperextended, that his or her nose and mouth be covered by the face mask, and that it is ascertained that the patient's thorax is moving with each respiration.
   b. Once spontaneous respiration returns, the patient is turned on his or her side to prevent aspiration in case of vomiting. The intravenous access is left in place in case it is needed in the recovery room.
   c. The physician records the relevant information related to the treatment procedures on the patient's individual ECT record as well as in the progress notes of the chart before beginning treatment on the next patient.
   d. Between 24 hours post-ECT and the next ECT treatment, the patient's response to treatment and cognitive function-

ing (including orientation and immediate, short-term, and long-term memory) are assessed and recorded. If therapeutic response is inadequate, modifications should be discussed with the ECT team, possibly including increasing stimulus (especially in unilateral ECT) or switching from unilateral to bilateral ECT. If cognitive functioning is severely affected, modifications should be considered, including increasing the time interval between treatments, decreasing the stimulus, or switching from right unilateral to left unilateral or from bilateral to unilateral treatment.

Complications of Treatment

1. *Laryngospasm* is evidenced by the patient's making rasping sounds without moving air into and out of his or her lungs. An immediate check to determine that there is no airway obstruction should be done. Vigorous mechanical respiration will often break the laryngospasm. If that fails, however, succinylcholine 10 mg iv should be administered and the patient given continuous respiration with 100% oxygen until spontaneous respiration returns.

2. Serious *cardiovascular complications* are rare. It is essential that a member of the ECT treatment team be certified in advanced cardiac life support (ACLS) and that all members of the team understand the principles and practice of cardiopulmonary resuscitation. Elevated blood pressures and pulse are common during the ECT-induced seizure and are often treated in compromised patients either before or after ECT with β-adrenergic blockers such as labetalol (Stoudemire et al. 1990). However, marked degrees of hypertension or hypotension and malignant arrhythmias may also occur, and it is important for a member of the treatment team to be trained to recognize and respond to such situations. Monitoring of oxygen and carbon dioxide blood levels is frequently done during anesthetic procedures and may prevent many arrhythmias. (For good reviews, see Abrams 1991 and Abrams 1992a.)

3. *Pseudocholinesterase deficiency* (actually, butyryl cholinesterase deficiency) is a homozygous recessive trait occurring in approximately 1 in 3,000 people. The individual who has this deficiency lacks the enzyme necessary to metabolize succinylcholine and thus may take several hours to return to spontaneous respiration after a standard dose of succinylcholine (Fink 1979; Pitts et al. 1968). The reaction would be noted the first

time a patient is given succinylcholine. Respiration may need to be supported for several hours and emergency anesthesiology consultation obtained.

4. *Prolonged seizures* (>3 minutes' duration) and *post-ECT confusion* are treated with 2–8 mg midazolam or 5–20 mg diazepam iv. Consideration should be given to administering these medications during subsequent ECTs just after the seizure ends and spontaneous respiration resumes.

Medications Used in ECT

■ Atropine and Glycopyrrolate

Atropine, a potent cholinergic-blocking agent of the antimuscarinic type, is useful in modifying the vagal response immediately after ECT. Thus, the bradycardia that occurs with ECT unmodified by atropine is prevented, as is the possibility of the arrhythmias that accompany bradycardia. In addition, atropine inhibits secretions of the upper airway and prevents bronchial constriction to some extent, thus decreasing the possibility of laryngospasm (Miller et al. 1987; Rich et al. 1969).

Intravenous administration of atropine immediately before ECT is as effective and safe as intramuscular or subcutaneous administration 30 minutes before treatment. Doses of more than 1.0 mg have no proven advantages in modifying bradycardia, and doses less than 1.0 mg are not as effective. The effects of atropine administered intravenously persist for 1–4 hours (Kramer et al. 1992; Rich et al. 1969).

Glycopyrrolate 0.4 mg may be used in place of atropine. This agent is preferred by some clinicians because it has substantial peripheral anticholinergic activity comparable to that of atropine but does not cross the blood-brain barrier, and hence has no CNS activity. One study indicated that glycopyrrolate caused less post-ECT confusion than atropine but was not as effective in preventing bradycardia and ectopy (Kramer et al. 1986).

There is some disagreement as to whether these agents should be routinely administered before ECT, although it is generally agreed that they should be given to patients who are receiving sympathetic-blocking agents or in whom it is medically important to prevent vagal bradycardia (American Psychiatric Association 1990). Because atropine and glycopyrrolate increase cardiac work (because of their effect on heart rate), it has been suggested that their use be avoided in patients at risk for ischemia (Welch 1993).

■ Methohexital

Methohexital is an ultra-short-acting barbiturate. It is administered intravenously after atropine and before succinylcholine. When given in a dose of 0.75 mg/kg, methohexital will cause most patients to fall asleep within 15 to 60 seconds. Higher doses may attenuate seizure duration and, perhaps, therapeutic efficacy. The mechanism producing sleep is unknown, but the rapid effect of the drug is a result of its swift penetration of the blood-brain barrier and high lipid solubility, with maximal brain concentrations requiring only two to three circulation times. The rapid (5–20 minutes) recovery from anesthesia is due, not to methohexital's metabolism, but rather to its redistribution from brain to muscle and fat tissue (Pitts et al. 1965; Woodruff et al. 1968).

Methohexital is preferred by most clinicians to thiopental, an ultra-short-acting barbiturate used with ECT in some treatment centers, because it has been demonstrated to cause fewer ECG abnormalities (Mokriski et al. 1992; Woodruff et al. 1968, 1969). However, not all studies concur with these findings (Pearlman and Richmond 1990).

Short-acting barbiturates are metabolized by the liver into inactive metabolites and hence should be used with caution in patients with severely compromised hepatic function.

Ketamine has been suggested as an anesthetic agent for use in ECT because of its ability to prolong seizure duration. However, this agent has the disadvantages of being associated with transient emergent psychosis and being relatively cardiotoxic. Ketamine's use is probably best reserved for patients in whom other procedures for potentiating seizures are ineffective or not tolerated (Weiner et al. 1991).

Propofol has also been used as an anesthetic for ECT because of its favorable emergence profile, but it attenuates seizures, and some authorities recommend that it not be used for this reason (Welch 1993). However, two recent randomized double-blind studies comparing propofol and methohexital in patients with major depressive disorder found that although propofol did lead to shorter seizure durations, it did not differ from methohexital in therapeutic efficacy, recovery time from anesthesia, effects on memory, or length of ECT course required (Fear et al. 1994; Martensson et al. 1994).

Etomidate was compared with methohexital in ECT in an open, randomized, crossover study. It was found to lead to a 24% longer wake-up time after ECT and to cause more pain at the injection site but to have equivalent effects on seizure duration (Kovac and

Pardo 1992). However, etomidate has also been reported in a small case series to be effective in inducing seizures in seizure-resistant patients and in prolonging seizures in patients with seizures of inadequate duration (Ilivicky et al. 1995). Etomidate may be an adequate substitute when a barbiturate anesthesia cannot be used.

■ Succinylcholine and Curare

Succinylcholine is administered intravenously immediately after sleep has been induced by methohexital. A dose of 0.5 mg/kg is given, which may need to be titrated up or down, depending on individual patient response. Succinylcholine produces rapid depolarization of the motor end plate, observed as fasciculations of large muscle groups. To prevent excessive muscle soreness, which is most commonly experienced by young, muscular males, curare 4.5 mg may be given before succinylcholine, in which case higher doses of succinylcholine may be necessary. Generally, paralysis with succinylcholine occurs at 60 seconds, is maximal at 2 minutes, and disappears at 5 minutes. The reason for giving this medication is to prevent fractures that could result from the tonic-clonic muscular contractions accompanying ECT-induced seizures. In general, the electrical stimulus can be applied 50–60 seconds after the administration of succinylcholine. Most clinicians prefer to wait for fasciculations to appear and disappear (or for plantar reflexes to disappear) before administering ECT (Pitts et al. 1968; Woodruff et al. 1969).

Metabolism by butyryl cholinesterase (pseudocholinesterase) is complete, as noted above, usually within 5 minutes. Apnea lasts between 2 and 4 minutes and requires immediate postseizure assisted respiration. In patients with pseudocholinesterase deficiency, atracurium, a nondepolarizing muscle relaxant, is an appropriate alternative to succinylcholine (Welch 1993).

References

Abraham FR, Kulhara P: The efficacy of electroconvulsive therapy in the treatment of schizophrenia—a comparative study. Br J Psychiatry 151:152–155, 1987

Abrams R: Is unilateral electroconvulsive therapy really the treatment of choice in endogenous depression? Ann N Y Acad Sci 462:50–55, 1986

Abrams R: Electroconvulsive therapy in the medically compromised patient. Psychiatr Clin North Am 14:871–885, 1991

Abrams R: Electroconvulsive therapy in the high-risk patient, in Electroconvulsive Therapy. New York, Oxford University Press, 1992a, pp 77–105

Abrams R: Technique of electroconvulsive therapy: theory, in Electroconvulsive Therapy. New York, Oxford University Press, 1992b, pp 140–177

Abrams R: Unilateral electroconvulsive therapy, in Electroconvulsive Therapy. New York, Oxford University Press, 1992c, pp 116–139

Abrams R, Taylor M: Catatonia: prediction of response to somatic treatment. Am J Psychiatry 134:78–80, 1977

Abrams R, Swartz CM, Vedak C: Antidepressant effects of high-dose right unilateral electroconvulsive therapy. Arch Gen Psychiatry 48:746–748, 1991

Acevedo AG, Smith JK: Adverse reaction to use of caffeine in ECT (letter). Am J Psychiatry 145:529, 1988

American Psychiatric Association: The Practice of Electroconvulsive Therapy (Task Force Report #14). Washington, DC, American Psychiatric Association, 1978

American Psychiatric Association: The Practice of Electroconvulsive Therapy: Recommendations for Treatment, Training, and Privileging. Washington, DC, American Psychiatric Association, 1990

Asnis G, Fink M, Safersein S: ECT in metropolitan New York hospitals: a survey of practice 1975–1976. Am J Psychiatry 135:479–482, 1978

Barton J, Mehta S, Snaith R: The prophylactic value of extra ECT in depressive illness. Acta Psychiatr Scand 49:386–392, 1973

Beale MD, Kellner CH, Pritchett JT: Stimulus dose titration in ECT: a 2-year clinical experience. Convuls Ther 10:171–176, 1994

Brandon S, Cawley P, McDonald C, et al: Electroconvulsive therapy: results in depressive illness from the Leicestershire trial. BMJ 288:22–25, 1984

Buchan H, Johnstone E, Palmer R, et al: Who benefits from electroconvulsive therapy? combined results of the Lancaster and Northwick Park trials. Br J Psychiatry 160:355–359, 1992

Clark CP, Alexopoulos G, Kaplan J: Prolactin release and clinical response to electroconvulsive therapy in depressed geriatric inpatients: a preliminary report. Convuls Ther 11:24–31, 1995

Clinical Research Centre Division of Psychiatry: The Northwick Park ECT trial: predictors of response to real and simulated ECT. Br J Psychiatry 144:227–237, 1984

Coffey CE: The role of structural brain imaging in ECT. Psychopharmacol Bull 30:477–483, 1994

Coffey CE, Figiel GS, Weiner RD, et al: Caffeine augmentation of ECT. Am J Psychiatry 147:579–585, 1990

Coffey CE, Weiner RD, Djang WT, et al: Brain anatomic effects of electroconvulsive therapy: a prospective magnetic resonance imaging study. Arch Gen Psychiatry 48:1013–1021, 1991

Coffey CE, Lucke J, Weiner RD, et al: Seizure threshold in electroconvulsive therapy, I: initial seizure threshold. Biol Psychiatry 37:713–720, 1995a

Coffey CE, Lucke J, Weiner RD, et al: Seizure threshold in electroconvulsive therapy (ECT), II: the anticonvulsant effect of ECT. Biol Psychiatry 37:777–788, 1995b

Colenda CC, McCall WV: A statistical model predicting the seizure threshold for right unilateral ECT in 106 patients. Convuls Ther 12:3–12, 1996

Consensus Conference: Electroconvulsive therapy. JAMA 254:103–108, 1985

Coppen A, Abou-Saleh M, Milln P, et al: Lithium continuation therapy following electroconvulsive therapy. Br J Psychiatry 139:284–287, 1981

Cronholm B, Ottosson JO: The experience of memory function after electroconvulsive therapy. Br J Psychiatry 109:251–258, 1963

Crow TJ, Johnstone EC: Controlled trials of electroconvulsive therapy. Ann N Y Acad Sci 462:12–29, 1986

Crowe R: Electroconvulsive therapy—a current perspective. N Engl J Med 311:163–167, 1984

Curran S: Effect of paroxetine on seizure length during electroconvulsive therapy. Acta Psychiatr Scand 92:239–240, 1995

d'Elia G: Unilateral electroconvulsive therapy. Acta Psychiatr Scand 215 (suppl):598, 1970

d'Elia G, Raotoma H: Is unilateral ECT less effective than bilateral ECT? Br J Psychiatry 126:83–89, 1975

DeBattista C, Mueller K: Sumatriptan prophylaxis for postelectroconvulsive therapy headaches. Headache 35:502–503, 1995

Decina P, Sackeim HA, Kahn DA, et al: Effects of ECT on the TRH stimulation test. Psychoneuroendocrinology 12:29–34, 1987

Devanand DP, Dwork AJ, Hutchinson ER, et al: Does ECT alter brain structure? Am J Psychiatry 151:957–970, 1994

Devanand DP, Fitzsimons L, Prudic J, et al: Subjective side effects during electroconvulsive therapy. Convuls Ther 11:232–240, 1995a

Devanand DP, Shapira B, Petty F, et al: Effects of electroconvulsive therapy on plasma GABA. Convuls Ther 11:3–13, 1995b

Elliott DL, Linz DM, Kane JA: Electroconvulsive therapy: pretreatment medical evaluation. Arch Intern Med 142:979–981, 1982

Farah A, McCall WV: Electroconvulsive therapy stimulus dosing: a survey of contemporary practices. Convuls Ther 9:90–94, 1993

Fear CF, Littlejohn CS, Rouse E: Propofol anesthesia in electroconvulsive therapy: reduced seizure duration may not be relevant. Br J Psychiatry 165:506–509, 1994

Fink M: Convulsive Therapy: Theory and Practice. New York, Raven, 1979

Fink M: Impact of the antipsychiatry movement on the revival of electroconvulsive therapy in the United States. Psychiatr Clin North Am 14:793–801, 1991

Fink M: Who should get ECT? in The Clinical Science of Electroconvulsive Therapy. Edited by Coffey CE. Washington, DC, American Psychiatric Press, 1993, pp 3–15

Fink M, Sackeim HA: Convulsive therapy in schizophrenia? Schizophr Bull 22:27–39, 1996

Fochtmann LJ: Animal studies of electroconvulsive therapy: foundations for future research. Psychopharmacol Bull 30:321–444, 1994

Freeman CPL, Basson JV, Crichton A: Double-blind controlled trial of electroconvulsive therapy (ECT) and simulated ECT in depressive illness. Lancet 1:738–740, 1978

Frith CD, Stevens M, Johnstone EC, et al: Effects of ECT and depression on various aspects of memory. Br J Psychiatry 142:610–617, 1983

Gangadhar BN, Kapson RL, Kalyanasundaram S: Comparison of electroconvulsive therapy with imipramine in endogenous depression: a double-blind study. Br J Psychiatry 141:367–371, 1982

Gangadhar BN, Janakiramaiah N, Subbakreshna DK, et al: Twice versus thrice weekly ECT in melancholia: a double-blind prospective comparison. J Affect Disord 27:273–278, 1993

Geretsegger C, Rochawanski E: Electroconvulsive therapy in acute life-threatening catatonia with associated cardiac and respiratory decompensation. Convuls Ther 3:291–295, 1987

Gleiter CH, Nutt DJ: Chronic electroconvulsive shock and neurotransmitter receptors: an update. Life Sci 44:985–1006, 1989

Greenblatt M, Grosser G, Wechsler H: Differential response of hospitalized depressed patients to somatic therapy. Am J Psychiatry 120:935–943, 1964

Grogan R, Wagner DR, Sullivan T, et al: Generalized nonconvulsive status epilepticus after electroconvulsive therapy. Convuls Ther 11:51–56, 1995

Guze BH, Liston EH, Baxter LR: Poor interrater reliability of MECTA EEG recordings of ECT seizure duration. J Clin Psychiatry 50:140–142, 1989

Hamilton M: Electroconvulsive therapy: indications and contraindication. Ann N Y Acad Sci 462:5–11, 1986

Hansen-Grant S, Tandon R, Maixner D, et al: Subclinical status epilepticus following ECT. Convuls Ther 11:134–138, 1995

Heshe J, Roeder E: Electroconvulsive therapy in Denmark. Br J Psychiatry 128:241–245, 1976

Heshe J, Roeder F, Theilgaard A: Unilateral and bilateral ECT: a psychiatric and psychological study of therapeutic effects and side effects. Acta Psychiatr Scand Suppl 275:1–181, 1978

Hickie I, Mason C, Parker G, et al: Prediction of ECT response: validation of a refined sign-based (CORE) system for defining melancholia. Br J Psychiatry 169:68–74, 1996

Hicks P, Matthews TK, Riggs M: Caffeine and ECT in the treatment of depression. Psychopharmacol Bull 30:106, 1994

Hinckle PE, Coffey CE, Weiner RD, et al: Use of caffeine to lengthen seizure during ECT. Am J Psychiatry 144:1143–1147, 1987

Ilivicky H, Caroff SN, Simone AF: Etomidate during ECT for elderly seizure-resistant patients. Am J Psychiatry 152:957–958, 1995

Imlah NW, Ryan E, Harrington J: The influence of antidepressant drugs on response to electroconvulsive therapy and on subsequent relapse rates. Neuropsychopharmacology 4:438–442, 1965

Jha AK, Stein GS, Fenwick P: Negative interaction between lithium and electroconvulsive therapy—a case-control study. Br J Psychiatry 168:241–243, 1996

Joffe RT, Sokolov S: The thyroid and electroconvulsive treatment. Psychopharmacol Bull 30:485–487, 1994

Johnstone EC, Deakin JFW, Lawler P, et al: The Northwick Park electroconvulsive therapy trial. Lancet 2:1317–1320, 1980

Kalinowsky L, Hippius H: Pharmacological, Convulsive and Other Treatments in Psychiatry. New York, Grune & Stratton, 1969, pp 229–249

Kamil R, Joffe RT: Neuroendocrine testing in electroconvulsive therapy. Psychiatr Clin North Am 14:961–970, 1991

Kantor S, Glassman A: Delusional depressions: natural history and response to treatment. Br J Psychiatry 131:351–360, 1977

Kapur S, Mann JJ: Antidepressant action and the neurobiologic effects of ECT: human studies, in The Clinical Science of Electroconvulsive Therapy. Edited by Coffey CE. Washington, DC, American Psychiatric Press, 1993, pp 235–250

Karliner W, Wehrheim H: Maintenance convulsive treatment. Am J Psychiatry 121:113–115, 1965

Kay D, Fahy T, Garside R: A 17-month double-blind trial of amitriptyline and diazepam in ECT-treated depressed patients. Br J Psychiatry 117:667–671, 1970

Kellner CH, Nixon DW, Bernstein HJ: ECT-drug interactions: a review. Psychopharmacol Bull 27:595–609, 1991

Kellner CH, Beale MD, Pritchett JT, et al: Electroconvulsive therapy and Parkinson's disease: the case for further study. Psychopharmacol Bull 30:495–500, 1994

Kelsey MC, Grossberg GT: Safety and efficacy of caffeine-augmented ECT in elderly depressives: a retrospective study. J Geriatr Psychiatry-Neurol 8:168–172, 1995

Kety S: Biochemical and neurochemical effects of electroconvulsive shock, in Psychobiology of Convulsive Therapy. Edited by Fink M, Kety S, McGaugh S, et al. Washington, DC, VH Winston, 1974, pp 285–294

Kopelman MD: Speech dominance, handedness, and electroconvulsions. Psychological Med 12:667–670, 1982

Kornhuber J, Weller M: Patient selection and remission rates with the current practice of electroconvulsive therapy in Germany. Convuls Ther 11:104–109, 1995

Kovac A, Pardo M: A comparison between etomidate and methohexital for anesthesia in ECT. Convuls Ther 8:118–125, 1992

Kramer BA, Allen RE, Friedman B: Atropine and glycopyrrolate as ECT preanesthesia. J Clin Psychiatry 47:299–300, 1986

Kramer BA, Afrasiabi A, Pollock VE: Intravenous versus intramuscular atropine in ECT. Am J Psychiatry 149:1258–1260, 1992

Kroessler D: Relative efficacy rates for therapies of delusional depression. Convuls Ther 1:173–182, 1985

Krystal AD, Weiner RD: ECT seizure duration: reliability of manual and computer-automated determinations. Convuls Ther 11:158–169, 1995

Krystal AD, Weiner RD, McCall WV, et al: The effects of ECT stimulus dose and electrode placement on the ictal electroencephalogram: an intraindividual crossover study. Biol Psychiatry 34:759–767, 1993

Lambourn J, Gill D: A controlled comparison of simulated and real ECT. Br J Psychiatry 133:514–519, 1978

Lerer B, Shapira B: Neurochemical mechanisms of mood stabilizations: focus on ECT. Ann N Y Acad Sci 462:366–375, 1986

Lerer B, Shapira B, Calev A, et al: Antidepressant and cognitive effects of twice- versus three-times-weekly ECT. Am J Psychiatry 152:564–570, 1995

Letemendia FJJ, Delva NJ, Rodenburg M, et al: Therapeutic advantage of bifrontal electrode placement in ECT. Psychol Med 23:349–360, 1993

Maletzky B: Multiple Monitored Electroconvulsive Therapy. Boca Raton, FL, CRC Press, 1981

Maletzky B, McFarland B, Burt A: Refractory obsessive-compulsive disorder and ECT. Convuls Ther 10:34–42, 1994

Manly DT, Swartz CM: Asymmetric bilateral right frontotemporal left frontal stimulus electrode placement: comparison with bifrontotemporal and unilateral placements. Convuls Ther 10:267–270, 1994

Mann JJ, Kapur S: Elucidation of biochemical basis of the antidepressant action of electroconvulsive therapy by human studies. Psychopharmacol Bull 30:445–453, 1994

Mann SC, Carnoff SN, Bleier HR, et al: Lethal catatonia. Am J Psychiatry 143:1374–1381, 1986

Martensson B, Bartfai A, Hallen B, et al: A comparison of propofol and methohexital as anesthetic agents for ECT: effects on seizure duration, therapeutic outcome, and memory. Biol Psychiatry 35:179–189, 1994

McAllister DA, Perri MG, Jordan RC, et al: Effects of ECT given two vs. three times weekly. Psychiatry Res 21:63–69, 1987

McCabe M: ECT and the treatment of mania: a controlled study. Am J Psychiatry 133:688–691, 1976

McCabe MS, Norris B: ECT versus chlorpromazine in mania. Biol Psychiatry 12:245–254, 1977

McCall WV, Shelp FE, Weiner RD, et al: Convulsive threshold differences in right unilateral and bilateral ECT. Biol Psychiatry 34:606–611, 1993

Medical Research Council, Cawley RH, et al: Clinical trial in the treatment of depressive illness. BMJ 1:881–886, 1965

Meduna L, Friedman E: The convulsive-irritative therapy of the psychoses. JAMA 112:501–509, 1939

Miller ME, Gabriel A, Herman G, et al: Atropine sulfate premedication and cardiac arrhythmia in electroconvulsive therapy (ECT). Convuls Ther 3:10–17, 1987

Milstein V, Milstein MJ, Small IF: Radiographic screening for ECT: use and usefulness. Convuls Ther 11:38–44, 1995

Minneman SA: A history of oral protection for the ECT patient: past, present, and future. Convuls Ther 11:94–103, 1995

Minter R, Mandel M: The treatment of psychotic major depressive disorder with drugs and electroconvulsive therapy. J Nerv Ment Dis 167:726–733, 1979

Mokriski BK, Nagle SE, Papuchis GE, et al: Electroconvulsive therapy–induced cardiac arrhythmias during anesthesia with methohexital, thiamylal, or thiopental sodium. J Clin Anesth 4:208–212, 1992

Mukherjee S: Combined ECT and lithium therapy. Convuls Ther 4:274–284, 1993

Mukherjee S, Sackeim HA, Schnur DB: Electroconvulsive therapy of acute manic episodes: a review of 50 years' experience. Am J Psychiatry 151:169–176, 1994

Nobler MS, Sackeim HA: ECT stimulus dosing: relations to efficacy and adverse effects, in The Clinical Science of Electroconvulsive Therapy. Edited by Coffey CE. Washington, DC, American Psychiatric Press, 1993, pp 29–52

Nutt DJ, Glue P: The neurobiology of ECT: animal studies, in The Clinical Science of Electroconvulsive Therapy. Edited by Coffey CE. Washington, DC, American Psychiatric Press, 1993, pp 213–234

O'Leary D, Gill D, Gregory S, et al: Which depressed patients respond to ECT? the Nottingham results. J Affect Disord 33:245–250, 1995

Ottosson JO: Seizure characteristics and therapeutic efficiency in electroconvulsive therapy: an analysis of the antidepressant efficiency of grand mal and lidocaine-modified seizures. J Nerv Ment Dis 135:239–251, 1962a

Ottosson JO: Electroconvulsive therapy: electrostimulatory or convulsive therapy? Journal of Neuropsychiatry 3:216–220, 1962b

Ottosson JO: Systemic biochemical effects of ECT, in Psychobiology of Convulsive Therapy. Edited by Fink M, Kety S, McGaugh J, et al. Washington, DC, VH Winston, 1974, pp 209–220

Pearlman C, Richmond J: New data on the methohexital-thiopental arrhythmic issue. Convuls Ther 6:221–223, 1990

Peppard J, Ellam L: Electroconvulsive Treatment in Great Britain. London, Gaskell, 1980

Perrin G: Cardiovascular aspects of electroshock therapy. Acta Psychiatr Neurol Scand 36:1–45, 1961

Perry P, Tsuang M: Treatment of unipolar depression following electroconvulsive therapy. J Affect Disord 1:123–129, 1979

Petrides G, Dhossche D, Fink M, et al: Continuation ECT: relapse prevention in affective disorders. Convuls Ther 10:189–194, 1994

Pettinati HM, Nilsen S: Missed and brief seizures during ECT: differential response between unilateral and bilateral electrode placement. Biol Psychiatry 20:506–514, 1985

Pettinati HM, Mathisen KS, Rosenberg J, et al: Meta-analytical approach to reconciling discrepancies in efficacy between bilateral and unilateral electroconvulsive therapy. Convuls Ther 2:7–17, 1986

Piper A: Tricyclic antidepressants versus electroconvulsive therapy: a review of the evidence for efficacy in depression. Ann Clin Psychiatry 5:13–23, 1993

Pitts F, Desmarais G, Stewart W, et al: Induction of anesthesia with methohexital and thiopental in electroconvulsive therapy. N Engl J Med 273:353–360, 1965

Pitts F, Woodruff R, Craig A, et al: The drug modification of ECT, II: succinylcholine dosage. Arch Gen Psychiatry 19:595–599, 1968

Post RM, Putnam F, Uhde TW, et al: Electroconvulsive therapy as an anticonvulsant. Ann N Y Acad Sci 462:398–410, 1986

Potter WZ: ECT methodologic issues. Psychopharmacol Bull 30:455–459, 1994

Price T: Short- and long-term cognitive effects of ECT, I: effects on memory. Psychopharmacol Bull 18:81–91, 1982a

Price T: Short- and long-term cognitive effects of ECT, II: effects on non-memory-associated cognitive function. Psychopharmacol Bull 18:92–101, 1982b

Prudic J, Sackeim HA, Devanand DP: Medication resistance and clinical response to electroconvulsive therapy. Psychiatry Res 31:287–296, 1990

Rasmussen K, Abrams R: Treatment of Parkinson's disease with electroconvulsive therapy. Psychiatr Clin North Am 14:925–933, 1991

Rasmussen KG, Zorumski CF, Jarvis MR: Possible impact of stimulus duration on seizure threshold in ECT. Convuls Ther 10:177–180, 1994

Reichert H, Benjamin J, Keegan D, et al: Bilateral and nondominant unilateral ECT, I: therapeutic efficacy. Canadian Psychiatric Association Journal 21:69–78, 1976

Rice EH, Sombrotto LB, Markowitz JC, et al: Cardiovascular morbidity in high-risk patients during ECT. Am J Psychiatry 151:1637–1641, 1994

Rich C, Woodruff R, Cadoret R: Electrotherapy: the effects of atropine on EKG. Diseases of the Nervous System 30:622–626, 1969

Riddle WJR, Scott AIF: Relapse after successful electroconvulsive therapy: the use and impact of continuation antidepressant drug treatment. Human Psychopharmacology Clinical Exp 10:201–205, 1995

Ries RK: Poor interrater reliability of MECTA EEG seizure duration measurement during ECT. Biol Psychiatry 20:94–119, 1985

Roemer RA, Dubin WR, Jaffe R, et al: An efficacy study of single versus double-seizure induction with ECT in major depression. J Clin Psychiatry 51:473–478, 1990

Rudorfer MV, Risby ED, Hsiao JK, et al: ECT alters human monoamines in a different manner from that of antidepressant drugs. Psychopharmacol Bull 24:396–399, 1988

Sackeim HA: Central issues regarding the mechanisms of action of electroconvulsive therapy: directions for future research. Psychopharmacol Bull 30:281–308, 1994a

Sackeim HA: Continuation therapy following ECT: directions for future research. Psychopharmacol Bull 30:501–521, 1994b

Sackeim HA, Rush AJ: Melancholia and response to ECT. Am J Psychiatry 152:1242–1243, 1995

Sackeim HA, Decina P, Prahovnik I, et al: Dosage, seizure threshold and the antidepressant efficacy of electroconvulsive therapy. Ann N Y Acad Sci 462:398–410, 1986

Sackeim HA, Decina P, Kanzler M, et al: Effects of electrode placement on the efficacy of titrated, low-dose ECT. Am J Psychiatry 144:1449–1455, 1987a

Sackeim HA, Decina P, Prohovnik I, et al: Seizure threshold in electroconvulsive therapy. Arch Gen Psychiatry 44:355–364, 1987b

Sackeim HA, Brown RP, Devanand DP, et al: Should tricyclic antidepressants or lithium be standard continuation to treatment after ECT? an alternative view. Convuls Ther 5:180–183, 1989

Sackeim HA, Prudic J, Devanand D, et al: The impact of medication resistance and continuation pharmacotherapy on relapse following response to electroconvulsive therapy in major depression. J Clin Psychopharmacol 10:96–104, 1990

Sackeim HA, Devanand DP, Prudic J: Stimulus intensity, seizure threshold, and seizure duration: impact on the efficacy and safety of electroconvulsive therapy. Psychiatr Clin North Am 14:803–843, 1991

Sackeim HA, Prudic J, Devanand DP, et al: Effects of stimulus intensity and electrode placement on the efficacy and cognitive effects of electroconvulsive therapy. N Engl J Med 328:839–846, 1993

Sand-Stromegren L: Unilateral versus bilateral electroconvulsive therapy. Acta Psychiatr Scand 240 (suppl):1–65, 1973

Sarkar P, Andrade C, Kapur B, et al: An exploratory evaluation of ECT in haloperidol-treated DSM-III-R schizophreniform disorder. Convuls Ther 10:271–278, 1994

Schwarz T, Lowenstein J, Isenberg KE: Maintenance ECT: indications and outcome. Convuls Ther 11:14–23, 1995

Scott AI: Which depressed patients will respond to electroconvulsive therapy? the search for biological predictors of recovery. Br J Psychiatry 154:8–17, 1989

Scott AI, Shering PA, Legros JJ, et al: Improvement in depression is not associated with altered release of neurophysins over a course of ECT. Psychiatry Res 36:65–73, 1991

Seager C, Bird R: Imipramine with electrical treatment in depression—a controlled trial. Journal of Mental Science 108:704–707, 1962

Segman RH, Shapira B, Gorfine M, et al: Onset and time course of antidepressant action: psychopharmacological implications of a controlled trial of electroconvulsive therapy. Psychopharmacology (Berl) 119:440–448, 1995

Shapira B, Lerer B, Gilboa D, et al: Facilitation of ECT by caffeine pretreatment. Am J Psychiatry 144:1199–1202, 1987

Shapira B, Lidsky D, Gorfine M, et al: Electroconvulsive therapy and resistant depression: clinical implications and seizure threshold. J Clin Psychiatry 57:32–38, 1996

Sikdar S, Kulhara P, Avasthi A, et al: Combined chlorpromazine and electroconvulsive therapy in mania. Br J Psychiatry 164:806–810, 1994

Small JG: Efficacy of ECT in schizophrenia, mania, and other disorders. Psychopharmacol Bull 22:469–471, 1986

Small J: EEG monitoring during ECT research. Convuls Ther 10:220–223, 1994

Small JG, Milstein V, Klapper MH, et al: Electroconvulsive therapy in the treatment of manic episodes. Ann N Y Acad Sci 462:37–49, 1986

Small JG, Klapper MM, Kellam JJ, et al: ECT compared with lithium in the management of manic states. Arch Gen Psychiatry 45:727–732, 1988

Small JG, Milstein V, Small IF: Electroconvulsive therapy for mania. Psychiatr Clin North Am 14:887–903, 1991

Small JG, Milstein V, Kellams JJ, et al: Hemispheric components of ECT responses in mood disorders and schizophrenia, in The Clinical Science of Electroconvulsive Therapy. Edited by Coffey CE. Washington, DC, American Psychiatric Press, 1993, pp 111–123

Sobin C, Sackeim HA, Prudic J, et al: Predictors of retrograde amnesia following ECT. Am J Psychiatry 152:995–1001, 1995

Squire LR: Memory functions as affected by electroconvulsive therapy. Ann N Y Acad Sci 462:307–314, 1986

Squire L, Slater P: Bilateral and unilateral ECT: effects on verbal and nonverbal memory. Am J Psychiatry 135:1316–1320, 1978

Squire LR, Slater PC: Electroconvulsive therapy and complaints of memory dysfunction: a prospective 3-year follow-up study. Br J Psychiatry 142:1–8, 1983

Steibel VG: Maintenance electroconvulsive therapy for chronically ill patients: a case series. Psychiatr Serv 46:265–268, 1995

Stephens SM, Greenberg RM, Pettinati HM: Choosing an electroconvulsive therapy device. Psychiatr Clin North Am 14:989–1006, 1991

Stephens SM, Pettinati HM, Greenberg RM, et al: Continuation and maintenance therapy with outpatient ECT, in The Clinical Science of Electroconvulsive Therapy. Edited by Coffey CE. Washington, DC, American Psychiatric Press, 1993, pp 143–164

Stevenson G, Georghegan J: Prophylactic electroshock. Am J Psychiatry 107:743–748, 1951

Stoudemire A, Knos G, Gladson M: Labetalol in the control of cardiovascular responses to electroconvulsive therapy in high-risk depressed medical patients. J Clin Psychiatry 51:508–512, 1990

Swartz CM, Larson G: ECT stimulus duration and its efficacy. Ann Clin Psychiatry 1:147–152, 1989

Swartz CM, Lewis RK: Theophylline reversal of electroconvulsive therapy (ECT) seizure inhibition. Psychosomatics 32:47–51, 1991

Swartz CM, Abrams R, Rasmussen K, et al: Computer automated versus visually determined electroencephalographic seizure duration. Convuls Ther 10:165–170, 1994

Taylor MA: Catatonia: a review of a behavioral neurologic syndrome. Neuropsychiatry, Neuropsychology, and Behavioral Neurology 3:48–72, 1990

Taylor PJ, Fleminger JJ: ECT for schizophrenia. Lancet 1:1380–1382, 1980

Vanelle JM, Loo H, Galinowski A, et al: Maintenance ECT in intractable manic-depressive disorder. Convuls Ther 10:195–205, 1994

Voelker R: Anesthesia-related risks have plummeted. JAMA 273:445–446, 1995

Warmflash VL, Stricks L, Sackeim HA, et al: Reliability and validity of measures of seizure duration. Convuls Ther 3:18–25, 1987

Warner MA, Shields SE, Chute CG: Major morbidity and mortality within 1 month of ambulatory surgery and anesthesia. JAMA 270:1437–1441, 1993

Weeks D, Freeman CPL, Kendell RS: ECT, III: enduring cognitive deficits. Br J Psychiatry 137:26–37, 1980

Weiner RD: ECT and seizure threshold: effects of stimulus wave form and electrode placement. Biol Psychiatry 15:225–241, 1980

Weiner RD: Electrical dosage, stimulus parameters, and electrode placement. Psychopharmacol Bull 22:499–502, 1986

Weiner RD: Treatment optimization with ECT. Psychopharmacol Bull 30:313–320, 1994

Weiner RD, Coffey CE, Krystal AD: The monitoring and management of electrically induced seizures. Psychiatr Clin North Am 14:845–869, 1991

Welch CA: The relative efficacy of unilateral nondominant and bilateral stimulation. Psychopharmacol Bull 18:68–70, 1982

Welch CA: ECT in medically ill patients, in The Clinical Science of Electroconvulsive Therapy. Edited by Coffey CE. Washington, DC, American Psychiatric Press, 1993, pp 167–182

West ED: Electroconvulsive therapy in depression: a double-blind controlled trial. BMJ 282:355–357, 1981

Woodruff R, Pitts F, McClure J: The drug modification of ECT, I: methohexital, thiopental, and pre-oxygenation. Arch Gen Psychiatry 18:605–611, 1968

Woodruff R, Pitts F, Craig A: Electrotherapy: the effects of barbiturate anesthesia, succinylcholine and pre-oxygenation on the EKG. Diseases of the Nervous System 30:180–185, 1969

Zielinski RJ, Roose SP, Devanand DP, et al: Cardiovascular complications of ECT in depressed patients with cardiac disease. Am J Psychiatry 150:904–909, 1993

13

Patient Advice

The patient advice monographs provided in this chapter are intended to provide information to patients and their concerned others regarding their medication. These monographs are not inclusive of all possible adverse effects; rather, they review *common* adverse effects. The health professional should discuss this information with the patient and modify the content as deemed necessary.

Amoxapine

Generic name: amoxapine
Trade name: _____
Strength: _____mg
Purpose: This medication is used to treat depression.
Directions: It is important to follow these directions:
Take _____ tablet(s) or capsule(s) by mouth _____ time(s) daily.
Your medicine should be taken at the following
time(s):_____

Tell your physician, nurse, and pharmacist if you

- Have allergies
- Are pregnant or plan to become pregnant
- Are breast-feeding
- Are taking other medicine, including nonprescription medicine such as antacids, aspirin, or cold medication
- Have other medical problems

Warnings:

- Do not give this medicine to others. It may harm them.
- Do not take more than the recommended amount of this medication, and do not stop taking it without the advice of your physician.
- Store this medicine as directed on the auxiliary label(s) on the bottle.
- Keep all medicines away from the reach of small children.
- It is best to avoid the use of alcohol.
- If you should miss a dose of this medicine, take it as soon as possible. However, if it is almost time for your next dose, skip the missed dose. Do not double doses.
- Do not drive a car or operate dangerous machinery until you know how this drug affects you.

Important information about your medication:

- It is very important that you take this medication as directed by your physician in order for it to help you. When taken regularly, this medication usually requires 2–4 weeks before the full effects are noticed.
- This medication does not produce euphoria (a high feeling) and is not addictive.

The following side effects may occur:

- Dry mouth—Chewing sugarless gum or sucking on sour, sugarless hard candy will help relieve this. Sucking on ice chips or rinsing your mouth with water might also help. This side effect may go away in several weeks. Brush your teeth regularly.

- Drowsiness—This side effect is usually a problem only during the first few days when you start taking the medication. If it is a problem, be very cautious in driving and operating dangerous machinery.
- Blurred vision—This effect is temporary and usually goes away with continued use of the medication. If it becomes severe, notify your physician.
- Constipation—A high-fiber diet (bran) and exercise may help to alleviate this problem.
- Dizziness—This may occur when you get up too quickly or rapidly change positions. It can be avoided by arising or changing positions slowly.
- Difficulty in passing urine—If this becomes a problem and continues, notify your physician.
- Allergic reactions (e.g., rash, itching)—These are rare. If these reactions are accompanied by a high fever, sore throat, or fainting spells, notify your physician
- Nausea and/or headache—If these persist or are severe, contact your physician.
- Sexual dysfunction—If a change in your sex drive or functioning occurs, contact your physician.
- Restlessness, tremors, stiffness, muscle spasms—These side effects can occur and can be treated by your physician. If they persist or get worse, contact your physician.
- Abnormal movements—If this medication is taken continuously for more than 6 months, the possibility exists of developing a condition known as tardive dyskinesia. This term refers to unwanted movements of the tongue, lips, arms, and legs. If the problem is noticed early and the medication changed or stopped, the condition goes away. If not noticed, however, it may become permanent, even if the medication is stopped. Therefore, inform your physician if you experience any of the following:
  - Continuous movement of the mouth, jaw, and/or tongue
  - Continuous movement of hands, arms, legs, or body
  - Other people telling you that they have noticed unusual or continuous movement of your mouth, jaw, tongue, hands, arms, legs, or body

Because people respond to medicines in very individual ways, you and your physician may have to go through a trying-out period before he or she finds the dose that works best for you.

If you feel you are having problems with your medication, notify your physician.

Anticholinergics

Generic name: _____
Trade name: _____
Strength: _____ mg
Purpose: This medication is used to treat the side effects of the antipsychotic medication (_____) you are taking.
Directions: It is important to follow these directions:
Take _____ tablet(s) or capsule(s) by mouth _____ time(s) daily.
Your medicine should be taken at the following
time(s): _____

Tell your physician, nurse, and pharmacist if you

- Have allergies
- Are pregnant or plan to become pregnant
- Are breast-feeding
- Are taking other medicine, including nonprescription medicine such as antacids, aspirin, or cold medication
- Have other medical problems

Warnings:

- Do not give this medicine to others. It may harm them.
- Do not take more than the recommended amount of this medication, and do not stop taking it without the advice of your physician.
- Store this medicine as directed on the auxiliary label(s) on the bottle.
- Keep all medicines away from the reach of small children.
- It is best to avoid the use of alcohol.
- If you should miss a dose of this medicine, take it as soon as possible. However, if it is almost time for your next dose, skip the missed dose. Do not double doses.
- Do not drive a car or operate dangerous machinery until you know how this drug affects you.

Important information about your medication:

- It is very important that you take this medication as directed by your physician.
- The medication does not produce euphoria (a high feeling) and is not addictive.

The following side effects may occur:

- Dry mouth—Chewing sugarless gum or sucking on sour, sugarless hard candy will help relieve this. Sucking on ice chips or rinsing your mouth with water might also help. This side effect may go away in several weeks. Brush your teeth regularly.

- Drowsiness—This side effect is usually a problem only during the first few days when you start taking the medication. If it is a problem, be very cautious in driving and operating dangerous machinery.
- Dizziness—This may occur when you get up too quickly or rapidly change positions. It can be avoided by arising or changing positions slowly.
- Blurred vision—This effect is temporary and usually goes away with continued use of the medication. If it becomes severe, notify your physician.
- Constipation—A high-fiber diet (bran) and exercise may help to alleviate this problem.
- Difficulty in passing urine—If this becomes a problem and continues, notify your physician.
- Allergic reactions (e.g., rash, itching)—These are rare. If these reactions are accompanied by a high fever, sore throat, or fainting spells, notify your physician
- Sexual dysfunction—If a change in your sex drive or functioning occurs, contact your physician.

Because people respond to medicines in very individual ways, you and your physician may have to go through a trying-out period before he or she finds the dose that works best for you.

If you believe you are having problems with your medication, notify your physician.

Antipsychotics (typical class)

Generic name: _____
Trade name: _____
Strength: _____mg
Purpose: This medication is used to treat a variety of psychiatric problems, such as overactivity, preoccupation with troublesome and recurring thoughts, and unpleasant and unusual experiences such as hearing and seeing things not normally seen or heard. This medication will reduce or stop these experiences and help you to remain outside the hospital.
Directions: It is important to follow these directions:
Take _____ tablet(s) or capsule(s) by mouth _____ time(s) daily.
Your medicine should be taken at the following
time(s):_____

Tell your physician, nurse, and pharmacist if you
- Have allergies
- Are pregnant or plan to become pregnant
- Are breast-feeding
- Are taking other medicine, including nonprescription medicine such as antacids, aspirin, or cold medication
- Have other medical problems

Warnings:
- Do not give this medicine to others. It may harm them.
- Do not take more than the recommended amount of this medication, and do not stop taking it without the advice of your physician.
- Store this medicine as directed on the auxiliary label(s) on the bottle.
- Keep all medicines away from the reach of small children.
- It is best to avoid the use of alcohol.
- If you should miss a dose of this medicine, take it as soon as possible. However, if it is almost time for your next dose, skip the missed dose. Do not double doses.
- Do not drive a car or operate dangerous machinery until you know how this drug affects you.

Important information about your medication:
- It is very important that you take this medication as directed by your physician in order for it to help you. When taken regularly, this medication usually requires 2–4 weeks before the full effects are noticed.
- This medication does not produce euphoria (a high feeling) and is not addictive.

The following side effects may occur:

- Drowsiness—This side effect is usually a problem only during the first few days when you start taking the medication. If it is a problem, be very cautious in driving and operating dangerous machinery.
- Dry mouth—Chewing sugarless gum or sucking on sour, sugarless hard candy will help relieve this side effect. Sucking on ice chips or rinsing your mouth with water might also help. This effect may go away in several weeks. Brush your teeth regularly.
- Blurred vision—This effect is temporary and usually goes away with continued use of the medication. If it becomes severe, notify your physician.
- Restlessness, tremors, stiffness, muscle spasms—These side effects can occur and can be treated by your physician. If they persist or get worse, contact your physician.
- Difficulty in passing urine—If this becomes a problem and continues, notify your physician.
- Dizziness—This may occur when you get up too quickly or rapidly change positions. It can be avoided by arising or changing positions slowly.
- Weight gain—Some patients experience an increase in weight after they start taking this medication. If this is not desired, exercise and dietary restriction may be of benefit.
- Severe sunburn—Avoid direct sunlight and, if you must be out in the sun, use a sunscreen lotion (Presun® or Pabafilm®). Regular suntan lotion is not protective against this type of sunburn.
- Abnormal movements—If this medication is taken continuously for more than 6 months, the possibility exists of developing a condition known as tardive dyskinesia. This term refers to unwanted movements of the tongue, lips, arms, and legs. If the problem is noticed early and the medication changed or stopped, the condition goes away. If not noticed, however, it may become permanent, even if the medication is stopped. Therefore, inform your physician if you experience any of the following:
  - ✦ Continuous movement of the mouth, jaw, and/or tongue
  - ✦ Continuous movement of hands, arms, legs, or body
  - ✦ Other people telling you that they have noticed unusual or continuous movement of your mouth, jaw, tongue, hands, arms, legs, or body
- Sexual dysfunction—If a change in your sex drive or functioning occurs, contact your physician.

Because people respond to medicines in very individual ways, you and your physician may have to go through a trying-out period before he or she finds the dose that works best for you.

If you feel you are having problems with your medication, notify your physician.

Anxiolytic-Hypnotics (benzodiazepines, zolpidem)

Generic name: _____
Trade name: _____
Strength: _____ mg
Purpose: This medication is used to help relieve anxiety and tension or to induce sleep.
Directions: It is important to follow these directions:
Take _____ tablet(s) or capsule(s) by mouth _____ time(s) daily.
Your medicine should be taken at the following
time(s):_____

Tell your physician, nurse, and pharmacist if you

- Have allergies
- Are pregnant or plan to become pregnant
- Are breast-feeding
- Are taking other medicine, including nonprescription medicine such as antacids, aspirin, or cold medication
- Have other medical problems

Warnings:

- Do not give this medicine to others. It may harm them.
- Do not take more than the recommended amount of this medication, and do not stop taking it without the advice of your physician. Stopping this medication abruptly may lead to trouble sleeping, increase in anxiety or nervousness, increased blood pressure, sweating, headache, nausea, diarrhea, and possibly convulsions.
- Store this medicine as directed on the auxiliary label(s) on the bottle.
- Keep all medicines away from the reach of small children.
- It is best to avoid the use of alcohol.
- If you should forget a dose, do not take the missed dose when you remember it, but instead omit it completely; then take the next dose at the regularly scheduled time.
- Do not drive a car or operate dangerous machinery until you know how this drug affects you.

Important information about your medication:

- It is very important that you take this medication as directed by your physician.
- The medication does not produce euphoria (a high feeling) and is not addictive.

The following side effects may occur:

- Drowsiness, dizziness, weakness, muscle incoordination—You should be careful about standing up quickly, going up and down stairs, and driving. Lie down or sit down at the first sign of dizziness.
- Confusion, memory problems, excitement, nightmares—Contact your physician if these occur.

Because people respond to medicines in very individual ways, you and your physician may have to go through a trying-out period before he or she finds the dose that works best for you.

If you feel you are having problems with your medication, notify your physician.

Bupropion

Generic name: bupropion
Trade name: _____
Strength: _____ mg
Purpose: This medication is used to treat depression.
Directions: It is important to follow these directions:
Take _____ tablet(s) or capsule(s) by mouth _____ time(s) daily.
Your medicine should be taken at the following
time(s): _____

Tell your physician, nurse, and pharmacist if you
- Have allergies
- Are pregnant or plan to become pregnant
- Are breast-feeding
- Are taking other medicine, including nonprescription medicine such as antacids, aspirin, or cold medication
- Have other medical problems

Warnings:
- Do not give this medicine to others. It may harm them.
- Do not take more than the recommended amount of this medication, and do not stop taking it without the advice of your physician.
- Store this medicine as directed on the auxiliary label(s) on the bottle.
- Keep all medicines away from the reach of small children.
- It is best to avoid the use of alcohol.
- If you should forget a dose, do not take the missed dose when you remember it, but instead omit it completely; then take the next dose at the regularly scheduled time.
- Do not drive a car or operate dangerous machinery until you know how this drug affects you.

Important information about your medication:
- It is very important that you take this medication as directed by your physician in order for it to help you. When taken regularly, this medication usually requires 2–4 weeks before the full effects are noticed.
- This medication does not produce euphoria (a high feeling) and is not addictive.

The following side effects may occur:
- Drowsiness—Although unlikely, this side effect may occur. Do not drive a car or operate dangerous machinery until you know how this drug affects you.

- Weight loss, nausea, decreased appetite—If these persist or are severe, contact your physician.
- Convulsions—These may occur with standard and higher doses. Follow the recommended dosing schedule.
- Dizziness—This may occur when you get up too quickly or rapidly change positions. It can be avoided by arising or changing positions slowly.
- Allergic reactions (e.g., rash, itching)—These are rare. If these reactions are accompanied by a high fever, sore throat, or fainting spells, notify your physician
- Sexual dysfunction—If a change in your sex drive or functioning occurs, contact your physician.

Because people respond to medicines in very individual ways, you and your physician may have to go through a trying-out period before he or she finds the dose that works best for you.

If you believe you are having problems with your medication, notify your physician.

Buspirone

Generic name: buspirone
Trade name: _____
Strength: _____ mg
Purpose: This medication is used to help relieve anxiety and tension.
Directions: It is important to follow these directions:
Take _____ tablet(s) or capsule(s) by mouth _____ time(s) daily.
Your medicine should be taken at the following
time(s):_____

Tell your physician, nurse, and pharmacist if you

- Have allergies
- Are pregnant or plan to become pregnant
- Are breast-feeding
- Are taking other medicine, including nonprescription medicine such as antacids, aspirin, or cold medication
- Have other medical problems

Warnings:

- Do not give this medicine to others. It may harm them.
- Do not take more than the recommended amount of this medication, and do not stop taking it without the advice of your physician.
- Store this medicine as directed on the auxiliary label(s) on the bottle.
- Keep all medicines away from the reach of small children.
- It is best to avoid the use of alcohol.
- If you should forget a dose, do not take the missed dose when you remember it, but instead omit it completely; then take the next dose at the regularly scheduled time.
- Do not drive a car or operate dangerous machinery until you know how this drug affects you.

Important information about your medication:

- It is very important that you take this medication as directed by your physician in order for it to help you. When taken regularly, this medication usually requires 2–4 weeks before the full effects are noticed.
- This medication does not produce euphoria (a high feeling) and is not addictive.

The following side effects may occur:

- Drowsiness—Although unlikely, this side effect may occur. Do not drive a car or operate dangerous machinery until you know how this drug affects you.

- Nausea and/or headache—If these persist or are severe, contact your physician.

Because people respond to medicines in very individual ways, you and your physician may have to go through a trying-out period before he or she finds the dose that works best for you.

If you believe you are having problems with your medication, notify your physician.

Carbamazepine

Generic name: carbamazepine
Trade name: _____
Strength: _____ mg
Purpose: This medication has several uses. When taken regularly, it helps prevent or reduce the severity of mood swings. This medication may also be used to prevent the recurrence of depression.
Directions: It is important to follow these directions:
Take _____ tablet(s) or capsule(s) by mouth _____ time(s) daily.
Your medicine should be taken at the following
time(s):_____

Tell your physician, nurse, and pharmacist if you

- Have allergies
- Are pregnant or plan to become pregnant
- Are breast-feeding
- Are taking other medicine, including nonprescription medicine such as antacids, aspirin, or cold medication
- Have other medical problems

Warnings:

- Do not give this medicine to others. It may harm them.
- Do not take more than the recommended amount of this medication, and do not stop taking it without the advice of your physician.
- Store this medicine as directed on the auxiliary label(s) on the bottle.
- Keep all medicines away from the reach of small children.
- It is best to avoid the use of alcohol.
- If you should forget a dose, do not take the missed dose when you remember it, but instead omit it completely; then take the next dose at the regularly scheduled time.
- Do not drive a car or operate dangerous machinery until you know how this drug affects you.

Important information about your medication:

- It is very important that you take this medication as directed by your physician in order for it to help you. When taken regularly, this medication usually requires 2–4 weeks before the full effects are noticed.
- This medication does not produce euphoria (a high feeling) and is not addictive.

The following side effects may occur:

- Drowsiness—This side effect is usually a problem only during the first few days when you start taking the medication. If it is a problem, be very cautious in driving and operating dangerous machinery.
- Dizziness—This may occur when you get up too quickly or rapidly change positions. It can be avoided by arising or changing positions slowly. Dizziness is usually a temporary side effect and will go away with continued use of the medication.
- Nausea and/or vomiting—These side effects can usually be prevented by taking your medication with food or milk. If they continue or become severe, notify your physician.
- Blurred vision, dry mouth, difficulty in passing urine—These side effects are usually temporary and go away after several weeks. If any of these effects continue or become severe, notify your physician.
- Allergic reactions (e.g., rash, itching)—These are rare. If these reactions are accompanied by a high fever, sore throat, or fainting spells, notify your physician.
- Other side effects not listed above may also occur in some patients. If you notice any other effects, consult your physician. Some physicians might obtain a white blood cell count for patients taking this medication.

Because people respond to medicines in very individual ways, you and your physician may have to go through a trying-out period before he or she finds the dose that works best for you.

If you feel you are having problems with your medication, notify your physician.

Clozapine

Generic name: clozapine
Trade name: _____
Strength: _____ mg
Purpose: This medication is used to treat a variety of psychiatric problems, such as preoccupation with troublesome and recurring thoughts, and unpleasant and unusual experiences such as hearing and seeing things not normally seen or heard. This medication will reduce or stop these experiences and help you to remain outside the hospital.

Directions: It is important to follow these directions:
Take _____ tablet(s) or capsule(s) by mouth _____ time(s) daily. Your medicine should be taken at the following time(s):_____

Tell your physician, nurse, and pharmacist if you
- Have allergies
- Are pregnant or plan to become pregnant
- Are breast-feeding
- Are taking other medicine, including nonprescription medicine such as antacids, aspirin, or cold medication
- Have other medical problems

Warnings:
- Do not give this medicine to others. It may harm them.
- Do not take more than the recommended amount of this medication, and do not stop taking it without the advice of your physician.
- Store this medicine as directed on the auxiliary label(s) on the bottle.
- Keep all medicines away from the reach of small children.
- It is best to avoid the use of alcohol.
- If you should forget a dose, do not take the missed dose when you remember it, but instead omit it completely; then take the next dose at the regularly scheduled time.
- Do not drive a car or operate dangerous machinery until you know how this drug affects you.

Important information about your medication:
- It is very important that you take this medication as directed by your physician in order for it to help you. When taken regularly, this medication usually requires 2–4 weeks before the full effects are noticed.
- The medication does not produce euphoria (a high feeling) and is not addictive.

- It will be necessary for you to have weekly blood counts performed to follow possible adverse effects of clozapine.
- You should notify your physician immediately if you develop a high fever, bruising, extreme tiredness, or an extremely sore throat. These may be signs of an infection that could be serious. It is necessary to have your blood count monitored each week to determine the effect of clozapine, if any, on your infection-fighting cells.

The following side effects may occur:
- Drowsiness—This effect can be very troublesome. It usually gets better after several weeks to months of continuous treatment.
- Drooling—This side effect may lessen over time. If it is bad at night and your pillow is wet in the morning, place a towel on your pillow to reduce your discomfort.
- Blurred vision—This effect is temporary and usually goes away with continued use of the medication. If it becomes severe, notify your physician.
- Restlessness, tremors, stiffness, muscle spasms—These side effects can occur and can be treated by your physician. If they persist or get worse, contact your physician.
- Difficulty in passing urine—If this becomes a problem and continues, notify your physician.
- Dizziness—This may occur when you get up too quickly or rapidly change positions. It can be avoided by arising or changing positions slowly.
- Weight gain—Some patients experience an increase in weight after they start taking this medication. If this is not desired, exercise and dietary restriction may be of benefit.
- Sexual dysfunction—If a change in your sex drive or functioning occurs, contact your physician.

Because people respond to medicines in very individual ways, you and your physician may have to go through a trying-out period before he or she finds the dose that works best for you.

If you feel you are having problems with your medication, notify your physician.

Disulfiram

Generic name: disulfiram
Trade name: _____
Strength: _____ mg
Purpose: This medication is an aid to the overall achievement of sobriety in that it helps you to keep from drinking. It is not effective against abuse of drugs other than alcohol.
Directions: It is important to follow these directions:
Take _____ tablet(s) or capsule(s) by mouth _____ time(s) daily. Your medicine should be taken at the following
time(s):_____

Tell your physician, nurse, and pharmacist if you
- Have allergies
- Are pregnant or plan to become pregnant
- Are breast-feeding
- Are taking other medicine, including nonprescription medicine such as antacids, aspirin, or cold medication
- Have other medical problems

Warnings:
- Do not give this medicine to others. It may harm them.
- Do not take more than the recommended amount of this medication, and do not stop taking it without the advice of your physician.
- Store this medicine as directed on the auxiliary label(s) on the bottle.
- Keep all medicines away from the reach of small children.
- It is best to avoid the use of alcohol.
- If you should forget a dose, do not take the missed dose when you remember it, but instead omit it completely; then take the next dose at the regularly scheduled time.
- Do not drive a car or operate dangerous machinery until you know how this drug affects you.

Important information about your medication:
- You must not drink ethanol while you are taking this drug. Ethanol, even in small amounts, may cause you to have an disulfiram reaction with flushing, dizziness, sweating, shortness of breath, throbbing headache, and nausea. The more you drink, the more severe the reaction will be.
- If you have a reaction, call your physician or go to the emergency department of the nearest hospital.
- You should make sure that any medicines you receive by prescription or without prescription do not contain alcohol. Examples of

products usually containing alcohol are elixirs, tinctures, fluid extracts, rubs, spirits, and some injections. If you are in doubt about the safe use of any medications with disulfiram, ask your physician, nurse, or pharmacist.

- There are external preparations such as aftershave lotions and colognes that contain alcohol. Since these products applied to the skin may cause reactions, they should be avoided.
- There are many foods, especially sauces, soups, and certain desserts, that contain enough ethanol to cause a reaction. When eating at home this can be avoided. Dining out requires caution and if you have doubts about a menu item, ask the waiter, waitress, or chef.
- There is still enough drug in your system to cause a reaction as long as 2 weeks after you have stopped taking disulfiram.

The following side effects may occur:

- Drowsiness—This side effect is usually a problem only during the first few days when you start taking the medication. If it is a problem, be very cautious in driving and operating dangerous machinery.
- During the first 2 weeks of taking disulfiram, you may experience a garlic- or metallic-like taste; this effect should disappear after several weeks on the medication.
- Nausea and/or headache—If these persist or are severe, contact your physician.
- Sexual dysfunction—If a change in your sex drive or functioning occurs, contact your physician.

Because people respond to medicines in very individual ways, you and your physician may have to go through a trying-out period before he or she finds the dose that works best for you.

If you feel you are having problems with your medication, notify your physician.

The following is a partial list of alcohol (ethanol)–free liquid products:

Analgesics
Liquiprin® drops

Antidiarrheals
Kaopectate®
Pepto-Bismol®

Antacids
All alcohol-free except
Basaljel®

Cold/allergy
Sudafed® syrup
Triaminic® syrup

Cough
St. Joseph's® cough
medicine
Delsym®

Mouthwash/gargle
Chloraseptic®
Green mint mouthwash

Lithium

Generic name: _____
Trade name: _____
Strength: _____ mg
Purpose: This medication has several uses. When taken regularly, it helps to prevent or reduce the severity of mood swings.
Directions: It is important to follow these directions:
Take _____ tablet(s) or capsule(s) by mouth _____ time(s) daily.
Your medicine should be taken at the following
time(s):_____

Tell your physician, nurse, and pharmacist if you

- Have allergies
- Are pregnant or plan to become pregnant
- Are breast-feeding
- Are taking other medicine, including nonprescription medicine such as antacids, aspirin, or cold medication
- Have other medical problems

Warnings:

- Do not give this medicine to others. It may harm them.
- Do not take more than the recommended amount of this medication, and do not stop taking it without the advice of your physician.
- Store this medicine as directed on the auxiliary label(s) on the bottle.
- Keep all medicines away from the reach of small children.
- It is best to avoid the use of alcohol.
- If you should forget a dose, do not take the missed dose when you remember it, but instead omit it completely; then take the next dose at the regularly scheduled time.
- Do not drive a car or operate dangerous machinery until you know how this drug affects you.

Important information about your medication:

- It is very important that you take this medication as directed by your physician in order for it to help you. When taken regularly, this medication usually requires 2–4 weeks before the full effects are noticed.
- This medication does not produce euphoria (a high feeling) and is not addictive.

The following side effects may occur:

- Nausea and/or vomiting—If you experience these symptoms, stop taking the medication and contact your physician. It is best to take your lithium doses with meals to prevent nausea and/ or vomiting.

- Diarrhea—If you experience this side effect, stop taking the medicine and contact your physician.
- Tremor of the hands—Often, this effect is transient and goes away with continued use of the medication. Occasionally, dosage adjustment by your physician will be necessary.
- Weight gain—Some patients experience an increase in weight after they start taking lithium. If this is not desired, exercise and dietary restriction may be of benefit.
- Increased thirst and urination—Some people notice a mild increase in thirst and urination while taking lithium. Usually this side effect goes away in several weeks. However, if it continues or worsens, mention it to your physician.
- Muscular weakness—This usually goes away with continued use of the medication.
- Drowsiness—This is a temporary problem that goes away with time. If you should experience this effect, be very cautious in driving or operating dangerous machinery.
- Memory problems—Contact your physician if these occur.
- If you perspire excessively, it is important that you replace the lost salt. This can be done by increasing your daily intake of table salt or by using salt tablets during times of excessive sweating. If you have hypertension (high blood pressure), it is important that you do not increase your salt intake; instead, contact your physician. Also, inform your physician if you have a diuretic (a drug to remove excess water) prescribed for you or are to have the dose of diuretic changed while you are receiving lithium. The lithium dose may need to be changed to avoid a drug interaction.

Because people respond to medicines in very individual ways, you and your physician may have to go through a trying-out period before he or she finds the dose that works best for you.

If you feel you are having problems with your medication, notify your physician.

Lithium blood levels:
- For lithium to help you, there must be a certain amount of the drug in your body at all times. For this reason, your physician will request that blood samples be taken so that he or she will know how much lithium is in your body. By knowing this, your physician can adjust your dose so that you receive maximum benefit with no or minimal side effects.

Directions for lithium blood test:

- Do not take your morning dose of lithium before the blood test. If you forget and do take it, mention this to your physician and the laboratory technician. Ideally, the blood sample should be drawn 12–14 hours after your last dose.
- After the test, you may take your lithium dose, preferably with food.

Maprotiline

Generic name: maprotiline
Trade name:_____
Strength:_____mg
Purpose: This medication is used to treat depression.
Directions: It is important to follow these directions:
Take _____ tablet(s) or capsule(s) by mouth _____ time(s) daily.
Your medicine should be taken at the following
time(s):_____

Tell your physician, nurse, and pharmacist if you

- Have allergies
- Are pregnant or plan to become pregnant
- Are breast-feeding
- Are taking other medicine, including nonprescription medicine such as antacids, aspirin, or cold medication
- Have other medical problems

Warnings:

- Do not give this medicine to others. It may harm them.
- Do not take more than the recommended amount of this medication, and do not stop taking it without the advice of your physician.
- Store this medicine as directed on the auxiliary label(s) on the bottle.
- Keep all medicines away from the reach of small children.
- It is best to avoid the use of alcohol.
- If you should forget a dose, do not take the missed dose when you remember it, but instead omit it completely; then take the next dose at the regularly scheduled time.
- Do not drive a car or operate dangerous machinery until you know how this drug affects you.

Important information about your medication:

- It is very important that you take this medication as directed by your physician in order for it to help you. When taken regularly, this medication usually requires 2–4 weeks before the full effects are noticed.
- This medication does not produce euphoria (a high feeling) and is not addictive.

The following side effects may occur:

- Dry mouth—Chewing sugarless gum or sucking on sour, sugarless hard candy will help relieve this. Sucking on ice chips or rinsing your mouth with water might also help. This side effect may go away in several weeks. Brush your teeth regularly.

- Drowsiness—This side effect is usually a problem only during the first few days when you start taking the medication. If it is a problem, be very cautious in driving and operating dangerous machinery.
- Blurred vision—This effect is temporary and usually goes away with continued use of the medication. If it becomes severe, notify your physician.
- Constipation—A high-fiber diet (bran) and exercise may help to alleviate this problem.
- Dizziness—This may occur when you get up too quickly or rapidly change positions. It can be avoided by arising or changing positions slowly.
- Difficulty in passing urine—If this becomes a problem and continues, notify your physician.
- Allergic reactions (e.g., rash, itching)—These are rare. If these reactions are accompanied by a high fever, sore throat, or fainting spells, notify your physician
- Sexual dysfunction—If a change in your sex drive or functioning occurs, contact your physician.
- Convulsions—These may occur with standard and higher doses. Follow the recommended dosing schedule.

Because people respond to medicines in very individual ways, you and your physician may have to go through a trying-out period before he or she finds the dose that works best for you.

If you feel you are having problems with your medication, notify your physician.

Monoamine Oxidase Inhibitors

Generic name: _____
Trade name: _____
Strength: _____ mg
Purpose: This medication is used to treat depression.
Directions: It is important to follow these directions:
Take _____ tablet(s) or capsule(s) by mouth _____ time(s) daily.
Your medicine should be taken at the following
time(s): _____

Tell your physician, nurse, and pharmacist if you
- Have allergies
- Are pregnant or plan to become pregnant
- Are breast-feeding
- Are taking other medicine, including nonprescription medicine such as antacids, aspirin, or cold medication
- Have other medical problems

Warnings:
- Do not give this medicine to others. It may harm them.
- Do not take more than the recommended amount of this medication, and do not stop taking it without the advice of your physician.
- Store this medicine as directed on the auxiliary label(s) on the bottle.
- Keep all medicines away from the reach of small children.
- It is best to avoid the use of alcohol.
- If you should forget a dose, do not take the missed dose when you remember it, but instead omit it completely; then take the next dose at the regularly scheduled time.
- Do not drive a car or operate dangerous machinery until you know how this drug affects you.

Important information about your medication:
- It is very important that you take this medication as directed by your physician. You must take it regularly. The full effect of this medication may not be noticed for 2–4 weeks.
- This medication does not produce euphoria (a high feeling) and is not addictive.
- You must follow the dietary instructions provided below for 1 day before starting, all during treatment, and for 14 days after stopping the medication to prevent a severe reaction (headache, increase in blood pressure).

- Do not eat/drink the following foods/beverages:
  + Aged and natural cheeses (blue, cheddar, Camembert, etc.). In general, avoid foods that are aged or fermented. Cream cheese, cottage cheese, and American cheese can be eaten safely.
  + Broad beans (Italian green beans or Fava beans)
  + Draft beer
  + Summer sausage
  + Fermented bologna
  + Salami
  + Pepperoni
  + Soy sauce
  + Marmite
  + Banana peel
  + Sauerkraut
  + Improperly stored or spoiled meats, fish, or poultry

- The following may be consumed in moderation:
  + Red or white wine (no more than two 4-ounce glasses per day)
  + Bottled or canned beer, including nonalcoholic (no more than two 12-ounce servings per day)

- Do not take the following medications:
  + Amphetamines
  + Oral decongestants such as phenylpropanolamine, pseudo-ephedrine, ephedrine
  + Nasal spray decongestants (Afrin®, etc.)
  + Methylphenidate (Ritalin®)
  + Meperidine (Demerol®)
  + Antidepressants such as paroxetine (Paxil®), sertraline (Zoloft®), fluoxetine (Prozac®), fluvoxamine (Luvox®), nefazodone (Serzone®), venlafaxine (Effexor®)

- It is important to inform any physician, nurse, pharmacist, or dentist that you are taking this medication. Consult your pharmacist, physician, or dietitian if you are in doubt about other foods or medications that may be used. While taking a monoamine oxidase inhibitor, do not start or stop any medication without first consulting a health professional.

The following side effects may occur:
- Dry mouth—chewing sugarless gum or sucking on sour, sugarless, hard candy will help relieve this. Sucking on ice chips or rinsing your mouth with water might also help. This side effect usually goes away in several weeks. Brush your teeth regularly.

- Dizziness—This may occur when you get up too quickly or rapidly change positions. It can be avoided by arising or changing positions slowly.
- Sexual dysfunction—If a change in your sex drive or functioning occurs, contact your physician.

Because people respond to medicines in very individual ways, you and your physician may have to go through a trying-out period before he or she finds the dose that works best for you.

If you feel you are having problems with your medication, notify your physician.

Naltrexone

Generic name: naltrexone
Trade name: _____
Strength: _____ mg
Purpose: This medication is used to help someone stop using narcotics or drinking alcohol. Naltrexone is only part of a program to help someone to not use these drugs.
Directions: It is important to follow these directions:
Take _____ tablet(s) or capsule(s) by mouth _____ time(s) daily.
Your medicine should be taken at the following
time(s):_____

Tell your physician, nurse, and pharmacist if you

- Have allergies
- Are pregnant or plan to become pregnant
- Are breast-feeding
- Are taking other medicine, including nonprescription medicine such as antacids, aspirin, or cold medication
- Have other medical problems
- Think that you may still be having withdrawal symptoms

Warnings:

- Do not give this medicine to others. It may harm them.
- Do not take more than the recommended amount of this medication, and do not stop taking it without the advice of your physician.
- Store this medicine as directed on the auxiliary label(s) on the bottle.
- Keep all medicines away from the reach of small children.
- Do not use alcohol.
- If you should miss a dose of this medicine, take it as soon as possible. However, if it is almost time for your next dose, skip the missed dose. Do not double the dose.
- Do not drive a car or operate dangerous machinery until you know how this drug affects you.

Important information about your medication:

- It is very important that you take this medication as directed by your physician.
- This medication does not produce euphoria (a high feeling) and is not addictive.

The following side effects may occur:

- Drowsiness—This side effect is usually a problem only during the first few days when you start taking the medication. If it is a problem, be very cautious in driving and operating dangerous machinery.

- Weight loss, nausea, decreased appetite—If these persist or are severe, contact your physician.
- Decreased sleep—Take doses of this drug before supper each day.
- Dry mouth—Chewing sugarless gum or sucking on sour, sugarless hard candy will help relieve this. Sucking on ice chips or rinsing your mouth with water might also help. This side effect may go away in several weeks. Brush your teeth regularly.
- Allergic reactions (e.g., rash, itching)—These are rare. If these reactions are accompanied by a high fever, sore throat, or fainting spells, notify your physician
- Headaches—These may occasionally occur. If they persist or are severe, contact your physician.
- Restlessness—If this continues or gets worse, contact your physician.

Because people respond to medicine in very individual ways, you and your physician may have to go through a trying-out period before he or she finds the dose that works best for you.

If you believe you are having problems with your medication, notify your physician.

Nefazodone

Generic name: nefazodone
Trade name: _____
Strength: _____ mg
Purpose: This medication is used to treat depression.
Directions: It is important to follow these directions:
Take _____ tablet(s) or capsule(s) by mouth _____ time(s) daily.
Your medicine should be taken at the following
time(s):_____

Tell your physician, nurse, and pharmacist if you
- Have allergies
- Are pregnant or plan to become pregnant
- Are breast-feeding
- Are taking other medicine, including nonprescription medicine such as antacids, aspirin, or cold medication
- Have other medical problems

Warnings:
- Do not give this medicine to others. It may harm them.
- Do not take more than the recommended amount of this medication, and do not stop taking it without the advice of your physician. Stopping this medication abruptly may lead to trouble sleeping, increase in anxiety or nervousness, increased blood pressure, sweating, headache, nausea, diarrhea, and possibly convulsions.
- Store this medicine as directed on the auxiliary label(s) on the bottle.
- Keep all medicines away from the reach of small children.
- It is best to avoid the use of alcohol.
- If you should forget a dose, do not take the missed dose when you remember it, but instead omit it completely; then take the next dose at the regularly scheduled time.
- Do not drive a car or operate dangerous machinery until you know how this drug affects you.

Important information about your medication:
- It is very important that you take this medication as directed by your physician in order for it to help you. When taken regularly, this medication usually requires 2–4 weeks before the full effects are noticed.
- This medication does not produce euphoria (a high feeling) and is not addictive.

The following side effects may occur:

- Drowsiness—This side effect is usually a problem only during the first few days when you start taking the medication. If it is a problem, be very cautious in driving and operating dangerous machinery.
- Allergic reactions (e.g., rash, itching)—These are rare. If these reactions are accompanied by a high fever, sore throat, or fainting spells, notify your physician
- Dizziness—This may occur when you get up too quickly or rapidly change positions. It can be avoided by arising or changing positions slowly.
- Nausea or upset stomach—If these persist or are severe, contact your physician.
- Prolonged, painful erection—This effect has been reported, not with this medication, but with a medication like it. Male patients who experience this effect should stop nefazodone and contact their physician immediately.

Because people respond to medicines in very individual ways, you and your physician may have to go through a trying-out period before he or she finds the dose that works best for you.

If you believe you are having problems with your medication, notify your physician.

Olanzapine

Generic name: olanzapine
Trade name: Zyprexa®
Strength: _____ mg
Purpose: This medication is used to treat a variety of psychiatric problems such as preoccupation with troublesome and recurring thoughts, and unpleasant and unusual experiences such as hearing and seeing things not normally seen or heard. This medication will reduce or stop these experiences and help you to remain outside the hospital.
Directions: It is important to follow these directions: Take _____ tablet(s) or capsule(s) by mouth _____ time(s) daily. Your medicine should be taken at the following time(s):_____

Tell your physician, nurse, and pharmacist if you

- Have allergies
- Are pregnant or plan to become pregnant
- Are breast-feeding
- Are taking other medicine, including nonprescription medicine such as antacids, aspirin, or cold medication
- Have other medical problems

Warnings:

- Do not give this medicine to others. It may harm them.
- Do not take more than the recommended amount of this medication, and do not stop taking it without the advice of your physician.
- Store this medicine as directed on the auxiliary label(s) on the bottle.
- Keep all medicines away from the reach of small children.
- It is best to avoid the use of alcohol.
- If you should miss a dose of this medicine, do not take the missed dose when you remember it. Omit it completely, then take the next dose at the regularly scheduled time.
- Do not drive a car or operate dangerous machinery until you know how this drug affects you.

Important information about your medication:

- It is very important that you take this medication as directed by your physician in order for it to help you. When taken regularly, this medication usually requires 2–4 weeks before the full effects are noticed.
- This medication does not produce euphoria (a high feeling) and is not addictive.

The following side effects may occur:
- Drowsiness—This can be very troublesome. It usually gets better after several weeks to months of continuous treatment.
- Blurred vision—This effect is temporary and usually goes away with continued use of the medication. If it becomes severe, notify your physician.
- Restlessness, tremors, stiffness, muscle spasms—These side effects can occur and can be treated by your physician. If they persist or get worse, contact your physician.
- Difficulty in passing urine—If this becomes a problem and continues, notify your physician.
- Constipation—If this becomes a problem and continues, notify your physician.
- Dizziness—This may occur when you get up too quickly or rapidly change positions. It can be avoided by arising or changing positions slowly.
- Weight gain—Some patients experience an increase in weight after they start taking this medication. If this is not desired, exercise and dietary restriction may be of benefit.
- Sexual dysfunction—If a change in your sex drive or functioning occurs, contact your physician.

Because people respond to medicines in very individual ways, you and your physician may have to go through a trying-out period before he or she finds the dose that works best for you.

If you feel you are having problems with your medication, notify your physician.

Propranolol

Generic name: propranolol
Trade name: _____
Strength: _____ mg
Purpose: This medication has several uses. Your psychiatrist may prescribe it for the treatment of anxiety disorders, agitation, acute panic attacks, or possibly to alleviate tremors. Other medical uses for propranolol include the treatment of high blood pressure, angina, cardiac arrhythmia, and migraine headaches. If you have any questions regarding why this medication has been prescribed for you, consult your physician.
Directions: It is important to follow these directions:
Take _____ tablet(s) or capsule(s) by mouth _____ time(s) daily. Your medicine should be taken at the following time(s):_____

Tell your physician, nurse, and pharmacist if you

- Have allergies
- Are pregnant or plan to become pregnant
- Are breast-feeding
- Are taking other medicine, including nonprescription medicine such as antacids, aspirin, or cold medication
- Have other medical problems

Warnings:

- Do not give this medicine to others. It may harm them.
- Do not take more than the recommended amount of this medication, and do not stop taking it without the advice of your physician.
- Store this medicine as directed on the auxiliary label(s) on the bottle.
- Keep all medicines away from the reach of small children.
- It is best to avoid the use of alcohol.
- If you should forget a dose, do not take the missed dose when you remember it, but instead omit it completely; then take the next dose at the regularly scheduled time.
- Do not drive a car or operate dangerous machinery until you know how this drug affects you.

Important information about your medication:

- Do not discontinue this medication abruptly, except on the advice of a physician. Your physician may want to taper you off the medication gradually before stopping completely. Some conditions may become worse if the medication is stopped suddenly. Also, it is important not to miss any doses.

- Check your pulse rate regularly. If it is much slower than your usual rate (or less than 50 beats per minute), consult your physician.

The following side effects may occur:

- Breathing difficulty, night cough, swelling of hands or feet—Contact your physician if these occur.
- Dizziness, drowsiness, lightheadedness, reduced alertness—If these persist or are severe, notify your physician.
- Dry mouth—Chewing sugarless gum or sucking on hard sugarless candy will help relieve mouth and throat dryness.
- Low blood sugar—This medication may cause your blood sugar levels to fall. Also, it may cover up signs of hypoglycemia (low blood sugar). If you have any questions about these potential effects, consult your physician.
- Sexual dysfunction—If a change in your sex drive or functioning occurs, contact your physician.

Because people respond to medicines in very individual ways, you and your physician may have to go through a trying-out period before he or she finds the dose that works best for you.

If you believe you are having problems with your medication, notify your physician.

Risperidone

Generic name: risperidone
Trade name: Risperdal®
Strength: _____ mg
Purpose: This medication is used to treat a variety of psychiatric problems, such as overactivity, preoccupation with troublesome and recurring thoughts, and unpleasant and unusual experiences such as hearing and seeing things not normally seen or heard. This medication will reduce or stop these experiences and help you to remain outside the hospital.
Directions: It is important to follow these directions:
Take _____ tablet(s) or capsule(s) by mouth _____ time(s) daily. Your medicine should be taken at the following
time(s):_____

Tell your physician, nurse, and pharmacist if you
- Have allergies
- Are pregnant or plan to become pregnant
- Are breast-feeding
- Are taking other medicine, including nonprescription medicine such as antacids, aspirin, or cold medication
- Have other medical problems

Warnings:
- Do not give this medicine to others. It may harm them.
- Do not take more than the recommended amount of this medication, and do not stop taking it without the advice of your physician.
- Store this medicine as directed on the auxiliary label(s) on the bottle.
- Keep all medicines away from the reach of small children.
- It is best to avoid the use of alcohol.
- If you should forget a dose, do not take the missed dose when you remember it, but instead omit it completely; then take the next dose at the regularly scheduled time.
- Do not drive a car or operate dangerous machinery until you know how this drug affects you.

Important information about your medication:
- It is very important that you take this medication as directed by your physician in order for it to help you. When taken regularly, this medication usually requires 2–4 weeks before the full effects are noticed.
- The medication does not produce euphoria (a high feeling) and is not addictive.

The following side effects may occur:

- Drowsiness—This side effect is usually a problem only during the first few days when you start taking the medication. If it occurs, be very cautious in driving and operating dangerous machinery.
- Dry mouth—This is usually a temporary side effect, and sugarless gum or hard candy is often helpful.
- Blurred vision—This effect is temporary and usually goes away with continued use of the medication. If it becomes severe, notify your physician.
- Restlessness, tremors, stiffness, muscle spasms—These side effects can occur and can be treated by your physician. If they persist or get worse, contact your physician.
- Difficulty in passing urine—If this becomes a problem and continues, notify your physician.
- Dizziness—This may occur when you get up too quickly or rapidly change positions. It can be avoided by arising or changing positions slowly.
- Weight gain—Some patients experience an increase in weight after they start taking this medication. If this is not desired, exercise and dietary restriction may be of benefit.
- Severe sunburn—Avoid direct sunlight and, if you must be out in the sun, use a sunscreen lotion (Presun® or Pabafilm®). Regular suntan lotion is not protective against this type of sunburn.
- Abnormal movements—If this medication is taken continuously for more than 2 years, the possibility exists of developing a condition known as tardive dyskinesia. This term refers to unwanted movements of the tongue, lips, arms, and legs. If the problem is noticed early and the medication changed or stopped, the condition goes away. If not noticed, however, it may become permanent, even if the medication is stopped. Therefore, inform your physician if you experience any of the following:
  + continuous movement of the mouth, jaw, and/or tongue
  + continuous movement of hands, arms, legs, or body
  + other people telling you that they have noticed unusual or continuous movement of your mouth, jaw, tongue, hands, arms, legs, or body
- Sexual dysfunction—If a change in your sex drive or functioning occurs, contact your physician.

Because people respond to medicines in very individual ways, you and your physician may have to go through a trying-out period before he or she finds the dose that works best for you.

If you feel you are having problems with your medication, notify your physician.

Selective Serotonin Reuptake Inhibitors
(fluoxetine, paroxetine, sertraline, fluvoxamine)

Generic name: _____

Trade name: _____

Strength: _____ mg

Purpose: This medication is used to treat depression.

Directions: It is important to follow these directions:

Take _____ tablet(s) or capsule(s) by mouth _____ time(s) daily.
Your medicine should be taken at the following
time(s):_____

Tell your physician, nurse, and pharmacist if you

- Have allergies
- Are pregnant or plan to become pregnant
- Are breast-feeding
- Are taking other medicine, including nonprescription medicine such as antacids, aspirin, or cold medication
- Have other medical problems

Warnings:

- Do not give this medicine to others. It may harm them.
- Do not take more than the recommended amount of this medication, and do not stop taking it without the advice of your physician.
- Store this medicine as directed on the auxiliary label(s) on the bottle.
- Keep all medicines away from the reach of small children.
- It is best to avoid the use of alcohol.
- If you should forget a dose, do not take the missed dose when you remember it, but instead omit it completely; then take the next dose at the regularly scheduled time.
- Do not drive a car or operate dangerous machinery until you know how this drug affects you.

Important information about your medication:

- It is very important that you take this medication as directed by your physician in order for it to help you. When taken regularly, this medication usually requires 2–4 weeks before the full effects are noticed.
- This medication does not produce euphoria (a high feeling) and is not addictive.

The following side effects may occur:

- Drowsiness—Do not drive a car or operate dangerous machinery until you know how this drug affects you.

- Weight loss, nausea, decreased appetite—If these persist or are severe, contact your physician.
- Decreased sleep—Take doses of this drug before supper each day.
- Dry mouth—Chewing sugarless gum or sucking on sour, sugarless hard candy will help relieve this. Sucking on ice chips or rinsing your mouth with water might also help. This side effect may go away in several weeks. Brush your teeth regularly.
- Blurred vision—This effect is temporary and usually goes away with continued use of the medication. If it becomes severe, notify your physician.
- Allergic reactions (e.g., rash, itching)—These are rare. If these reactions are accompanied by a high fever, sore throat, or fainting spells, notify your physician
- Headaches—These may occasionally occur. If they persist or are severe, contact your physician.
- Sexual dysfunction—If you experience a decrease in your sex drive or an inability to achieve orgasm or (in men) an erection, contact your physician.
- Restlessness—If this effect continues or gets worse, contact your physician.

Because people respond to medicines in very individual ways, you and your physician may have to go through a trying-out period before he or she finds the dose that works best for you.

If you believe you are having problems with your medication, notify your physician.

Trazodone

Generic name: trazodone
Trade name: _____
Strength: _____ mg
Purpose: This medication is used to treat depression.
Directions: It is important to follow these directions:
Take _____ tablet(s) or capsule(s) by mouth _____ time(s) daily.
Your medicine should be taken at the following
time(s):_____

Tell your physician, nurse, and pharmacist if you
- Have allergies
- Are pregnant or plan to become pregnant
- Are breast-feeding
- Are taking other medicine, including nonprescription medicine such as antacids, aspirin, or cold medication
- Have other medical problems

Warnings:
- Do not give this medicine to others. It may harm them.
- Do not take more than the recommended amount of this medication, and do not stop taking it without the advice of your physician.
- Store this medicine as directed on the auxiliary label(s) on the bottle.
- Keep all medicines away from the reach of small children.
- It is best to avoid the use of alcohol.
- If you should forget a dose, do not take the missed dose when you remember it, but instead omit it completely; then take the next dose at the regularly scheduled time.
- Do not drive a car or operate dangerous machinery until you know how this drug affects you.

Important information about your medication:
- It is very important that you take this medication as directed by your physician in order for it to help you. When taken regularly, this medication usually requires 2–4 weeks before the full effects are noticed.
- This medication does not produce euphoria (a high feeling) and is not addictive.

The following side effects may occur:
- Drowsiness—Do not drive a car or operate dangerous machinery until you know how this drug affects you.

- Weight loss, nausea, decreased appetite—If these persist or are severe, contact your physician.
- Dry mouth—Chewing sugarless gum or sucking on sour, sugarless hard candy will help relieve this. Sucking on ice chips or rinsing your mouth with water might also help. This side effect may go away in several weeks. Brush your teeth regularly.
- Dizziness—This may occur when you get up too quickly or rapidly change positions. It can be avoided by arising or changing positions slowly.
- Allergic reactions (e.g., rash, itching)—These are rare. If these reactions are accompanied by a high fever, sore throat, or fainting spells, notify your physician
- Nausea and/or headache—These may occasionally occur. If they persist or are severe, contact your physician.
- Prolonged, painful erections—Male patients who experience this effect should stop trazodone and contact their physician immediately.

Because people respond to medicines in very individual ways, you and your physician may have to go through a trying-out period before he or she finds the dose that works best for you.

If you believe you are having problems with your medication, notify your physician.

Tricyclic Antidepressants

Generic name: _____
Trade name: _____
Strength: _____ mg
Purpose: This medication is used to treat depression.
Directions: It is important to follow these directions:
Take _____ tablet(s) or capsule(s) by mouth _____ time(s) daily.
Your medicine should be taken at the following
time(s):_____

Tell your physician, nurse, and pharmacist if you
- Have allergies
- Are pregnant or plan to become pregnant
- Are breast-feeding
- Are taking other medicine, including nonprescription medicine such as antacids, aspirin, or cold medication
- Have other medical problems

Warnings:
- Do not give this medicine to others. It may harm them.
- Do not take more than the recommended amount of this medication, and do not stop taking it without the advice of your physician.
- Store this medicine as directed on the auxiliary label(s) on the bottle.
- Keep all medicines away from the reach of small children.
- It is best to avoid the use of alcohol.
- If you should forget a dose, do not take the missed dose when you remember it, but instead omit it completely; then take the next dose at the regularly scheduled time.
- Do not drive a car or operate dangerous machinery until you know how this drug affects you.

Important information about your medication:
- It is very important that you take this medication as directed by your physician in order for it to help you. When taken regularly, this medication usually requires 2–4 weeks before the full effects are noticed.
- This medication does not produce euphoria (a high feeling) and is not addictive.

The following side effects may occur:
- Dry mouth—Chewing sugarless gum or sucking on sour, sugarless hard candy will help relieve this. Sucking on ice chips or rinsing

your mouth with water might also help. This side effect may go away in several weeks. Brush your teeth regularly.

- Drowsiness—This side effect is usually a problem only during the first few days when you start taking the medication. If it is a problem, be very cautious in driving and operating dangerous machinery.
- Blurred vision—This effect is temporary and usually goes away with continued use of the medication. If it becomes severe, notify your physician.
- Constipation—A high-fiber diet (bran) and exercise may help to alleviate this problem.
- Dizziness—This may occur when you get up too quickly or rapidly change positions. It can be avoided by arising or changing positions slowly.
- Difficulty in passing urine—If this becomes a problem and continues, notify your physician.
- Allergic reactions (e.g., rash, itching)—These are rare. If these reactions are accompanied by a high fever, sore throat, or fainting spells, notify your physician
- Sexual dysfunction—If a change in your sex drive or functioning occurs, contact your physician.

Because people respond to medicines in very individual ways, you and your physician may have to go through a trying-out period before he or she finds the dose that works best for you.

If you feel you are having problems with your medication, notify your physician.

Valproate (valproate, valproic acid, divalproex sodium)

Generic name: _____

Trade name: _____

Strength: _____ mg

Purpose: This medication has several uses. When taken regularly, it helps prevent or reduce the severity of mood swings. This medication may also be used to prevent the recurrence of depression.

Directions: It is important to follow these directions:

Take _____ tablet(s) or capsule(s) by mouth _____ time(s) daily. Your medicine should be taken at the following time(s):_____

Tell your physician, nurse, and pharmacist if you

- Have allergies
- Are pregnant or plan to become pregnant
- Are breast-feeding
- Are taking other medicine, including nonprescription medicine such as antacids, aspirin, or cold medication
- Have other medical problems

Warnings:

- Do not give this medicine to others. It may harm them.
- Do not take more than the recommended amount of this medication, and do not stop taking it without the advice of your physician.
- Store this medicine as directed on the auxiliary label(s) on the bottle.
- Keep all medicines away from the reach of small children.
- It is best to avoid the use of alcohol.
- If you should forget a dose, do not take the missed dose when you remember it, but instead omit it completely; then take the next dose at the regularly scheduled time.
- Do not drive a car or operate dangerous machinery until you know how this drug affects you.

Important information about your medication:

- It is very important that you take this medication as directed by your physician in order for it to help you. When taken regularly, this medication usually requires 2–4 weeks before the full effects are noticed.
- This medication does not produce euphoria (a high feeling) and is not addictive.

The following side effects may occur:

- Drowsiness—This side effect is usually a problem only during the first few days when you start taking the medication. If it is a problem, be very cautious in driving and operating dangerous machinery.
- Dizziness—This may occur when you get up too quickly or rapidly change positions. It can be avoided by arising or changing positions slowly. Dizziness is usually a temporary side effect and will go away with continued use of the medication.
- Nausea and/or vomiting—These can usually be prevented by taking your medication with food or milk.
- Allergic reactions (e.g., rash, itching)—These are rare. If these reactions are accompanied by a high fever, sore throat, or fainting spells, notify your physician
- Other side effects not listed above may also occur in some patients. If you notice any other effects, consult your physician.

Because people respond to medicines in very individual ways, you and your physician may have to go through a trying-out period before he or she finds the dose that works best for you.

If you feel you are having problems with your medication, notify your physician.

Venlafaxine

Generic name: venlafaxine
Trade name: _____
Strength: _____ mg
Purpose: This medication is used to treat depression.
Directions: It is important to follow these directions:
Take _____ tablet(s) or capsule(s) by mouth _____ time(s) daily.
Your medicine should be taken at the following
time(s):_____

Tell your physician, nurse, and pharmacist if you

- Have allergies
- Are pregnant or plan to become pregnant
- Are breast-feeding
- Are taking other medicine, including nonprescription medicine such as antacids, aspirin, or cold medication
- Have other medical problems

Warnings:

- Do not give this medicine to others. It may harm them.
- Do not take more than the recommended amount of this medication, and do not stop taking it without the advice of your physician.
- Store this medicine as directed on the auxiliary label(s) on the bottle.
- Keep all medicines away from the reach of small children.
- It is best to avoid the use of alcohol.
- If you should forget a dose, do not take the missed dose when you remember it, but instead omit it completely; then take the next dose at the regularly scheduled time.
- Do not drive a car or operate dangerous machinery until you know how this drug affects you.

Important information about your medication:

- It is very important that you take this medication as directed by your physician in order for it to help you. When taken regularly, this medication usually requires 2–4 weeks before the full effects are noticed.
- This medication does not produce euphoria (a high feeling) and is not addictive.

The following side effects may occur:

- Drowsiness—This side effect is usually a problem only during the first few days when you start taking the medication. If it is a

- problem, be very cautious in driving and operating dangerous machinery.
- Weight loss, nausea, decreased appetite—If these persist or are severe, contact your physician.
- Decreased sleep—Take doses of this drug before supper each day.
- Dry mouth—Chewing sugarless gum or sucking on sour, sugarless hard candy will help relieve this. Sucking on ice chips or rinsing your mouth with water might also help. This side effect may go away in several weeks. Brush your teeth regularly.
- Constipation—A high-fiber diet (bran) and exercise may help to alleviate this problem.
- Dizziness—This may occur when you get up too quickly or rapidly change positions. It can be avoided by arising or changing positions slowly.
- Allergic reactions (e.g., rash, itching)—These are rare. If these reactions are accompanied by a high fever, sore throat, or fainting spells, notify your physician
- High blood pressure—If you have high blood pressure, you should have your blood pressure checked frequently while your dose is being increased.
- Sexual dysfunction—If a change in your sex drive or functioning occurs, contact your physician.

Because people respond to medicines in very individual ways, you and your physician may have to go through a trying-out period before he or she finds the dose that works best for you.

If you believe you are having problems with your medication, notify your physician.

Index

*Page numbers printed in **boldface** type refer to tables or figures.*

selective serotonin reuptake
inhibitors, 167
tricyclic, 132
barbiturates. *See* Barbiturates;
specific drugs
benzodiazepines. *See*
Benzodiazepines (BZDs);
specific drugs
β-adrenergic-blocking agents as.
See β-Adrenergic-blocking
agents
miscellaneous, 339–340
efficacy of, 339–340
patient advice regarding,
655–656
Anxiolytic withdrawal, 569, **570,**
571–587
presentation of, 571–577
high-dose withdrawal
symptoms, 574–577
low-dose withdrawal
symptoms, 572–573
rebound symptoms, 571
rebound and, 569
relapse and, 569
treatment of, 577–587
for high-dose withdrawal,
580–587
for low-dose withdrawal,
577–580
Appetite
decrease in. *See* Anorexia
increase in, with nefazodone,
196
Aprobarbital, dose equivalent and
half-life classification for, 570
Arrhythmias
with anticholinergic overdose,
treatment of, 541
with antidepressant overdose,
treatment of, 514–515
with antipsychotic overdose,
treatment of, 509–510
with carbamazepine, **265**
with monoamine oxidase
inhibitor overdose,
treatment of, 518
Artane. *See* Trihexyphenidyl
Asendin. *See* Amitriptyline

Asthenia
with imipramine, **193**
with nefazodone, **196**
with trazodone, **193**
with venlafaxine, **193**
Ataractics. *See* Antipsychotics;
Typical antipsychotics;
specific drugs
Ataxia
with carbamazepine, **265,**
268–269
with flurazepam, **380**
Atenolol, efficacy of
for generalized anxiety disorder,
330
for social phobias, 331
Ativan. *See* Lorazepam
Atrial fibrillation, with
carbamazepine, **265**
Atropine
for arrhythmias, with
antidepressant overdose,
515
for electroconvulsive therapy,
629, 630, 634
Attention-deficit/hyperactivity
disorder, miscellaneous
antidepressant efficacy for,
178
Atypical antipsychotics. *See*
specific drugs and drug types
Atypical depression
monoamine oxidase inhibitor
efficacy for, 157–158
selective serotonin reuptake
inhibitor efficacy for,
169–170
Atypical mania, lithium carbonate
efficacy for, 223–224
Autonomic reactions. *See also*
specific reactions
to amoxapine, 185–186
to clozapine, 70–72
to imipramine, **193**
to maprotiline, 189
to olanzapine, 85
to pimozide, 90
to selective serotonin reuptake
inhibitors, **174**

Hallucinations
  with antidepressant overdose,
    treatment of, 515
  with flurazepam, **380**
Haloperidol
  adverse effects of, **33,** 36
  for borderline personality
    disorder, 8–9
  for delirium, 11
    with lorazepam, 11
  dosage of
    for agitated patients, 14–15
    for delirium, 19–20
    maintenance, 17
    for nonagitated patients, 13
    supranormal, 15
  drug interactions of
    with barbiturates, 460
    with β-adrenergic-blocking
      agents, 460–461
    with buspirone, 488
    with carbamazepine, 461
    with fluoxetine, 462
    with guanethidine, 454
    with nefazodone, 473
  pharmacokinetics of, 29–30
  product information for, 105–106
  for schizophrenia
    nonrefractory, 93
    refractory, 5, 94
Haloperidol decanoate
  dosage of, 22–24, **24**
    fluphenazine decanoate dosage
      conversion and, 25
    intervals for, 25
    loading, 23–24
    maintenance, 17–18
    non-loading-dose approach
      to, 23
  injection technique for, 25–26
  pharmacokinetics of, **28,** 30
  product information for, 106
Haloperidol hydrochloride,
    pharmacokinetics of, **28**
Haloperidol lactate,
    pharmacokinetics of, **28**
Hangover
  with flurazepam, **381**
  with triazolam, **381**

Headache
  with electroconvulsive therapy,
    624
  with flurazepam, **381**
  with imipramine, **193**
  with nefazodone, **196**
  with risperidone, 100
  with selective serotonin
    reuptake inhibitors, **174**
  with trazodone, **193**
  with triazolam, **381**
  with venlafaxine, **193**
Health Care Financing
    Administration, 10
Heart rate, with monoamine
    oxidase inhibitors, 162
Hematological reactions. *See also
    specific reactions*
  to amoxapine, 186
  to β-adrenergic agents, 333
  to carbamazepine, 267–268
  to clozapine, 74–76
  to lithium carbonate, 247
  to olanzapine, 86
  to tricyclic antidepressants,
    151–152
  to typical antipsychotics, 39
  to valproate, 278–279
Hemodialysis, lithium carbonate
    dosage during, 230
Hepatic reactions. *See also specific
    reactions*
  to carbamazepine, 268
  to clozapine, 76
  to disulfiram, 432–433
  to lithium carbonate, 247
  to olanzapine, 86
  to risperidone, 98
  to tricyclic antidepressants,
    152
  to valproate, 279
Hepatotoxicity
  of typical antipsychotics,
    39–40
  of valproate, 279
Heroin, withdrawal from,
    presentation of, 560–561
Hexobarbital, pharmacokinetics
    of, **377**

Typical antipsychotics, adverse
  effects of *(continued)*
  dermatological, 36–37
  endocrinological, 37–38
  extrapyramidal. *See*
      Extrapyramidal side
      effects (EPS)
  hematological, 39
  hepatic, 39–40
  metabolic, 40
  neuroleptic malignant
      syndrome. *See*
      Neuroleptic malignant
      syndrome (NMS)
  ophthalmological, 53–55
  psychiatric, 55
  seizure threshold reduction,
      53
  sexual, 55–57
  temperature regulation and,
      57
  teratogenic and in breast
      milk, 58
  urinary, 58–59
  dosages for, 12–26
  for cognitive disorders, 18–20
  of decanoate esters, 21–26
  equivalent doses and, 12
  of hydrochloride/lactate salts,
      20–21
  maintenance, 15–18
  oral–parenteral dose
      equivalents and, 20–21
  potency classification and,
      12–13, **13**
  for psychotic depression, 18
  for schizophrenia, mania, and
      schizoaffective and
      schizophreniform
      disorders, 13–15
  supranormal, 15
  efficacy of, 2–12
  for anxiety disorders, 12
  for cognitive disorders, 9–11
  for drug-induced psychosis,
      11–12
  for mania, 7–8
  for personality disorders, 8–9
  for psychotic depression, 9

  for schizoaffective disorder, 8
  for schizophrenia, 2–7
  for schizophreniform disorder,
      8
  indications for, 2
  mechanism of action of, 12
  patient advice regarding,
      652–654
  pharmacokinetics of, 26–27, **28,**
      29–31
  sampling time and, 26
  rapid neuroleptization and,
      14–15
  rational prescribing of, 59–60
  withdrawal from, 34–35
Tyramine, hypertensive crisis and,
      163

Ulcers, peptic, tricyclic
      antidepressants for, 132
Unipolar depression
  carbamazepine efficacy for, for
      maintenance treatment,
      260–261
  lithium carbonate efficacy for,
      for maintenance
      treatment, 229
  valproate efficacy for, for
      maintenance treatment,
      274
Urinary alkalinizers, drug
      interactions of, with lithium,
      476
Urinary incontinence, with typical
      antipsychotics, 58
Urinary retention
  with tricyclic antidepressants,
      149–150
  with typical antipsychotics, 34,
      59
Urogenital reactions. *See also*
      specific reactions
  to anticholinergics, 409
  to clozapine, 82
  to imipramine, **193**
  to risperidone, 100
  to trazodone, **193**
  to typical antipsychotics, 58–59
  to venlafaxine, **193**